PENGUIN BOOKS

THE RUNNER'S HANDBOOK

BOB GLOVER is founder and president of Robert H. Glover and Associates, Inc., a sports and fitness consulting firm. Since he founded the program in 1978, Glover has directed the running classes for the 32,000-member New York Road Runners Club. More than 2,000 students participate each year in these classes at the beginner, advanced beginner, intermediate, basic competitive, competitive, and advanced competitive levels. Glover also directs the training clinics for the New York City Marathon. His Official New York City Marathon Training Program is followed annually by thousands of runners. Each year since its founding in 1990, Glover has directed over 1,000 boys and girls aged five to fourteen in the City-Sports-For-Kids track-and-field program sponsored by the New York Road Runners Club and the Asphalt Green. A high school (Dansville, NY) county champion at 2 miles and a three-time gold medalist at the Hue Sports Festival during the Vietnam War, he has competed for more than thirty years at distances ranging from the quarter-mile to the 50-mile ultra-marathon, and has completed over thirty marathons. He now places frequently in local races as a masters runner competing for the Westchester Track Club. Glover has coached three women athletes to U.S. top ten rankings in the marathon event, and has coached his running teams to several national titles at a variety of distances in both the open and masters categories. With more than twenty years' experience coaching all levels of runners, he gains his greatest satisfaction helping beginner runners, beginner racers, and beginner marathoners increase their enjoyment of the sport. More than 50,000 runners have participated in his classes and nearly a million runners have followed his training program in his books since *The Runner's Handbook* was first published and became an immediate national best-seller in 1978. He and his wife, Shelly-lynn, live in North Tarrytown, New York, where they love to run together along wooded trails. They often win awards together in couples races.

JACK SHEPHERD is the author of nine books, including the national best-sellers *The Adams Chronicles*, and (co-authored with Bob Glover) *The Runner's Handbook*. Shepherd graduated from Haverford College and Columbia University and, twenty-five years later, earned his Ph.D. at Boston University. He began his career as an international journalist and has covered assignments in forty-eight of the fifty states, in the Far East, Europe, the Middle East and sub-Saharan Africa. Following this, Shepherd became a foreign policy specialist at the Carnegie Endowment for International Peace in Washington. After receiving his doctorate, Shepherd taught at Dartmouth College for five years. He now directs an international program at the University of Cambridge, England, where he also teaches in the Faculty of Social and Political Sciences. In December 1975, after returning from an assignment in East Africa, Shepherd joined Bob Glover's running class which, he quickly realized, deserved to be the subject of this book. Shepherd not only survived the beginner's program, he also graduated to become a convinced lifetime intermediate runner who has completed two New York City Marathons. Shepherd and his wife, Kathleen, currently live in Cambridge, but they maintain a permanent home in Norwich, Vermont, where they enjoy running, hiking, rowing, and cross-country skiing for fitness. To commemorate his twenty years of running under Bob Glover's care and influence, in 1995 Shepherd began training for the Coast-to-Coast hike across England. He is using his running and weight-training as a form of cross-training to condition him for this difficult trek.

SHELLY-LYNN FLORENCE GLOVER is an exercise physiologist with a master's degree from Columbia University as well as certification as a fitness professional from the American Council on Exercise and Marymount Manhattan College. She has an undergraduate degree in journalism. As a researcher, she has been active in several studies involving runners. Her work involving "critical velocity" as a means of predicting marathon times was accepted for publication and was presented at the 1995 American College of Sports Medicine Conference in Minneapolis. As an athlete, she was the captain of her high school (Canisteo, NY) soccer team and a member of her college's first women's cross-country team. As a veteran of twenty years of racing, she competes for the Westchester Track Club and frequently wins awards in local races ranging in distance from 5K to the marathon. She is founder and president of Great Strides, a personal trainer consulting firm. She also founded and coaches Mercury Masters—a running team for athletes who are over the age of fifty. As program director for Glover and Associates, she coaches with the New York Road Runners Club's City-Sports-For-Kids youth track program and running classes, where she directs the beginner- and intermediate-level runners who are the focus of this book.

ALSO BY BOB GLOVER

The Competitive Runner's Handbook
The Runner's Handbook Training Diary
The Injured Runner's Training Handbook
The Family Fitness Handbook

The Runner's Handbook

The Best-selling Classic Fitness Guide for Beginner and Intermediate Runners

Bob Glover, Jack Shepherd and
Shelly-lynn Florence Glover

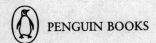 PENGUIN BOOKS

PENGUIN BOOKS
Published by the Penguin Group
Penguin Books USA Inc., 375 Hudson Street, New York, New York 10014, U.S.A.
Penguin Books Ltd, 27 Wrights Lane, London W8 5TZ, England
Penguin Books Australia Ltd, Ringwood, Victoria, Australia
Penguin Books Canada Ltd, 10 Alcorn Avenue, Toronto, Ontario, Canada M4V 3B2
Penguin Books (N.Z.) Ltd, 182–190 Wairau Road, Auckland 10, New Zealand

Penguin Books Ltd, Registered Offices: Harmondsworth, Middlesex, England

First published in the United States of America by The Viking Press 1978
Revised and updated edition published in Penguin Books 1985
This second revised and updated edition published in Penguin Books 1996

1 3 5 7 9 10 8 6 4 2

A NOTE TO THE READER
The ideas, procedures, and suggestions contained in this book are not intended to substitute for medical or other professional advice applicable to specific individuals. As with any activity program, yours should be prepared in consultation with a physician or other qualified professional person.

The authors acknowledge with thanks *The New England Journal of Medicine* for permission to adapt material from an article by Dr. Melvin Herskowitz that appeared in the January 20, 1977 issue.

LIBRARY OF CONGRESS CATALOGING IN PUBLICATION DATA
Glover, Bob.
The runner's handbook: the bestselling classic fitness guide for
beginner and intermediate runners / Bob Glover, Jack Shepherd, and
Shelly-lynn Florence Glover.
p.   cm.
"All new."
Includes index.
ISBN 0 14 04.6930 3
1. Running—Training.   2. Running—Physiological aspects.
I. Shepherd, Jack, 1937-   .   II. Glover, Shelly-lynn Florence.
III. Title.
GV1061.5.G56   1996
796.4'26—dc20   95-25847

Printed in the United States of America
Set in Sabon
Designed by Jessica Shatan

Dedication

So many men and women have contributed to the development of running for fitness and competition that it is difficult to choose the single man or single woman who have had the most profound influence. For me, however, it was an easy choice. Both the third edition of *The Runner's Handbook* and the third edition of *The Competitive Runner's Handbook* are proudly dedicated to two good friends who contributed the most to my career as a running coach and writer. For many reasons they can be called "The Marathon Man" and "The Marathon Woman."

Fred Lebow died in 1994, just four weeks prior to the twenty-fifth anniversary of his pride and joy, the New York City Marathon. When Fred took the reins as president of the New York Road Runners Club, the organization had fewer than 200 members. When he died, the NYRRC was over 30,000 strong. A charismatic, innovative leader, Fred's most publicized accomplishment was his direction of the New York City Marathon. In a bold move in 1976, he took the event from the confines of Central Park out onto the streets of all five boroughs. He brought the marathon to the people. His concept excited the media, which further promoted the sport and helped fuel the big running boom of the late 1970s. Just as important, thousands of spectators caught up in the excitement took up running themselves—first running for fitness and then training to run the marathon itself. Cities around the world started marathons through their streets and sought out Fred and his staff for advice. Fred's fame spread and spread as three U.S. presidents met with him at the White House and even the pope had an audience with him. Despite all this, Fred remained a dedicated middle-of-the-pack—and later, as he battled cancer, back-of-the-pack—runner. He immediately endorsed and promoted the many ideas that I presented to him concerning expansion of the NYRRC's educational services to runners. Together, we started running clinics years before anyone else was doing them. More programs followed: Saturday morning group fun runs, long runs for marathon training, brochures on training for all levels of runners, the official New York City Marathon training schedule. Two programs that we developed remain very special. While he was in the hospital the first time in his battle with cancer, Fred gave the go-ahead to start our very successful City-Sports-For-Kids track-and-field program. From a humble beginning with 23 kids in our first session, we expanded to include over 1,000 boys and girls ages five to fourteen in our fun-and-fitness program each year. Fred loved to stop by and cheer the kids on. Ironically, I was at this program, started from his hospital room, when I learned that Fred had died. Through misty eyes I looked around the field and saw over 300 kids having fun at Fred's sport—running. Back in 1978, I approached Fred with the idea of starting classes for running. To our knowledge at that time, such a thing did not exist. Coached workouts were for high school and college teams and a few elite adult runners, not for the average man and woman. "Even if one person shows up, we should try," was Fred's command. We started with 25 runners—including Fred—and now get as many as 750 runners per ten-week session; more than 2,000 students per year. Fred made it to the classes as often as he could, fighting it out with the intermediates during speed workouts. He was always ready to offer encouragement to even the slowest runner in the class. His advice to runners entering his races was the same whether it was a back-of-the-packer or a world record holder: "Whatever you do, just do your best." All of these programs, and this book, remain as a legacy to Fred's commitment to the average runner.

Nina Kuscsik is a pioneer athlete and a leader in the women's running movement. More important, she has been a good friend for more than two decades and is my heroine. Nina has completed more than eighty marathons, which, to my knowledge, is more than any other woman in the world. She was a world-class marathoner who was ahead of her time as an athlete. Until 1971, women were still trying to break the three-hour barrier for the marathon, and Nina was one of the few athletes competing back then capable of such a feat. That year in the New York City Marathon she came within a minute of becoming the first woman in the world to race a marathon under three hours—Beth Bonner held off her challenge to win in 2:55:22 to Nina's 2:56:04. This was a remarkable achievement considering that the event consisted of four loops of hilly Central Park. The following spring, Nina became the first official women's finisher of the Boston Marathon, and in the fall won New York to become the first woman to win both of these prestigious races in the same year. She won New York again in 1973 to become the first athlete—male or female—to win consecutive titles in this event. Nina went on to win several marathons and lower her time to 2 hours, 50 minutes. I was there to cheer her on—again over those Central Park hills—when she set an American record for 50 miles. Nina's many contributions to running were far from restricted to her racing accomplishments. She was politically active in the sport back when men said that women were inferior and could harm themselves by running too far. Thus, women were banned from competing in distances longer than a mile on the track and were outlawed by Boston Marathon officials. But Nina attacked this thinking with her body and her mind, proving that women can run long and fast, and boldly challenged the rules at boring meeting after meeting with crusty AAU officials. By 1972, Boston officials finally gave in and stood by shaking their heads as Nina not only led the women to the finish line, but finished well ahead of the majority of the "superior" men. The battleground shifted that fall to the New York City Marathon, which that year was the National AAU championship. The unenlightened AAU agreed to sanction women to run that race, but ruled that they couldn't start with the men—they were to begin ten minutes earlier. Ladies first. Nina fixed that! She spearheaded a well-publicized protest: the women sat down at the starting line and refused to budge until the men started. Nina organized a civil rights lawsuit against the AAU for discrimination in a public place.

The AAU was forced to give in to Nina's demands. But the battle still wasn't over for women marathoners: they were not allowed to compete in the Olympic Games at a distance longer than 1500 meters. Nina became the national chairman of the women's subcommittee of The Athletics Congress (TAC), the governing body for running in the United States, and used this position to lobby with the fuddy-duddies who controlled the running events in the Olympic Games. She even pulled a trick on the international president of the ruling body for the sport of running by placing a pin on his lapel that read, "I support fast women." At last, in 1984, women were allowed, by the men, to compete in the Olympic Marathon and Nina served as chairperson for the first U.S. Olympic Trials Marathon for women. Nina has been on the board of directors of the New York Road Runners Club for more than twenty years, and one of her staunchest supporters throughout her campaigns to promote the rights of women's running was Fred Lebow. Thus, it was fitting that, at the 1995 Road Runners Club of America national convention, Nina was presented with the first Fred Lebow Women's Running Award. Thus, the "Marathon Man" and the "Marathon Woman" were honored together—with that award and with this book.

—BOB GLOVER

Acknowledgments

Dozens of men and women have influenced my career—and thus contributed to this book. There are far too many to name, however some deserve special mention.

Bob Elia, executive director of the Enterprise, Alabama, YMCA, was my first employer when I returned from the Vietnam War. He guided me into "people work." George Goyer hired me as fitness director of the ambitious, new Rome, New York, Family Y despite my lack of experience (I did not lack enthusiasm). He taught me the basics of fitness programming. The late Bill Coughlin, then athletic director at Rome Free Academy, served as my Sports-Fitness Committee chairman and provided expertise and friendship that proved invaluable.

Alexander Melleby has been my role model as a fitness leader and was perhaps the finest physical education instructor in the long history of the YMCA's service. He hired and trained me to be his fitness director at one of the largest and most active Y's in the United States, the 5,000-member West Side YMCA in New York City. Al encouraged my enthusiasm for running and invited the fledging 200-member New York Road Runners Club to move into our building and forge a close working relationship. His professional training and friendship have shaped me and are deeply appreciated.

Much of the fitness philosophy in my work and writing is based on the teaching and research of Dr. Hans Kraus—to whom the first edition of this book was dedicated. Hans codeveloped with Al Melleby the Y's Way to a Healthy Back program and recruited me as one of his first instructors. As the author of several books, founder of the President's Council on Physical Fitness, and fitness adviser to Presidents Eisenhower and Kennedy, he has provided a wealth of knowledge for me in my career. Most important, Hans has served as my "guru" in the area of physical fitness and has been a valued personal friend.

Dr. Richard Schuster has been a pioneer in the field of sports podiatry and a good friend. He developed orthotics for my feet that saved me from injury. Without his professional and personal encouragement I wouldn't be running today. Dr. Murray Weisenfeld is the author of *The Runner's Repair Manual* and my coauthor for *The Injured Runner's Training Handbook*. His advice on running injuries is a key part of the injury chapter in this book. Murray's work as my personal sports podiatrist and friendship continues to be much appreciated. Dr. Norbert Sander, a former winner of the New York City Marathon, has contributed immensely to our sport and guided me through my initial treatment for a herniated disk. Dr. Brian Halpern, an orthopedist and director of the Athlete's Choice program at New York City's Hospital for Special Surgery, teamed with physical therapist Jimmy Dempsey to direct and encourage my rehabilitation after my serious back injury.

Two runner-writers inspired and encouraged me at the start of my career: Joe Henderson was a guiding light as editor for *Runner's World* well before the running boom, and the late Dr. George Sheehan gave freely of his advice in sports medicine.

Several key members of the New York Road Runners Club have been influential in my career. Nina Kuscsik and the late Fred Lebow are honored in the dedication of this book. NYRRC founders Joe Kleinerman and Ted Corbitt helped pave the way as did the late Kurt Steiner and the late Harry Murphy. NYRRC board member Peter Roth was one of the first instructors in my beginner running classes and board member Dick Traum, founder of the Achilles Track Club, was one of my first students. Later, Dick helped me start my business as did longtime friend John Eisner.

Board member Andy Kimerling, owner of the Westchester Road Runner store in White Plains, New York, is to be thanked for his review of the shoe and apparel chapters of the book.

Allan Steinfeld, Fred Lebow's successor as president of the New York Road Runners Club, is to be thanked for picking up the baton and keeping it going forward. His work for many years as the technical director of the New York City Marathon is the model for such events around the world. His staff of dedicated workers is to be thanked, too, for putting on so many great events and servicing the needs of over 32,000 members—that's 160 times the number of members we had when I first started my association with the NYRRC more than two decades ago. Fred's best friend, Brian Crawford, is to be thanked not only for his many years of service to the running community despite not being a runner himself, but for being there for Fred over the last few years.

A special thanks to Liz Feinberg and Brian Florence who ran countless intervals with Shelly and me over our favorite running trails in sub-freezing weather while photographing the cover of this book.

Last, but not least, I want to thank the thousands of runners of all levels who have participated in my running classes over the past two decades and the one million runners who have read my various running books. Your feedback is what keeps me going and what keeps improving this book. After all, a coach is never too smart to learn from his students.

—BOB GLOVER

Contents

Introduction:
Down the Road to Fitness

When Jack Shepherd entered my fitness office in September 1975, he looked like any other out-of-shape American. He had just finished *The Adams Chronicles*, which became a national best-seller and a television series, and he was paunchy and very tense from months of writing and meeting deadlines. He talked nervously as he changed into his shorts and sneakers for his first fitness test. He wanted to begin a jogging program. He was thirty-seven years old, and some friends of his had already died from heart attacks.

I had heard this story hundreds of times before, and since. Shepherd looked fit, or almost fit, and ready to run a mile or more. But in fact, he was dangerously out of shape. He couldn't pass any of my flexibility tests. When I took his resting heart rate, it was 108 —far above the normal range of 60 to 80 beats per minute. His blood pressure was measured at 160/90, also above normal, and I couldn't even test him for cardiorespiratory endurance on the bicycle ergometer because his heart rate would shoot up too fast.

Shepherd became a man of distinction: He was the first person to flunk my fitness test! Worse, when he mentioned it to his wife and friends, they laughed. How can anyone flunk a fitness test for a beginner's class?

From this undistinguished beginning grew a successful long-term collaboration in friendship and fitness: *The Runner's Handbook*. After it was published in 1978, that book made everybody's national best-seller list and even reached the number one position on some. It was followed by *The Runner's Handbook Training Diary* in 1978, *The Competitive Runner's Handbook* in 1983, *The Injured Runner's Handbook* in 1985, and *The Family Fitness Handbook* in 1989. Together, this series of fitness books has sold almost one million copies worldwide. More importantly, it has enabled us to help thousands of men, women, and children start fitness programs—just as I started Shepherd down the road to fitness—and to enjoy running, to complete their first marathons, and to improve their race times from distances of one mile to 50 miles. Further, it has enabled them to enjoy the fun and fellowship that comes with a good running and fitness program.

During the decades since 1975, Shepherd and I have learned a great deal about the fitness needs of our readers. Many of you have written to us; others stop us for chats about running, to tell us your stories or to exchange tips or ask questions about training. More than 50,000 runners—from raw beginners to elite marathoners—have participated in my running classes, teams, and clinics. This, plus my own research and reading, has kept me in touch with your needs and fitness goals. Your many questions at my clinics and classes have also provided me with a wealth of knowledge about what you want to know that is not available in the research laboratory or your local bookstore. Your many successes and efforts in my running programs give me information and experience unmatched by coaches more distant from large numbers of runners.

This edition of *The Runner's Handbook* is filled with your names, experiences, enthusiasms, victories, and struggles. This is not a book written by elite athletes or coaches of elite athletes who may water down their training concepts to what they think the average runner needs. This is a book about my basic training program, experiences, and ideas, tested over more than two decades. It is written by an experienced coach, an accomplished writer, and a dedicated exercise physiologist—all with plenty of mileage on the running paths. *The Runner's Handbook* is a book by and about all of *us*—the novice runner, the back-of-the-pack racer, the aspiring marathoner. At its heart, it is simply a book about how we all get in shape and work to stay in shape.

Who are we? Shepherd is a sort of Everyman. When he came into my office, he exemplified the average middle-aged American. He wasn't aware of how out of shape he had gotten, but he knew he couldn't run the length of a city block or climb a flight of stairs without becoming breathless. He was the epitome of Dr. Thomas Cureton's warning: "The average middle-age man in this country is close to death. He is only one emotional shock or one sudden exertion away from a serious heart attack—this nation's leading cause of death." Cureton's warning, made in 1974, still rings true.

Shepherd is now aging into a feisty old runner full of vigor and bite. What did he do? First, I sent him to his doctor, who gave him a stress test and a twenty-four-hour outpatient, ambulatory electrocardiogram (ECG). A minor heart condition was discovered and a medical conclusion similar to mine was reached: Jack was grossly out of shape. Start exercising!

In December 1975, Shepherd entered my beginner's fitness class in New York City's West Side YMCA. For the next ten weeks, he and the men and women in his class followed my beginner's running program. This is the one I still use, and is detailed in Chapter 10. At first, like many other sedentary Americans, Shepherd couldn't run for 20 consecutive minutes. So he ran for one minute, walked one minute, ran one, walked one for the 20-minute period. After ten weeks, however, he was out of the gym and into Central Park, where he ran one mile and then 2 miles nonstop. By the end of six months, he was running 5 miles. His resting heart rate was down to 75 beats per minute, and his blood pressure had dropped to normal. By 1980, Shepherd had completed two New York City Marathons—his times are divulged only over expensive dinners. Today, he has been running for more than twenty years and has run with readers of *The Runner's Handbook* all over the United States, in England (where in 1996 he was working at the University of Cambridge), and in Africa.

Joining Shepherd and me in this edition is Shelly-lynn Florence Glover. With an undergraduate degree in journalism, a master's degree in exercise physiology from Columbia University, ten years of coaching experience, and twenty years of running and racing, she adds an important perspective as a female athlete and runner. Like many girls and women in the seventies, she was discriminated against in sports. In fact, she wasn't allowed to play on the Little League baseball team in her home town because she wasn't a boy. She went on to participate on the girls' soccer and track teams at her Canisteo (New York) High School. Her college had a men's cross-country team, but not one for women. So she helped get one started. Now she coaches a boys' baseball team (as well as several girls' and co-ed sports programs) with me and beats most of the men who line up against her in road races, myself included. Shelly directs the beginner and intermediate levels of our New York Road Runners Club running classes, coaches many runners with her personal training services, and has won many trophies in local races from 5K to the marathon. More important to me, she is not only my valued running partner, she is also my partner in business and in life. Without her support I would never have made my comeback to running and racing after a debilitating herniated disk or survived to the finish line of this book.

After working myself back into shape just the way each of you (and Shepherd) have to do, I am back on the road to fitness once again. The exercise method I prefer is running. I was hooked on it as a teenager. In 1963, while a junior in high school, I went out for track, ran the half-mile, and won fifth place for the Dansville (New York) Mustangs in the Livingston County Championships. The next year marked the most important achievement of my life because it gave me the knowledge that hard work pays off and the confidence to try to be the best at whatever I do. I won the county championship at the 2-mile distance! I can still remember every detail of the race and feel the glow that comes with such an accomplishment—just like you will feel when you complete your first mile of running and, perhaps, even your first marathon.

The next year I injured both knees while competing for my college team and the doctors gave me the worst verdict possible for a runner: I would never be able to run again! I never realized how much I loved to run, for the fun of it not just for the competition, until I couldn't. So, I cheated: I played basketball and baseball in college, and later in the U.S. Army. I snuck in a few runs here and there until my knees hurt again. I even won a 400-meter race while helping to direct the Hue Sports Festival during the peak of the Vietnam War. But I missed running. When I started working as the fitness director of the Rome, New York, Family YMCA in 1971, the Y didn't have any fitness classes at all. Runners were few and far between back then.

But in Rome I was quickly challenged by Carl Eilenberg, a local radio announcer and later city mayor, to run/walk 20 miles in a walkathon for YMCA youth, which we cochaired. Carl, a former fat guy who ran himself skinny (and some say silly) announced on the air (without my knowledge) that if we both didn't make it—running all the way—we couldn't collect the pledge money. More than $1,000 was "bet" against us: the former fatso and the feeble-kneed. I had started running again when I began teaching fitness classes at the Y, but could I run 20 miles when I had never, ever run more than 5? My pride was on the line and youth was on my side. We made it, but Carl, who was nearly twice my age, ran off and left me at the halfway point and never let me forget it.

The next year I saw Frank Shorter win the Olympic Marathon on TV. It motivated me to make another attempt at long-distance running—though I never thought I'd start it in quite this way. I was visiting my late, good friend Mike Wiley, a former hurdler, in his Kansas University apartment, where we spent a whole night drinking beer with a group of track runners. There was a marathon the next day, and as the beer went down the challenges went up. More beer, more challenges; when dawn broke I agreed (as I remember) to run. A case of beer was bet on me. A few hours later I found myself, a little furry around the tongue, at the starting line of the Kansas Relays Marathon. Despite enduring rain, then sleet, and then hail, I managed to win my bet as I finished in about three and a half hours—a time I would lower by nearly an hour within six years! I couldn't walk for three days, and had to call in to work and take a few more vacation days. This is not the way I recommend to train for a marathon: I was only running a few miles a week before being lured into this challenge. Still, the experience left me determined to train for and compete in the Boston Marathon.

What about those bad knees? Dr. George Sheehan's writings about podiatrist Dr. Richard Schuster's pioneer work with orthotics for runners led me to Schuster's office. Then came the great discovery: My knee pain didn't require surgery, just exercises and orthotics to correct for pronation. It worked, and I was off on a running path that would carry me through more than thirty marathons and earn me many awards for placing in local races. I also became a proselytizer of running and fitness. The more I ran, the more I spread the word to others about its benefits. I helped start the Roman Runners club at the Rome Y and encouraged hundreds of Y members to start running and racing.

In 1975, I became fitness director of the largest YMCA (then 12,000 members) in America—on New York City's West Side. I was actually recruited by Alexander Melleby, one of the country's foremost physical educators, because I was an enthusiastic runner. He felt that my enthusiasm for running and fitness was just what was needed to upgrade a program that had emphasized the sixties concept of fitness: "calisthenics drills" with plenty of push-ups, sit-ups, and jumping jacks along with a few wind sprints. Relaxation and stretching were ignored as were aerobic or endurance exercises. Few women ventured into the classes. I was challenged to turn things around and get the membership fit.

So I slowed everybody down, wrote a manual for the instructors, started fitness testing, and began fitness classes based on running. Within a year and a half I had tested more than 1,000 men and women and gotten 2,000 started in beginner's running classes. Even Shepherd joined in. Soon, over 5,000 people were involved with my fitness classes. Next, Melleby encouraged me to hook up with Fred Lebow and his then 200-member (now 32,000-member) New York Road Runners Club. Soon, Fred moved his office out of his apartment into the back of my fitness complex, and together we plotted how we could recruit even more people to join us in our sport.

It was then that Shepherd had THE GREAT IDEA. Why not share our experiences and knowledge about running and fitness with the thousands of men and women around the country that couldn't take part in my classes? So we teamed up to write *The Runner's Handbook*. Just about the time the first edition of this book was released in 1978, I started running classes for beginner and competitive runners through the New York Road Runners Club. Now we have anywhere from 300 to 800 students per session; each year, over 2,000 runners participate in the program, which serves as the primary research tool for my running books. In addition, the official training program for the New York City Marathon, which is sent to each of the more than 30,000 participants each year, is based upon these books and these classes.

The Runner's Handbook was revised in 1985 and has been completely rewritten here. *The Competitive Runner's Handbook*, which was revised in 1988, is also being completely rewritten. Why?

First, this allows us the opportunity to update information that has changed because of scientific and technological advances. High-tech running clothing and running shoes, for example, have replaced the canvas running shoes, old T-shirt, and baggy gray sweatpants that I trained in as a high schooler. Sports drinks and sports bars and increased knowledge about carbohydrate-loading and rehydration have led to improved, safer running performances. Exercise physiologists and medical researchers have published countless studies that have changed and enhanced our knowledge of health, fitness, and running performance.

Second, running has become an important part of a healthy lifestyle for most of us rather than just a sport. Thus, we have turned this book into as much of a fitness handbook as a runner's handbook. We have added several chapters on wellness: the combination of health and fitness. Here we have included the most recent recommendations on such important topics as nutrition, weight management, and stress. We also discuss ways to prevent or minimize heart disease, cancer, asthma, osteoporosis, arthritis—and many other diseases—with exercise and wellness habits. As more and more Americans reach middle age and beyond, running and fitness can help us live longer and live better. Shepherd and I have shared our experiences with aging and running as well as the benefits and advice offered by researchers. More and more women run and exercise each year and we have updated and expanded this important area throughout the book with Shelly's experiences and direction. More of us have even busier schedules than before, so we've added sections on travel and time management and updated the chapter on balancing the "runner's triangle"—work, family, and running. We have also further emphasized two important components of fitness—flexibility, and muscular fitness—with updated and expanded chapters on stretching and strengthening. To show that we don't just run, and recommend that all of you enjoy the benefits of more than just one type of aerobic exercise, we have added a full chapter on cross-training—biking, swimming, in-line skating, cross-country skiing, and more—to enhance your overall fitness program.

Third, and most important, this rewrite allows us the opportunity to update and expand training information based on our experiences with several thousand more runners in our various programs over the years since our last revision. A coach is only wise if he or she learns from his students and thus improves his services. The following pages do not represent new and modern training techniques. Rather, they offer practical training advice that can be easily understood and used by runners of all ability levels. They work because they have been tested and improved upon by

men and women runners of all sizes, shapes, and running paces—
people just like you.

This rewrite of *The Runner's Handbook* was a three-year ultra-
marathon effort. Each of the 700-plus pages of this encyclopedia
of running—double the size of the first two editions—went
through a vigorous workout. First, Shelly and I did exhaustive research on each topic. Then I wrote a first draft. It was then reviewed by Shelly, the exercise physiologist, and sent off to Jack,
the professional writer, for a rewrite. Then it was reviewed again
by Shelly and myself for further updates. Off it went to the pub-
lisher for editing and back again to Shelly and me—two more
times—for final review and updates.

Our team of coach–writer–exercise physiologist is available, in
this book, to guide you to a healthier, happier, more energetic life.
Read each section carefully and then keep the book handy and
continually refer back to it. I've had many runners tell me that they
read the book often; others say they go to bed with it every night.
One of my greatest pleasures is to hear stories of how runners have
read and referred back to *The Runner's Handbook* so many times
that it's dog-eared. Go ahead, abuse our book and pass it on to a
friend. But whatever you do, get out the door and start—and
continue—running down the road for health and fitness, and perhaps even a little competition.

Part I

Fitness

Why Exercise?

Remember the fitness boom that began in the mid-1970s? More and more men and women started running for health and exercise as the decade progressed. They bought running clothes, shoes, and books. In 1978 alone, three books about running—including *The Runner's Handbook*—were among the top ten books sold in the United States.

And the boom continued! According to a Gallup Poll, in a two-year period, from November 1984 to November 1986, approximately 25 million Americans started exercising for the first time. During that same period, the percentage of Americans who exercised increased from 54 to 68 percent—more than two-thirds of all U.S. adults. In the 1988 edition of *The Competitive Runner's Handbook*, I announced: "These trends are expected to continue into the nineties."

Wrong. The fitness boom went bust. Why?

For one thing, many people who said they were exercising weren't. They just wanted to feel as though they were part of the action. Or, if they were actually exercising, they didn't stick with it. The word "sweat" was just not in their vocabularies. The rate at which people started exercise programs leveled off.

This happened in the late 1980s just as an increasing number of medical research studies began reporting what runners already knew: Exercise is good for you and brings significant health benefits. Despite this knowledge, large numbers of Americans actually took several giant steps backward on the road to fitness!

In 1980, the Public Health Service (PHS) sought to have 60 percent of all Americans—six out of ten of us—exercising regularly by 1990. That was a commendable and seemingly attainable goal. The result? By 1990, the PHS had convinced only 20 percent of us—two out of ten—to exercise regularly; one-third of their goal. They tried again. The PHS set a Healthy People 2000 goal. They *lowered* the target for regular exercisers by half—from the 60 percent by 1990 to 30 percent by the year 2000. In the second decade of their plan, the PHS sought to add only one more American out of every ten to their list of exercisers—from 20 percent to 30 percent. In addition, the PHS also wanted to reduce inactivity—this is the couch potato constituency—to 15 percent of all Americans over age six (down from about 24 percent in 1990).

The efforts by the Public Health Service are highly laudatory. Wouldn't you think that in the 1990s—with all the supportive medical research, the healthy low-fat diet and antismoking campaigns, the publicity about health and exercise—finding three Americans out of every ten who would exercise three or more times a week would be a lock? Yet at the halfway mark to the year 2000, PHS statistics reveal the following physical activity profile:

- Only 12 percent of Americans are vigorously active

- 10 percent are regularly active

- 54 percent are irregularly active and would benefit from more exercise

- 24 percent are completely sedentary and badly in need of more exercise. These are the hard-core couch potatoes that the government wants to trim to less than 15 percent by the year 2000. They have a better chance of getting the couch out for a run: This core of inactive Americans has remained about the same percentage since 1985—one out of every four of us.

▪ Only 22 percent of us—compared to the goal of 60 percent by 1990 and the retreating goal of 30 percent by 2000—get sufficient exercise; 78 percent do not. In short, about two Americans out of ten get sufficient exercise today; nearly eight out of ten do not. This is true despite studies which show that sedentary and irregularly active men and women are at the highest risk of heart disease and other illnesses and would benefit most from even small increases in physical activity.

Our children aren't any better: The National Children and Youth Fitness Study indicates that at least half of today's youth do not engage in physical activity appropriate to promoting long-term health. Our couch-potato adults are reproducing themselves!

Excuses

Shepherd and I have heard a lot of excuses in our time. We've been known to use a few of the best ones ourselves! When a Gallup poll asked: "What are the two or three most important reasons you don't exercise?" it compiled the following list of excuses. It's as good as any:

No time (see Chapter 26, Time Management)	40%
Get enough exercise at home or work (most likely not true)	20%
Too lazy (points here for honesty!)	15%
Health problems (but most are helped with exercise)	15%
No interest; exercise is boring (look for a fun activity)	13%
Too old (you're never too old; see Chapter 29)	12%
It's not necessary (no comment!)	10%
Too tired (no comment II)	9%

Do any of these excuses sound familiar to you? They are to us. Believe it or not, even some runners and exercisers occasionally fall back on almost all of those excuses. But we also overcome them.

We don't let work, boredom, age, fatigue (usually from work-related stress which is directly relieved by exercise), minor health pains or other excuses delay us. We know the benefits of exercise.

So come on and get started. We only ask that you take the first steps down the road to fitness. You're the one who will benefit most. We ask you to run (or do other exercises) along with us following the guidelines in this book.

Why Do People Start Running?

Many people start running for health and fitness reasons: to lose or control weight, firm up the body, allay the fear of heart disease. I know runners who exercise daily for only one reason: so they can better enjoy eating *and not have to worry about weight gain*. Others start off running because they have a family history of heart disease or obesity and choose to combat these risks with exercise, or because their doctor advised them to start exercising to improve their health. A few have told me that they actually don't like running at all. But, like brushing their teeth, they do it faithfully because they know it's good for them. Some run to keep from getting depressed or anxious—they like the way running makes them feel better and relieves stress. Many people run just because it makes them look good, perhaps allowing them to fit into the clothes they want to wear or attract the type of men or women they want. Many run to give themselves more strength and energy for work and daily tasks. There are those who take up running and fitness to expand their social horizons—it's a great way to make and maintain friends and many romances begin on the running paths. I've had several students in my running classes admit that they come to my program to meet potential dates more than to improve their running speed. Some people take up running to improve their fitness for other sports, such as tennis and basketball.

Jack Shepherd took up running because, back in 1975, he was overstressed and worried about his health. He started for medical reasons but runs today because he found that he enjoys it. Shelly-lynn Florence Glover started running as a fifteen-year-old so she could get home in time to meet her parents' curfew: The faster she ran, the later she could stay out. She discovered that she liked it and has been running ever since. I started running as a fifteen-year-old when I found myself staring at the track team workout while my baseball coach was giving a boring lecture. I can still hear his words: "Hey, Glover, go ahead over there and run with the track team if you can't pay attention to your baseball." Always one to meet a challenge, I accepted his invitation and jumped into a one-mile time trial for the track team—running in full baseball uniform, including cleats. I beat them all and discovered that not only did I like running, I liked racing. More than thirty years later I run because I, too, enjoy it. Not only that, as a fifty-year-old I ran a 2-mile race in almost exactly the same time as I did as an eighteen-year-old. How's that for motivation to keep running?

The Benefits of Running

Why should you start a running and fitness program? Here are a dozen good reasons, all of which are detailed in the following chapters.

1. *Health.* Running and other forms of aerobic exercise reduce the risk of heart disease and some forms of cancer. Running improves blood cholesterol levels, increases immunity to illness, and helps control high blood pressure, osteoporosis, diabetes, arthritis, asthma, and other health problems. Runners and others who get and stay fit also report an enhanced sex life (45 percent of those in the Gallup survey). Those who follow a regular exercise program are more likely to change other health habits— 64 percent of new exercisers polled by Gallup also started eating a healthier diet (compared to 47 percent of nonexercisers) and 43 percent lost weight (compared to 31 percent of nonexercisers).

2. *Fitness.* Running strengthens your cardiorespiratory, respiratory, and musculoskeletal systems, giving you more energy to carry out daily tasks and leisure activities. Sixty-two percent of the galloping Gallup exercisers feel they have more energy throughout the day than they did before they started exercising.

3. *Weight management.* Running is a high-energy burn off. You'll burn about 100 calories per mile of running, which will not only help you control your weight but will also reduce your percentage of body fat as you build firm, lean running muscles.

4. *Longevity.* Research shows that those who exercise vigorously on a regular basis will live longer. Just as important, you'll be more likely to live those years in better health and with fewer

disabilities. Studies show that the largest drop in death rates occur in the group going from sedentary to moderately active exercise.

5. *Aging.* Although it isn't an unending fountain of youth, running and exercise will help slow the aging process so that we can have more quality years. Exercise can slow the loss of stamina, strength, flexibility, bone density, metabolic rate, and general enthusiasm for being active that seems to go with getting older. Not only does exercise help us age with better health, but fitness levels decrease much more slowly for runners and other vigorous exercisers.

6. *Women.* Exercise helps prevent osteoporosis and health problems and discomfort associated with menstruation, pregnancy, and menopause.

7. *Sleep.* Regular exercise promotes sound sleep, leaving you feeling more refreshed to start each day. (Staying up late writing a book on running, however, doesn't.)

8. *Stress.* The impact on our health of the many stresses in our lives is significant. Running helps us relax (as reported by two-thirds of the Gallup exercisers), makes us feel organized, and builds self-esteem—all of which help us manage stress. Regular exercise also gives a sense of commitment and control—two positive mental attitudes that help counteract stress.

9. *Psychological.* Running promotes good mental health, including increased confidence and self-esteem, positive mood, general well-being, and less anxiety and depression. Exercisers report being more alert, able to think more clearly and solve problems more efficiently. Thirty-seven percent of the Gallup survey exercisers reported feeling more creative at work than they did before they started on a fitness program. Running makes you feel physically and mentally better and might even give you a mystical "runner's high."

10. *Financial.* Bill Horton, president of Fitness Systems, a company that plans and manages on-site health and fitness programs for businesses, made a survey of the financial benefits of exercise.

One example, printed in the Dartmouth College *Alumni Magazine*, cites the case of Tenneco, where male employees who exercised regularly averaged medical claims of just $561 a year; those who did not exercise made medical claims of $1,003 a year. Among the corporation's women exercisers, the average medical claim was $639 annually. The nonexercising women averaged $1,535. In a time of skyrocketing health care costs and insurance premiums, Horton's survey carries great significance for corporate America—and all of us.

Rand Corporation researchers determined that runners and other vigorous exercisers miss 32 percent fewer workdays, reduce group life insurance fees because they live one and a half years longer, and have one-third fewer hospital admissions than nonexercisers. Again, fitness saves corporate America money. Finally, there is this statistic from *Shape* magazine: For every mile you walk or run, you could add 21 minutes to your life and save twenty-four cents in health care costs.

11. *Competition.* Running offers an important outlet for competition. After you graduate from the beginner level you may decide to try racing. You may compete against yourself—improving your distances and times—or against others. You may even take on the challenge of the marathon.

12. *Fun and fellowship.* Running is a great way to meet other people and to expand friendships. Forty-six percent of new exercisers reported to the Gallup folks that sports or exercise have "helped me make new friends," yet only 2 percent said that exercise "has left me less time for a social life." And 20 percent reported that workouts actually makes close relationships closer (see Chapter 27, "The Runner's Triangle," for guidelines on running and relationships). Best of all, if you follow a sensible training program and have the support of others, it can be lots of fun. But not everyone enjoys running, so find the physical activity or activities that bring you the most pleasure and get out there and exercise, and reap the benefits of a physically active lifestyle.

So, what's your excuse? Let's get running!

TWO

What Is Fitness?

If you are well-coordinated, or good at sports, does this mean that you are physically fit? If you pass all the fitness tests in the next chapter, does that mean you are in good health?

Most people confuse being athletic with being physically fit. At any age, a person may be very good in sports but not very fit. Just watch a big but overweight kid or adult hit a long ball in baseball and then huff and puff trying to run the bases. This is one of the serious weaknesses of the competitive team sports so revered in our country. Most of them don't promote the type of exercise that improves fitness. On the other hand, one can be very fit but not very athletic. Which skills define fitness? Hitting a ball out of the park, shooting a basketball with great accuracy, or being able to run a few miles in comfort?

Just what is physical fitness? The physicians of the American Academy of Pediatrics (AAP), concerned that kids today are exposed to competitive sports but not to fitness activities, warn:

Our concept of what "physical fitness" means has undergone a major change. Traditionally, the "physically fit" child was one who had obvious motor (or athletic) abilities, ordinarily defined by such parameters as muscle strength, agility, speed and power. But the high levels of power, speed and agility necessary for success in most competitive sports have little or no relevance in the daily lives of most adults. Today, the words "physical fitness" imply optimal functioning of all physiological systems of the body, particularly the cardiovascular, pulmonary and musculoskeletal systems.

The American College of Sports Medicine (ACSM) defines fitness as "the ability to perform moderate to vigorous levels of physical activity without undue fatigue and the capability of maintaining such ability throughout life." The ACSM also states: "Physical fitness refers to your ability to carry out daily tasks without being overly tired. People who are fit have energy not only to complete everyday work, but also to participate in planned and unplanned activities outside the home or workplace."

The American Alliance for Health, Physical Education, Recreation and Dance (AAHPERD) defines fitness as "a physical state of well-being that allows people to perform daily activities with vigor, reduce their risk of health problems related to lack of exercise, and establish a fitness base for participation in a variety of physical activities."

There are key words and phrases in these statements: "perform moderate to vigorous" physical activity; carry out our daily tasks "without being overly tired"; create "well-being" and reduce health problems; build "a fitness base." What this means, and what we need, is a lifelong exercise program that leaves us fit, healthy, and full of vigor from childhood through our retirement years. We are not likely to play football or baseball throughout our lives. But we certainly can run, walk, bike, swim, and enjoy other vigorous exercise that will allow us to live longer, healthier lives. Thus the primary goal is to participate in "health-related" fitness programs that improve our cardiorespiratory and musculoskeletal systems, help manage weight, and promote the many health benefits of exercise detailed in the previous chapter. A secondary goal is to improve our fitness level so that we can perform better in physical tasks whether at work, at home, or in sports, including running.

As we detail in the wellness section of this book, a fitness program alone will not guarantee good health. You can be fit but not healthy. The term "wellness" refers to the combination of fitness (exercise) with good health practices—sound nutrition, stress management, and weight control—to improve the quality of our lives.

Health-Related Fitness Components

The American College of Sports Medicine—a professional group of over 12,000 exercise scientists, physicians, educators, and fitness professionals—emphasizes that fitness has four different components. No single exercise will result in total fitness. It is important to develop a balanced exercise program—including exercises such as running, stretching, and weight training—that will result in improvements in all aspects of fitness. The four fitness components as defined in *The ACSM Fitness Book* are:

- Cardiorespiratory fitness: the heart's ability to pump blood and deliver oxygen throughout your body

- Muscular fitness: the strength and endurance of your muscles

- Flexibility: the ability to move your joints freely and without pain through a wide range of motion

- Body composition: concerned with the portion of your body weight made up of fat.

Throughout this book I refer to cardiorespiratory fitness as aerobic fitness since the term "aerobic," which means "promoting the supply and use of oxygen," has been popularized by the fitness industry. Anaerobic fitness is the ability to produce energy with no oxygen. This really isn't a health-related fitness component, but anaerobic training is important to race performances. The faster you run, the more your body is working anaerobically and the less it is working aerobically. As beginner and intermediate runners, you will run almost exclusively at aerobic levels. You may run anaerobically if you race or do more intense workouts to train for races. You can improve your anaerobic fitness with speed training as introduced in Chapter 15.

Body composition is discussed in detail in Chapter 41, "Weight Management." A lean body can best be reached and maintained by following a program combining aerobic exercise, weight training, and a healthy diet. The more overweight you are, the more body fat you will store. You will be less healthy and less able to perform to your maximum ability as a runner.

Total fitness can't be obtained by just running, which reduces rather than increases flexibility and contributes little to upper-body muscular fitness. Flexibility training will not improve aerobic or muscular fitness. Resistance training, such as weight lifting, is the best way to improve muscular fitness, but it isn't the most effective way to improve flexibility or aerobic fitness, although it may contribute to a certain extent.

To be physically fit you need to include all the major fitness components in your exercise program. Running and other aerobic exercise combined with stretching to promote flexibility and weight training to develop muscular fitness will give you a balanced program. This will not only leave you leaner and healthier but also better able to perform as a recreational or competitive runner.

Chapter 3 offers a variety of ways to test your fitness levels in the important areas of aerobic fitness, muscular fitness, and flexibility. But first, let me detail some fitness components:

Aerobic (Cardiorespiratory) Fitness
Aerobic or cardiorespiratory fitness is measured in terms of aerobic capacity (also known as maximal oxygen uptake or max VO_2). The AAHPERD defines that as the ability to perform large-muscle, whole-body physical activity of moderate to high intensity over extended periods of time. We are talking about endurance and stamina. This kind of exercise, called aerobic exercise, helps the heart get bigger and stronger, which allows you to be more active, have more energy, reduce risk to heart disease and other illnesses, and remove stress from your cardiorespiratory system and your life.

Dr. Kenneth Cooper popularized aerobic exercise beginning in the late 1960s with a series of best-selling books. In one of them, *The Aerobics Program for Total Well-Being*, Dr. Cooper writes:

> Aerobic exercises refer to those activities that require oxygen for prolonged periods and place such demands on the body that it is required to improve its capacity to handle oxygen. As a result of aerobic exercise, there are beneficial changes that occur in the lungs, the heart, and the vascular system. More specifically, regular exercise of this type enhances the ability of the body to move air into and out of the lungs; the total blood

volume increases; and the blood becomes better equipped to transport oxygen.

Your aerobic capacity can be improved by consistent, progressive aerobic endurance exercise. There are many kinds of aerobic exercises other than running—biking, swimming, walking, cross-country skiing, skating, and so on. These are discussed in Chapter 35, "Cross-Training." The basic idea is to exercise your body steadily and vigorously over a period of at least 20 to 30 minutes at least three to five times a week. The result of such a regular program will be an aerobically fit individual. Aerobic capacity can be measured in a laboratory while running on a treadmill; aerobic fitness can be estimated by using walking and running tests such as those discussed in the following chapter. Aerobic capacity is expressed as the amount of oxygen consumed in relation to the weight of an individual (milliliters of oxygen per kilogram of body weight per minute [ml/kg/min]). Thus, you can improve your aerobic fitness both by improving the amount of work you can do and by losing weight. Generally, the higher the aerobic capacity the more fit you are and the better your race times. Such factors as anaerobic capacity, efficiency of running form and mental toughness also contribute to your performance.

Muscular Fitness
Muscular strength. This is defined as the maximum amount of force a muscle or muscle group can produce during a single contraction or exertion. The ACSM defines strength as how much weight you can safely lift. This is usually measured in fitness tests by how much you can lift in one all-out effort. All movements require a certain amount of muscle strength. To be able to carry out daily tasks in a safe manner, or to perform efficiently as a runner or other athlete and to minimize injury, you need a certain amount of muscular strength.

Muscular endurance. This is the ability to sustain repeated productions of force at low to moderate intensities over extended periods of time. The ACSM defines endurance as how many times you can lift or how long you can hold an object without fatigue. A typical fitness test for endurance would be how many sit-ups or push-ups you could do in one minute.

Muscular fitness enhances both health and athletic performance.

Abdominal muscle fitness helps you achieve good posture and decreases the incidence and severity of low-back pain. Upper-body muscle fitness helps us perform daily tasks like taking out the trash, mowing the lawn, lifting a child, changing a tire, moving furniture, and lifting, pulling, or pushing objects. Strong legs, abdominals, and upper body also contribute to an improved running form, more power to run at a faster pace and up hills, and decreased chance of injury. Further, resistance training as in weight lifting helps to slow the loss of muscular fitness due to aging. It also builds and maintains dense bones, thus helping to prevent osteoporosis, stress fractures, and other bone injuries.

Chapter 36, "Strengthening," details exercises to improve muscular fitness.

Flexibility

Flexibility is the ability of the muscles to move a joint through its full range of motion. A supple, flexible body, while of no direct benefit to your cardiorespiratory function, does allow you to exercise aerobically with greater ease and more readily perform daily tasks requiring reaching, twisting, and turning your body. It also reduces your chance of injury and of developing back problems. And if you are injured, you cannot exercise. Despite the obvious importance of flexibility, most people who engage in vigorous exercise, especially runners, often neglect it.

Unlike weight training, which works muscles against resistance, flexibility exercises involve stretching the muscles. Work on your flexibility before and after your runs and weight training sessions, as well as throughout the week. Guidelines for safe exercises to improve your flexibility are detailed in Chapter 37, "Stretching."

In summary, run, weight train, stretch, and be fit.

THREE

How Fit Are You? Check Your Progress

You have now read about the benefits of exercise and the components of physical fitness. But what about *your* fitness level? If you want to find out, read on. If you already know that you huff and puff going up the stairs, strain to carry a bag of heavy groceries, or that you haven't been able to bend down and touch your toes since you were in the sixth grade, then you already know the answer: You need to improve.

In truth, Shepherd thinks this chapter shouldn't be in the book at all. "Drop it," he said. "It's too competitive and too discouraging for the Beginner Runner. Or stick it way in the back somewhere, out of sight."

I told him: "That's because you can't do any of the tests!"

"I hate pushups," Shepherd responded. "I don't run to improve my time, but for fun! Chapter 3 is too early for Beginner Runners to start measuring their fitness levels. Get 'em started running, not deciding whether or not they're fit—or they'll quit on you."

Okay, okay. We leave the choice to you. I say, read this chapter and measure your fitness. Then start getting into shape. Shepherd says, skip this chapter and get right into the running program. He didn't need charts to tell him he was out of shape in 1975!

So, if you don't want to know the details of just how far out of shape you are—or more positively how far you need to go to get into shape—then read no further. Skip to the next chapter and get started with your exercise program. Perhaps, after you've made fitness gains, you'll come back and assess yourself with the simple tests in this chapter. If you've already been following a good exercise routine, these tests will be a good measure of where you are at and will serve as goals to motivate you to improve.

The tests in this chapter are designed to enable you to measure the basic fitness components—flexibility, muscular fitness, and aerobic fitness—defined and discussed in the previous chapter. Additional evaluations and goal setting should be established for body composition. Chapter 41 establishes guidelines for body fat percentages, weight goals, and so forth.

If you choose to do so, assess your fitness level now, and then reassess with the same tests after a period of fitness training—at least eight weeks—to check your progress.

Two cautions:

1. Consult the medical clearance guidelines in Chapter 4 prior to taking these vigorous tests and before starting a running and fitness program.

2. Practice the test skills before taking the tests; for example, practice doing sit-ups at a relaxed pace. After getting your doctor's approval, walk briskly a few times a week for a few weeks prior to taking the walking test. Don't take the running test until you can comfortably run 1.5 miles nonstop. Before taking the tests, warm up; then cool down afterward. (See guidelines in Chapter 7.) Be conservative in your first tests. Don't go all out. (After all, you want to leave some room for improvement!).

Use these tests as motivating tools. View the tests as an opportunity to know more about yourself and to set a baseline from which to start your journey to improved fitness and health. Although I have detailed in the previous chapters the level of unfitness in the United States, do not feel as though you are competing against that mark. Do not compete against other family members or peers either. Instead, focus on competing against—and improving—yourself. Every step you take toward fitness runs along your own personal path; you compete only against the "old" you.

Don't be discouraged if you score poorly on these tests. In our unfit society, most adults would do just as badly (as do most kids on youth fitness tests). Remember Shepherd's first test! Don't think the tests are too hard; they measure where we should be. They are goals. You may score "excellent" or "high" in one fitness component but "poor" or "low" in another. To be physically fit, you should score at least at the average-good level of fitness in all components.

After assessing yourself, follow the training guidelines in the following chapters to improve your fitness levels in each of the key components. If you score poorly, set a goal to reach average levels. If you score "average," aim to meet "good" standards.

The following fitness assessment program includes information from a variety of testing programs. I have selected and pieced together highlights from many programs to provide a comprehensive, simplified assessment requiring a minimum of equipment and time. Remember, the tests are optional. You may choose to do all of them, some of them, or none of them. Don't feel intimidated by them—only you need to know the results. If you are brave enough to be honest with yourself, the results can be used to guide you down that road to fitness.

So let's get started!

How do you score in flexibility, muscular fitness, and aerobic fitness? You can take these tests alone or with friends or family members. Here's what you should do:

1. After getting your doctor's go-ahead and practicing the test skills a few times, find an appropriate place to do the tests. Then, after warming up, take them one at a time. You should take breaks between each one.

2. Establish fitness baseline scores for each test and record them.

3. Establish goals to improve each test score.

4. Follow the fitness training program, as detailed in the following chapters, to achieve your individual goals.

5. After eight or more weeks, reassess all items to monitor progress and record your scores. Continue with your fitness program. You may wish to reassess a few times each year.

Except for the half-mile walking test for aerobic endurance, the following tests are from the *ACSM's Guidelines for Exercise Testing and Prescription* with data provided by the Institute for Aerobics Research in Dallas, Texas.

Flexibility Test

No single test can measure your overall body flexibility. You might be flexible in some areas but not in others. For example, you might be flexible in your shoulder area but inflexible in the ankles. Individuals who are inflexible in the lower back, hip, and hamstring area are more prone to back problems. Running strengthens these muscle groups yet inhibits flexibility. People who sit for long periods are also likely to be tight in these areas. The YMCA and the American College of Sports Medicine developed and recommend the following sit-and-reach test (also called a trunk flexion test) since it measures lower back and hamstring flexibility and loosely correlates with overall body flexibility.

Because your muscles need to be relaxed and limber before you can test them properly, warm up for this test with 5 to 10 minutes of walking and gentle relaxation and stretching exercises, particularly for the low back and hamstring muscles. Include some gentle sit-and-reach movements prior to your first test attempt. To improve your scores for your retest, follow the stretching program recommended in Chapter 37.

Place a yardstick (or measuring tape) on the floor. Take off your shoes and socks and sit with the yardstick between the legs with the zero end towards you. Keep the legs straight and flat on the floor. Your heels should be 12 inches apart and even with the 15-inch mark of the yardstick. (A strip of tape at a right angle to the yardstick at the 15-inch mark will make it easier to line up your heels.) If available, a partner should hold your knees down by gently pushing on your thighs while making sure not to impede your movement.

The test: Slowly reach forward with both hands overlapped, palms facing the floor, tips of middle fingers on top of each other. Do not jerk or bounce—that's cheating and you might injure yourself.

Exhale slowly and drop your head as you reach forward, sliding your fingertips along the yardstick. Reach out with your fingertips and touch as far up the yardstick as possible without lifting your knees. Hold this position for 3 seconds. Record, to the nearest inch, your best score in three attempts. *Caution:* Do not get competitive. This test should be performed in a slow, safe manner.

If you can't reach to your heels while keeping your legs flat on the floor as you reach forward, you are in need of improvement. It should be noted that women are naturally more flexible than men. Also, we lose flexibility as we age (but the loss can be minimized with a good stretching program).

Figure 3.1 gives the standardized norms by age and gender as developed by the Institute for Aerobics Research (scores listed to the nearest inch):

Muscular Fitness Tests

Muscular strength and endurance are generally tested simultaneously. No single test can measure your overall muscular fitness. Two important areas of muscular fitness in terms of general health are the abdominals and the upper body, thus they are commonly used in fitness assessment. Your abdominal muscles relate to lower back strength (and pain) and your upper body muscles relate to good posture and your ability to lift, carry, and push objects. Abdominal strength and endurance are measured by sit-ups; upper body strength by push-ups. Warm up carefully with some gentle stretching prior to starting the following tests.

The Sit-up Test: This test measures your abdominal and hip flexor muscular endurance. The idea is to see how many sit-ups you can do within a minute.

To begin the sit-up test, lie on your back on a carpet or mat, knees bent, heels about 18 inches from your buttocks, feet flat on the floor about shoulder-width apart. Have someone hold your ankles firmly or anchor them under a couch or other heavy piece of furniture. Place your fingers next to your ears.

While exhaling, curl up to a sitting position. Alternately touch the inside of one knee with the opposite elbow—left elbow to right knee and return to starting position, right elbow to left knee and return to starting position. While inhaling, slowly recline until your shoulders, but not necessarily your head, touches the floor.

FIGURE 3.1: SIT-AND-REACH TEST FOR FLEXIBILITY (MEN)

%	<20	20–29	30–39	40–49	50–59	60+	
99	>23.4	>23.0	>22.0	>21.3	>20.5	20.0	
95	23.4	23.0	22.0	21.3	20.5	20.0	S
90	22.6	21.8	21.0	20.0	19.0	19.0	
85	22.4	21.0	20.0	19.3	18.3	18.0	
80	21.7	20.5	19.5	18.5	17.5	17.3	E
75	21.4	20.0	19.0	18.0	17.0	16.5	
70	20.7	19.5	18.5	17.5	16.5	15.5	
65	19.8	19.0	18.0	17.0	16.0	15.0	
60	19.0	18,5	17.5	16.3	15.5	14.5	G
55	18.7	18.0	17.0	16.0	15.0	14.0	
50	18.0	17.5	16.5	15.3	14.5	13.5	
45	17.3	17.0	16.0	15.0	14.0	13.0	
40	16.5	16.5	15.5	14.3	13.3	12.5	F
35	16.0	16.0	15.0	14.0	12.5	12.0	
30	15.5	15.5	14.5	13.3	12.0	11.3	
25	14.1	15.0	13.8	12.5	11.2	10.5	
20	13.2	14.4	13.0	12.0	10.5	10.0	P
15	11.9	13.5	12.0	11.0	9.7	9.0	
10	10.5	12.3	11.0	10.0	8.5	8.0	
5	9.4	10.5	9.3	8.3	7.0	5.8	VP
1	<9.4	<10.5	<9.3	<8.3	<7.0	<5.8	

Data provided by the Institute for Aerobics Research, Dallas, TX (1994). S, superior; E, excellent; G, good; F, fair; P, poor; VP, very poor. Score in inches.

Each time you come up counts as one sit-up. Score the number of sit-ups you can complete with correct form within one minute.

Caution: Do not attempt to grind out more sit-ups than you can do with reasonable comfort, especially if you haven't been doing sit-ups lately. Do not bounce, jerk with your arms, pull on your head, or arch your back in an attempt to improve your score. That's cheating and may result in injury. Don't hold your breath: Exhale as you sit up and inhale as you lie down.

The protocol for this test uses full sit-ups. However, it is recommended that modified sit-ups (commonly referred to as crunches) be used for strength training for the abdominals since full sit-ups may place too much strain on your back. To improve your score for your retest follow the guidelines for crunches and other abdominal exercises in Chapter 36, "Strengthening."

FIGURE 3.1: SIT-AND-REACH TEST FOR FLEXIBILITY (WOMEN)

			AGE				
%	<20	20–29	30–39	40–49	50–59	60+	
99	>24.3	>24.0	>24.0	>22.8	>23.0	>23.0	
95	24.3	24.5	24.0	22.8	23.0	23.0	S
90	24.3	23.8	22.5	21.5	21.5	21.8	
85	22.5	23.0	22.0	21.3	21.0	19.5	
80	22.5	22.5	21.5	20.5	20.3	19.0	E
75	22.3	22.0	21.0	20.0	20.0	18.0	
70	22.0	21.5	20.5	19.8	19.3	17.5	
65	21.8	21.0	20.3	19.1	19.0	17.5	
60	21.5	20.5	20.0	19.0	18.5	17.0	G
55	21.3	20.3	19.5	18.5	18.0	17.0	
50	21.0	20.0	19.0	18.0	17.9	16.4	
45	20.5	19.5	18.5	18.0	17.0	16.1	
40	20.5	19.3	18.3	17.3	16.8	15.5	F
35	20.0	19.0	17.8	17.0	16.0	15.2	
30	19.5	18.3	17.3	16.5	15.5	14.4	
25	19.0	17.8	16.8	16.0	15.3	13.6	
20	18.5	17.0	16.5	15.0	14.8	13.0	P
15	17.8	16.4	15.5	14.0	14.0	11.5	
10	14.5	15.4	14.4	13.0	13.0	11.5	
5	14.5	14.1	12.0	10.5	12.3	9.2	VP
1	<14.5	<14.1	<12.0	<10.5	<12.3	<9.2	

Data provided by the Institute for Aerobics Research, Dallas, TX (1994). S, superior; E, excellent; G, good; F, fair; P, poor; VP, very poor. Score in inches.

Figure 3.2 gives the standardized norms by age and gender as developed by the Institute for Aerobic Research.

The Push-up Test: This is a simple assessment of strength and endurance in your arms, shoulders, and chest. The idea is to see how many push-ups you can do within a minute.

The testing protocol for men is the traditional push-up. Lie on your stomach, place your hands, palms down, under your shoulders, fingers pointing straight ahead. Get into the push-up position: Rest your weight on your hands with arms fully extended and on your toes with your legs parallel to each other. Keep your body straight and your head aligned with your spine throughout the test. Lower yourself to the floor until your chest lightly touches it. Then, push yourself up to the starting position. Straighten your arms fully at the top of the push-up. Keep your back and legs straight and

FIGURE 3.2: SIT-UP TEST FOR MUSCULAR FITNESS (MEN)
1 Minute Sit-up: Number

%	<20	20–29	30–39	40–49	50–59	60+	
			Age				
99	>62	>55	>51	>47	>43	>39	
95	62	55	51	47	43	39	S
90	55	52	48	43	39	35	
85	53	49	45	40	36	31	
80	51	47	43	39	35	30	E
75	50	46	42	37	33	28	
70	48	45	41	36	31	26	
65	48	44	40	35	30	24	
60	47	42	39	34	38	22	G
55	46	41	37	32	27	21	
50	45	40	36	31	26	20	
45	42	39	36	30	25	19	
40	41	38	35	29	24	19	F
35	39	37	33	28	22	18	
30	38	35	32	27	21	17	
25	37	35	31	26	20	16	
20	36	33	30	24	19	15	P
15	34	32	28	22	17	13	
10	33	30	26	20	15	10	
5	27	27	23	17	12	7	VP
1	<27	<27	<23	<17	<12	<7	

Data provided by the Institute for Aerobics Research, Dallas, TX (1994). S, superior; E, excellent; G, good, F, fair; P, poor; VP, very poor.

knees off the ground throughout the push-up. Arching of the back is not allowed. You should not touch your knees or stomach to the floor, only your chest.

For women, the testing protocol is the modified push-up. On a carpet or mat, get down on your hands and knees, ankles crossed, knees bent, palms down, under your shoulders, fingers pointing straight ahead. Get into the push-up position: Rest your weight on your hands with arms fully extended and on your knees. Lower your upper body to the floor until your chest lightly touches it. Then, push yourself up to the starting position. Keep your knees in contact with the floor while keeping your back straight and your head aligned with your spine. Straighten your arms fully at the top of the push-up.

For both men and women: Exhale as you push up and inhale as you come down. Do not hold your breath. No rest periods are

FIGURE 3.2: SIT-UP TEST FOR MUSCULAR FITNESS (WOMEN)
1 Minute Sit-up: Number

%	<20	20–29	30–39	40–49	50–59	60+	
99	>55	>51	>42	>38	>30	28	
95	55	51	42	38	30	28	S
90	54	49	40	34	29	26	
85	49	45	38	32	25	20	
80	46	44	35	29	24	17	E
75	40	42	33	28	22	15	
70	38	41	32	27	22	12	
65	37	39	30	25	21	12	
60	36	38	29	24	20	11	G
55	35	37	28	23	19	10	
50	34	35	27	22	17	8	
45	34	34	26	21	16	8	
40	32	32	25	20	14	6	F
35	30	31	24	19	12	5	
30	29	30	22	17	12	4	
25	29	28	21	16	11	4	
20	28	27	20	14	10	3	P
15	27	24	18	13	7	2	
10	25	23	15	10	6	1	
5	25	18	11	7	5	0	VP
1	<25	<18	<11	<7	<5	0	

Data provided by the institute for Aerobics Research, Dallas, TX (1994). S, superior; E, excellent; G, good; F, fair; P, poor; VP, very poor.

allowed. Do as many push-ups as you can until you can no longer do them with proper form, or until a minute elapses. Score one push-up each time you fully extend in the up position with proper form. To improve your score on your retest, follow the guidelines in Chapter 36, "Strengthening."

Figure 3.3 gives the standardized norms by age and gender as developed by the Institute for Aerobics Research.

Aerobic Fitness Tests

The most accurate way to measure maximal aerobic fitness is in a special laboratory on a treadmill. There, exercise physiologists will have you run to your limit while measuring your heart rate (with an electrocardiogram) and your oxygen consumption (with gas analyzers). This is called a maximal exercise test since it measures a

FIGURE 3.3: PUSH-UP TEST FOR MUSCULAR FITNESS (MEN)
1 Minute Push-up: Number

%	20–29	30–39	40–49	50–59	60+	
99	>62	>52	>40	>39	>28	
95	62	52	40	39	28	S
90	57	46	36	30	26	
85	51	41	34	28	24	
80	47	39	30	25	23	E
75	44	36	29	24	22	
70	41	34	26	21	21	
65	39	31	25	20	20	
60	37	30	24	19	18	G
55	35	29	22	17	16	
50	33	27	21	15	15	
45	31	25	19	14	12	
40	29	24	18	13	10	F
35	27	21	16	11	9	
30	26	20	15	10	8	
25	24	19	13	9.5	7	
20	22	17	11	9	6	P
15	19	15	10	7	7	
10	18	13	9	6	4	
5	13	9	5	3	2	VP
1	<13	<9	<5	<3	<2	

Above the age columns: AGE

Data provided by the Institute for Aerobics Research, Dallas, TX (1994). S, superior; E, excellent; G, good; F, fair; P, poor; VP, very poor.

person's maximal aerobic capacity (VO$_2$ max) and requires a total effort to the point of voluntary exhaustion.

Fortunately, exercise scientists have come up with submaximal tests that don't require a lot of expensive equipment and an exhaustive run, and thus are safer. I've chosen two types of these tests that fairly accurately predict aerobic fitness: a half-mile walk, and a 1.5 mile run. If you are not already running at least 1.5 miles with comfort, start with the walking test. Again the warning: If you have not been exercising vigorously on a regular basis, check with your doctor before attempting these tests.

Wear comfortable, loose-fitting clothing and a good pair of running shoes for the tests. Don't attempt these tests on a hot or windy day as the weather conditions will affect your score. Also, make sure you are well rested for the tests. It will help if you can bring a friend along to time you and cheer you on.

FIGURE 3.3: MODIFIED PUSH-UP TEST FOR MUSCULAR FITNESS (WOMEN)
1 Minute Push-up: Number

%	20–29	30–39	40–49	50–59	60+	
99	>45	>39	>33	>28	>20	
95	45	39	33	28	20	S
90	42	36	28	25	17	
85	39	33	26	23	15	
80	36	31	24	21	15	E
75	34	29	21	20	15	
70	32	28	20	19	14	
65	31	26	19	18	13	
60	30	24	18	17	12	G
55	29	23	17	15	12	
50	26	21	15	13	8	
45	25	20	14	13	6	
40	23	19	13	12	5	F
35	22	17	11	10	4	
30	20	15	10	9	3	
25	19	14	9	8	2	
20	17	11	6	6	2	P
15	15	9	4	4	1	
10	12	8	2	1	0	
5	9	4	1	0	0	VP
1	<9	<4	0	0	0	

Data provided by the Institute for Aerobics Research, Dallas, TX (1994). S, superior; E, excellent; G, good; F, fair; P, poor; VP, very poor.

Before doing these tests, you must warm up properly with a brisk 5- to 10-minute walk and moderate stretching exercises. The ideal place to test yourself is your local high school or college track, which should be a quarter-mile in length (or 400 meters, only about 3 yards short of a quarter-mile). You can design a course anywhere, but try to keep it level. If you measure a course with your car or if you take your test on a computerized treadmill, be aware that the calibrations may not be completely accurate. After finishing each test, be certain to cool down with a 5- to 10-minute walk and a series of stretching exercises.

Half-Mile Walking Test
This half-mile walking test is recommended for those not yet prepared to take the running test. It was developed for Merrell foot-

wear by cardiologist and exercise physiologist Dr. James Rippe at the Center for Clinical and Lifestyle Research affiliated with Tufts School of Medicine. This simple test can be completed in less than 10 minutes by most people—thus it is called the Merrell® Ten-Minute Challenge. For more information about The Merrell Rugged Walking Program write to P.O. Box 4249, Burlington, VT 05406.

If you wish to try a more sophisticated assessment, the one often used by fitness specialists is the Rockport Fitness Walking Test, which covers a full mile in distance and factors in your exercise heart rate. You can obtain a copy by writing to the Rockport Walking Institute, P.O. Box 480, Marlboro, MA 01752.

Half a mile is two laps of a standard-sized track. Thus, after one lap you'll be at the midpoint of the test and will know what pace you are on. Step out at a brisk and steady pace. Walk the distance as fast as you can with reasonable comfort. Push yourself just a little if you are a beginner in fitness, but push harder if you are in good shape. Time yourself for the half-mile and then compare your time in minutes and seconds to those in Figure 3.4, which is broken down by age and gender. Here's a good challenge: My father, Ross Glover, stepped off the half-mile in under 6½ minutes—at age seventy!

1.5 Mile Running Test

This running test was designed by Dr. Kenneth Cooper and associates at the Aerobics Center in Dallas, Texas. This distance is six laps of a standard quarter-mile track, thus you can pace yourself with the time "splits" you get after each lap. Because this test requires a strong effort, only persons who are healthy and at least moderately active should try it. Again, you should be able to run at least 1.5 miles in comfort prior to taking this test. The goal is to run at a brisk, steady pace. Do not run to exhaustion. Pace yourself; don't start too fast. Take walk breaks or terminate the test if necessary. Push yourself just a little if you are not experienced at running hard in tests or races. Push yourself harder if you are in good shape and are an experienced racer. Time yourself for 1.5 miles and then compare your time in minutes and seconds to Figure 3.5 which gives the standardized norms by age and gender as developed by the Institute for Aerobics Research.

FIGURE 3.4: HALF-MILE WALKING TEST FOR AEROBIC FITNESS
MERRELL® TEN-MINUTE CHALLENGE

AGE	20–29	30–39	40–49	50–59	60+
WOMEN					
High	<5:37	<5:55	<6:17	<6:40	<7:07
Above Avg.	5:37–6:27	5:55–7:00	6:17–7:21	6:40–7:53	7:07–8:31
Average	6:28–7:31	7:01–8:05	7:22–8:45	7:54–9:16	8:32–10:29
Below Avg.	7:32–8:59	8:06–10:09	8:46–10:29	9:17–11:12	10:30–12:04
Low	>9:00	>10:10	>10:30	>11:13	>12:05
MEN					
High	<5:14	<5:37	<5:55	<6:09	<6:24
Above Avg.	5:14–6:12	5:37–6:27	5:55–7:00	6:09–7:21	6:24–7:31
Average	6:13–7:21	6:28–7:31	7:01–8:18	7:22–8:45	7:32–9:00
Below Avg.	7:22–8:31	7:32–8:45	8:19–9:49	8:46–10:09	9:01–10:49
Low	>8:32	>8:32	>9:50	>10:10	>10:50

FIGURE 3.5: 1.5 MILE RUNNING TEST FOR AEROBIC FITNESS (MEN)

%	Age 20–29	30–39	40–49	50–59	60+	
99	7:29	7:11	7:42	8:44	9:30	S
95	8:13	8:44	9:30	10:40	11:20	
90	9:09	9:30	10:16	11:18	12:20	
85	9:45	10:16	11:18	12:20	13:22	
80	10:16	10:47	11:44	12:51	13:53	E
75	10:42	11:18	11:49	13:22	14:24	
70	10:47	11:34	12:34	13:45	14:53	
65	11:18	11:49	12:51	14:03	15:19	
60	11:41	12:20	13:14	14:24	15:29	G
55	11:49	12:38	13:22	14:40	15:55	
50	12:18	12:51	13:53	14:55	16:07	
45	12:20	13:22	14:08	15:08	16:27	
40	12:51	13:36	14:29	15:26	16:43	F
35	13:06	13:53	14:47	15:53	16:58	
30	13:22	14:08	14:56	15:57	17:14	
25	13:53	14:24	15:26	16:23	17:32	
20	14:13	14:52	15:41	16:43	18:00	P
15	14:24	15:20	15:57	16:58	18:31	
10	15:10	15:52	16:28	17:29	19:15	
5	16:12	16:27	17:23	18:31	20:04	VP
1	17:48	18:00	18:51	19:36	20:57	

Data provided by the Institute for Aerobics Research, Dallas, TX (1994). S, superior; E, excellent; G, good; F, fair; P, poor; VP, very poor.
Time in minutes, seconds.

FIGURE 3.5: 1.5 MILE RUNNING TEST FOR AEROBIC FITNESS (WOMEN)

	AGE				
%	20–29	30–39	40–49	50–59	60+
99	8:33	10:05	10:47	12:28	11:36
95	10:47	11:49	12:51	14:20	14:06 S
90	11:43	12:51	13:22	14:55	14:55
85	12:20	13:06	14:06	15:29	15:57
80	12:51	13:43	14:31	15:57	16:20 E
75	13:22	14:08	14:57	16:05	16:27
70	13:53	14:24	15:16	16:27	16:58
65	14:08	14:50	15:41	16:51	17:29
60	14:24	15:08	15:57	16:58	17:46 G
55	14:35	15:20	16:12	17:14	18:00
50	14:55	15:26	16:27	17:24	18:16
45	15:10	15:47	16:34	17:29	18:31
40	15:26	15:57	16:58	17:55	18:44 F
35	15:48	16:23	16:59	18:09	18:54
30	15:57	16:35	17:24	18:23	18:59
25	16:26	16:58	17:29	18:31	19:02
20	16:33	17:14	18:00	18:49	19:21 P
15	16:58	17:29	18:21	19:02	19:33
10	17:21	18:00	18:31	19:30	20:04
5	18:14	18:31	19:05	19:57	20:23 VP
1	19:25	19:27	20:04	20:47	21:06

Data provided by the Institute for Aerobics Research, Dallas, TX (1994). S, superior; E, excellent; G, good; F, fair; P, poor; VP, very poor.
Time in minutes, seconds.

Part II

Getting Fit

FOUR

Getting Started

Running is such a simple sport, you'd think it would be easy to get started. Not so. At least half of all adult men and women who attempt to start a running program fail. Even a quarter of the beginners in my running classes give up and don't graduate.

Why? Most beginners try to do too much too soon and become frustrated or feel defeated. They don't get started on the right foot. Or, they lack the commitment and motivation to change.

Why should you start running? There are many reasons why running is good for you—just look them up in the first chapter. But don't run only because it is good for you. Running should be enjoyable. Try the motivational techniques in the following chapter. Most of us enjoy running once we overcome the initial obstacles we face as beginners: our out-of-shape bodies and our too-hurried daily schedules.

Most people who give running a chance learn to love it. I feel running is the best way to get in shape and keep in shape since it is relatively inexpensive (only a good pair of running shoes is essential) and you don't have to find a pool or a bike to work out. It's portable—you can run anywhere you travel. Just put on your shoes and head out the door. You can exercise alone, or run and chat with others. You can run in your favorite parks, along wooded trails, at your school track or just go exploring. You can even stay indoors in really hot or cold weather and run on a treadmill. Running is one of the most effective ways to burn calories and thus lose weight. Running isn't the only answer to fitness, but it is an excellent choice for many men and women who wish to get in shape.

If you're beginning a running program it will help to follow my eight steps to getting started successfully:

1. Make a commitment.

2. Check with your doctor.

3. Establish your starting point.

4. Set reasonable, but challenging, goals.

5. Select the proper equipment.

6. Follow a sensible training program.

7. Set up a support network.

8. Keep motivated and stay with it.

Commitment

You need to be committed to your running and fitness program—whether you are just beginning or whether you are heading for your fortieth year of running like me. This is extremely important because lack of commitment and motivation are the primary reasons people don't exercise. If overweight, you should also make a commitment to lower your caloric intake and lose the excess baggage.

It probably took you years to get out of shape. It will take more than a few days (but not more than a few weeks) to start getting back in shape. At first, even my very easy running-walking program may seem like hard work and it may take time away from the rest of your life. But you'll soon realize that the hardest part is getting out the door a few times a week and coaxing yourself to get running. Unfortunately, as I detailed in Chapter 1, excuses are easy to come by. Discipline yourself to set aside the excuses.

Commit yourself to exercising at least three times a week for ten weeks. Be prepared to struggle a little, if need be, through the early stages until definite results are achieved. Make me—and yourself—a promise that you will carry out this commitment for the full ten weeks. If you do, and follow my sensible training program, you will have learned that the benefits of running outweigh the inconveniences. And as the running gets easier, it gets much more enjoyable.

You need to run at least three times a week, approximately every other day. Each workout, including warm-up and cool-down, will only take about an hour. Make your exercise hour "sacred" and free from interference. Pick the best time of day for you and stick to it.

I am only asking you to set aside three hours a week at the start. But you may complain, "I don't have the time." You do. In fact, you can easily find 3 hours out of the 168 hours in every week. Here's how:

Make a firm commitment that you will set aside one hour every other day for exercise. That's roughly one hour from every 48. You're sleeping 16 hours out of those 48, and working 16 hours or so. That still leaves 16 hours for other things, and one of those hours can be set aside for exercise. On a weekly basis, 3 hours out of 168 hours in every week takes only 1/56th of your time for exercise. Best of all, what you do with the remaining 55/56ths will be enhanced and invigorated by what you do in that 1/56th of time.

You need to plan exercise into your day. As previously emphasized, not having enough time is the most common excuse for not starting and sticking with an exercise program. You can make time for anything you are committed to doing. Make an appointment to exercise. Take out your calendar or day planner at the end of each week and identify the best times you have available for the coming week. Actually write your running appointments into your daily planner.

Your schedule should be firm, yet slightly flexible. Find the days and times that work best for you and *stick to it!* Set a priority. You do, however, have to be somewhat flexible. If I know I can't run at noon because of a business trip, I may get up early and do a short run in the morning, for example. In other words if your schedule changes, don't use that as an excuse not to keep your running commitment. Adapt. Be flexible, re-schedule your run.

When you start exercising, you'll want to maintain a balance between your fitness program, career, and family and social responsibilities. There is no need to become a fanatic about running. What is important here is to work fitness into your life. The commitment you make to take the time to exercise will be one of the best investments you'll ever make.

Check with Your Doctor

Whatever your age, if you are apparently healthy but have been inactive for any length of time it would be a good idea to get your doctor's okay before starting a running and fitness program. The American College of Sports Medicine (ACSM) advises that any man age forty and older, and any woman age fifty and older, should have a complete medical examination prior to starting any exercise program that includes a vigorous activity such as running. This also applies to people the ACSM considers to be at high risk—those who have two or more major coronary risk factors (family history of cardiovascular disease in parents or siblings prior to age fifty-five, high blood pressure, elevated cholesterol levels, smoking, diabetes); and/or symptoms suggestive of cardiopulmonary or metabolic disease such as pain or discomfort in the chest, unaccustomed shortness of breath, shortness of breath with mild exertion, dizziness, palpitations, tachycardia, or a known heart murmur. You may be advised to take an electrocardiogram (ECG)-monitored exercise stress test before starting. The ACSM advises a thorough medical evaluation before starting an exercise program for all individuals with known cardiovascular, pulmonary, or metabolic diseases (diabetes, thyroid disorders, renal or liver disease, etc.).

Discuss with your doctor any physical limitations you may have because of orthopedic problems, such as a bad back, foot problems, or old injuries, as well as any other health problems, such as allergies or asthma, which may affect your exercise program. If your doctor isn't enthusiastic about your starting a fitness program, or knowledgeable about the benefits of exercise, consider switching to a doctor who understands and promotes exercise for his or her patients and can advise you on how to start exercising safely.

Beginners often injure themselves by doing too much too soon and thus putting too much stress on muscles that have been underexercised. Even my conservative program may lead to aches and pains in some people who have been very inactive. If you develop any muscular or skeletal problems that don't go away after a few days' rest, see an experienced sports medicine professional. Don't try to keep running despite an injury—you'll just make it worse. By starting with a conservative training program, and by "listening to your body" for warning signs (pain), you will greatly reduce injuries.

Establish Your Starting Point

If you know how fit—or unfit—you are now, then it is easier for you to get started safely on an exercise program. Otherwise, you might start off running and doing exercises that are too easy or too hard for you. You might want to use the fitness tests in the previous chapter to establish your baseline—the starting point for your running and fitness program. If you are already active, perhaps in aerobic exercise classes or biking, then you still need to ease into your running since the pounding it involves will cause additional stress on your muscles and bones. You may be able to start with my advanced beginner or intermediate program.

Set Reasonable, But Challenging, Goals

As you start on a running and fitness program why not challenge yourself with some goals? Base them on your fitness tests results. Make sure the goals can be attained with a *reasonable amount of training*. Set a time period that is short enough to motivate you, but long enough to allow for results. Some examples:

- Lose 3 pounds in one month, 10 pounds in four months.

- Increase the number of push-ups you can do in one minute by 10 within two months.

- Improve your flexibility score by 2 inches within two months.

- Be able to run 20 minutes nonstop within ten weeks; 30 minutes within four months.

See Chapter 5 for more information on goal-setting.

Select the Proper Equipment

The only major equipment you need is a good pair of running shoes. Although you could get by for the first few sessions with an old pair of basketball sneakers or cross-trainers, it would be wise to make the commitment to start safely by investing in quality running shoes. They'll make your running safer and more enjoyable. See Chapter 16 for guidelines for choosing your first (but not last!) pair of running shoes.

At first you may choose to wear whatever clothing you have available that is comfortable on the run. See Chapter 17 for guidelines for various choices of clothing that will make you look and feel better as you run down the road to fitness and good health.

Follow a Sensible Training Program

Most often when beginners don't enjoy running or fail to achieve success, it is because they are not exercising correctly. It is extremely important to follow a sensible training program. *Do not* follow programs made up by friends who happen to run or coaches who are only experienced at coaching elite runners. Don't try to emulate the schedules of more experienced or accomplished runners. You must follow a conservative program to ease yourself gently into running. The key is learning how to run enough, but not too much. As a beginner, more is not better. If you try to run too fast, too often, or too long, you are likely to become injured, exhausted, frustrated. Typical mistakes are trying to run a full mile or more nonstop, or thinking that you have to run every day to see progress. Ease into running with a program that alternates running with walking and includes off days for rest. If you are overweight or way out of shape, you should walk briskly for 30 to 60 minutes several times a week for at least four weeks before you start to run.

Consider enrolling in a quality, supervised start-up fitness program at your local Y, fitness club, or running club that will help you get started on the right foot. In fact, my beginner and intermediate level classes with the New York Road Runners Club are the basis for the training programs in this book.

The methods I use for cautiously, systematically guiding beginners to minimal levels of fitness have been tested successfully on thousands of out-of-shape men and women of all sizes, shapes, ages, and fitness levels—just like you. They even worked on Shepherd! Follow the programs outlined in this book to ease your body through the stages of a beginning runner.

Give your running program a chance.

Set Up a Support Network

Making a lifestyle change as important as starting or upgrading your exercise program is quite a challenge. It will be difficult to succeed without a lot of help from others. Develop a support system to help you get started on the path to improved fitness. You can enlist two types of people: those who can sometimes serve as your running partners, and those who may not exercise with you but can be morale boosters (whether runners or nonrunners). Both types of supporters will help you through the pitfalls of starting and staying with your running program. Chapter 5 discusses the motivational advantages of running with others.

Keep Motivated and Stay With It

Getting started isn't easy. After all it takes admitting that you are out-of-shape and making a commitment to do something about it. And that involves hard work and sweat. You have to be motivated to get started on a running program. It may be any of the usual reasons: to lose weight, look better, feel better, improve health. But getting started is one thing, staying with it is another. Many people drop out on the way to fitness, or get in shape only to give up. Some runners drop out after running for a few months or even a few years. They've conquered the challenge of getting in shape and maybe even running their first race or first marathon. Why? They lack the motivation to stay with it. You need to keep it fun, keep it rewarding. This is such an important topic that I've set aside the next chapter to keep you running!

FIVE

Motivation: Staying with It

Rah-Rah-Rah-Sis-Boom-Bah, Go-Go-Go, Run-Run-Run!

Did that motivate you? All of us need a good cheer every once in a while to keep on running. This is true both for the beginner runner and the Olympic Marathoner. Motivation involves having the incentive to keep on going—staying with it. You need better reasons to continue than excuses to quit.

How Not to Be a Dropout

Why do runners become ex-runners? Psychologist Lynn McCutcheon, author of *Psychology for Runners*, conducted a survey and found that the five main reasons for stopping were:

1. *Time constraints.* This was also the number one reason given to Gallup pollsters for not starting an exercise program. True, as you start a family or progress in school or in your career, it is harder to find the time for running. But the Gallup poll also stated that only 6 percent of those who exercise regularly found that it took a lot of planning and effort to find the time to ex-

ercise. Again, set aside an hour at least three times each week for exercise and enjoy it. Look forward to it. Justify the time spent as an investment that will improve all the other aspects of your life.

2. *Bad weather*. We are basically talking about the hot and the cold of it here. Sure, I know plenty of runners who gave up running when it got hot and sticky, or when old man winter brought us lots of snow and plenty of cold weather. They just hung up their running shoes when the weather gets bad and never put them back on again when conditions improved. Remember that if you give up for a few days, the next thing you know it'll be a few weeks. You'll most likely regain lost weight and lose much of your conditioning. You'll have to work hard again just to get back to where you were. Protect your investment! The odds are high that if you give up your exercise program for even a few weeks you won't go back to it. Once good exercise habits are broken, inactivity is the easier choice. All those excuses start to add up.

To conquer bad weather you need to be prepared. Dress properly, adjust your training, and get out there. Look at it as a challenge. You'll soon find that the hardest part is just getting out the door. But sometimes we need to be flexible about running in bad weather. Facing too many days in a row of lousy conditions will sap the enthusiasm of even the most dedicated runner. Therefore I suggest taking a few breaks during long stretches of bad weather. Take a day or two off from exercise, or alternate running one day with the next day off to ride out a heat wave or a freeze.

You may also benefit from switching to other activities for a few days. When my running trails are snow-covered and I'm bored with running around and around a plowed parking lot, I'll strap on my cross-country skis or snowshoes and head for the woods. In the heat of the summer, I'll hop on my mountain bike late in the evening, turn on my headlights, and head for the hills. The air resistance created as I whiz along helps to keep me cooler than if I were running. Shepherd dives into one of those cool Vermont ponds and swims during his allotted running time on very hot days. These alternative workouts are also psychologically uplifting—instead of giving in to Mother Nature and quitting, we can accept her gifts as an opportunity to expand our exercise activities. It's not running, but it will keep you in shape and it can be lots of fun.

You don't have to go outdoors to exercise. Even if the weather is very bad outside—hot, cold, rain, air pollution—you can do your workout indoors. You can continue your stretching exercises to improve and maintain flexibility, and you can work on your muscular fitness with push-ups, crunches, and other simple at-home exercises. Many runners have learned the value of keeping an aerobic exercise machine at home. My exercise bike comes in handy as a bad weather backup. Or, I'll go to my air-conditioned fitness club and challenge the computerized bikes and stair-climbers when I need a break from too many days of running in heat and humidity. I'll even jump on the treadmill or cross-country ski machine if I've gone too many days in a row slipping and sliding on ice and snow.

So, if you want to be a wimp and skip a run or two because it's raining out, or it's too hot or too cold, go right ahead. I won't say a word. But if you skip more than a day or two then I'll call you a quitter. How's that for motivation!

3. *Preference for another type of exercise.* Okay, but before you leave us, why not review the motivational tips within this chapter to see if they will help you have more fun with your running. I certainly promote the value of cross-training, as clearly emphasized in Chapter 35. Alternating running with other types of exercise may be a good way for you to keep your overall fitness program going. If you do leave our sport entirely, be sure to stick with a good aerobic alternative and follow the general exercise guidelines in this book.

4. *Inability to stick with a schedule.* Whether you are training to complete your first fitness mile or to improve your marathon time, you need a training schedule that follows the behavioral principle known as "shaping." This is a process in which a target behavior is broken up into a series of progressive steps that lead eventually to the desired goal. You should start with simple, easily performed tasks and add gradual, attainable progressions that will enhance your self-confidence and motivation to continue. If you try to follow a schedule that is too advanced, you won't be able to stick with it. On the other hand, if your schedule is too easy you won't be motivated to keep working.

5. *Lack of running partners to keep you company.* If you like running with others, join a running club or group, travel to local parks or tracks where lots of others run, or make appointments with friends on a regular basis. I'll discuss this important topic more later in this chapter.

Other major reasons for dropping out include illness (back off and start back conservatively when you feel healthy again) and injury (this is a reason I hear quite often and it's usually caused by doing too much too soon). By the way, of the fifty-six dropout cases in McCutcheon's survey, half said they intended to return to running.

According to studies by John Martin and Patricia Dubbert at the University of Mississippi at Jackson, the most critical factors characterizing the exercise program dropout are:

Overweight. The more overweight you are the harder it is to run. In running, you are picking up your body weight and moving it forward with your own power. You hit the ground with three times your body weight with each footstrike, so the more you weigh the more likely you are to become injured and quit. If you are more than 20 percent above your recommended healthy weight, then running might not be the best activity for you—yet. Start with a healthy diet to cut back on the calories you take in combined with a non-weight-bearing, calorie-burning exercise such as swimming or biking combined with a walking program. If you first lose some weight and improve your fitness prior to starting a running program, you'll be less likely to become a dropout.

Low self-motivation. Many runners can easily come up with ways to motivate themselves (such as losing weight for improved health). Others just aren't the self-motivating type—they need to find external sources of motivation, such as praise by others, or tangible rewards, like a gift or trip for achieving goals.

Anxiety. If you fear that you won't be successful at running or racing, you won't be. There is nothing to fear except staying out of shape. You only need to compare yourself to one person—yourself. Running will improve your feelings of self-esteem and help control anxiety and depression.

No spousal support. As detailed in Chapter 27, "The Runner's Triangle," it is important to make your family part of your exercise program, and not only your spouse but your kids as well. Share your interest in running with them and convert them into cheerleaders if not running partners. Make them aware that they, too, will benefit if you look and feel better. Consider family and household responsibilities when you schedule your running. Reward them for their support: Take them along for a short vacation when you run a race, or buy them a nice present when you go shopping for running shoes or clothing for yourself. I'm real fortunate here in that Shelly and I can enjoy being together on training runs several times a week. We train at the same pace; we have to keep in shape so as not to let the other down. How's that for motivation!

Inconvenient exercise facility. Hey, you don't need a club or pool. Just head out the door and run. If you don't have safe, enjoyable places near you to run, then this could become an obstacle. Check out good spots to run in your area that are within a reasonable traveling distance. Join a fitness club that can be home base to runs in desirable areas. Or do what I did. I checked out houses in the suburbs when I moved out of New York City and told the real estate agent to find us a nice place within a short run of the wooded trails that we love. Now I can take a run with the deer, rabbits, and chipmunks within five minutes after heading out the door. If exercise is important to you, consider it when choosing the location of your next apartment or house.

Exercise intensity that is too high. The "no pain, no gain" philosophy doesn't apply to fitness running. You should run at a nice easy pace at which you can carry on a conversation. Running too fast or too far will soon become a burden. Slow down and enjoy your run. Give yourself time to smell the flowers.

No social support during and after exercise. This subject is so important to staying motivated that it pops up again on this list. I'll discuss this critical need later in this chapter.

Coach Bob Glover's Motivational Tips

The key to staying with a running program is the three "F" philosophy: Keep it Fun, provide Fellowship, and Fitness will follow. Here are my top motivational tips:

Have fun. If you don't enjoy running, you won't stay with it. True, some people run regularly and hate it. They do it because they know it's good for them. Not many of us work that way. Running may not necessarily be fun for you at the start. Persist. Your body may scream: "Why did I let Glover talk me into this?" But once you're beyond that, your body will adjust to the work and you will begin to feel the physical and psychological benefits and increased energy. If you hang in there for a few weeks you will start developing that feeling of "I want to run." You'll begin to truly enjoy it. At this stage you might get hooked for life.

Run at a relaxed pace and enjoy life around you. Or just tune out and escape from the pressures. Maybe you'll even enjoy that euphoric state called a runner's high as discussed in Chapter 42. Doesn't that sound like fun?

Don't make running another stress in your life. Don't overtrain. If you do, you'll burn out and running won't be fun. So train, don't strain. Smile, don't frown. Instead of thinking "no pain, no gain," think "no run, no fun." Dr. Jerry Lynch in his book *The Total Runner: A Complete Mind-Body Guide to Optimal Performance*, emphasizes, "There needs to be more joy experienced while *on the run*, not just when it is over. Runners tend to be rather spartan about having fun and their social life goes on hold. If your motivation is low, perhaps there's a paucity of *fun* in your training program. I always said that when running is no longer a joy, I would quit out of choice. I make sure to build into my life of motion enjoyable episodes and experiences. Many ex-runners' major complaint is that it ceased to be enjoyable."

Some runners enjoy listening to music while on the run. But the police swear that running with headphones may be dangerous (see Chapter 24). A study at Springfield College in Massachusetts indicates that people who listen to music exercise longer. They tested twenty-six exercisers riding stationary bikes both while listening to music and without music. They found that while listening to music the exercisers pedaled on the average 30 percent longer before feeling discomfort from their workouts. Why? If you enjoy music then it stands to reason that combining it with exercise will make your workout more fun, too. Shepherd listens to tapes on a headset while working out on a rowing machine. Many runners talk enthusiastically about how listening to music helps keep them motivated and on the run. It doesn't do anything for me; I'd rather listen to the birds singing or carry on a conversation with others while on the run. But if it motivates you, then give it a try at least once in a while to add some variety and fun to your runs.

Below are some tips for enjoying running. Add to them: The amount of fun you can have is only limited by your creativity and your enthusiasm.

Fellowship: run together. With the huge growth of our sport we don't have to train in solitude. Most runners will improve not just their fitness but also their enjoyment of running by teaming up with others. Even though this requires some planning, it's well worth the effort considering all the benefits you can derive from it.

Starting a program alone can be very demanding. You need the support of others. Our beginner level classes with the New York Road Runners Club get twenty to fifty men and women of all ages with each ten-week session. The fact that they have to show up once or twice a week to run with their new friends encourages them to get out at least two more times during the week for "homework" runs in order to be able to keep up with the progress of their classmates. You will be motivated to stick it out if you're committed to keeping up with the gradual progression of a class. For many of our students the fellowship becomes as important as fitness. They enjoy talking to one another as they walk and run in Central Park. After a few weeks they talk so much and so fast that they sound like a group of kindergarten kids heading out to the playground. The hundreds of experienced, faster runners in our intermediate- and competitive-level classes also enjoy the camaraderie of working out together—even through my sometimes grueling workouts. Again, many of them come to our classes as much for fellowship reasons as for fitness. They hang out and socialize before, during, and after class. I often have to remind some of them that if they are chatting away having a good time during speed workouts they really aren't going to reach their potential. Many of them come to class even if they are injured or coming off a race just so they won't miss the party. And then there is the dedicated pizza crowd. They work hard in class so they can eat guilt free afterward with "the gang."

If you can't find a beginner's running class in your area (unfortunately, they are very rare), then as you get under way, try to encourage a friend to start with you. The two of you (the more the merrier) will support each other when the weather turns bad, or when excuses blow in the wind.

Running with others will greatly reduce the mental strain that comes with training and will help keep you motivated and fit. If you make an appointment with your running partner you are much more likely to get out the door and enjoy a good run. Many runners set a standing date for a few running friends to get together at least once a week. It is a good idea, however, to include a few new running partners from time to time to add variety and thus enjoyment to your schedule. Shelly and I are fortunate in that we can run with our classes on Tuesday and Thursday evenings and we run together from our home two or three times a week. She also works out with her team—the Westchester Track Club—twice a week. And we often enjoy informal group runs on weekends with members of the Westchester Road Runners through the woods in "Sleepy Hollow," along the paths where Ichabod Crane was last seen with the Headless Horseman in pursuit. For many of these runners the most important part is the postrun brunch. Again, socializing is a great motivator.

After you get past the beginner stage you may enjoy joining a team. But for now at least look for one of the many clubs that stress fun and support, not serious training and racing. Each year the New York Road Runners Club sponsors a club race. Lots of teams show up—from fast ones to very slow ones—and then have a picnic afterward. Often teams organize exciting trips to races, regular social gatherings, and newsletters full of race results and team gossip. The biggest benefit from running with a team: the support members give each other.

But you don't have to be part of an official team to enjoy running with a group. Many towns and cities, running clubs and Y's, have informal group runs that are open to anyone. I used to lead one at New York City's West Side YMCA. We'd get as many as 100 runners, and more than a few of us would head to the local bar afterward to eat, drink, and be merry. One of our regulars who helped keep running in perspective was Robin Williams— back when he was a pretty good runner and an aspiring actor.

Finding individuals or groups to run with is especially important to those runners putting in those mind- and body-taxing long runs in preparation for running a marathon. Running with others is also a good idea for safety: Statistics show that the vast majority of crimes against runners occur when the runner is alone.

Whether you are running with a group or with an individual training partner, be sure to observe a few important rules. Don't get in over your head. If you get carried away with the fun and fellowship—or, if not careful, the competitive nature of some runners—you could end up running too fast or too far. Time and miles fly by when you're running and talking. Ideally, find people to run with who will stick to the conversational pace of the slowest runner in the group. After all, if you can't run alongside your running partners and talk, why should they want to run with you? However, if you run much slower than your ideal pace in order to run with a friend, you won't gain in fitness as much as you could.

Many runners find the perfect training companion has four legs. Run with your dog for pleasure and safety. Your dog needs exercise, too, but also remember that he or she also must ease into training just like you. And don't forget the water breaks. Unfortunately, our dogs, Knickerbocker and Kibbie, are sprinters, not distance runners.

If you can't find people—or dogs—going your pace or distance, try to hook up with others for a section of your run. Or plan a few runs at a location and time of day when lots of others will be out exercising; just having other runners around will make your run more enjoyable than always running alone. You can also have friends or family keep you company by riding along on a bike or on in-line skates. Nonexercisers can help motivate you by meeting you at various points along your course to give you drinks and encouragement. Afterward, you can celebrate your accomplishment by taking your helper out to eat.

Use your spouse or friends as cheerleaders. It is a cheerleader's job to help you become a graduate of your beginner running program—and then to stick with it—by being available to listen to you brag and complain about your daily running and offer cheerful encouragement. But beware! Don't let a spouse or friend who is not experienced and qualified at coaching become your coach. Use them as motivational cheerleaders, not running experts, or they could innocently lead you astray.

Group support and group pressure can be key factors in your development as a runner. Whether you run together for reasons of fellowship, safety, family, or to improve your racing performances, take the time to enjoy your running with your friends. You will all reap the benefits.

Set fitness goals. Goals are fundamental to improvement. They mark our progress, they motivate us—in short, they keep us going—and nowhere is that truer than in running. Whether you are training to run your first mile or your first marathon or to improve your race times, your goals and your desire to achieve them serve as motivation to train consistently despite the constraints that time, career, and family life may present.

The value of setting goals is cumulative, too. As you reach your first ones, you gain confidence and become inspired to challenge yourself further and work toward higher ambitions. Through short-term goals, you can move step by step toward seemingly unreachable long-term objectives.

Goals should be challenging but realistic. Too often I hear runners of all levels complain about not reaching their goals. Unrealistic objectives set the stage for frustration and failure. If you can't obtain your goals you will lose desire, enjoyment.

In planning goals, it's a good idea to choose both short-term and long-term objectives. The most important goal you set is the one for a year from now. It should be changed as you improve, but it should always be a year away—a carrot dangling out of reach that guides you in the direction of improvement and enjoyment. By reserving a goal or two for the future (such as completing your first marathon), you won't be in a rush to try to do too much too soon.

Coach Glover's Three-Goal System

I recommend a three-tier system to help runners set goals. For each challenge or race, I encourage runners to establish an "acceptable goal," a "challenging goal," and an "ultimate goal."

The acceptable goal represents a minimum. For example, improving your previous race time by a small amount, or increasing the distance you can run nonstop in comfort by a few minutes.

The challenging goal represents a significant improvement. It is a tough but realistic goal that requires you to put in solid training and a strong effort. It is also a goal that you can reach if everything goes well. This may be, for example, improving your 10K time by 5 minutes or running 20 minutes nonstop after ten weeks of training following my program in Chapter 10.

The ultimate goal is your dream—a race time or running accomplishment (such as running the 6-mile loop of New York City's

Central Park for a beginner runner) that represents a major break-through. This goal may be reachable in six months to a year.

To be effective, goals need to be specific and measurable. Also, set up a target date for accomplishing your goals. Write your goals down in advance and adjust them as you record your actual results. Use your training diary for this purpose, or make a simple chart for your goals and place it where you can see it often. Post your goals in phrases ("affirmations") that motivate you. For example, place a note by your mirror that states: "I am going to lose 10 pounds and run for a half-hour nonstop by June," or "I am going to finish the New York City Marathon next year."

Adjust your goals as you improve or as changes in your training and environment dictate. With hard work, patience, and the real-ization of small goals along the way, you will progress steadily toward your long-term objectives as a runner and racer.

Seek variety. As the saying goes, variety is the spice of life. If you do the same thing over and over, whether at work or at play, it will get boring. It will cease to be fun. You don't have to run all the time to be a runner. You might enjoy some cross-training with other aerobic sports such as swimming, rowing, biking, cross-country skiing, and skating. Taking a few aerobics classes where you exercise to lively music may add a dash of fun to your fitness routine.

Many runners travel the same course, at the same time of day, for the same distance day after day. Although such a routine adds discipline, it would be more enjoyable to vary the routine. Run short some days and longer on others; faster some days, slower on others. Run with people some days (and run with new friends at times, too), alone others. I have a basic 8-mile course—down to the pond, around it, and back—that I stick to most of the time because it is simple, scenic, and takes about an hour. But a few times a week I'll follow different routes for anywhere from 5 miles to 15 miles. You can even vary the same course by running it in the opposite direction—it's amazing how different things look.

Another trick I use to motivate myself is the use of my heart rate monitor. I'll go several days, even weeks, without using it and then I'll strap it on and head for the trails. When my heart rate reading is lower than it was the last time I monitored it over the same course at the same pace, then I've proof that my training is paying off. Further, it keeps me company. If I've been training alone too much, bringing along the heart rate monitor provides me with a running partner. I'll look at it frequently to see if I'm going too fast or too slow, to see how my heart responds to the hills. Sometimes I'll race it—trying to keep above a certain number. Other times I'll test myself to see if I can keep below a certain number. It is a challenge to see if I'm in tune with my body. This test provides me with a different element for my run, variety from slugging along alone.

Each session of our running classes we try to do at least one workout that's different. We always get an enthusiastic response. Sometimes it is a relay race where the runners make up fun names for their teams. Shelly-lynn has her students run holding potato chips to make them concentrate on keeping their hands relaxed (don't squeeze and break them!). Or we practice running while drinking water out of cups. These workouts produce lots of laughs. One of the most enjoyable runs we do with our running classes is when we go exploring, like a bunch of kids. We go sightseeing, we play. We get off the main paths in Central Park and run up and down grassy hills, around flower gardens, through the zoo, around ponds—I've even taken them to playgrounds for a quick trip down a slide. It's fun to act like a kid again!

I often leave my trusty routes through the country woods to explore new areas. Where does that road lead to? What is at the top of that hill? Whether you are at home or traveling, it's fun to just go out exploring. Later you can enjoy it again by bringing along a friend and showing him or her your new route. Then, look for new horizons to explore.

Vary your training, your running partners, and your environment. Only your imagination limits the ways you can spice up your running routine.

Find new challenges. Believe it or not, I know lots of people who started running only because they needed a ridiculous challenge to motivate them to begin exercising: completing the New York City Marathon. That's a great challenge, but for most beginners I'd recommend setting it for at least one year away. Other new challenges could include completing a 50-mile bike ride, or swimming across the local pond. If you've conquered the challenge of the marathon, look to improve your times at shorter distances.

Head for the races. You don't have to run in races to be inspired by them. Just watching them gets you pumped up. I often run in the opposite direction during races and cheer on my friends and students. Then I'll congratulate them afterward—the enthusiasm at races is infectious. You may choose to challenge yourself in races, too. Many races are basically "fun runs," where the emphasis is on participation rather than competition. Many communities have annual events that all the locals look forward to. Even my little hometown of Dansville, New York, has a 10K run that my father enjoys. He likes to show off and strut his stuff—now past his seventieth birthday, he leaves many youngsters in the dust in the walking division. Whether your goal is just to finish a new distance, or to better your times, having a race to train for adds zip to your workouts. While the strain of running a race isn't always fun, the postrace glow that can be shared with many others brings pleasure. Many runners aren't that serious about races. They run through them with friends chatting away from start to finish. They just love the excitement of being at races and being with so many other runners. Don't be intimidated by the fast folks up front—they are in the minority.

Be aware that overracing makes people stale. I've found that overracing is particularly common when people start to improve and they don't want to miss the feeling of doing well. They race too often, even every week. They are vulnerable to injury, to burnout. Race a few times a year for motivation, but not more than twice a month.

Keep a diary. Keep track of your running in a daily diary. If you have to write in your diary, you will be less likely to skip several runs in a row. You would mess up your careful bookkeeping with all those blank spaces. This record will help you maintain consistency with your training. Being able to finish off another week of training on schedule and writing it into your diary gives you a sense of accomplishment. You can look at it and feel good, proud that you had the motivation to keep on running. Chapter 9 details how you can use your personal diary to improve your running.

Reward yourself. Have a spouse or friend promise you a special gift—perhaps a nice trip or dinner at your favorite restaurant—once you reach a special goal, such as graduating from my beginners running program or completing your first race. Reward yourself, too. How about a trip to the local running store for a new winter or summer running wardrobe as a treat for all your hard work. Wearing your nice new duds will also make you feel better about yourself, reinforce your commitment, and further motivate you to keep on running.

Remember the health benefits. Most runners start for reasons of improving their health—the way they look and feel. Periodically remind yourself of the improvements you have made. Check your resting heart rate and blood pressure, your weight, measure your waist and hips—how much better are you now? Are you able to fit into clothes you couldn't fit into before? My friend Carl Eilenberg in Rome, New York, lost more than 100 pounds due to his running program. To remind himself of the importance of his running, he keeps a pair of pants from his fatso days where he can look at them often. He can fit into one pant leg now!

Can you wear sleek outfits that you wouldn't dare be seen in before you started running? Think about how much more energy you have now, how much better you can handle stress. These benefits can continue to be enjoyed, and enhanced, as you continue down the road to fitness. If you cut back, or quit, you'll begin to lose what you gained with hard work and sweat. Isn't that a good motivator to keep with it?

Dr. Lynch suggests making a list of the many physiological benefits of running, posting it and reading it daily. If you do, he says, "your movement to the front door will replace your movement to the cupboard door."

Run away or quit running. Got your attention didn't I? One of my biggest motivators is to occasionally run away. I'll go on a trip and run with new people and explore new places. Some runners enjoy running away to the many running camps for adults that are available in such great running locations as Maine, Vermont, and Colorado. There, you can run with new friends and get inspired by camp coaches. But be careful; you don't want to get too enthused and run too much or too fast and get injured. Most camps include lots of fun nonrunning activities, too. As I was finishing this book I traveled to the island of San Salvador in the Bahamas, where I led morning group runs at a Club Med Health and Fitness Week. The runners ran for fun as a group each morning and then enjoyed other exercise classes, biking, tennis, water sports, and more the rest of the day. They returned home reinvigorated about their running.

Got the mid-winter blues? Along about February most runners I know are losing their desire to run in the cold, dark days of winter. So take a break and head to Florida, Arizona, the Caribbean, or other exciting locations with plenty of sunshine and no ice or snow underfoot. When you return, spring will be that much closer. Many vacation resorts provide facilities so you can keep your exercise program going. But I'm basically a homebody. After a day or two away from my favorite trails I can't wait to get back to them. And I return with increased enthusiasm.

Sometimes I need to stop running for several days because of illness, injury, or just plain burnout from work. I can't or don't want to run. All the tricks described above stop working. So I quit. After a few days my body starts twitching. My mind gets restless. I get more and more irritable until finally the urge to run returns. Your spouse may even force you to run to improve your disposition! When I'm back running I appreciate it even more. Just like many things in life, you don't know how good it is until you don't have it anymore.

So run away, quit and come back, or just keep running toward reasonable goals. Whatever you do, remember that the key to keeping motivated is to run for fun. Enjoy!

SIX

Basic Exercise Principles

Training methods are based on established principles. Some are determined by physiological research. Others come from the personal experiences of runners and coaches. Each runner "borrows" hints from this person or that person and processes them through trial and error. The result is different applications of the same basic knowledge. We are greatly indebted to those pioneer coaches, runners, and scientists who contributed to the resource bank we draw on. Other books or other coaches may tell you to train differently—they are neither right nor wrong. They have simply interpreted the basic exercise principles in a different way.

The following ten principles of exercise will serve as the backbone of your running program:

Principle 1: Overload Gently

To improve your level of fitness, you must increase the amount of work your cardiorespiratory and musculoskeletal systems have to do and allow them to adapt. This is sometimes incorrectly translated by runners and coaches as "no pain, no gain."

You do need to increase your exercise level as you gain in fitness. Increase the stress load on the body, but not by excessive amounts, in order to bring about a training effect. This means that during aerobic exercise, you will need to work your heart and lungs harder by increasing pace or distance—but not necessarily both. During strength training, you increase the resistance or the number of repetitions performed—that is, you may need to do more push-ups. For flexibility exercises, you gently increase, over time, the amount of stretch placed on your muscles and connective tissues. Overload gently following the progressive training principle below and your body will adapt and be prepared for the next overload as you run down the road to fitness.

The acronym FIT sums up the three key components of increased exercise training: Frequency (how often), Intensity (how fast), and Time (how far). I've devoted Chapter 8 to these critical factors in the exercise prescription.

Principle 2: Progressive Stress—Train, Don't Strain

The body is a remarkable organism and will surprise you in its ability to get stronger. But it can also surprise you by breaking down if it is overstressed. Follow the principle of overload, but don't overtrain. The workout load should not be too light or too heavy. The body and mind gradually adapt to increasing levels of exercise stress. But that level must be delicately balanced to be intense enough and regular enough to promote adaptation to a higher level of fitness—the "training effect."

If the stress is too much, you overtax the adaptation system and cause fatigue, poor performance, or, worse, injury. "Train, don't strain" is the principle I support. You should train hard enough to improve your fitness level, no more. Don't train to the point of strain, which defeats improvement. More—harder and longer—exercise isn't always better.

Slow, steady progression will result in increased fitness. For example, my beginner's running program starts with alternating running with walking. Week by week I increase the amount of time spent running and decrease the walking period. As you adapt, you will walk less and run more until you don't need to walk at all—you will run the entire 20-minute period even though at the beginning you only ran a minute at a time!

As your fitness improves, you will be able to handle a greater training load with the same effort. You may wish to gradually increase the frequency, intensity, and time of your exercise program, but not all the variables should be increased at once. Instead, increase one variable at a time. A good rule of thumb is to never increase how much you exercise by more than 10 percent from one week to the next, or one month to the next.

For the beginner runner and racer, progress comes fairly rapidly with visible results: You can run farther and faster. Students in our classes often see their times improve by several minutes. But as you approach your maximum potential, or the maximum amount of time and energy you choose to devote to your training, it is harder to keep improving so dramatically. You may even reach a point where you plateau. You have a choice: (1) stay there and maintain fitness while enjoying your running, or (2) dedicate yourself to improving your training to seek further improvements in your running results.

It is amazing how much you can progress week after week, month after month, year after year if you allow for gradual training increases. I remember when my goal was to finish a 2-mile race in high school; by my senior year I was the county champion. Once my greatest dream was to run under a 6-minute-per-mile pace for 5K (3.1 miles); a few years later, I could run that pace and faster for the full 26.2-mile marathon distance. My goal after finishing my first marathon was to break three and a half hours to qualify for the Boston Marathon; a few years later, my goal was to run over an hour faster than that. But those results didn't happen overnight. I trained following the principle of progressive stress.

Runners of all levels are finding that by pushing themselves progressively farther and faster, they are reaching performances they never dreamed possible. If I can improve that much with limited natural talent, why can't you improve dramatically, too?

You can, but you need to take it one step at a time. Train by the principle of progressive stress.

Principle 3: Recovery—The Hard-Easy Method

It is essential to alternate your stress and recovery periods, what is called the "hard-easy method." In your day-to-day schedule, you should alternate your hard days (if you even need any) and easy ones. Hard days are runs that are faster or longer than usual. Easy days are short or medium runs over not too difficult courses at a comfortable, conversational pace. What is easy for one runner may be difficult for another. For beginners, an easy day is a day off from running. The older we get, the longer it takes us to recover. Also, it may take some runners longer to recover after certain runs.

Perhaps you ran your workout too hard, your course was unusually hilly, it was a very hot day, or you were short on sleep and long on stress.

Sometimes your body tricks you. You may feel very strong the day after a hard workout or race and, pumped up from the excitement of doing well, you may be tempted to run hard again. Don't! You will pay for it the next day. Beware of the "two-day lag," where, two days after an intense run that leaves you feeling high and proud, your body finally crashes as the principles of physiology finally catch up to you. If you ignore this principle of recovery, you could dig yourself into a very deep hole.

The human body responds best to the stress of exercise if it is allowed to recover and adapt. Stress applied on top of stress equals breakdown. Stress followed by recovery equals progress. Exercisers at all levels may wisely choose to recover from strenuous exercise with a day off or with "active rest" the following day (or days) rather than an easy run. This could be an exercise such as walking or swimming that is gentle to the musculoskeletal system.

For beginner runners the ideal program alternates an exercise day with a day off or a very easy day to allow for recovery. This can be done best if you exercise three or four times a week. If you run a race, take it easy for a few days if it was a short race; a few weeks if it was a marathon. Recover, allow the body and mind to regenerate.

The basic rule here is *listen to your body* and recognize its warning signs—sore muscles, aches and pain, and fatigue. Take a few days off when your body complains. (You should *not* be exercising so much that your body hurts.) Hard-easy training involves mixing the distance and speed of your runs in such a way as to induce the right amount of stress, and the needed types of both stress and recovery, that will help you in your running. I will teach you how to plan your training schedule safely and wisely by balancing how far, how fast, and how often you run. Follow this simple formula: Vigorous exercise plus rest equals improved fitness.

Principle 4: Specificity
You have to do specific exercises to get specific fitness benefits. Different exercises might particularly benefit different sets of muscles, such as crunches for the abdominals or push-ups for the upper-body muscles. These exercises may improve your overall exercise program, but they will not improve your aerobic fitness. You

need specific exercises for this: running, biking, swimming, and other vigorous activities. Even if running is the activity you want to do your best in, you will benefit from other aerobic exercises, but most of your training should be specific. The best way to train your body for running is by running. No matter how many hours you spend swimming, biking, or lifting weights, you still won't be using the same muscles the same way as you do in running. And you need to train as a distance runner, not as a sprinter if your goal is to increase endurance. Specific exercise brings about specific adaptations resulting in specific training effects.

You also will benefit by training specifically for specific situations. For example, you need to train in the heat in order to be able to race well in the heat. You should train on hills to be able to run better up hills. You need to train with long runs to prepare for running longer in races; to train sometimes at race pace and faster to improve race times at any distance.

Principle 5: Regularity

To maintain basic levels of fitness, you should work out at least three times a week, year-round. If you take too much time off between workouts, you will lose some of the fitness you have worked so hard to gain. In general, your body builds fitness slowly and loses it rapidly: It takes three times as long to gain aerobic endurance as it does to lose it. With complete inactivity, aerobic fitness may decline almost 10 percent per week. Strength and flexibility decline more slowly, but you will lose fitness over time if inactive.

John Quincy Adams, our sixth president and an avid exerciser (and a favorite subject of Shepherd in two of his books, including his best-seller *The Adams Chronicles*), maintained that there were three rules to living well: (1) regularity, (2) regularity, and (3) regularity. We can learn from his example. Adams got up every morning at five o'clock and either went for a swim in the Potomac River (wearing only goggles and bathing cap—imagine the media coverage today if we had a skinny-dipping president) or for a vigorous walk of between 4 and 6 miles at a pace that, according to his diaries, raised a sweat. Nothing stopped him—not even the winters he spent as the first U.S. ambassador in St. Petersburg, Russia!

As I fought back into shape after my back injury, I gradually—following the three principles above—worked myself up to 40 miles a week of training. Then, as I was finishing this book, I reeled off twenty straight weeks of exactly 40-mile training weeks. In my prime racing years I once ran twelve straight 100-mile weeks in preparation for a marathon.

I challenge myself to be consistent because regularity is the key to fitness. But it requires discipline. Make that appointment with yourself—and keep it. Be regular, consistent. By planning your fitness routine, and following it, you will come to understand John Quincy Adams's simple basic rule and why it is essential for living well. But leave some room for being flexible. You should be prepared to adapt to weather conditions, available facilities, your health, and family obligations. Alter your training to fit your needs—be stubborn, but practical.

Principle 6: Individuality

Not everyone has the same capacity to adapt to a training program. To a large extent heredity determines how well your body adjusts to training, and how good you can be as a runner. All exercise must be flexible and adapted to the specific needs of the individual. Find out what exercise routines work best for you. Find out, too, which motivational tips discussed in the previous chapter help you. Not every training method or psychological method works equally well on all people.

A coach or a book shouldn't establish a single training schedule for all runners. Each of us has personal likes and dislikes, strengths and weaknesses. Your ability level and training goal are unique to you.

We are all different. Yet the basic training principles discussed here apply to all of us. We just need to determine how to best adapt them for our individual needs. Some runners, for example, may find that my beginner's training schedule is too slow for them and they should move ahead by a few weeks; others may find that they can't keep up and should stick to the level they can handle before moving ahead.

Principle 7: Patience

Fitness will not come overnight. But then you didn't get out of shape overnight either. Success in reaching your fitness goals should be measured in weeks and months, not days. Generally, an adult needs eight to ten weeks to get into fairly good shape after being sedentary. Beyond that, each day you put more miles in the bank and build for the future. Every day that you exercise means that you are moving one more day away from the old you and toward a newer and better-fit you. In fitness, the tortoise beats the hare. Regularity, adaptability, and patience pay off. Take your time, enjoy your running and life, and steadily get into better shape and stay there.

Principle 8: Moderation

Too much of anything—food, drink, work, book writing, sex, exercise—isn't good. You need to be moderate in your approach to life. Balancing the major stresses—work, school, family, friends—with exercise is as important as balancing the individual parts of your exercise program. See Chapter 27, "The Runner's Triangle," for more information on this important concept.

Principle 9: Reversibility

You need to keep working at a certain level to maintain your fitness level, and work at an even higher level to improve it. But if for some reason you stop exercising, your fitness will go into reverse and slip away. If you stop exercising completely, most or all of your conditioning will be lost in five to ten weeks. Use it or lose it!

Principle 10: Share the Flowers

A year from now, when you can feel and see the difference in yourself, pause. Remember the eighty-five-year-old woman who said if she had her life to live over she would take the time to smell more flowers and walk barefoot earlier in the spring. Take that time to smell the flowers when you run. In addition, look around and find someone else—child, spouse, parent, friend—who is not exercising and would benefit from it. Gently bring that person into your runner's world. Share the flowers.

SEVEN

Warm-up, Run, Cool-down

An essential ingredient to your exercise program is the warm-up and cool-down program. Many runners I know lace up their running shoes and head out the door full speed. "Don't have time for a warm-up," they say. And when they return they also don't take the time to stretch tired muscles, or even let their heart rates gradually lower. You should follow the "1-2-3 approach" to exercise: warm-up, peak work, cool-down. Peak work would include not only your running program but also other aerobic exercise and weight training. Treat the warm-up and cool-down as part of a three-step process that you incorporate into every workout, and you will help avoid injury and improve the quality of your workouts. These routines help move your mind and body from your hectic life into running and calmly back again.

1. The Warm-up

Warm-ups let your body gradually adjust to exercise, preparing you for harder work to come and actually making that work easier. You need to prepare your musculoskeletal and cardiorespiratory systems for vigorous exercise. Warming up raises your body temperature, which brings more oxygen and blood to the muscles. This results in improved muscle efficiency, increases in the speed of nerve impulses resulting in improved coordination, and increases in muscular elasticity as well as in the flexibility of tendons and ligaments. The warm-up allows your heart rate and breathing rate to gradually make the transition from the resting state to vigorous exercise. Warming up will increase blood flow to the heart. This reduces the risk of heart attack. In summary: The warm-up will help improve your performance, lessen the strain on your heart, and may reduce the risk of injury.

This phase is extremely important, but unfortunately often ignored. The proper warm-up consists of three steps: relaxation, mild stretching, and, the most important step, cardiorespiratory buildup.

Relaxation

Ideally, begin your warm-up routine with a few minutes of relaxation exercises to loosen up muscles that are tense (see Chapter 37). These exercises should help ease the tension out of your mind and body. They will calm you and prevent you from carrying tension with you on the run. Unscrew the "hurry head" and prepare yourself for an enjoyable run. This is an optional but recommended step.

Stretching

Next, 5 to 10 minutes of gentle limbering and stretching exercises will prepare your muscles and tendons for exercise and guard against injury. Many experts suggest skipping this phase, since muscles should be "heated up" with some moderate exercise to enable a more thorough, safe stretch to take place. They say to hold off on the stretching completely until after the run. I agree, and I disagree. Yes, save the more advanced stretches for after your run when your muscles will be well warmed and more receptive to stretching. But some *gentle* stretches before your run will prepare you. So limber up but don't overstretch here. My tight muscles sure appreciate some gentle stretches before I start my runs. When I rush out the door and skip them they yell at me for a few miles.

Some experts recommend that you run for 5 to 10 minutes and then stop to stretch prior to continuing your run. This may work fine for a team working out on the school track, but for most runners this is unrealistic. It would be especially difficult in cold weather. Here is a compromise if you wish to warm the muscles prior to your prerun stretch: a few minutes of stationary biking or walking may be added to the routine before stretching. While this will warm up your muscles and make them easier to stretch (chapter 37 has detailed guidelines for relaxation and stretching exercises), you'll still need time for the cardiorespiratory warm-up after you stretch and directly before you start your run.

Cardiorespiratory Warm-up

This 5–10 minute phase is the critical part of the warm-up routine because it is here that the body actually warms up. It may be ok to skip the pre-run relaxation and stretch, but this part is essential. The key to beneficial warm-ups is to gradually increase the body temperature by one or two degrees Celsius so that you produce perspiration. A one-degree increase in muscle temperature during warm-up will make your muscles 13 percent more efficient. A warm muscle contracts more forcefully and relaxes more quickly, enhancing speed and strength and minimizing injury. How hard do you need to work during your warm-up? The intensity and duration of work should gradually increase to produce mild perspiration without fatigue.

Before starting your vigorous peak workout—whether it be a run, biking, or weight training session—you should always spend at least 5 minutes in cardiorespiratory warm-up (walking briskly, biking easily, etc.) to gradually increase your resting heart rate toward your target aerobic heart rate (this concept is detailed in the following chapter). After a 5–10 minute walking warm-up, start running slowly, gradually increasing your pace for 5 to 10 minutes until you level off at a steady rate. Please note: If I can't get you to do a walking warm-up before you run, then at least be sure to start your run at a slow pace. You may require a longer period to warm-up and feel loose on a cold day than on a hot day. Also, early morning exercisers may require a longer warm-up than those who have been up and moving for part of the day.

During the warm-up routine, your heart starts to pump faster, blood flow and respiration rates increase, body temperature rises causing you to perspire, and your muscles heat up and become more limber; you prepare, gradually, for vigorous exercise.

You can compare it to warming up your car on a cold day. You don't just jump into your car, start it, and take off at 60 miles an hour down the highway. Well, you could, but it would strain your car's engine and you wouldn't have a very efficient ride. Rather, it is recommended that you turn on the car and let it warm up for a few minutes before you drive it. Then start off gradually before reaching your cruising speed. If you stay there at a steady rate, but not too fast, you will get better gas mileage—improved performance just like runners who warm up gradually. Most of us treat our car's engine better than our own. Respect your heart; warm it up gently prior to vigorous exercise.

My warm-up routine is very important to me since I have to ward off two obstacles: asthma and back problems. My muscles, bones, and lungs require a gradual warm-up. I might get started slowly and carefully, but if I do this, then once I get going few people anywhere near my age will keep up with me. If I'm feeling especially tight I start off by cheating. I'll take a warm shower massage while doing first some relaxation exercises and then some mild stretching. The heat of the shower is relaxing in itself and it helps to warm the muscles. I'll play the pulsating stream up and down my back and legs. Then I'll dry off and put on my running clothes. I'll lay down and do more relaxation exercises, followed by some gentle stretches. Here I'll cheat some more. I'll take the dogs for a 10- to 20-minute walk. This is called "time management," since they would need their walk anyway. They give me plenty of company for a walking warm-up that isn't that much fun alone when I want to get running. Then I'm off and running at a nice slow pace. Since I have to go up some hills to get into the woods I have to start slow anyway. By 10 minutes into the run I'm into my groove, cruising at my vigorous but comfortable training pace.

So warm up before you run. If you don't have the time or aren't in the mood to stretch first, at least start off with a brisk walk or slow jog to break into a mild sweat (but promise to stretch adequately when you finish to work on that flexibility!). Your engine and your chassis will appreciate it. And don't forget to warm up prior to any physical exertion—for example, shoveling snow or chopping wood.

2. Peak Work (Run)

Warm-up routines prepare you for both aerobic and strength training. You may wish to incorporate some strength training exercises into your daily routine as I do. After stretching, I do a few sets of push-ups and sit-ups prior to starting my run. That way I'm sure to get in some work on those important muscle groups several times a week. To prepare for strength training sessions not integrated with your run, such as training with weights, do a 5-minute (or longer) cardiorespiratory warm-up followed by stretching. When I go to my fitness gym to work out with weights, I bike, or walk on the treadmill briskly prior to starting my strength workout.

3. The Cool-down

Many runners can't resist the urge to sprint to the finish of the run and then head for the easy chair or couch to recover. Sorry, your body needs to cool down first and then you can just hang out. Don't sit down—keep moving. The cool-down is the warm-up in reverse and is equally important. Stopping an activity abruptly may cause the pooling of blood in your extremities and the slowing of waste product removal in your system. It may also cause cramps, soreness, dizziness, or an abnormal strain on your heart. The majority of exercise-related heart abnormalities among adults occur not during the aerobic phase but following exercise. These may be avoided by gradually cooling down your body. Never sit immediately or enter a warm shower or sauna without first properly cooling down.

The purpose of the cool-down is to help your body return to its preexercise level. Cooling down helps your heart rate and breathing return to normal and keeps your muscles from becoming sore and stiff. Why do you think they walk prize racehorses after workouts and races? Take care of your prize body, too.

After your run or other aerobic workout, keep moving at a slow pace for at least 5 minutes. This will allow your heart rate and breathing to gradually return to near your preexercise level. Walking slowly is usually the best cardiorespiratory cool-down. The important thing is to keep moving around so that blood is pumped from your extremities, especially your legs, back into the central circulatory system. Before moving on to your stretching exercises, you should be breathing normally and you should feel relaxed; your heart rate should be within 20 beats of your prerun level. If not, walk around some more until you have properly recovered from the workout. I usually let the dogs out when I return from my run and chase them around and play with them in the yard as I cool-off. It is nice to look forward to such an enthusiastic welcoming committee at the end of a run.

Your stretching routine should last 10 to 15 minutes (or more).

You may repeat the same exercises that you do during the warm-up, or add others. You may wish to follow my sample routine in Chapter 37. It is important to stretch all major muscle groups, in particular those that you used during the workout. This is a good time to work on your flexibility, since it is easier and safer to stretch warm muscles. Thus, you can do more advanced stretches than you did during your warm-up, or if you do the same stretches you may try to comfortably stretch your muscles a little farther.

End your cool-down with relaxation exercises. Properly done, they should leave you feeling very relaxed and energized instead of fatigued. You should no longer be sweating. Your heart rate should be close to normal and your muscles fully relaxed.

EIGHT

The FIT Prescription:
How Often? How Fast? How Far?

The most common questions runners of all levels ask are: How often should I run? How fast should I run? How far should I run? I am asked those three questions more than any others, and the answers form the basis of my exercise program.

The acronym "FIT" is used by fitness experts to sum up the three key components of a recommended exercise prescription: "F" is for frequency (how often); "I" is for intensity (how fast); "T" is for time (how long a time period or how far a distance). In short, to achieve and maintain aerobic fitness you need to exercise often enough, at an appropriate pace, and for a sufficient length of time.

So what are my recommendations for getting fit with the FIT exercise prescription? Same as they were back in 1978 when the first edition of this book became a runaway national best-seller. To get in shape and stay in shape you should run (or perform other aerobic exercises):

- *Frequency:* at least three times a week (preferably at least five times a week);

- *Intensity:* at a brisk but conversational pace within your training heart rate range (see Figure 8.1);

- *Time:* for at least 20 to 30 consecutive minutes.

To achieve cardiorespiratory fitness, you need to follow the FIT exercise prescription for at least eight to ten weeks. Once fit, in order to maintain minimal fitness, you must continue to exercise aerobically at least three times a week. To increase your fitness level, you must increase the frequency, intensity, and/or duration of your exercise. In other words, improvement comes by exercising aerobically more often and for longer periods of time. You will also naturally increase the speed of your runs as you become more fit, yet remain within your training heart rate range. But don't change more than one of the key variables of the FIT exercise prescription at a time or you may overdo it.

Fitness gains are not proportionately as large after the first ten weeks. Yet you will continue to improve. You will be able to run farther and faster with less effort if you train progressively and wisely.

Frequency: How Often Should I Run?

You should perform some form of aerobic exercise at least three times a week to gain and then maintain a minimal level of fitness. But this doesn't mean that you can run three or four days in a row and then take the rest of the week off! Spread the exercise out over the entire week. Most runners can easily find the time to exercise on the weekend but have trouble getting out during the week. Don't be a "weekend warrior" and try to cram in all your exercise on Saturday and Sunday. That will set you up for injury. As a minimum goal for these runners I suggest the following: run Saturday and Sunday, then schedule at least one more run during the week.

Should I run every day? Some so-called experts argue that you must run every day to build a habit you won't break: It's too easy to take more days off if you give in and take one, they say. This is nonsense! I feel, and studies back me up, that your body needs at least one, and perhaps two, days off a week to recover. Regenerate. The average beginner and intermediate runner should run three or four days a week, gradually move up to five, and later, if he or she wishes, increase to six. Running every day is not recommended unless you are a very experienced runner.

Should I run every other day? Many coaches and runners advocate running every other day, even for more experienced runners. More recovery between runs minimizes the chance of injury and allows you to feel fresher for your next run. Because of time restraints, or susceptibility to injury, you might find this system helpful. You may fill in some of the off days with cross-training such as biking or swimming to help keep your aerobic endurance up.

But many of us enjoy running more often. We run as much for the pleasure or stress management as we do for fitness. Runners often feel very antsy if they don't get in their daily run. My legs get twitchy and I can't sleep if I take off two days in a row. But I always take off at least one day a week from the pounding of running. I recommend that you do, too.

Frequency is important in terms of building fitness and race performances. Studies show that those who exercise more often are less likely to become fitness dropouts. A study of British women marathoners in the *Journal of Sports Science* indicated that the frequency of runs better predicted superior racing times than any other variable, including weekly mileage and years of running experience. Consistently getting out the door and running pays off if you listen to your body and don't overdo it.

Run at least three times a week, preferably at least five times. Take at least one if not two days off per week to rest and recover.

Intensity: How Fast Should I Run?

The answer to this question is easy: not too fast, but not too slow.

Most people start out training too fast. They get injured, exhausted, or frustrated and quit. Slow down! You want to run fast enough to gain fitness but slow enough for it to be comfortable and enjoyable.

Several simple checks can be used to monitor the intensity of aerobic exercise. These include:

1. Training heart rate

2. Talk test

3. Perceived exertion

4. Pace per mile

The most commonly used monitor of intensity in fitness programs is the training heart rate, which measures how your heart responds to exercise. But your body basically knows what level of exercise is good for it. If you listen to it—following the talk test and your perceived exertion—you will probably be exercising at the appropriate intensity within your training heart rate range. Most veteran runners measure intensity by their pace per mile for training runs, speed workouts, and races. You can use the various monitors of intensity individually or in combination.

Heart Rate

This is the best monitoring system for anyone starting an exercise program. The heart rate check uses your own heart to follow how your body responds to training. Four types of heart rates are important in developing a safe aerobic training program: the resting, maximum, training, and recovery heart rates.

Your heart rate is the number of times your heart beats per minute. Generally, the faster it beats during exercise, the harder you are working out. The slower it beats in response to your vigorous exercise, the better shape you are in. For example, before you become well-conditioned, your heart rate may go up to 140 beats per minute when you run at a pace of 12 minutes per mile. After perhaps two months of training, it may rise to only 130 beats per minute at the same speed. And you will be able to hold that same pace for a longer distance, too.

Finding your heart rate. You can measure your heart rate at several places on your body including the left side of your chest (directly over your heart) or at your upturned wrist (directly below the index finger). Use your fingers to take this measure but not your thumb, which has its own pulse. The most common place to count your heart rate is your carotid artery, which is found just in front of the large vertical muscle along the sides of your neck beneath your jaw. Gently feel for a heartbeat there with the tips of your first two fingers. Don't press too hard.

When you feel your heartbeat—and everyone has a heartbeat, although some have a hard time finding it!—count the number of beats for 10 seconds and multiply by six. That will give you your heart rate per minute. For example, if you count 20 beats in ten seconds and multiply by six, that will give you an approximate heart rate of 120.

It may be more difficult to count your exercise heart rate than your heart rate at rest. As a beginner, check your heart rate a few times during your run and again at the end. You may need to stop briefly to do this. You should count it immediately after stopping or your heart rate may drop too quickly to give you an accurate measure. It isn't necessary to jog in place while measuring your heart rate. Move gently back into your run as soon as you have checked it. At first, you may want to monitor your heart rate three or four times during a run. Later, when you develop a feel for your pace, you may choose to monitor your heart rate halfway through your workout and immediately at the end of your run.

Monitoring your heart rate by touch is inconvenient and inexact. It is hard to stop quickly and then count your heartbeats when you are huffing, puffing, and sweating. Further, if you are not exercising, your heart rate is dropping quickly while you are counting. A study at the University of Massachusetts Medical School found that 60 percent of exercisers could not take their heart rates accurately by touch.

Heart rate monitors. The most efficient, simplest way to monitor your heart rate is to wear a heart rate monitor. These are very easy to use. A lightweight transmitter is strapped across your chest with an adjustable elastic belt. Electrodes sense your heart's electrical signals from your skin and the transmitter then sends this information to a wrist monitor. The wrist monitor is just like a wristwatch except that besides time of day and running time, it can also flash your heart rate—at rest, while exercising, while recovering, or anytime.

With a heart rate monitor you don't have to stop exercising to check your heart rate—just look down at your watch and read the numbers. Further, you can look at it several times during your run to see how your heart rate is reacting to hills, heat, change in pace, and so on. You get instant, accurate feedback. The fancier models, made by Polar, will even set off alarms if you go above or below a set training heart rate range, and give you all kinds of data including: your average heart rate for the run, how many minutes you ran above and below your range, and the highest and lowest heart rate you reached during the run. I highly recommend a heart rate monitor, especially for beginning runners. They make great gifts. I got one for my dad and he thinks it is the most fun toy he's had since Santa Claus last visited him. Shepherd is staying with his fingers!

I don't wear my monitor on each and every run, however; that to me is too stressful. It takes the pure joy out of the runs. But I do run with it a few times a week—it keeps me company and gives me something to think about. Other runners find the monitors as valuable as their running shoes and bring them along on every run. Some runners even race with them so they can better judge the intensity of their effort, keeping them from starting too fast or slowing too much during the race without realizing it. An excellent guide for using heart rate monitors as a training tool is *The Heart Rate Monitor Book* by Sally Edwards.

Resting heart rate (RHR). This is your heart rate when you are at rest—either when you wake up in the morning (before getting out of bed) or when you are very relaxed during the day. Take your RHR several times over a period of a few days and average it out. Do not measure your preexercise heart rate and think that is the same as your resting heart rate. Because your body anticipates getting called into action, your preexercise heart rate will be higher than when you are relaxed. The average RHR for men is 60 to 80 beats per minute; for women, 70 to 90. Sedentary individuals may have resting heart rates that exceed 100 beats per minute. RHR usually increases with extremes in temperature and altitude. It may also increase or decrease with various medications.

A well-conditioned adult's heart rate may be around 60 or below. Serious endurance athletes often have resting heart rates in the 40- to 50-beat-per-minute range; some elite athletes have even been measured as low as 28 beats per minute. When I was marathon training in my prime and running 100 miles a week, my RHR was 42 beats per minute. Now, at half that mileage and two decades later, my heart is still quite efficient with a RHR of 52.

This base heart rate is helpful in several ways. First, you can chart your resting heart rate over the course of months or years as a measure of how you are progressing in your fitness. Check your RHR each morning and record it in your diary. Generally, as you get into better shape, your RHR lowers. On the average, sedentary individuals who start on a vigorous exercise program will decrease their RHR by one beat per minute per week over the first ten weeks of training. Thus, if your RHR is now 85 beats per minute and you follow my ten-week beginner's running program outlined in the next chapter, then your RHR is likely to drop to around 75 beats per minute at the end of the program. How's that for proof that running is making your heart stronger!

Second, your RHR may serve as a warning signal of overtraining. A higher than usual morning resting heart rate (by more than a few beats) may indicate that you are training too hard, not sleeping well or long enough, or are overstressed. You should take a day or more off from running, or at least exercise less until the rate returns to normal.

You should not quickly increase from your resting heart rate up to your training heart rate. As discussed in the previous chapter, use a good cardiorespiratory warm-up of brisk walking and slow running to make a safe transition into your training pace.

Maximum heart rate (MHR). This is at or near your level of exhaustion, where your heart "peaks out" and cannot meet your body's demand for oxygen or cannot beat faster. MHR cannot be improved with exercise like the resting heart rate. It can't be increased, but it does decrease with age—by about one beat per year for adults.

The only accurate way to measure MHR is in a fitness laboratory where you run on a treadmill while monitored by an electrocardiogram (ECG). Very experienced, fit runners can estimate their MHR by running an all-out half-mile, or running hard for 1½ to 3 minutes up a steep hill and then, when they feel they have reached maximum effort, monitoring their heart rate. The highest heart rate you are able to reach is your MHR; to get it you may need to repeat the test after a short rest period (one more time for the half-mile, up to four more for the hills). This exhausting method is not recommended for beginner and intermediate runners.

Fortunately, exercise scientists have come up with formulas to estimate your maximum heart rate. Unfortunately, they aren't precise. The most commonly used method is to subtract your age from the figure 220. For example, a forty-year-old would subtract his or her age from 220 to get an estimated maximum heart rate of 180. This is not a goal figure. Do not try to test yourself to see if you can reach or exceed this heart rate level. That would place a severe stress on your cardiorespiratory and musculoskeletal systems.

Remember, this is just an estimate based on average values. Your actual maximum heart rate is likely to be 5 to 10 beats (or more) higher or lower. Research at Ball State University in Indiana indicates that the standard "220 minus age formula" may work for most fitness runners, but not for well-trained athletes. They found that between ages 26 and 48 there was only a minimal decline in MHR for highly competitive runners. Thus the standard formula would result in an underestimation of their MHR and thus a training heart rate range too low for maximum fitness gains. The running test described on page 74 will provide these runners with a more accurate estimation of MHR. Since determining your MHR is an inexact task for most runners, determining your training heart rate based on the MHR will also be less than accurate. Still, it can be a valuable aid for most runners.

Training Heart Rate (THR). You should exercise at an intensity high enough to bring about a sufficient training effect, but not so high as to overstress the body. Thus, to achieve sufficient and safe aerobic training, you should exercise at a continuous rate within your estimated training heart rate range. This range falls between two numbers—a minimum and a cutoff heart rate. Fitness experts don't all agree on either the recommended lower or upper limit for the THR range.

Some argue that 50 percent of your estimated MHR is high enough to promote fitness—it is for those who need to start with a low-intensity program such as easy walking. The American College of Sports Medicine (ACSM) recommends a minimum THR limit of 60 percent of MHR. Many experts maintain that this minimum rate should be 70 percent of your MHR. At this level of intensity both your heart and lungs are working vigorously; between 70 and 80 percent of your maximum heart rate is where aerobic conditioning improves the most.

What about the upper limit? Even the ACSM experts have varied their recommendations between 80 and 90 percent of maximum. Others recommend 85 percent as the upper limit. Somewhere between 80 and 90 percent of maximum heart rate is where aerobic training phases into anaerobic training—that is, you will be running so fast that your heart can't pump enough oxygen to the body to meet the demands of exercise. At this level of training you are no longer able to pass the "talk test" and your "perceived exertion" is now above "hard" (both of these monitors are described soon). Once you exercise above 80 percent of your maximum heart rate you will begin to spend a great deal of extra effort (and agony) and risk injury, with little additional aerobic fitness value.

Why would anyone need to exercise that intensely? Only to train their bodies to perform well in races. So, you can pass on this higher intensity level until you are ready to train for racing as fast you can run. Most runners work at between 85 and 95 percent of their maximum heart rate when doing hard workouts and races.

Okay, forget all the numbers! How fast should I run? In previous editions of *The Runner's Handbook*, I recommended a training heart rate range of 70 to 85 percent of estimated maximum. But too many runners—especially beginners—are in too much of a hurry; they are running too fast for it to be enjoyable. Too many runners get injured or frustrated because they push the pace too much, too often. So I'll agree with the THR range recommended in the *ACSM Fitness Handbook*: 60 to 80 percent of estimated maximum heart rate.

The key here is to keep your heart rate in the target area— between those minimum and cutoff figures—during your run. After your cardiorespiratory warm-up you should settle into a pace. When this vigorous but not too strenuous pace is held constant, heart rate will increase for about a minute or two until it levels off. At this rate—called "steady state"—your cardiorespiratory system works efficiently to meet the demand of your exercise. By slowing the pace (even walking briskly) you can lower your heart rate; by picking up the pace you can raise it. Thus, you can, and should, make adjustments during your run to keep within your THR range. Here again is the value of having one of those fancy heart rate monitors that can help keep you on target.

You should at least reach and maintain the 60 percent of maximum heart rate figure during your run. This minimal intensity level (a range of 60 to 70 percent) is adequate for beginners to start to get a training effect. After you get into better shape, I still recommend the goal of at least reaching the 70 percent figure (except for easy days and long training runs), which will result in increased aerobic fitness training. The goal is not to reach or exceed the 80 percent upper figure. Rather, consider this the level you stay below unless you are a very experienced, fit runner in serious training.

If you find that your training heart rate is higher than normal for your effort, then search for the reasons. Heat, wind, and hills are obvious ones. Others include dehydration from previous runs, lack of recovery from hard or long runs, overtraining (too much too soon), first sign of illness coming on, taking medications or caffeine, stress, and lack of sleep. Slow the pace, shorten the run, or take off a day or more from running until you are able to return to your usual training pace within your training heart rate range.

If you run with someone who is not your age, don't think that you should both have the same heart rate at the same pace. For example, Shelly-lynn and I train and race at nearly the same pace. But when we both wear our heart rate monitors for training runs my heart rate will be lower than hers even if we are both running at a similar effort. That is because maximum heart rates decrease with age. If we both train at 70 percent of our estimated maximum, my heart rate will be approximately 120 and hers will be about 130 beats per minute (due to the fact that I am fifteen years older than she). This points out the importance of not comparing your THR to that of others.

Note: As mentioned, THR is based on a predicted maximum heart rate and thus some error is possible. You may find that you can exceed your cutoff without breathing hard. Or you may be tired at the minimum level of your range. This system is a general training target based on averages of many subjects. It works quite well for most runners. Some runners won't fit the averages. Don't be a slave to it. Let your body tell you what is best. When in doubt, rely on the talk test system described later in this chapter.

If you want to do the math, here then is the formula for determining your training heart rate range:

1. Subtract your age from 220 (220 minus 40, for example) to determine your estimated maximum heart rate (180 in this case). Some experts recommend that women should be subtracting their age from the higher figure of 226 to determine MHR—that is, women have a higher MHR than men at the same age according to some studies. Later research at Ball State University, however, indicated that women actually have lower MHR's than men. So I'll stick with the original formula (220 minus age) for both men and women until more conclusive evidence is presented.

2. Multiply your estimated maximum by 60 percent to determine the lower range of your training heart rate zone (60 percent of 180 is 108).

3. Multiply your estimated maximum by 80 percent to determine the upper range of your heart training zone (80 percent of 180 is 144).

FIGURE 8.1 TRAINING HEART RATE RANGE*

Age	60 Percent	70 Percent	80 Percent	Maximum
15–19	123–121	144–141	164–161	205–201
20–24	120–118	140–137	160–157	200–196
25–29	117–115	136–134	156–153	195–191
30–34	114–112	133–130	152–149	190–186
35–39	111–109	129–127	148–145	185–181
40–44	108–106	126–123	144–141	180–176
45–49	105–103	122–120	140–137	175–171
50–54	102–100	119–116	136–133	170–166
55–59	99–97	115–113	132–129	165–161
60–64	96–94	112–109	128–125	160–156
65–69	93–91	108–106	124–121	155–151
70–74	90–88	105–102	120–117	150–146
75–79	87–85	101–99	116–113	145–141

Beats per minute as percentage of estimated maximum heart rate. Heart rate ranges listed correlate with age range listed. Interpolate to estimate your training range if you are between the age ranges.

4. Train aerobically between those numbers—this is your estimated training heart rate range. In our example, train at a rate of at least 108 beats per minute, but not above 144 beats per minute. As you become fit, a good goal would be to train at least at 70 percent of maximum; for our example, that would be 126 beats per minute. Be aware of any factors, such as medications, that may alter your heart's response to exercise and consult your doctor about their effects on your running program.

If you don't want to do the math, I've put together Figure 8.1 for your use in determining your THR. Figure 8.2 summarizes my recommendations for the various training heart rate ranges used by runners.

Recovery heart rate. A proper cool-down is essential following all exercise as emphasized in the previous chapter. The goal of the cool-down is to get your heart rate down to within 20 beats of your pre–warm-up resting heart rate. If it takes a long time for your heart rate to drop, you may be exercising too hard or you haven't cooled down properly. It may take longer for your heart rate to recover when running in hot weather or at higher altitudes. The more fit you are, the sooner your heart rate will recover after exercise.

FIGURE 8.2: RECOMMENDED TRAINING HEART RATE RANGES

PERCENT OF MAXIMUM HR	RECOMMENDED FOR:
50–60	Easy walking and other moderate activity to introduce sedentary people to exercise, lose some weight, and promote health benefits.
60–70	Training range for beginner runners; also for experienced runners on easy recovery days and for easy long training runs. A good range for promoting weight loss.
70–80	Recommended training range for maximum aerobic fitness for experienced runners.
80–90	Threshold between running aerobically and anaerobically; somewhere in this range you can't talk comfortably while running.
85–95	Hard training range and racing range.

The Talk Test: Conversation and Perspiration

Instead of taking your heart rate, here you *listen to your body—*that is, exercise according to how you feel. You should be able to carry on a conversation as you run, or hum a tune if you run alone. If you cannot do this, you are exercising too hard. You haven't passed the talk test. (Most likely you are exercising above your heart rate.) If you can say a few words but not full, coherent sentences, you are running too fast for aerobic training.

Listen to your body. If it yells at you that you are getting breathless, tiring, or feeling overheated or uncomfortable, slow down and even walk briskly until you feel ready to run again at a more moderate pace. There is no shame in taking brisk walk breaks to keep you going.

Generally, when you are perspiring and breathing fairly hard, you are running fast enough to benefit. No sweat, no gain. Some people don't sweat easily or very much, but most of us can tell when we are exercising vigorously. Most err on the too-fast side: They strain to run and strain to talk. If you are running with friends, make sure the pace is slow enough that you can chatter back and forth. After all, why bother to run with others if you can't socialize? The formula here is simple: run fast enough for perspiration, but slow enough for conversation.

It is a good idea to take your training heart rate often when you are first starting as a beginner runner and at least occasionally once you are an experienced runner. This will teach you what your body feels like when you run within your THR range. Once you have a good feel for your range, you can use the talk test method and periodically recheck your heart rate to confirm your training level. But if you are running within your THR range and yet feel tired and can't talk comfortably, ignore the heart rate numbers and cut back.

Perceived Exertion

This is similar to the talk test method. But it involves a rating scale designed by Swedish psychologist Dr. Gunnar Borg of the University of Stockholm, who devised a way to exercise at the appropriate level by monitoring something called ratings of perceived exertion (RPE). He created a measuring device, called the Borg Scale. The scale runs from six to twenty. At six, you are at rest. At twenty, you are at total exhaustion.

On the Borg Scale, the equivalent intensity of the recommended 60 to 80 percent of maximum heart rate would be to reach a RPE of between twelve and fifteen (from just below the "somewhat hard" rating of thirteen to the "hard" rating of fifteen). This is a simple idea. You perceive how you are reacting to your running intensity, and you try to maintain it near the somewhat hard range. In other words, "listen to your body."

Interestingly, several studies have demonstrated that both active and sedentary adults will select an exercise pace that not only falls within this RPE range but also within the training heart rate range of 60 to 80 percent of maximum heart rate. As exercise scientist Rod Dishman summarized in an article in *Medicine and Science in Sports and Exercise*, "this indicates that individuals tend to self-select an intensity that will improve fitness." He termed this "preferred exertion."

Figure 8.3 shows the Borg Scale ratings of perceived exertion.

Training Pace

In deciding how fast to run, most runners think in terms of pace per mile, not heart rate. But your training heart rate will reflect such factors as heat, fatigue, hills, and head winds that would be neglected if you measure only your exertion at pace per mile. The safest bet is to learn what your heart rate feels like at various paces: for example, a 12:00- to 12:15-minute-per-mile pace may keep you within your training range at a steady 140–145 beats per minute under normal conditions and on a flat course. Be flexible enough

FIGURE 8.3: RATINGS OF PERCEIVED EXERTION (RPE)

BORG SCALE	PERCEIVED EXERTION
6	at rest
7	very, very light
8	
9	very light
10	
11	fairly light
12	
13	somewhat hard—lower end of training range
14	
15	hard—upper end of training range
16	
17	very hard
18	
19	very, very hard
20	total exhaustion

to adjust to environmental conditions and other stresses. The bottom line should not be to stick stubbornly to a prearranged training pace but rather to keep your perceived exertion constant and your heart rate within your training range. Remember that as you become more fit, you will be able to handle the same pace-per-mile effort at a lower heart rate (assuming similar conditions).

Uphills and head winds slow the pace, just as downhills and tail winds may help you temporarily pick up the pace. Heat, fatigue, slippery footing, and other factors may cause you to run at a slower pace per mile for your entire workout.

Most veteran runners will have a good idea of what their pace per mile should be and how their body feels at that effort—in terms of heart rate, talk test, and perceived exertion. If you know some of the mile markers along your course, you can measure your pace to monitor your intensity—just like you would in a race. Or if you run the same course or courses regularly and know the approximate distance, you can establish landmarks along the way that let you know if you are running faster or slower than usual.

I normally run at an 8:30- to 9:00-minute-per-mile pace on my easy days, at an 8:00 to 8:30 pace on moderate-paced days, and at a 7:30 to 8:00 pace on brisk runs. Faster than that and I'm running a hard day. On my 8-mile course through the woods I know that I normally hit the edge of the deer meadow in 10 minutes, the duck pond in 24 minutes, finish the pond loop at 34 minutes, greet the cows at the top of the hill by the red barn in 45 minutes, and be welcomed back home by the dogs in 64 minutes. If I'm wearing my heart rate monitor I check it at these landmarks to measure my intensity that way, too. If I'm much slower than my normal checkpoints then I'm probably tired and need an easy day. When I find that I'm hitting all my landmarks at a faster pace yet within my THR, then I have proof that my fitness has improved. I don't play this game every day. I may get lured into being competitive, racing against myself rather than running for fun and fitness.

I suggest you do as I do, learn to monitor your intensity by all the methods described. Effective monitoring of intensity requires a simultaneous monitoring of heart rate, subjective feeling, and pace. When in doubt as a beginner or intermediate runner, slow down the pace, take it easy. Keep your running enjoyable.

Time: How Far Should I Run?

For the beginner, how far you should run is measured in time, not distance. When you first start running your goal is to run 20 and then 30 minutes nonstop. The goal is to train the heart and lungs to work hard for a half hour, thus strengthening them and improving your level of fitness. For minimal fitness, mileage means nothing—you must train the cardiorespiratory system for the recommended time period. The minimum length of time of your workout in order to build fitness is 20 minutes, preferably at least 30 minutes.

This does not mean that the beginner runner starts out running for a full 20–30 minutes. Rather, you start by walking briskly, alternating with slow running if you can, for 20 consecutive minutes. Gradually build up to running the entire 20 minutes nonstop as detailed in Chapter 10. Advanced beginner and intermediate runners should build to running at least 30 minutes nonstop and then increase from there if they wish to further improve their aerobic fitness.

If you go out and run around the block and stop, or even run a full mile and stop, you aren't exercising long enough to improve and condition your cardiorespiratory system. If you run for 5 or 10 minutes, but then sit down or walk slowly and then run again, you are not conditioning yourself properly. The idea is to move briskly, by fast walking or slow running, for the entire 20- to 30-minute period or more. The goal is to burn at least 300 calories, which would take about 30 minutes of continuous exercise.

Once you are averaging 30 minutes of nonstop running at least three to five times a week and are starting to ease into longer runs, you may wish to start counting daily and weekly mileage instead of minutes run. Most runners eventually switch to counting mileage, since most of their friends do and all races and most training for races are measured in miles run. Chapter 12 details how to gradually increase weekly mileage as an intermediate runner. But if you wish to continue measuring your runs by minutes rather than miles, then that's fine with me, as long as you get out there for at least half an hour at a time.

How much do you need to exercise for minimal fitness? Aerobic fitness pioneer Dr. Kenneth Cooper recommends that you cover, in your chosen form of exercise, at least this mileage per week:

Running	6.0 miles per week
Biking	30.0 miles per week
Walking	15.0 miles per week
Swimming	1.5 miles per week

Cooper recommends that you don't need to run more than 15 miles a week unless you are doing so for reasons other than good health and physical fitness.

How much you run, if at all, beyond those 6 to 15 miles per week, or 30 minutes at a time at least three to five times a week, depends on a number of things: your goals, what distances you train to race, what you can tolerate, your running experience, how much time you can set aside for it, and, most importantly, whether you enjoy running farther and more often. As you'll see in Chapter 14, you may even build to 30 miles a week or more if you take on the challenge of training for your first marathon.

Some experts feel the more you exercise, the better. Epidemiologist Paul Williams, Ph.D., a researcher at the Lawrence Berkeley Laboratories in Berkeley, California, analyzed several major studies on exercise and gathered information from *Runner's World* readers and at several road races. He concluded that the benefits of exercise increase more-or-less continuously with increasing levels of exercise. His data shows that the risks of heart disease decrease as mileage increases to 50 miles per week. His data wasn't sufficient to project beyond this level of training.

ACSM's Exercise Prescription

For years, the American College of Sports Medicine's recommended exercise prescription was to train at least three to five days a week for at least 20 to 60 continuous minutes at an intensity level of 60 to 90 percent of MHR. This guideline was the model followed by most fitness programs in the country, including mine.

But in 1993, the ACSM joined forces with the President's Council on Physical Fitness, the U.S. Centers of Disease Control and Prevention, the American Heart Association, and numerous other scientific and public health groups in promoting new recommendations about how we should exercise. They made the minimal recommendations much easier.

According to the new guidelines:

Every American adult should accumulate 30 minutes or more of moderate-intensity physical activity over the course of most days of the week.

Hold on here! The experts are now saying that you can exercise for 5 or 10 minutes or so here and there and add them up at the end of the day rather than have to exercise continuously for 20 to 30 minutes or more? Is this true?

Studies do show that you may get almost the same benefit from three 10-minute workouts as one 30-minute workout. Researchers at Stanford University had one group of subjects run at an intensity of approximately 60 to 70 percent of MHR for 30 minutes at a time, five days a week. A second group divided the run up into three separate 10-minute runs—that is, they ran the same frequency, intensity, and time, but they didn't run continuously. They had at least a four-hour rest period between runs. Which method of exercise was best?

Following this training schedule for eight weeks brought about desirable results for *both groups*: On average, the runners improved aerobic endurance by 12 percent, lowered their resting heart rates by 6 percent, and lost 4 pounds. The researchers summarized that a 30-minute continuous workout isn't necessary since you get almost as much fitness benefit from running in three, 10-

minute sessions. The continuous runners, however, did have an important advantage. Their aerobic capacity was boosted by 14 percent compared to 8 percent for the other group.

Why? As Owen Anderson, Ph.D., summarized in *Runner's World*: "That's because the first 2 minutes of any run barely count; it takes that long for increased amounts of oxygen to move through the blood. Two minutes amounts to 20 percent of a 10-minute run but only 7 percent of a 30-minute run. The resulting higher percentage of aerobic running time during the 30-minute run (93 percent vs. 80 percent) is what builds up your aerobic capacity." Besides wasting aerobic time when you break up your runs into several small daily stints, you spend a lot more time changing clothes and showering. Also, you should warm-up and cool-down for each of the runs, which takes even more time.

If you only have 10 or 15 minutes to spare, go ahead and run. You will still gain from it. But for the most part, continuous runs of 30 minutes or longer are your best choice. And running continuously also means not stopping for extended breaks (other than a brief water stop), which would lower your heart rate below your training range, and then restarting your run. Brisk walking breaks during your run, however, are not only acceptable but recommended if needed.

The revised ACSM guidelines state that exercise needs only to be moderate—as in such everyday "lifestyle" activities as walking the dog, gardening, mowing the lawn, raking leaves, walking up stairs, and walking all or partway to work. No need to break a sweat running vigorously? What gives here? Did the experts soften their stand in frustration over the poor fitness of most Americans?

Basically, yes, they did. According to Russell Pate, Ph.D., president of the American College of Sports Medicine, "It may be that the current low rate of participation is due, in part, to the public's perception that they must engage in vigorous, continuous exercise to reap health benefits. But actually, the scientific evidence shows that even moderate physical activity can also provide substantial health benefits."

According to the experts, then, it is better to give sedentary people an easier goal in an attempt to at least get them up and moving and to provide some fitness and health benefits. So what about those previous guidelines? "The lower guidelines are meant to complement and not supersede the previous fitness guidelines," assured Dr. Pate, himself a former national class marathoner. He suggested that the ACSM's previous exercise recommendation was a good one and should still be followed when possible. I agree.

The ACSM's position is that it's best if you exercise vigorously for fitness, but if you can't, you should at least be active. Okay, I'll go along with that. Let's get the couch potatoes moving around more so they'll appreciate the activity and reap some of the health benefits. Then they may be motivated to get into even better shape with running!

Moderate exercise, such as walking and gardening, at 50 to 60 percent of MHR will result in health-boosting benefits including lowering your cholesterol, blood pressure, and weight. You will feel and sleep better and have more energy. Moderate exercise can also have disease-busting benefits. It can help fight off heart disease, obesity, diabetes, and osteoporosis. Many studies indicate that even moderate exercise can increase longevity. Moderate-intensity exercise will also lead to fitness gains for the sedentary. But if your goal is to significantly improve your aerobic fitness level you will need to exercise vigorously at 70 to 80 percent of MHR. Many of the psychological benefits of exercise may not occur unless you exercise continuously and vigorously. And studies of Harvard University alumni by Dr. I-Min Lee show that vigorous exercise prolongs life more than moderate exercise.

Dr. Kenneth Cooper cautions: "Don't confuse health with physical fitness. Health has to do with reduction in disease and increase in life span. That's different from fitness. Health enables me to enjoy a long life, but fitness enables me to enjoy a long life plus a quality life." He adds: "I've always said that you exercise for three reasons: (1) rest and relaxation, (2) muscle building or figure contouring, and (3) cardiovascular-pulmonary conditioning." After his research center in Dallas demonstrated with a study of over 13,400 people that you can derive health benefits from moderate-intensity exercise, he added a fourth reason: health and longevity. Dr. Cooper noted: "Number three and number four are not the same. With number three you get all the benefits of number four, but with number four you don't get all the benefits of number three. I'm not about to cut back to number four, because number four sure won't prepare me for climbing to the top of a 14,000-foot mountain as I did a couple of weeks ago in Colorado (at age 59). I'm interested in fitness, not just health." Me, too! I'll add a fifth and perhaps the most important reason to exercise: It's fun!

So if you want to look better, feel better, and perhaps live longer, accumulate at least 30 minutes of moderate-intensity exercise most days of the week. But if you want to look and feel even better, get physically fit so you can live an active lifestyle, and perhaps live even longer—as well as learn to enjoy your exercise time—then work out vigorously for extended periods of time. Run.

The best exercise solution in my opinion is to follow both guidelines. I run at least five times a week, but I also get in as much "lifestyle" exercise as possible: mowing the lawn with a push mower, walking the dogs, taking the stairs rather than elevators whenever possible, walking rather than riding when doing most of my daily errands. Make physical activity part of your life with both planned exercise and lifestyle exercise.

Okay, it's time to get fit with the FIT exercise prescription. The chapters in Part III are my training programs for beginner, advanced beginner, and intermediate runners. Work hard but take it easy. Enjoy the benefits of running. Have fun!

Part III

Training

NINE

The Training Diary

Shepherd, Shelly, and I keep training diaries. We strongly recommend that you do, too. Why? Your training diary—or running log or journal—becomes a record of your fitness program. In it you can enter your day-to-day training record; weekly, monthly, and yearly mileage; best races and PRs (personal records); and favorite running courses.

Over time, your training diary becomes a significant and accurate record of your progress up (and down and back up) the training ladder. You'll refer to it regularly. What did I weigh just before the holidays? How did I train for that last marathon? What was my PR for that 10K two years ago? How did I overcome that injury? What shoes did I run the New York City Marathon in? Your training diary will have a record of your glories and your agonies. Everything.

Well, not *everything*. You may not need to write down the details of every run or even every race. You'll soon get the hang of what is important. Record weight, heart rate, shoes, injuries, weather, course and distance, time (if important), time of day— that kind of stuff. Remember that you may be referring back to this from time to time, most likely when you are preparing for a similar race, coming back from illness or injury, or trying to regain fitness or lose weight.

In effect, you are creating a record of your life. Okay, okay, maybe not your whole life—although we know runners who do indeed write down *everything*. In addition to a record, you are able to use the diary to set goals and to plan your training. You write into it what you did, why, and how it felt. The diary contains the facts and feelings of your training. It doesn't leave them to memory.

Many runners don't keep diaries at all. Others record only their training and races; some keep only race preparation and race diaries. Still others, like Shepherd and me, are obsessive. We hoard away records of shoes, weight, sleep, pulse rates, favorite runs, cross-training, race times and *feelings* that would make an archivist's eyes glaze over. I have a closet full of extremely detailed diaries going back three decades. Shepherd follows the KISS theory: Keep It Simple, Stupid. He spends fewer than 3 minutes on each diary entry, but faithfully records the most essential figures and comments of each day. Why bother? Well, once you do this recording, and then refer back to it, you will swear by the training diary forever.

For example, one year, Shepherd suddenly pulled up on a training run all gimpy in his right leg. Pain shot down the leg from the knee to the toe. He kept running. Over several days the pain started to migrate. He still kept running. (Did he call Coach Glover? Nooooooooo.) After a week of run-rest-run he had pain from the small of his back to his right big toe. He literally could not walk more than 100 feet without resting. Being a calm and rational fellow, he thought he probably had cancer. (Did he call Coach Glover yet? Noooooooo. He took aspirin and kept running.)

This went on for several weeks, a month, then several months. He'd rest, run, rest. The pain would subside for a while during the runs—"Ah ha!" he thought. "Running eased the pain, therefore running is *good* for me!" This run-rest-run-rest and serious pain continued for—no kidding!—five months. Finally, just before leaving the United States to direct the Dartmouth College Foreign Study Program in Kenya, he called me.

"Check your running diary, Shep," I told him.

He looked back through his running diaries. He noticed that ten years earlier he had suffered the same problem, same leg. He had even written the injury and its solution into the updated version of this book published in 1985.

And what did Shepherd's training diary tell him? His right leg is slightly shorter than his left—a common condition—and when his right shoe wears down it accentuates this imbalance. This, in turn, causes pinching on the sciatic nerve. Shepherd had been using Shoe Goo to build up the heels on both shoes, but had run out. When he didn't build up the heel and kept running, the heel wore down. (Talk about *cheap*!) The pain started. Solution? His training diary noted that his pain subsided as soon as he did one simple thing: Buy new shoes. He did—and entered into his training diary this entire new episode.

If you are a beginner runner you will want to record and measure your training and progress. The diary itself will be encouraging. You will actually see your progress over the course of several months. The training record won't lie: your weight will drop, your heart rate will fall, your distance will increase. Read it and cheer!

Intermediate runners will find the training diary a splendid way of establishing a base of running fitness and building on it. It will help you set new goals. As you train for your first race, or your first marathon, the diary will help you train regularly and gradually. Its accurate recording of your workouts will be there when you start preparing for your next race. Afterward, you can review the diary to see what you did right (and wrong) in preparing for a race or reaching a fitness level. You can then repeat the training program (or at least the pattern), and avoid past mistakes.

Here are some tips in keeping your training diary:

▪ Be consistent. Fill it in after each workout. It is easier to motivate yourself to get the minimal mileage required if you record it each day. Nobody likes to see too many unplanned zeros. But don't become a slave to recording mileage. Remember, fitness or performance is the goal, not accumulating mileage in your diary. By keeping a diary you can be sure you do enough—not too much.

▪ Use the diary as a training partner. It should provide you with goals, feedback, and a sense of continuity and encouragement over the long haul. Being well organized, planning and recording your runs, is one of the secrets of success for most runners.

• Include the basics: date, course, distance, time. You may wish to expand the diary to include the details from the samples that follow. You may want to write into it personal things like birthdays or encounters with friends. Why not make it an interesting record?

The diary also gives you perspective. It is sometimes difficult to see the successes and failures of your training while they are going on. But if you look back on the training weeks or even years later, you can see the pattern and the outcome; you will be able to understand what causes success and failure. And by looking back at the good times while you are struggling to retain them, you become encouraged.

A training diary is a document of hope. Keep a diary over several years and you will see the gradual rise and fall and rise again— the peaks and valleys—of your training routines and fitness levels. It's reassuring. You will see that you can come back from illness or injury, or that attaining peak fitness for an important race is indeed possible. Perhaps more important, you will see a clear pattern and purpose to your life.

The training diary kept over the years also offers you the opportunity to look back and reflect over a long running career. I find an old training diary wonderful reading. Reviewing my past successes as a competitive runner in the good ol' days makes me feel more assured about my running as a masters competitor. I also feel more motivated to help others improve their running and racing. Perhaps best of all, the training diary is a record of inspiration: that you can recover, that you can come back, that you created goals and achieved them.

The diary can be a simple wall calendar or a more formal log or book. Some are available in running stores. Or you can create your own. Figure 9.1 is a sample.

I have many fond memories stored in my diaries. Your diary, like any good coach or running friend, should be a motivator, not an overbearing creator of stress. Joe Henderson, one of the original running gurus, writes that his running log "gives a sense of substance and permanence to efforts that otherwise would remain as invisible and temporary as footprints on a hard road.

"Logs store old memories where you can see and touch them again. A feeling of accomplishment grows as the records of past runs accumulate. You put every minute and mile onto those pages, and each fact tells a story worth remembering.

"Days of running leave behind only individual footprints in a diary. You can't take much direction from them. But weeks, months and years of running line up in a trail that points two ways: where you have been and where you might go next."

Good luck in writing your personal book of running!

How to Use Your Training Diary

Week

Start your training week on any day you choose (many diaries begin on Sunday). I generally recommend starting on Mondays for several reasons. First, Monday is the beginning of most work or school weeks. So why not start your running week on Mondays, too? Since Monday is often the toughest day at work after a get-away weekend, and your training is usually heaviest on weekends, it makes more sense to view Monday as a day to start off the week. Second, if you end one week on Saturday and start a new one on Sunday, you may just flip the diary page and not pay close attention to the need to rest after a hard or long day on Saturday. Third, starting your diary on a Sunday often encourages runners to do too much back-to-back on the weekend, since they think of Sunday as starting a new week. If you end your week with a full weekend, you have more flexibility to tally up your weekly total. It is easier to make up a few miles spread out over the weekend than just on Saturday. Finally, most races are held on Sunday. It is better to plan your week in your diary going into races than to plan a week starting with a race. This will help you focus better on a good performance and help you emphasize the prerace taper.

Time of Day

By noting what time of day you run, you can better monitor how comfortable you feel at various times. You may find that too many early morning runs result in fatigue, or that too many late evening runs interfere with sleep or meals. Midday runs may leave you short on mileage if you are not able to set aside an appropriate length of time. You may see that you feel better in warm weather by running earlier or later, but that in cold weather you feel better running during the day when it is lighter and warmer. A pattern relating to injuries may be detected in your diary. For example,

FIGURE 9.1: SAMPLE RUNNER'S DIARY

WEEK _____

DAY _____ Time of day: _____ Weather: _____
Pace/Type of workout: _____
Course: _____ Shoes: _____
Health: _____ Sleep: _____
Comments: _____ Cross-training: _____
_____ Distance or time: _____
_____

DAY _____ Time of day: _____ Weather: _____
Pace/Type of workout: _____
Course: _____ Shoes: _____
Health: _____ Sleep: _____
Comments: _____ Cross-training: _____
_____ Distance or time: _____
_____

DAY _____ Time of day: _____ Weather: _____
Pace/Type of workout: _____
Course: _____ Shoes: _____
Health: _____ Sleep: _____
Comments: _____ Cross-training: _____
_____ Distance or time: _____
_____

DAY _____ Time of day: _____ Weather: _____
Pace/Type of workout: _____
Course: _____ Shoes: _____
Health: _____ Sleep: _____
Comments: _____ Cross-training: _____
_____ Distance or time: _____
_____

DAY _____ Time of day: _____ Weather: _____
Pace/Type of workout: _____
Course: _____ Shoes: _____
Health: _____ Sleep: _____
Comments: _____ Cross-training: _____
_____ Distance or time: _____
_____

DAY _____ Time of day: _____ Weather: _____
Pace/Type of workout: _____
Course: _____ Shoes: _____
Health: _____ Sleep: _____
Comments: _____ Cross-training: _____
_____ Distance or time: _____
_____

DAY _____ Time of day: _____ Weather: _____
Pace/Type of workout: _____
Course: _____ Shoes: _____
Health: _____ Sleep: _____
Comments: _____ Cross-training: _____
_____ Distance or time: _____
_____

SUMMARY _____ Total distance or time: _____
_____
_____ Weight: _____
_____ Resting heart rate: _____
_____ Longest run: _____
Goals for next week: _____ Days off: _____
_____

shin pain throughout the day following early morning runs may not appear as often or as intense in runs later in the day. You should especially monitor how you feel on early morning runs since this is the time of day where you are more prone to injury.

Weather

Record the temperature and weather conditions as they are during your workout. This includes humidity, rain or sun, snow or wind. The weather has a strong influence on how well you run. By tracking your feelings you can better monitor how well you are able to handle all kinds of weather. Also, if you are comparing times for various training courses or races, you will have a more accurate comparison if you can also compare weather conditions.

Heart Rate

Review Chapter 8, which describes how your heart rate reacts to your training. At least a few times per week, especially the day after a hard workout or when you feel tired, take your resting heart rate when you wake up in the morning, prior to getting out of bed. This early morning heart rate will tell you if you're getting adequate sleep and if you've recovered from the previous day's workout. In my diary, I note the resting heart rate with the letter "R." As you get in better shape, you will most likely see that your resting heart rate will become lower and your training heart rate will also be lower for the same workout. You may wish to check your heart rate during training a few times a week to see if you are staying within your training heart rate range. In my diary, I note the training heart rate with the letter "T."

Weight

By recording your weight regularly, you can measure weight fluctuations, which may indicate problems. For example, you may be eating too much (gaining weight) or overtraining or dieting too strictly (losing too much weight). It is best to weigh yourself at the same time of day each time, generally when you first get up in the morning (after emptying your bladder and bowels). Recording your weight once or twice a week is generally sufficient to track any trends. However, it is a good idea to weigh yourself the day after hard workouts or long runs on hot days. A morning weight loss of more than a pound or two may indicate dehydration. Chapter 41 details weight management and exercise.

Sleep

There is generally a correlation between the number of hours you sleep and the quality of your workouts. You may notice that as you get in better shape you require a little less sleep, and that you sleep more soundly. On the other hand, you may find that if you train harder you require more sleep and at times have trouble sleeping well. Note how many hours you slept and any important factors relating to your sleep, such as a late workout, late bedtime, or earlier wakeup. If you note any problems you have with the pattern of your sleep, you may detect a trend. For example, working out or eating too close to bedtime may be a pattern demonstrating why you are having trouble sleeping. Also, getting up earlier than normal to run may throw off your sleep for several days. The relationship of sleep and exercise is examined in Chapter 38.

Shoes

As detailed in Chapter 16, after 300 to 500 miles your shoes lose their cushioning properties. Thus, it is a good idea to track the mileage on your shoes to minimize the chance of injury. Mark your shoes if you wear more than one pair. For example, "NB-1" and "NB-2" would refer to your two marked pairs of New Balance shoes. You can sum up the total miles in each pair of your running shoes in the weekly summary section.

Distance/Time

You can log the distance you ran, the amount of time you ran, or both. Some runners prefer to track only total minutes in their diary, but most runners are interested in tracking mileage. Don't be obsessed with trying to run faster times over your course distances. This is racing, not training, and will lead to injury or burnout or both. If you find yourself prone to this, just log either the distance or time traveled for your run. Don't be concerned about exactly measured courses every time out. You can just run, keeping track of time. When you finish, estimate your mileage based on the pace per mile you felt you ran.

Pace

You can note your approximate pace per mile for your run even if you don't measure your course accurately or monitor your elapsed running time. If the pace, for example, felt like 9 minutes per mile then it was probably close to that. Just mark it down: "approx. 9 min. per mile." At least occasionally you may wish to measure accurately the time and distance of your runs so that you can monitor your fitness. Of course, you should note that the pace may be slower compared to the effort if the course is hilly or if it's hot or windy.

Course/Workout
By noting the exact course you ran, you can monitor how you feel running a given pace over the same route. Note the terrain: hilly, icy, dirt trails, track, asphalt, and so on. You may wish to include your warm-up and cool-down program here, too. If you did a speed workout you would write here all of the details: length and time of each run, recovery, etcetera. You may also note here who ran with you. This section may be used to record information for your races: split times for each mile, average pace, finish time, and place.

Exercise Comments
Describe how you felt during (and after) your workout. Words like sluggish, stiff, sore, and heavy can describe a less-than-ideal run. And great, peppy, awesome, and terrific help describe a good workout. You may add comments such as "started too fast," "tired at end," "terrible on hill," or "stitches after third interval" to further detail your experience.

Rating
You may choose to grade your run. For example, you may score "A" for an excellent workout, "B" for a good one, "C" for an average run, "D" for a fair one, and "F" for a run you'd like to forget. Be sure to note why you felt you had a bad run and what the symptoms were. Don't expect to have a great run every time you go out. Shelly tells her clients that for every five runs, most runners can expect to have one excellent run and one that is fair or worse. The other three will be average or good.

Health
This section allows you the opportunity to note the various health factors that may affect your running, or be caused by it: illness, injury, stress, and so on. Note here what the health problem is and what you are doing about it. For example, icing a sore Achilles or

taking medication for allergies. By noting warning signs of illness and injury you may be able to prevent them from happening. Women may wish to track their menstrual cycle and note how the different phases affect training.

Cross-training

Note here whatever aerobic training workouts you did this day. Note how many minutes you exercised aerobically, your effort, and whatever other particulars would be valuable to record. Don't forget to assign Running Equivalent values (see Chapter 35).

Weight Training

Note the basic details of your workout for future comparison, including which strength exercises you accomplished and the weight or resistance used.

Week's Summary

This is the place for totals and comments that summarize your week's exercise program. This section can serve as a quick progress check as you flip through the pages and review trends in your training.

Total Distance/Time for Week

By monitoring these weekly figures you can guard against doing too much too soon, overtraining, and undertraining.

Total Distance/Time for Month

If you monitor your monthly totals as well as your weekly totals you may discover trends that you might have missed. Monthly mileage goals give you more flexibility to reach your training goals. Compare month-to-month totals and also compare them to the same month in previous years.

Total Distance/Time for Year

Charting this figure is fun because the number keeps getting larger and larger. This is very motivating. Compare your data with that of previous years to monitor your progress. If you are behind, for whatever reasons, note it here.

Longest run
By reporting your longest run of the week you will know how well prepared you are to tackle upcoming races. This is especially valuable when marathon training.

Days off
The best way to make sure you include some rest days each week, but not too many, is to record them in your diary.

Rating for the Week
Compare your overall rating from week to week, year to year.

Comments for Week
Summarize here the highlights and low points for your week.

Goals for Next Week
Increase mileage, lose another pound, or add more stretching or weight training. By writing your goals in your diary you are more likely to achieve them.

TEN

The Beginner Runner's Training Program

Joan Benoit Samuelson was the winner of the first Olympic Marathon for women in the 1984 Olympics in Los Angeles. She began running along the country roads in her home state of Maine. She remembers: "When I started running, I was so embarrassed I'd walk when cars passed me. I'd pretend I was looking at the flowers."

"I'm just a beginner." I hear that statement almost every day. You don't need to feel inadequate and you don't need to feel embarrassed. It's okay to be a beginner runner. All of us started as beginners, and we can tell some pretty good stories about the stupid mistakes we made as novices. We can also proudly tell you about our many successes and how much we benefit from our running. You should feel proud that you have made the commitment to get fit and improve your health. In just a few short weeks, following the program in this chapter, you will have graduated and become a full-fledged runner!

Before you read any further, let's first make sure you are in the right training group. There is a wide range of people who think they are beginners. I'm always amazed at how many people register for my classes with the New York Road Runners Club and think they are beginners even if they are already running 3 or 4 miles at a time. They sure feel better about themselves when I congratulate them on how much they can run and tell them that they are way too advanced for the beginner class! On the other end are the people who feel they are complete nonathletes and aren't even good enough to be beginners. Almost anyone can learn to run and to enjoy it. You don't need talent, just common sense, patience, and discipline. And a good training program!

My definition of a beginner runner is: *someone who can walk briskly for at least 20 minutes but can't comfortably run a full mile.*

If you can't walk briskly for 20 minutes in reasonable comfort then stick to a walking program until you are fit enough to start with the following beginner running schedules. If you can already run comfortably for a mile you should move on to the next chapter, which is about the advanced beginner. If you can run for 30 minutes, or for 3 miles at a 12-minute-per-mile pace or faster, then move on to Chapter 12, the intermediate runner.

If you have been active in other sports and are just starting a running program, be careful. Your heart and lungs may be ready to take on more running than your muscles and bones can handle. Because you are aerobically fit, it may be best for you to start in the advanced beginner program or, especially if you are young and active, in the intermediate program.

Whatever your background, select the category that *best* describes you. Don't inflate your value: You want to select the best training program for you at your *present* fitness level (be careful here if you are an ex-runner who is restarting), and work up from there.

My beginner-, advanced beginner–, and intermediate-level training schedules are the exact same programs used successfully for two decades by thousands of runners in my New York Road Runners Club classes. They have proven to be effective over and over. But just as in our classes, you need to be flexible. Start out in the group that makes the most sense for you. Be a little conservative. You can always move up or down a group any time you want. You be the coach here.

Before starting on one of the following beginner training schedules, review Chapters 4 thru 7 for tips on getting started, motivation to stay with it, exercise principles, and the importance of the warm-up and cool-down. Chapter 8 details the FIT exercise prescription, and this is where beginner runners make their biggest mistakes. It is therefore important to summarize them again here:

Too often. Don't run every day. Every other day may be best for you now. Run at least three days a week, but take off at least one or two days a week.

Too fast. Here is where most beginners go wrong! Say no to "no pain, no gain" and instead "train, don't strain." Remember the talk test concept and the training heart-rate range theory. Run slow enough for conversation and fast enough for perspiration. Beginners should start their running program at a training heart rate below 70 percent of their maximum heart rate. You will start with a program of alternating walking fast with running slow. Another strain similar to too fast is too hilly. Running up hills will add stress to your cardiorespiratory and musculoskeletal systems. Save that challenge for when you get past the beginner stage. Design your courses so that you avoid hills. If you have to include hills, walk them until you are strong enough to run them.

Too far. Many runners set a goal of running a mile their first time out. That may be too much. Also, don't fall into the game of comparing mileage with other runners. Run for minutes, not miles, as a beginner. Your first goal is to build up to running for 20 minutes nonstop. You can do that in ten weeks if you stick to my program.

Run Like a Pig

Right now, you might have second thoughts about this running stuff. "What is Glover getting me into," you say. You may feel that you won't ever get into shape. You may feel as if you're stuck in the mud, like a pig. Listen to this:

Dr. Max Sanders, an exercise physiologist at the University of California at San Diego, studied the value of exercise on the human heart. His laboratory animals were pigs, whose heart structure closely resembles that of humans. At first, Dr. Sanders used dogs. "But you take the average dog on the street," he said. "And put him on a treadmill, and he can run for two straight hours at a reasonable rate. That's far longer than any sedentary human—or pig—could do. When we started working with the pigs, they could run for only a few minutes at a time."

Dr. Sanders had half his pigs jog and the other half "just standing around all day, like most people." The jogging pigs ended up healthier and had less heart disease than the sedentary pigs. He got the pigs running up to 5 miles a day. Dr. Sanders noted that a well-trained pig can run a mile in less than 8 minutes.

The way I figure it, if a hog can get into shape, anybody can.

Walking: The Preconditioning Program

Walk before you run. If you are just beginning, start first with walking. Older or overweight persons, anyone with joint problems, or someone who has been inactive for a long time, should start with a walking program. Think of it as a preconditioning program.

Some of you may find that walking is a sufficient exercise in itself. My father can't run due to an old World War II injury. I was able to convince him to start walking when the first edition of this book came out in 1978 and he hasn't stopped since. Now past the age of seventy, he still walks briskly for an hour or more most days of the week.

Start with an easy-paced walk for 20 to 30 minutes every other day. Then gradually make your walks more brisk. Slow down if you find yourself out of breath. Don't stop. Keep moving. By pumping your arms as you walk, and really stepping out, you can increase your heart rate to a level nearly equivalent to a slow run.

Once you can walk briskly for 20 to 30 consecutive minutes, you can add slow running breaks to your brisk walking program. You are ready to start one of the following beginning running programs.

Four Training Programs for Beginner Runners

I use four training programs for beginner runners. These are conservative, progressive systems based on the principles discussed in Chapter 6. These programs work very much the same way. They all require you to run at least three times a week (preferably at least five times) at a conversational pace, building up to at least 20 minutes of nonstop running.

They differ only in how they are structured. Pick the one that fits your needs and goals the best. The first two programs allow more freedom to select how far you run before taking a walk break and more flexibility for increasing your run-walk ratio. And there isn't a ten-week time limit on reaching 20 minutes of nonstop running. Take all the time you need to reach that goal. These two methods are particularly good for those beginners at the extremes—those who need more time to build up their running than is allowed with the more structured programs; and those who have been active in other physical activities who may need less time to move up to 20 minutes of consecutive running. Others just prefer this less structured approach to running.

The last two programs are very structured. I have found that many runners benefit from the discipline and motivation of such a precise program. I prefer these programs for most beginner runners.

Whichever program you follow, I suggest that you invest in a runner's watch. They are inexpensive and provide you with a digital read-out of your running time, which will make it much easier for you to monitor your progress. If you want to splurge, get a heart rate monitor that includes a chronograph mode. I still find it quite amazing that I can be running along and in one glance at my watch know the time of day, my elapsed running time, and my heart rate!

The 20-Minute Run-Easy Program

This is the simplest, easiest program of them all. After your 5- to 10-minute walking warm-up, just start running easily until you feel like taking a brisk walking break. Just *run easy*. When your body signals you to slow down—this may be shortness of breath, inability to talk in complete sentences, weakness in the legs, and so forth—then walk. Keep walking briskly until you feel like running easily again. What could be more simple! Follow this program three to five days a week.

Be conservative. Take several walk breaks during your run: approximately every 1 to 5 minutes, depending upon what kind of shape you were in prior to starting this program. Resume running when your body feels ready, ideally after 1 to 3 minutes of walking. Keep moving. Don't quit and sit down.

The goal is to alternate brisk walking with easy running to keep within your training heart rate range. Walking too slowly may lower your heart rate below your range; running too fast may raise it over the training range, and you may not pass the talk test. Don't forget the key here is conversation and perspiration!

Follow this routine continuously for 20 minutes. Then walk for 5 to 10 minutes to cool down. Gradually, over a period of several weeks, shift the ratio of run-walk so that you are progressively running more and walking less. The goal is to run the full 20 minutes nonstop at a conversational pace. The average beginner will take eight to twelve weeks to reach this goal. If you are older, overweight, or have been quite inactive it may take you longer. Don't be in a hurry, but don't be too soft on yourself either. If you have been involved in other vigorous activities, or if you are younger, then you may advance in less time. Again, don't be in a hurry. Even if you have been swimming, for example, several times a week, and are aerobically fit, your musculoskeletal system needs time to adapt to the different work and the pounding of the running. Don't do too much too soon or you may injure yourself.

Since you are exercising within a *time* measurement—20 minutes—it doesn't matter how much *distance* you cover. Your goal is to keep your heart rate in your training range for a specific period of time.

Don't be concerned if a friend goes faster or further than you for the 20 minutes. If you are both working within your training heart rate ranges, you will have gained equal benefit. Most important, you are not competing with anyone—except that old, previously out-of-shape you. That's someone you can improve on every time you lace up your running shoes and go out the door.

This run-easy system is based upon my belief that running should be easy, simple, fun. Running at an easy pace, you'll find that your body will gently move into a new life with a minimum of discomfort. Consistency and endurance, not speed, are the key to success as a beginner. Be determined—but also patient. Muscles and wind won't return in two weeks, but they will return.

The 1.5-Mile Run-Easy Program

This program is almost the same as the previous one. The only difference is that instead of alternating walking briskly and running easy for *time* (20 minutes), you alternate walking briskly with running easy for *distance*. The key here is to pick a distance that will take approximately 20 to 30 minutes to run. Review all the tips I suggest for the 20-Minute Run-Easy Program since they will all apply here, except substitute a distance goal for a time goal.

Actually, this was the very first beginner's program I used over twenty years ago. I had our beginner runners work out on the 1.5-mile cinder track around the reservoir in New York City's Central Park. Their goal was to finish the loop, complete with a wonderful view of the Big Apple's midtown skyline. This gave them a physical, tangible goal: building up to that glorious day when they could run all the way around the reservoir without stopping! This method may work best for you if you prefer a distance goal to a time goal.

First, pick your goal course. It should be a distance of at least a mile but not more than 2 miles. The 1.5-mile distance is about right since it would take most beginners approximately 20 minutes to run that far. Of course you have to build up to running this distance nonstop. Start by alternating walking and running just like in the 20-Minute Run-Easy Program. But your finish line for each workout isn't when you reach 20 minutes but rather when you complete your course. Gradually, you will run more and walk less—progressing according to how you feel. I'll never forget the day our first group of beginners ran their first loop of the reservoir nonstop—you could hear their whoops of joy throughout the park!

You may find it helpful to break up your run into segments. This can be done two ways. First, set some goals for how many minutes you can run nonstop before you take a walk break. Be conservative, but progress to longer time periods of running. Run timed segments within your overall goal to alternate running and walking for your goal distance.

Second, set some physical goals. Pick out landmarks and run to them. Gradually increase the distance you run nonstop by choosing landmarks that are farther away. This is how Shelly-lynn Florence Glover started running as a fifteen-year-old. Behind her house in Canisteo, New York, is a dike that is a mile long. Her overall goal was to run the length of it and back—2 miles. She started out running from one dam to the next, progressing to running two dams at a time. Then she added more landmarks, such as a rabbit hole and a big rock. (This worked well until the rock moved—it was a woodchuck!) Her big breakthrough came when she was able to run the length of the dike—one mile—without stopping. Then she was motivated to be able to run out a mile and continue running all the way back to her house. Of course, it helped that she had a training partner with her every step of the way—Buffy, the Labrador retriever. Every time Shelly-lynn returns home to visit she runs that out-and-back course along the dike and smiles as she reflects on how she got started running. You will have fond memories of your first runs, too.

Here are some suggestions for setting a distance goal (approximately 1.5 miles, an exact distance isn't necessary) for your program:

■ Walk-run a loop in a local park.

■ Walk-run from your house to a friend's.

■ Walk-run a specific number of laps (six laps for 1.5 miles) of a local high school or college track.

■ Walk-run a loop or an out-and-back course in your neighborhood.

■ Walk-run home from work.

You may wish to set a goal distance at first for 1 mile, then 1.5 miles, and then 2 miles. This will work as long as you don't set a goal of running that first mile nonstop. Work up to it by following the run-walk system. Follow the same guidelines for frequency (three to five times a week) and intensity (run at a conversational pace, between 60 to 70 percent of your maximum heart rate) as for the 20-Minute Run-Easy Program.

Caution: Do not combine time with distance yet. Either run 20 minutes, or run a distance that approximates that time (perhaps 1.5 to 2 miles). If you start timing your runs each day to see how fast you're running, you'll be racing yourself. This will result in additional pressure to start running faster than conversation pace, or to run too long before taking walk breaks.

The New York Road Runners Club Run-Easy Program

Most beginner runners benefit from a structured program. "Just tell me what to do each day and I'll do it," they say. The ten-week program that I have developed for our New York Road Runners Club classes has been tested successfully by thousands of runners over the last twenty years. It is ridiculously easy. We start out running only one minute at a time!

True, most of you can run more than that at first. But we start out for just one minute. Very gradually, we increase that amount to running 20 minutes without stopping—a level that comes after ten weeks of training at least three times a week. I've made some

FIGURE 10.1: TEN-WEEK BEGINNER RUNNER'S PROGRAM

Week	Run-Walk Ratio (minutes)	Total Run Time
1	Run 1, walk 2. Complete sequence 7 times.	7
2	Run 2, walk 2. Complete sequence 5 times.	10
3	Run 3, walk 2. Complete sequence 4 times.	12
4	Run 5, walk 2. Complete sequence 3 times.	15
5	Run 6, walk 1½. Complete sequence 3 times.	18
6	Run 8, walk 1½. Complete sequence 2 times.	16
7	Run 10, walk 1½. Complete sequence 2 times.	20
8	Run 12, walk 1, run 8	20
9	Run 15, walk 1, run 5	20
10	Run 20 minutes nonstop	20

Warm up with 5 to 10 minutes of brisk walking. Cool down with 5 to 10 minutes of slow walking. Run segments at a conversational pace. Walk break segments should be brisk.

slight adjustments in the schedule since the previous edition of this book, but the goal remains the same: build from one minute of continuous running to 20 minutes of running.

Such a program cuts to almost zero your chances of injury—or discouragement. All running should be done at an easy conversational pace, and all walking should be done briskly. Review all the guidelines I detailed under the 20-Minute Run-Easy Program. They all apply here. The programs are exactly the same except that here, instead of you choosing when to run and when to walk, a precise schedule is laid out for you to follow. Just pretend that Coach Glover is out there telling you when to start running and when to start walking. Don't be too zealous and don't be a wimp—or you may hear my voice reprimanding you in your dreams!

The ten-week schedule shown in Figure 10.1 starts conservatively. You can even fall a little behind schedule (if you are ill or need to rest a slight injury, for example) and still easily get back on track. Once you reach the halfway mark, however, you will find it difficult to keep up unless you run faithfully at least three, and preferably five, times a week.

Most runners will benefit from following the schedule exactly. If you are overweight, older, or were very inactive prior to starting the program, you may need to progress more slowly. Thus, it may take you longer than ten weeks to complete the program. That's okay, just don't give up. If you can't keep up, or lose time from illness or injury, don't panic. Stay at the level you can handle (or

FIGURE 10.2: TEN-WEEK PYRAMID BEGINNER RUNNER'S PROGRAM

WEEK	RUN-WALK RATIO (MINUTES)	TOTAL RUN TIME
1	Run 1–1–2–2–1–1 (2-minute brisk walk breaks between runs)	8
2	Run 1–1–2–3–2–1 (2-minute brisk walk breaks between runs)	10
3	Run 1–2–3–3–2–1 (2-minute brisk walk breaks between runs)	12
4	Run 2–5–5–3 (1½-minute brisk walk breaks between runs)	15
5	Run 2–5–8–3 (1-minute brisk walk breaks between runs)	18
6	Run 2–3–10–3 (1-minute brisk walk breaks between runs)	18
7	Run 4–12–4 (1-minute brisk walk breaks between runs)	20
8	Run 3–14–3 (1-minute brisk walk breaks between runs)	20
9	Run 2–16–2 (1-minute brisk walk breaks between runs)	20
10	Run 20 minutes nonstop	20

Warm up with 5 to 10 minutes of brisk walking. Cool down with 5 to 10 minutes of slow walking. Run segments at a conversational pace.

go back a level) until you are ready to move on. This may mean it will take twelve or sixteen or more weeks to build up to running 20 minutes nonstop. So what! Don't worry. Don't hurry. Just remember how many years it took you to get out of shape; take your time getting back into it. Your goal is to run 20 minutes nonstop —smiling and talking all the way. It doesn't matter if you take four weeks or four months to reach that goal. For most, ten weeks is a good goal.

If you find that the program is too easy, simply adjust by moving up to a level that is more challenging for you, but not too difficult, and continue from there. If you have been quite active prior to starting this schedule, you may find that you can start, for example, at Week 3. Or you may start at Week 1, but skip a level or two if you progress quickly. Just don't be in a hurry; don't set yourself up for injury or failure. It is better to be conservative and progress slowly. *Warning:* It is better to be cautious than to be macho and try to go too far too fast. Runners who go too far too fast end up being sedentary whiners!

The Pyramid Run-Easy Program

Here is a variation of the previous structured ten-week program. Shelly-lynn Florence Glover favors this method when she works with her personal training clients through her company, Great Strides. Instead of running the same time sequence throughout the workout, she favors having the beginner runner warm up to the task with shorter run segments prior to moving to longer ones at the peak of the workout, and then tapering down to shorter ones at the end when he or she is tired.

She feels that this method works well psychologically for her clients. The first few runs and the last few runs are shorter, and thus easier. Try it out and see if it works better for you. You are still starting off with one-minute runs at the beginning and building to 20 minutes of nonstop running after ten weeks.

Use the same guidelines as described in the 20-Minute Run-Easy Program and the New York Road Runners Club Run-Easy Program. Figure 10.2 summarizes Shelly-lynn's Pyramid Run-Easy Program.

After completing one of these programs, you will be running 20 minutes at a time nonstop. Congratulations! You may now graduate from my beginner's program, with honors! You're ready for the next step—moving up to running 30 minutes nonstop with my advanced beginner's program in the following chapter.

ELEVEN

The Advanced Beginner Runner's Training Program

There are two types of advanced beginner runners: those who have just graduated from the beginner's program, and those who are starting running at a slightly higher level. My definition of an advanced beginner runner is: *someone who can comfortably run a full mile nonstop but can't comfortably run for 30 minutes nonstop.*

The advanced beginner runner should review Chapters 4 through 7 for guidelines on starting out, motivation, and exercise principles before starting the training program below.

Remember those guidelines in Chapter 8 for the FIT exercise prescription? *Frequency* remains the same for the advanced beginner as for the beginner—run at least three times a week, preferably five times. My recommended *intensity* may be adjusted slightly from that of the beginner. You should still run at a conversational pace, but now it's okay for you to run a little faster in order to get a little more aerobic benefit. I now widen the training heart rate range from the beginner's recommendation of 60 to 70 percent of maximum heart rate to 60 to 80 percent (with a target of 70 percent). In addition, the goal now is to increase the amount of *time* that you can run nonstop from the 20-minute goal for beginners to 30 minutes.

Moving Up

If you have just completed the beginner's program in the previous chapter and are now running comfortably for 20 minutes nonstop, you are now almost ready to move up. I say almost ready because you are actually going to level off or even take a step back before moving up. Why? First, you shouldn't continually add more and more running time to your program. Give your body a chance to adapt to running for 20 minutes nonstop by remaining at the same level for a few weeks. Second, the goal now is to slightly quicken the pace of your runs, but you shouldn't do that while also increasing the distance. In our New York Road Runners Club classes, we also start to ease our advanced beginner runners up a few hills. This presents a new challenge and further strengthens their legs, hearts, and lungs. Ease into the hills—don't make them too steep, too long, or run them too often. We actually divide our advanced beginners into two groups, one for those not yet up to running for 30 minutes and one for those who can run that long but need to work on improving their pace.

We use the program outlined in Figure 11.1 in our classes to ease graduates of our beginner program into our advanced beginner program. We actually go back to Week 7 of the beginner's schedule and work back up to 20 minutes of running nonstop. Then, we gradually build to 30 minutes of nonstop running within the ten-week program. Thus, we take a raw beginner up to 20 minutes of consecutive running in ten weeks, and to 30 minutes after twenty weeks.

Other beginner programs that you may come across build up to 30 minutes of running within the first ten weeks. If you feel that you can safely progress that quickly, then just move up a few weeks on my schedules and enjoy yourself. But for those people going from complete nonrunner to an active lifestyle, my conservative program works well. Again, what's the hurry to get into shape after being out of shape for so long?

Figure 11.1 is my official New York Road Runners Club Advanced Beginner Runner Program. If you prefer not to move back to 10-minute runs at the start of the program, then go ahead and

FIGURE 11.1: TEN-WEEK ADVANCED BEGINNER RUNNER'S PROGRAM

WEEK	
1	Run 10 minutes, walk 1½ minutes, then repeat once
2	Run 12 minutes, walk 1 minute, run 8 minutes
3	Run 15 minutes, walk 1 minute, run 5 minutes
4	Run 20 minutes nonstop
5	Run 20 minutes nonstop
6	Run 22 minutes nonstop
7	Run 25 minutes nonstop
8	Run 28 minutes nonstop
9	Run 30 minutes nonstop
10	Run 30 minutes nonstop

Warm up with 5 to 10 minutes of brisk walking. Cool down with 5 to 10 minutes of slow walking.

stay at 20 minutes of running for the first five weeks before picking up my schedule at Week 6.

Starting at Advanced Beginner

Sometimes young men and women and even some of us older folks who keep themselves together somewhat can bypass the beginner program and start with the advanced beginner schedule. This is especially true if you were a former athlete or if you have kept in reasonably good shape in other physical activities such as aerobics classes, biking, walking, tennis, rowing, basketball, and swimming. You may already be running a little here and there and can run at least a mile in comfort.

But be cautious! It's better to start at too low a level and work up, than to start too high and drop out. If you get injured or fatigued, or cannot progress on a gradually increasing plane, you may not make it. Let common sense and caution guide you, not your ego or your competitive friends.

I recommend that you start with Week 1 of the ten-week advanced beginner program unless you can very comfortably run at least 20 minutes at a time. In that case, start with Week 6 of the program.

What's Next?

After completing this ten-week program, you will be running 30 minutes at a time nonstop at least three times a week. Congratulations! You are no longer an advanced beginner, you have graduated to fitness runner.

What's next? Here's the good news. This is all you need to run to achieve and maintain fitness. When you reach this point, pause. Hold your running at this level for at least a month. Reflect back on the progress you made since you started out. Think about how much better you look and feel. Consider all the benefits you have derived from your running program. Most of all, smile. Isn't it fun to run and be fit!

Now the struggle isn't to get started and build fitness, but to stay with it and maintain your newfound fitness. As your body gets into shape, the challenge of running may start to fade. This may be a good time to review once again my motivational tips for staying with it in Chapter 5.

You can decide if you want to remain at this minimal fitness level or if you want to move on to the intermediate level in the next chapter. You might even look ahead to the beginner racer level in Chapter 13. Some will even choose the ultimate goal at this point and turn to Chapter 14, "The Beginner Marathoner."

But remember: Once you have reached this fitness runner level, and can faithfully run 30 minutes at least three times a week, you do not need to progress any further. You have achieved the level of fitness runner, and only need to hold there. Many runners do advance—largely because the challenge and enjoyment is there and they want to be in excellent shape. But at this fitness level you can sightsee on runs in any city you visit, work out with friends, or just enjoy the running experience by yourself. You like the way you look and feel. You are more graceful, more comfortable on the run. You have become a runner.

TWELVE

The Intermediate Runner's Training Program

This chapter is for the runner who has graduated from the beginner's and advanced beginner's program or is already running enough to be termed a fitness runner. My definition of an intermediate runner is: *someone who can comfortably run for 30 minutes nonstop at a pace of 9 minutes per mile or slower.* If you run faster than this you are ready for the basic competitor training program in *The Competitive Runner's Handbook.*

The intermediate level is where most runners arrive, full of enthusiasm, and where they stay. They run forever at this level of fitness. That's fine. You may choose to stay at 30 minutes of running or you may increase how far you run to add to your fun and fitness program. You may choose to move on to the challenge of racing, or even take on the challenge of the marathon.

The intermediate sometimes forgets the lessons of the beginner. Review Chapters 5 to 7 before starting the training program below. Read again those important guidelines in Chapter 8 for the FIT exercise prescription. *Frequency* remains the same for the intermediate runner as for the beginner—run at least three times a week. But if you intend to move up to racing you will need to run four to six times a week in order to be strong enough to reach the finish line.

My recommended *intensity* for the intermediate runner is still conversational pace (THR of 60 to 80 percent) for most runs. Some easy runs at 60 to 70 percent of maximum heart rate are recommended; this will also be the pace that is best if you add some longer runs. Most of your other runs should be at 70 to 80 percent of your maximum heart rate (with a target of 70 percent) in order to increase your aerobic fitness. You may run at an intensity above 80 percent—above your conversational pace—if you ease into speed training (see Chapter 15) to prepare for race efforts. In our classes at the New York Road Runners Club, we gently move runners into speed and hill workouts. It is amazing to watch the men and women get faster and faster as their confidence grows with each session. Once you know that you can run faster for short distances, you can keep up a faster pace in races. Some runners just want to learn how to run faster without any intention of entering races. They just like the feeling of moving along quickly and gracefully. If you decide to try racing for fun and challenge, your first few races should be run within your training heart rate range (below 80 percent). Then you will learn to push at faster paces and a higher heart rate (80 to 90 percent or more of maximum) in order to improve your times as you become more fit.

At the intermediate level, many runners begin to increase the *time* of some of their runs beyond the 30-minute level. Most runners at this point make the switch from counting how many minutes they run to how many miles they run. The intermediate training program outlined here is measured by mileage, but you are welcome to continue measuring your runs by minutes like many other intermediates.

Go easy here as you start to run for mileage and work to increase it. This is a serious and important transition. Keep your easy days at 30 minutes per run (about 3 miles). Gradually add one day a week of longer runs (6 to 8 miles). The remaining running days will be medium-distance runs of 4 to 5 miles. Don't forget to include at least one day off.

Most intermediates run 10 to 15 miles a week. This is all you need to get the fitness and health benefits of exercise. And it gives you a minimal endurance base for training for a few short races.

FIGURE 12.1: SAMPLE INTERMEDIATE BUILD-UP SCHEDULE
(from a 10-mile-a-week base to 20 miles)

WEEKS	MON.	TUES.	WED.	THUR.	FRI.	SAT.	SUN.	TOTAL
Base	Off	3	Off	2	Off	3	2	10
1	Off	3	Off	3	Off	3	2	11
2	Off	3	Off	3	Off	3	3	12
3	Off	3	Off	3	Off	4	3	13
4	Off	3	Off	3	Off	4	3	13
5	Off	3	2	3	Off	4	3	15
6	Off	3	2	3	Off	4	3	15
7	Off	3	3	3	Off	5	3	17
8	Off	3	3	4	Off	5	3	18
9	Off	3	4	4	Off	5	3	19
10	Off	3	4	4	Off	6	3	20

This is a sample schedule; Saturdays and Sundays are interchangeable days; you may switch the workouts to accommodate long runs, resting and races.

How much mileage you need beyond that level depends on your goals as a runner. Many of us enjoy running so much that we prefer running at least 20 miles a week. Others increase their mileage to improve their performance at races. Chapters 13 and 14 detail mileage guidelines for various racing distances from 5K (3.1 miles) to the marathon (26.2 miles).

Sample Training Schedule

Figures 12.1 and 12.2 are examples of how you can distribute your mileage over the course of a week (including off days, short easy days, medium days, and long runs) and how you can gradually increase your mileage from week to week. One sample schedule builds gradually from a base level (held for at least three to four weeks) of 10 miles per week to 20; the other builds from 20 to 30 miles per week. If you choose to level off at any point (or cut back), just use a sample week for that mileage model. For example, follow Week 5 for a 15-mile training week if you want to plateau at that level.

Remember, 10 to 15 miles a week is all you need for fitness running. If you run 15 to 20 miles a week following my schedule, you should be able to safely run races of 5K (3.1 miles) to 10K (6.2 miles). For races up to the half-marathon (13.1 miles), the

FIGURE 12.2: SAMPLE INTERMEDIATE BUILD-UP SCHEDULE
(from a 20-mile-a-week base to 30 miles)

WEEKS	MON.	TUES.	WED.	THUR.	FRI.	SAT.	SUN.	TOTAL
Base	Off	3	4	4	Off	6	3	20
1	Off	3	4	4	Off	6	4	21
2	Off	3	4	4	Off	7	4	22
3	Off	3	4	4	Off	5	4	20
4	Off	3	4	4	Off	8	4	23
5	Off	3	4	5	Off	8	4	24
6	Off	3	4	5	Off	8	4	24
7	Off	3	5	5	Off	8	4	25
8	Off	3	4	4	Off	6	3	20
9	Off	3	4	5	3	8	4	27
10	Off	3	4	6	4	8	5	30

This is a sample schedule; Saturdays and Sundays are interchangeable days; you may switch the workouts to accommodate long runs, resting and races.

25- to 30-mile-per-week schedules will allow you to run with at least modest success. These programs can be used as a base for marathon training, but longer runs will have to be added over the four months going into the big race (follow the marathon training guidelines in Chapter 14).

Please note: These are *sample schedules*. Use them as a model for designing a program that works best for you.

Be a Fitness Runner Forever

Once you've reached that 30- to 60-minute per run, three to five days per week intermediate level, you'll have plenty of company, including Jack Shepherd. Many of you may follow his pattern. After starting with my beginner running class back in 1975, he progressed to the advanced beginner– and then intermediate-level classes. He then ran his first race and his first two marathons. Two decades later, he seldom races. He's done that. Now he runs for fitness and fun day after day, week after week, month after month, year after year. And as he runs past his sixtieth birthday, he's a great example of how running and fitness can keep your body and mind young.

Jack's total fitness program is a good model for all of you. He runs 3, 5, or 7 miles at a time—running every other day. That's about 15 to 20 miles per week. On alternate days he lifts weights and uses a rowing machine for 15 minutes. The way I look at it, if out-of-shape, overstressed Jack Shepherd could get into shape—and stay there for over twenty years—why can't you do it, too?

Part IV

Racing

THIRTEEN

The Beginner Racer

I love converting runners to racers. Why? It's fun and inspiring to watch fitness runners set challenges to run farther or faster, reach those goals, and then raise them again. "Hooray! I did it, Coach Glover!" you can exclaim.

Racing isn't for everyone. But I think every runner should try at least one or two races to see what it's like. For one thing, the era of the "fun racer"—the average runner—has emerged. For most of the runners in most of the races, the race is not to win, but to better personal goals and to have fun doing it. After all, in most races today there are hundreds, perhaps thousands of runners, but only a handful of them are top athletes. The rest of you battle not against the leaders but against yourselves. And you win by meeting realistic goals, such as simply finishing the race with a smile.

In the average 5K (3.1 miles) or 10K (6.2 miles) race, less than 10 percent of the runners (the "front of the pack") will race at better than 6 minutes per mile. The "middle of the pack" group that makes up the majority of the field will cover the distance at 9 to 10 minutes per mile. The "back of the pack"—consisting of just as many runners as the speedy front pack—will finish the race in 10 to 12 minutes per mile and slower. So you can see that once you have progressed to my intermediate runner training program you will fit the profile of the average racer. You will have plenty of company at your pace. And remember this: The first and foremost goal of all runners in a race, from the front to the back of the pack, is the finish line. We all have that common bond.

Some runners don't want to race. They dislike the competition. They run for the pleasure of it. My good friend Nina Kuscsik, the first women's division winner of the Boston Marathon, doesn't think of racing as competition but as running with other people "to show off what you can do." Following are some of the many reasons, besides "showing off," why you should consider moving on to racing:

- It gives your running life a goal, a focus. You circle the race date on your running calendar and train for that day. This helps you get "over the hump" that some runners face who are having trouble moving through dull periods in their running. Thinking of your upcoming race motivates you to get out the door and get going with your training.

- You make friends. Races give you the opportunity to meet other runners. You may meet potential running partners, or even runners who become close friends. I know many runners who met their spouses at races. You can exchange training tips and experiences with other runners at races. Most of all, you can enthusiastically offer each other encouragement to meet goals.

- It's fun. Races are a large social gathering, a party in running shorts. For every runner that grunts and groans, huffs and puffs in an all-out effort to win a trophy, there are hundreds behind him or her that are chatting away with friends or perfect strangers, smiling all the way from start to finish. Of course, if you want to run your best times, you may need to save the chatter till after you've crossed the finish line with a personal record. Then you can laugh and smile!

In fact, the best part of the race for most runners isn't the race itself, but the after-race party. Most events provide refreshments and a gathering area where runners can bask in their glory, brag and complain, exchange excuses for not running faster (too hot, too hilly, started too fast, started too slow . . .), compare blisters, look for old friends, or even check out the runner with the nice legs that passed you with a mile to go. It's this atmosphere that often hooks runners on the whole idea of racing.

▪ You can test yourself. Racing gives you a way to measure your progress toward some specific goal. Finishing a race is a great achievement: You have set a goal and accomplished it; you may also get satisfaction from doing something physical, especially if you have not been successful in athletics in the past. At this early racing level, your competition is entirely against the "old you." Racing lets you discover the new you. As you see your racing distances and times improve, you will feel better physically and mentally. You will feel proud, ready to take on new challenges in running—and in the rest of your life.

▪ You have a dream of someday running the big one—the marathon. This is the super-fitness goal for thousands of runners (but you can still be a successful, happy runner without running a marathon). Your first race, which should not be the marathon, is a stepping-stone along the path toward running the "ultimate challenge." You must start with shorter races to build experience and fitness.

▪ It's exciting. We overcome discomfort, and that's exhilarating. And we discover an honest flirtation with danger that must be respected. The race excites because it makes us play the edges, challenge boundaries, yet follow common sense. You may choose to race to see how far or how fast you can run. Taking a chance at success or failure is a heart-thumping, mind-numbing experience. But if you train properly, race wisely, and set reasonable but challenging goals, you can charge to the finish line and win "your race."

Like many runners, I have a love-hate relationship with racing. I love to train for races, I thrive on the challenge it presents. But as race day approaches I start to wonder, "Why am I doing this?" After all, I'm asking my mind to push my aging body to its limits once again. "What happened to running for fun and fitness?" I ask myself. But during the race, at the starter's gun, a new surge of confidence pumps my blood and drives me onward! How do I feel during a race? I hate it. I want to quit over and over. But I love it, too, so I keep going. The challenge of defeating fatigue, of reaching beyond my potential keeps me going forward. When I finish, I look back at the discomfort I experienced as mere fleeting moments. Instead of dwelling on how much work it was, I glow with the feeling of accomplishment. I'm motivated, inspired to race once again to improve myself.

We suffer individual hardships together in races. All of us, you and me, the winner and the final finisher. We test ourselves against ourselves and against the elements and, if we wish, against each other. The racer wins by sharing his or her unique personal experience. Enjoy your first race experience and beyond, but most of all share it with others. That way we can motivate one another to run to loftier goals, and provide the fellowship that will keep running and racing fun.

Shelly-lynn and I shared a very special experience with a beginner racer as we raced to bring this book to the finish line. Our sister-in-law, Caylee Nychis-Florence, decided to run her first race. Why? She said that she was "intrigued with how much we glowed when we talked about racing." But as she prepared for the local 5K event, she became ill and wasn't able to run. So she cheered for us on the sidelines and promised to run it the next year. A few months later it was discovered that her illness was caused by stomach cancer. Nevertheless, she decided that she would run the upcoming annual race on Labor Day despite the cancer and the chemotherapy treatments.

She now had a new reason to run her first race. She stated, "I felt that, symbolically, if I can finish a race then I can also finish my race against cancer." Caylee reviewed the final draft of this chapter and prepared her race strategy. She started off with her friend, Sasha Bowers, who was running her second race. This gave her more confidence to get started. She stationed her husband, Brian (a former high school running whiz now making a running comeback), and three-year-old son, Spencer (who always beats me when we race sprints), near the finish line. This gave her more incentive to make it all the way.

How did she feel at the starting line? "I was so overwhelmed by the sense of community among the hundreds of runners around me that I became very excited, and I got that glow that I had seen in Bob and Shelly." Caylee started back in the pack at a comfortable pace with her friend. Along the way she made a friend, another cancer patient. A veteran marathoner who was near the end of his chemo treatments, he singled Caylee out since she was the only bald woman in the field. "We bonded right away," said Caylee, "we were there for the same reason."

After I crossed the finish line of the race, the New Haven (CT) 5K, I headed out to look for her. I admit to feeling nervous. Would her strength hold up after three chemo treatments? A half a mile from the finish line I saw her running along with a big smile on her face. She invited me to join her for her special "party," so I ran along. She was bubbling with enthusiasm and told me that she stopped to walk for half a block when her stomach became queasy. I assured her that was okay. As we neared the finish line the crowd became larger and noisier. She felt as if they were cheering just for her. They were rooting her on, and they'll be there cheering for you too at the finish line of your races. To top off the excitement, the announcer read off her name as she crossed the finish line in 34:18. Way to go Caylee!

She said that it was a moment she'll cherish forever. I was so inspired by her accomplishment that I presented her with a trophy with the inscription: "Caylee's First Race." And Caylee was so inspired by her feat that she vowed to fight her cancer with renewed strength and confidence.

If you're running at the intermediate training level as outlined in the preceding chapter, you are ready to train for your first race. So, "On your mark, get set, *go!*"

On Your Mark: Selecting Your First Race

Pick a race (or a series of races). The distance should be long enough to challenge you but short enough to be completed with a reasonable amount of effort. I recommend a distance between 2 miles and 5K (3.1 miles), but not more than 10K (6.2 miles). These are popular racing distances so you should have a number of events to choose from in your area. It is best to choose a local race— traveling adds to your excitement and stress. Besides, you can be a "hometown hero" finishing in front of friends and family if you race in your town or city. Pick a low-key event such as a "fun run," which do not give out awards for running fast but rather are just for fun. Often these runs are benefits for local charities.

If you can't find a fun run for your first race (or races), then be sure to avoid very serious races that don't include lots of runners of your speed and experience. To avoid being alone and frustrated at the tail end of a small race, pick a mass-participation event with plenty of novice and casual racers. Think this way: Rather than counting how many runners finish ahead of you, seek comfort in the fact that the more runners there are at the starting line, the more will be behind you at the finish line. Don't be afraid; you'll soon find that most of the runners in the race are more like you than those sleek, skinny runners up front. If possible, stay away from very hilly courses and avoid hot weather for your first race experience. In other words, minimize your obstacles. Women may prefer women-only races at first.

Get Set: Training for Your First Race

If you are now running at least for 30 minutes at a time, at least three to five times a week, you are ready to train for your first race. You should concentrate on building your endurance to the point where you can run and finish a race distance comfortably.

You need a minimum amount of mileage and long runs to be able to race and reach the finish line with reasonable comfort. My basic guidelines are the following:

- Your weekly mileage should be at least two to three times the distance of the race itself (I prefer three). For example, 12 to 18 miles per week for a 6-mile race. This formula is altered for marathon training (see the following chapter).

- Hold that mileage for at least four to eight weeks prior to the race itself.

- Complete at least three long runs, which cover at least two-thirds of the race distance, in the eight-week period prior to the race. For example, a 4-mile-long run for a 6-mile race. If you are able to safely build up to long runs equal to or beyond the race distance, that is even better.

Never try to cram mileage in during the last weeks before a race. Build gradually. Remember the hard-easy system and all the other basic training principles detailed in Chapter 6. Alternate your three types of conversational endurance runs—long, short, medium. Do not concern yourself yet with speed work. Your goal is to merely hold your normal, conversational running pace to the finish line of your first race. After you have experienced the thrill of finishing your first race, you may then decide to work on increasing the intensity of a few of your training runs so that you can run faster

FIGURE 13.1: EIGHT-WEEK TRAINING PROGRAM
FOR YOUR FIRST RACE (5K–4 miles)

Week	Mon.	Tues.	Wed.	Thurs.	Fri.	Sat.	Sun.	Total Mileage
1	Off	2	2	2	Off	2	Off	8
2	Off	2	2	2	Off	2	2	10
3	Off	2	2	2	Off	2	2	10
4	Off	2	3	2	Off	2	3	12
5	Off	2	3	2	Off	2	3	12
6	Off	2	3	2	Off	2	3	12
7	Off	2	3	2	Off	2	3	12
8	Off	2	2	2	Off	2	race (5K–4 miles)	8 + race

in races (see Chapter 15). Run up and down a few hills if the race route includes them.

Taper for your race. This means take it easy over the last few days going into the race. Take some days off, and when you do run, run short and easy. Also cut back on all other physical activity. No additional amount of training will help at this point, but it could hurt your race performance. It is too late to get in better shape for the race. Let your body rest up for the big effort.

Refer back to Figures 12.1 and 12.2 in the previous chapter for the sample schedules for gradually increasing your mileage from 10 to 20 miles per week, and from 20 to 30 miles per week. Choose the level you feel you can safely build up to for your race and use it as your model. Hold at that level for at least six weeks and then taper off over the last week prior to your race.

Figures 13.1 and 13.2 are sample first race training schedules for you to use. One is a specific eight-week training program, including a tapering week, for the 5K to 4-mile race distance; the other is for a 10K race distance. Please note that these schedules are designed to help you make it to the finish line with a minimal amount of training. If your goal is to improve your fitness and race times beyond this level, then move on to the more advanced training guidelines in *The Competitive Runner's Handbook*.

Go! Running Your First Race

Your goal is simple: finish.

Experience your first race, don't race it. Your first race should

FIGURE 13.2: EIGHT-WEEK TRAINING PROGRAM
FOR YOUR FIRST RACE (10K)

Week	Mon.	Tues.	Wed.	Thurs.	Fri.	Sat.	Sun.	Total Mileage
1	Off	2	3	3	Off	2	4	14
2	Off	2	3	3	Off	2	4	14
3	Off	3	3	3	Off	2	5	16
4	Off	3	4	3	Off	3	5	18
5	Off	3	4	4	Off	3	4	18
6	Off	3	4	3	Off	3	5	18
7	Off	3	4	3	Off	2	4	16
8	Off	4	2	2	Off	2	race (10K)	10 + race

be slightly longer or slightly faster than your normal run. *Run* your first race. Later you can *race*. You will be a hero just for finishing, so don't put pressure on yourself by announcing a time goal. Look at it this way: The slower you run the distance, the easier it will be to show off by improving your time the next race!

Tips for Your First Race
Organize yourself. The day *before* your race, carefully plan everything you will need. Double check the start time of the race, how to get there, and how long it will take you to get to the race start. Listen to the weather report and set out the clothes and shoes you'll wear for the race as well as your runner's stopwatch. Also set aside clothing to change into when you finish and a towel to dry off with. Stick some money into your racing shoe just in case you need it for emergency transportation, food, or drink.

Put on your number. If possible, register in advance of the race and pick up your registration materials prior to race day. Put your number on your T-shirt or singlet way before the race starts. If you are able to get it early, you might even do this the night before the race. Otherwise, pin it on as soon as you pick it up on race morning. That way you won't lose it in your last nervous prerace moments. Also, you'll get used to the feel of it being pinned to the *front* of your shirt (on the lower third). Adjust how your number is pinned on well before the race starts. And relax. Think of this as a training run only you're wearing a number.

Wear your trusty shoes. Wear your faithful, well-cushioned, well-broken-in training shoes. You don't need a fancy new pair just for the race, nor are you ready for lightweight, flimsy racing shoes. See Chapter 16 for guidelines on shoes.

Don't overdress or underdress. Beginner racers usually wear too much clothing. You should start the race feeling slightly under-dressed. Your body will heat up during the race, and even clothing that was comfortable for training runs may now feel too warm. If the weather is cold you should dress in layers. In the heat, cover the body with a minimal amount of lightweight, light-colored, loose, breathable clothing. See Chapters 17, 21, and 22 for guidelines on how to dress for racing in hot or cold weather.

Eating. On race day, don't eat or drink anything out of the ordinary. This is not the time to experiment. Do not eat for two to three hours before the race. Carbohydrate-loading is only for experienced runners and long racing distances such as the marathon. See Chapter 19 for guidelines for fueling up for racing.

Drinking. Pour fluids into yourself before, during, and after the race—especially on hot days. You should be used to drinking from your training runs. See Chapter 20 for guidelines on drinking and racing.

Warm-up and cool-down. Walk around and jog slowly for a few minutes to prepare your heart and lungs for the race, just as you do in your training runs. Do a few light stretches, but be careful not to overstretch while you are pumped up and nervous. Don't forget to cool down after all runs and races with a slow walk and a thorough stretching routine.

Run with a partner. If possible, run with a friend who is also running his or her first race so you can help each other along. Make a promise not to race each other but to finish together, no matter what. If an experienced racer volunteers to run with you, make him or her promise to go at your pace. Find someone who is willing to chat with you all the way, holding you back at the start, and supporting you at the end when you feel like quitting. If you can't bring along a friend, just make runners around you aware that it is your first race and you'll soon have plenty of new friends to cheer you on.

Walk if necessary. You can walk during a race if you wish. If someone gives you a hard time just tell them Bob Glover said it was okay. Nowhere on the race application does it say you can't walk. Be tough and try to run all the way, but be smart and walk if necessary so that you can finish. As a beginner racer, you might need a light breather here and there, or the hills or heat may be too much for you. If your heart rate or body temperature soars, or you can't "catch" your breath and run at conversation pace, or your legs tire, take brisk walk breaks. But keep moving toward that finish line. Cheat: Since you should drink water at the stations, walk with your cup of water as you slowly drink it. Everyone will think you are only walking so you can drink! And if you walk up steep hills, I can guarantee you won't be alone. Avoid walking across the finish line; take your walk break earlier, and run across smiling.

Fear not. Afraid of finishing last? That's unlikely if you are well prepared and following these guidelines. Some runners start too fast and struggle in last, or attempt to run the distance without proper mileage "in the bank" beforehand.

Gain confidence by planning your race strategy in advance; break the course down into small sections, and know where key landmarks, mileage markers, and hills are located. Run from mile marker to mile marker. Be confident in knowing you have prepared well and properly. Everyone is nervous before a race, especially me. Turn your nervousness and fear around and use this energy to help you get to the finish line. Look forward to this opportunity to show off. After all, you only get to run your first race once.

Race day. Here you are. The morning of your first race may find your heart pounding. Prerace nerves strike the fast and the slow. You may take your leisure in the bathroom, eat toast, drink orange juice (if that's your style), and read the paper. Carefully pack your bag (actually you might be wise to pack the night before and then recheck it in the morning): foot powder or petroleum jelly to prevent blisters, sunscreen and sunglasses if it's a bright day, options for clothing for the race (depending on weather conditions) and for after the race (keeping dry after the race is especially important in cold weather), toilet paper (very important since supplies often run out at races or you need to improvise due to long lines at the toilets), an extra pair of shoelaces, postrace first-aid equipment, a hat and gloves in case it's cold, a hat in case it's sunny, a bottle of water, inhalers if you need them. When in doubt about what you might need, stick it in. My bag is stuffed so full you'd think I was going away for a week instead of just heading to a local race. But when I need something, I'm sure to have it.

Before checking your bag, put on the clothes (with race number attached) and shoes (double knot the laces to prevent them from untying) you will race in so you know for sure where they are. You might think this all sounds stupid, but believe me, as the race approaches, runners get nervous and they don't always think clearly. My biggest error was when I packed only one of my racing shoes for an out-of-town marathon and didn't notice it until an hour before the start. I ended up running the race in my heavy training shoes (lesson: pack an extra pair of shoes just in case). I was very upset about it, but then I got so pumped up when the gun sounded that I forgot about it until I took my shoes off after crossing the finish line in my all-time best marathon performance. So if you do forget something, forget about it. Don't let it ruin your day. Go ahead and run with confidence.

Arrive at least an hour before race time so you can check in, warm up, make the compulsory anxious trips to the toilet, find out information about the course (where are the hills!), and of course chat with the other runners. If you haven't signed up for the race in advance, make sure they take race-day entries before you leave the house—actually, you should do this a couple of days or better yet a few weeks—before race day. Late-day entries put a strain on the race volunteers and on you (the wait in line is longer) so please register in advance.

It is now time for last-minute preparations. Apply a dab of petroleum jelly to your toes, heels, and bottoms of your feet (or use foot powder) and perhaps nipples to prevent blistering. With a half hour to go, start your warm-up with a walk, then light stretching, and then jog for a few minutes. If possible, run a few minutes into the finish area to get a feel for it. Think positively. Practice running the race in your mind. This is called visualization. Actually "see" and "feel" yourself starting off, reaching key landmarks, conquering hills, holding pace, and finishing with a smile. See the following chapter for detailed guidelines on visualization.

With 15 minutes to go, it is time for a cup or two of water or sports drink and one more trip to the toilet. At this point I have some toilet paper tucked into my shorts in case I need it before—or during—the race. (Actually, I use paper towels, since regular tissue paper doesn't hold up well when it gets wet with sweat or water dousings.) Peel off any clothing you're wearing that is non-essential for racing and place it in your easily recognized, tagged bag or hand it to a friend or family member. On a hot day I'll give myself one final psychological boost—I pour a cup or two of cold water over my head to help me think cool.

Lining up. Position yourself in the very back so you won't get trampled by the speedsters, or get dragged out at too fast an early pace. Let as many people start ahead of you as possible. This will help ensure that you start slowly, and instead of having lots of people passing you during the race, there'll be plenty of people for you to pass.

Standing there among a crowd of runners who all look younger, sleeker, and faster than you, you may begin to feel all alone, insecure, intimidated. Be assured, all runners go through this—even the elite. Before you panic and look for escape routes, think about all the good training you did to prepare for this first race experience. You can do it! Give yourself a good pep talk. Soon it will be too late to chicken out—you will be saved by the starter's horn.

You're off! The blast of the starter's horn propels you along with the flowing mass of runners down the road. "Why did I let Bob Glover start me on this madness?" your inner voice screams. But you're off. You fight adrenaline and hold back. Begin slowly; after a while, if you feel good, pick up your pace. Start slowly and let as many runners get ahead of you as possible. (If you start too fast, they'll pass you later anyway.) Then, toward the end of the race, if you feel good, pick up your pace and pass some of them; you're the tortoise passing the hares who went out too fast. This gives you confidence and the excitement of passing runner after runner over the last mile or two of the race.

Maintain a comfortable, slightly slow pace. Find a group of runners going at your pace and join them. Remember, you aren't out there to beat people. Your goal is to finish. Don't race against anyone who passes you or whom you pass—you'll lose your sense of an even pace. Chat with the runners around you, wave to your fans, laugh, have fun. This is a fun race for you, not a serious race, as it is for those up ahead. Hang in there; set goals to run from one landmark to the next. Take frequent water breaks and, if necessary, brisk walking breaks. But keep on moving toward that finish line.

Don't be a hot dog, finishing the race with a face-twisting, arm-whirling sprint. Finish in good form. Be in control. Make sure to look good as you cross the finish line in case someone takes a photo of you completing your first race.

Now comes the fun: You can brag to everyone in sight (and then go home and call all your friends) about how great you felt in your first race. After you cool down by walking and stretching, you can cheer the top runners as they receive their trophies, and know that you, too, are a winner.

Most runners remember their first race vividly, and each of their tales is instructive and often inspiring. My first race was as a sixteen-year-old. For the first time, high schoolers in New York State (boys only, girls weren't yet allowed to run long distances) were being allowed to run longer than a mile. In preparation for the 2-mile event being added to the high school track program the following season, the folks in Hornell, New York, added to their adult 7-mile Memorial Day road race a 2-mile road race for boys. One of my best friends, Bob Elliott, challenged me to do it with him. I was very nervous about running my first road race. Not only that, this would be the first time I had ever run 2 miles! I finished with a lot left, passing a lot of experienced distance runners. Afterward, all my friends in school called me "marathon man." They thought 2 miles must be a marathon, and they certainly had never heard of anyone back in those days who could run that far. Little did I know back then that I would one day run the 26.2 miles of a marathon at a faster pace per mile than I ran my first 2-miler. Who would have dreamed that I would run 2 miles faster as a fifty-year-old than as a sixteen-year-old? This very event helped shape the rest of my life. The following track season at Dansville High School I became a pioneer—the first ever Livingston County 2-mile champion. I found something to give me the confidence to excel in whatever I chose to do. Perhaps you, too, will be inspired by finishing your first race.

Recover. After the race, take it easy the next few days with less and slower running. Even though you will not be racing hard, you will still be under a lot of stress from the excitement and exertion of your first race. Recover carefully.

Analyze the results, what's next? For some runners, one race experience is enough. They can say they met the challenge and will return to running for fitness and pleasure. Most of us, however, get hooked on all the excitement and can't wait to see how much more we can improve. The first step is to analyze your first race.

Now that you have won *your* race, think it over. What went well? What problems did you have, and why? What worked and what didn't in terms of equipment, starting pace, finish, and so forth? Do you need more work on hills? Did you drink enough fluids? Use the experience as background to help you prepare for your next race. Reevaluate your training program and select new racing goals. Make them either farther or faster, but not both— not yet.

Here are some goals that you can set for yourself:

1. The safest, least competitive goal is to extend the distance of your longest race. If you have run a 5K, enter a race that's 4 miles or 10K, then 10 miles, then the half-marathon, then perhaps a marathon. Finishing will continue to be a reward; only now the distance will be tougher. However, you don't have to keep racing longer and longer distances, and if you aren't properly prepared for them, you shouldn't.

2. Another goal is to improve your time over the same distance, then improve your time over a variety of distances. You'll soon hear other runners talk about setting PRs (personal records). Record your PR for different race lengths and then set a goal of improving those times. Don't forget that as you get older, you should set your PRs all over again as you move up to a new five-year age group. I keep three sets of PRs: my all-time best at each distance (which, like my youth, I'll never see again), my best time within my present age group, and my comeback PRs (my best races since coming back from racing retirement and injury).

3. A third, but more competitive, goal is to aim for a certain place (overall or within your age and/or gender category) in a race, like the top 100 or even the top 10,000. I faintly remember

the days when I always aimed for the top ten. Or, aim for finishing within a certain percentage of the field, or your age group. In my comeback I can now aim for the top 10 percent of the field—including the youngsters. Percentages sometimes sound better when you want to brag. Instead of saying that you finished 15,132d in the New York City Marathon, you can say that you finished in the top 60 percent!

Your individual goals should meet your individual needs at the time. For most of us, that means goals based on individual improvement. Let the elite run against each other.

Take your future races, as you take your training, step by step. Your times will gradually improve. But eventually your times may not get any better. You may need to train harder to improve, or just relax and enjoy running races at your level of fitness.

Don't be in a hurry to make the transition from beginner racer to a more serious racer, or to move up to the marathon distance (if you even choose to accept this challenge). The "too much too soon" syndrome will leave you injured or frustrated or both. You can constantly set new goals, and you will surprise yourself when you see how far you've come. In this instance, do look back. You'll be pleased. Remember you can level off at any time. You can back down a step or more. You can progress at a slower pace.

If your next step is the marathon, just follow my guidelines in the next chapter. If you would like to improve your race times by adding speed training, then turn to Chapter 15 for an introduction to competitive training. If you are ready for more advanced training guidelines for distances ranging from a mile to the ultramarathon, then you are ready to graduate to *The Competitive Runner's Handbook*.

FOURTEEN

The Beginner Marathoner

Every year for over twenty years I have been the speaker for a series of training clinics for the New York City Marathon. We always have a standing-room-only crowd of over 500 people. At the start of each lecture I always ask the same question: "How many of you are on the lunatic fringe?" Then, I smile and add, "That is, how many of you are preparing for your first marathon?" I'm amazed year after year when I ask the beginner marathoners in the crowd to stand, because over 90 percent of the audience consists of first-timers. So if you are thinking of running your first marathon, be assured that you have a lot of company. Also, take heart in the fact that my Official New York City Marathon Training Program, which is included in this chapter, is sent to every marathon entrant, and we have a better than 95 percent finishing rate each year.

Why would anyone want to run a marathon? It involves a lot of time and effort. But the glamour and tradition of "the classic distance" captures the imagination. It is the ultimate fitness challenge. It is "there," like the highest mountain or the tallest building. As the longest, most grueling, and most unpredictable of mainstream running events, it symbolizes fitness and performance. It is agony—and it is ecstasy.

The marathon is the longest and most difficult run most runners ever attempt. It is also a popular challenge. Dick Traum has completed a dozen marathons with an artificial leg and each year enters over 100 physically challenged runners in the New York City Marathon from his Achilles Track Club (see Chapter 30 for inspiring stories of some of these remarkable marathoners). According to Traum, "Anyone who honestly takes the time to train can finish a marathon. You don't have to be much of an athlete, just patient and disciplined. You have to put in the time." And you're never too old to run your first marathon—more than half of the novice marathoners each year in the New York City Marathon are over the age of forty, and some are twice that.

The standard marathon event of 26.2 miles (42.195 kilometers) is run through the streets of almost every major city in the United States and the world. It has become a vacation attraction offered by travel agents in such exciting spots as San Francisco, Honolulu, New York, Boston, Los Angeles, London, Rome, Tokyo, Berlin, Paris, Montreal, Madrid, Stockholm, Rio de Janeiro, Athens, Moscow, and even around the pyramids of Cairo. What a way to see a city! Even Mickey Mouse and Goofy have joined the act as the hosts of the Disney World Marathon in Orlando, Florida.

A marathon, says the dictionary, is any test of endurance. But almost every marathon runner knows the story of the fierce battle on the plains near the small Greek town of Marathon in 490 B.C. The invading Persian army was caught by surprise by the outmanned Athenians, who charged into their ranks and saved the Greek empire. Pheidippides, a Greek soldier, was ordered to run to Athens with the news of victory. His run of about 24 miles from the battlefield of Marathon is considered the first "marathon," but poor Pheidippides wasn't as fit as modern-day marathoners. He entered Athens, exclaimed "Rejoice, we conquer!," collapsed, and died. In honor of his feat, the marathon was added to the first modern Olympic Games held in Athens in 1896, and was won by a Greek, Spiridon Loues.

The first New York City Marathon was held in 1970, when 126 men and one woman toed the starting line in Central Park. Fifty-five men finished, including Fred Lebow. Nina Kuscsik, the sole female starter, didn't finish, but she went on to complete over eighty marathons and speaks with me each year at our clinics as a former winner of the event. In 1976, Lebow came to me with the crazy idea of running the marathon course through the streets of all five boroughs of the city. I told him it was impossible, but I would help him anyway. I then went on vacation, and when I returned I discovered that he had turned my office into the marathon headquarters and put my secretary to work for him full time! More than 2,000 runners, including myself, enjoyed that first marathon through the streets of New York City. Fred became known as the "marathon maestro," and his concept of taking the event to the people in the streets was copied in cities around the world. Now, some 30,000 marathoners run New York every year and thousands more are turned away (don't even think of calling me to help you get in!). The Boston Marathon, run every year since 1896, has passed its hundredth birthday and remains the oldest continuous marathon in the world.

The distance of the marathon varied in its early years. From 1896 to 1908, the Olympic Marathon distance was unset—it varied from the 24 miles run by Pheidippides to about 25 miles. In the 1908 London Olympics, the marathon began at Windsor Castle and ended at the new White City Stadium. An English princess, so the story goes, wanted to watch the start of the race from her castle window and then view the finish from her seat at the stadium. The distance, set to please royalty, was 26 miles, 385 yards. That was about 2 miles longer than previous marathons, but it became the standard distance. As you puff along those last few miles, all obscenities should be uttered to "Her Royal Highness," whose vanity created the distance.

In the Munich Olympics of 1972, Frank Shorter, Kenny Moore, and Jack Bachelor finished 1, 4, and 9 for the greatest American Olympic Marathon performance to date. Millions of excited Americans watched on television. This American triumph in an event previously dominated by other nations signaled the start of the marathon boom in this country. Within an hour of our country's greatest marathon moment, I was on the roads training seriously for the first time in eight years. I had one goal in mind: finish a marathon. And a lot of other Americans joined me over the next three decades.

Most first-timers take on the marathon to prove that their minds and bodies can meet the challenge, and their only goal is to finish.

Then they set time goals and train toward them. They search to find their limits and reach beyond them.

As a veteran of more than thirty marathons and as the coach of thousands of first-timers, I've learned many "secrets" of survival, although I never guarantee that any one of you will ever experience that beautiful, pain-free, fast marathon of runners' dreams. The marathon event is a true test of the runner. Proper training, diet, race experience, pacing, and so forth are important, but among the elusive elements that make the marathon special are the combination of Mother Nature and Lady Luck, and your mental ability to overcome the physical demands of 26 miles, 385 yards of roadway. The marathoner learns to discover the peace inside of pain.

Can you do it? Are you up to the challenge? Here's the message I pass on in my lectures to first-time marathoners: "Once you've crossed the finish line of the marathon, there isn't anything you can't do." Time and again I've heard stories about runners who were so inspired after conquering their first marathon that they then had the confidence to make significant career and life decisions. Success breeds success.

If you are running at the intermediate training level discussed in Chapter 12 and have experienced your first race, you are ready— if you wish—to train for your first marathon.

Selecting Your First Marathon

Don't pick a hot one, a hilly one, or a race that won't include a lot of spectators to cheer you on and plenty of novices running at your pace to keep you going. Choose a marathon near your home, when possible, to avoid the excitement of both travel and a race in an unfamiliar environment. Another key factor: If you run near home, you'll have that many more friends and family available to support you during the race and congratulate you after you finish!

Training for Your First Marathon

Before training for your first marathon, you should have at least six months of running logged in your diary, preferably a year or more. I know many runners who start running because they want to run a marathon. This may be a great motivator for getting off and running, but don't rush into marathon training. Your body needs time to adjust to the stress of your training. Once you have built up to running 15 to 20 miles per week for several weeks, then you may be ready to start a four- to six-month program to prepare for your first marathon.

The key is balancing the right amount of mileage, long runs, and practice races. Some controlled speed and hill training may also help. Avoid the temptation to overtrain. If you train too much, you won't make it to the starting line. If you train too little, you won't make it to the finish line. The percentage of marathon starters who cross the finish line is much higher than the percentage of runners who start marathon training and make it to the starting line. My minimum and maximum training guidelines below will help you survive both marathon training and the marathon itself.

Mileage

Beginner marathoners should gradually increase weekly mileage to a base level of at least 15 to 20 miles a week and hold there for at least four weeks. After adjusting to this base, you will be ready for one of my sixteen-week buildup programs outlined in Figures 14.1 and 14.2. Consistency of training—"putting miles in the bank"—is the key. Use your training diary (Chapter 9) to help keep you on schedule.

Beginners and experienced "casual" marathoners should then gradually build from this base to a peak of 30 to 45 miles per week. Hold at this level for at least six to eight weeks, then taper down over the last two or three weeks prior to race day. As you get stronger, you will increase your weekly mileage from the base level at a rate of not more than 10 percent, or about 2 or 3 miles per week. You do not have to increase mileage every single week. It's good to plateau at certain levels—for example at 30 miles—for a few weeks to allow your body a chance to adjust to the training load. You may also benefit from cutting back the mileage by about 5 miles (sometimes more) for a week every three or four weeks to give your mind and body a break. This may be especially valuable when coming off a race, tough long run, stressful times at work or home, or illness or minor injury.

Be sure to take good care of your body as you increase your workload—you will need plenty of sleep, carbohydrates and fluids, and well-cushioned training shoes in good repair. Handling high mileage is a strain. Review Chapter 5 for tips on how to stay with it—training partners, group runs, change your running courses, and so on. Most of your running should be at conversational pace, within your training heart rate range. Review Chapter 8 for guidelines on training pace.

You will benefit little from additional mileage during your two- or three-week tapering period prior to the race. In fact, you will benefit most by doing less mileage, since that minimizes the chance of injury, gives your mind and muscles an opportunity to rest up for a big effort, and allows your body to stock up on carbohydrates to energize your marathon effort. Cramming in last-minute mileage will do more harm than good—it is too late for any physiological benefit.

The sample training programs in this chapter include all four of these important training concepts: a gradual, progressive weekly mileage buildup from the base level to the peak level; periodic periods of holding mileage steady; a few cutback weeks to recover; and tapering weeks in the countdown to marathon day.

A key to success is to start four to six months in advance of the marathon and to develop a large reservoir of endurance from which to draw in case you need to lose a few days—or even a week or two—along the way to baby an injury or illness, or to attend to other responsibilities. Each year I get several frantic calls from runners who are concerned about missing some training time for one reason or another. "Can I still finish?" they ask. Sure, as long as you don't take off too long; you have been faithfully running on schedule up to that point, so you can ease back into your schedule. If you lose a week or two, don't just start again where you would have been. Rather, move *back* a week or two from the highest mileage level you reached, and then gradually catch back up to the program. Don't panic. A long-term schedule allows you to miss even a few weeks and still make it to the starting line. If you miss a month or more and don't keep in shape with aerobic cross-training, seriously consider postponing your first marathon for later when you can be better prepared. The New York City Marathon will guarantee your spot for the following year if you notify them far enough in advance that you wish to postpone until the next year.

Besides just totaling up your weekly mileage, it is also important to learn to properly distribute runs of varying distances and paces. Alternate your three types of conversational endurance runs—long, short, medium—as well as off days and speed work. Remember the "hard-easy" system and all the other basic training principles detailed in Chapter 6. An easy day or two should come before and after any hard day.

The following are "hard" days:

- Long runs

- Races

- Speed training or any run faster than conversational pace

The following are "easy" days:

- Short runs of 2 to 4 miles at conversational pace

- Medium runs for your average daily distance of about 4 to 6 miles at conversational pace

- Off days, which may include some light cross-training such as biking or swimming

Long Runs

The single most important ingredient to marathon success is the long run. "Going long" is a hallowed weekend tradition that is despised and loved, feared and revered, bragged about and complained about. Whether you like long runs or not, one thing remains clear: You have to run them if you want to maximize your potential on marathon day. The long run can make you physically and psychologically stronger or it can destroy you, turning running into a painful task. The long run mirrors the marathon itself: it demands attention and respect.

The long run provides the marathoner with several critical benefits:

- It improves the capacity of your muscles to utilize fat as fuel, sparing glycogen. Long runs teach your body to utilize both fats and glycogen in producing muscular energy. If you only burned glycogen you would run low and "hit the wall" somewhere between 1½ hours of running and the finish line. By utilizing some fat, and not depleting your glycogen storage, you have sufficient energy reserves to keep a good pace in the late stages of a marathon. The long run combined with carbohydrate-loading and intelligent marathon pacing allows you to push back the wall. Practice the carbohydrate-loading technique detailed in Chapter 19 for some of your long runs of 18 to 20 miles (without tapering your mileage). Not only will it enable you to find what foods work best for you, this will allow you to feel more comfortable during the late stages of training runs lasting beyond two or three hours.

■ It improves your nervous system's ability to recruit muscle fibers. During the first 15 to 20 miles of the marathon you're using primarily slow-twitch (endurance-oriented) muscle fibers. They become exhausted late in a marathon, contributing to leg fatigue. Long runs train your body to search for help from fast-twitch (speed-oriented) muscle fibers, which can be trained to assist slow-twitch fibers for a marathon effort.

■ It strengthens the heart muscle and oxygen delivery system because you spend two to three or more hours running aerobically within your training heart rate range.

■ It teaches you to stay relaxed and run with efficient form for long periods despite fatigue.

■ It allows you the opportunity to test your body's reaction to water, sports drinks, potential racing shoes and clothing, prerun eating habits, etcetera under marathonlike conditions.

■ It teaches you to be patient—a very important virtue when running long distances. Most marathoners succeed in direct proportion to how well they can hold back and run wisely. Since you will run long at a slower pace than your short and medium distance training runs, you become accustomed to a leisurely pace.

■ Above all, the long run is for the mind. Forcing yourself to get out the door and running for three or so hours in all kinds of weather involves discipline. Your reward for this effort is increased confidence and mental toughness. Watching your long runs build from 10 to 20 miles, you have measurable proof that your training is making you stronger. This motivates you to keep up your rigorous training schedule. By experiencing what it feels like to keep running when tired, you're not afraid of having to run the last few miles of the marathon while tiring. You learn the difference between fatigue and exhaustion by forcing your body to finish long runs. These runs teach you to finish despite the objections of the mind and body. Once you can handle 20 miles, you know you can handle the whole distance.

How far and how often do you need to run long? Beginner marathoners gradually build up the distance of the long runs from a base of 6 to 10 miles and *complete at least three runs of 18 to 20 miles prior to the marathon.*

For the 10K and other shorter racing distances, I recommend long runs at race distance or longer. For the marathon, however, that would require runs of 26 miles or more. Although some experienced marathoners (yet few of the elite marathoners) put in a few runs of that length, the average runner would suffer more than he or she would benefit from such a practice. A few coaches suggest that even first-time marathoners should build up to 26-mile training runs. Along with most coaches and exercise physiologists, I strongly disagree. Some runners may do well with this strategy, but most would not. This would put you on your feet—often alone and in the heat—for four to six hours. Long runs cause wear and tear on the musculoskeletal system. Past 20 miles, fatigue accumulates rapidly and running form deteriorates. Additional pounding greatly increases chance of injury as each stride pounds the pavement with three times the force of your body weight. Runs beyond 20 miles seriously deplete energy reserves, leaving marathon hopefuls not only very tired but susceptible to illness. Further, attempting such long runs will leave you more vulnerable to failing to finish, or finishing exhausted, leaving you wiped out for days. This would be a severe psychological blow.

Thus, my recommended long run limit for beginner marathoners is 20 miles—22 to 23 miles for experienced marathoners. The potential gain beyond 3½ to 4 hours (my recommended time limit no matter what the mileage) isn't worth the risk. Save the destructive effects of such lengthy runs for the marathon itself or you may not make it to the starting line. Save the excitement of running those last few long miles for when you have plenty of support from spectators, fluid station volunteers, and your fellow marathoners. Don't worry, on race day your mileage base and the excitement of the crowd will carry you over the last 6.2 miles to the finish line.

Too many runners make the mistake of concentrating on weekly mileage but not getting in a sufficient number of long runs. I've heard many runners brag about their 40-mile weeks but then grow quiet when I ask about their long runs. You are not training to run 30 or 40 miles in a week, you are training to run 26.2 miles at once. To do that, you need long training runs. Just as you gradually increase your weekly mileage by not more than 2 or 3 miles at a time, you need to also follow that same progressive pattern for building up your long runs.

As you get up to runs of the half-marathon distance and more, alternate running long every other week to minimize the physical and mental fatigue associated with the long run. Besides, your family will be happy to know that you won't ruin every weekend for them. In some cases, due to scheduling difficulties, you may need to "go long" two weeks in a row. If so, at least try to go long on a Saturday the first weekend and then on the following Sunday to give yourself an extra day of rest. To do this occasionally may not be too much for you. If you plan well in advance, you can get in an adequate number of long runs by running two per month rather than forcing yourself to squeeze in weekly long runs as the marathon looms ahead.

Take an easy day before and after your long run. If you are very sore and tired the day after a long run, take a day off. However, a short bike ride, swim, or walk later in the day or the day following a long run may help you minimize stiffness and aid recovery.

Your last long run should be two or three weeks prior to marathon day to minimize the risk of injury and maximize recovery time. The weekend before the marathon, the long run should be no farther than 6 to 8 miles. Taper your long runs as you taper your weekly mileage.

The long run can be something to look forward to, or it can be drudgery. Here are some tips to make them more enjoyable and thus more productive:

■ Control the pace. You should start your long runs at a slower speed than you run for short and medium distance runs. If you run too fast on your long runs you'll fatigue much sooner. The recommended pace for your long runs is 60 to 70 percent of your maximum heart rate. This may be a little slower than your daily training heart rate range, which would be in the 60 to 80 percent range. Better to err by starting too slow than too fast.

What pace per mile should you run? Approximately 1½ to 2 minutes per mile slower than your 10K race pace.

▪ Find someone to run with you, otherwise you may get quite lonely. Make sure your running partner is willing to run at your conversational pace. If your friend can't run the whole distance with you, it is preferred to have him or her hook up with you for the last miles of your run to give you a welcomed boost of energy. You might even be able to form a relay of friends who take turns keeping you going. If you can't find a running partner, ask your spouse, child, or a friend to ride along on a bike. If you're lucky, you might find a club that organizes group long runs. The New York Road Runners Club offers such a program for the New York City Marathon; they divide hundreds of runners up into groups based on their training pace. The distraction of social chattering will make your runs more manageable, even fun.

▪ Avoid, if possible, heat, hills, and head winds. Start your runs early in the morning or late in the day to avoid the heat, and seek courses that offer shade. You should incorporate some hills into your long run course to toughen you, but avoid too many killer hills—long runs are taxing enough as it is! In the winter, plan your runs to avoid freezing head winds, or at least run into the wind on the way out rather than facing it (and potential frostbite) when you are tired and sweat-soaked on the way back.

▪ If the weather is very bad, consider postponing your long run until the next day or even the next weekend. Abort your long run if the weather is too bad. Be tough, but be reasonable. You don't have to force yourself to be uncomfortable and endanger your health.

▪ Run long on Saturday if possible so you can rest on Sunday. That will make it easier on you when you have to go to work Monday morning.

▪ In general, you are wise to stick to a few trusty courses where you know the distance and where to get fluids. As a change of pace, you may wish to run with a partner over terrain that you have never covered. This may require a short trip to get there, but it would be worth it if it leaves you invigorated.

- Beware of running long on slanted surfaces—that is, most roads—as it leaves you prone to injury. If you must run on crowned roads, change direction (and the slant) every few miles. I run long on dirt trails that absorb the pounding much more than pavement. Try to run at least some of each run off the pavement to be kind to your legs. Avoid congested areas and potholes—especially late in the run when dodging cars, bikes, people, and other obstacles is not easy because of physical and mental fatigue.

- Take walk breaks if needed, especially when it is hot or when hills are causing your heart rate to soar. But keep moving. It is okay to stop running for a few minutes to drink fluids or use the toilet, but if you stop for too long and stand around or sit down you will stiffen up.

- Drink, drink, and drink on long runs—at least every 30 minutes, ideally every 15 to 20 minutes. You need more fluids on long runs than you will for your daily run—especially in hot weather, although fluids are still essential for long runs in cooler weather, too. Refer to Chapter 20 for guidelines.

- Do not attempt to run long if you are not fully recovered from illness or injury. Bail out of long runs if you feel an injury coming on, or if you turn an ankle, fall and bang a knee, and so on. Favoring an injury over the course of a long run will likely cause additional injury. Stubbornly pushing ahead may cause you to lose several days of training—or worse. When returning from injury, you may be able to ease back into long runs by combining a run with a bike ride or swim for a long aerobic workout totaling two or three hours.

- Wear well-cushioned, well-broken-in (but not broken down) shoes. The effect of inadequate shoes is greatly exaggerated over the course of a long run.

■ Replenish your body with fluids and carbohydrates (see Chapter 19 and 20) immediately after running since you will be dehydrated and low on stored glycogen.

■ Be flexible. If you have properly built up your mileage and long runs well in advance, you can skip a long run here and there and not lose out. Don't panic if you miss a long run due to unforeseen circumstances. A poor run when too tired or too hot can lead to a negative feeling rather than building fitness and confidence. One run won't make a difference if you have at least three long runs under your belt prior to marathon day. With proper depth of training, you can take a few days off and miss a few long runs without guilt or loss of fitness.

Many runners look forward to their long runs. It is a time to relax and just run slow and easy. You can do plenty of deep thinking on solitary runs or enjoy the company of others. If you look at the long run as something to savor rather than a dreaded task that you must get out of the way, it will be easier to do it.

Speed Training

Beginner marathoners benefit from some speed training to improve running form, ability to run hills, sense of pacing, and mental discipline. More than 500 marathoners, many first-timers, take our New York Road Runners Club speed classes in preparation for the New York City Marathon each year for this reason.

Ease into these workouts. You don't need to run them full speed to benefit. Experienced marathoners often attempt to race a marathon at a faster pace than their daily runs of 5 miles or so. They need to learn to push the pace. But first-timers will most likely run the marathon distance at a pace slower than their daily runs, so they don't need to push hard in speed training. Workouts should be at your 10K race pace or faster in order to build fitness and confidence. Don't attempt fast running if you haven't fully recovered from your long run or if you are feeling tired from high mileage.

Marathoners should emphasize longer speed workouts such as three to five repeats of one mile at 10K race pace with a 3-minute rest in between. Brisk repeats of 200 to 400 yards up a hill will also strengthen your mind and body for hills on the marathon course. Run six to ten of these, recovering with a slow jog back down. The following chapter introduces speed training for competitive running. For more detailed guidelines on speed workouts for marathoners refer to *The Competitive Runner's Handbook*.

Buildup Races

Many first-time marathoners do not race at all in preparation for their marathons. A few practice races are recommended so you can learn how to handle pacing, prerace meals, fluid replacement, shoes and clothing choices, and so on. They also break up the monotony of training by giving you intermediate goals. Races are also a great place to meet other marathoners and share experiences—even add a training partner.

Races can be used three ways:

1. To get in long training runs—with water stations and split times along the way to help you learn pacing. You get to run with lots of people, which is great if you've been running long all alone. I have New York Road Runners Club members in my program run two half-marathons and then the New York City Marathon Tune-Up 30K (18.6 miles) as part of their marathon buildup. You can create a more beneficial long run by running a few training miles prior to a race of any distance and then running the race at training pace. For example, run 10 miles prior to the start of a 10K race and then run through the race (remember to register so you can use the water stations) for a total run of 16.2 miles. This is sure easier than going long alone. If you prefer, you can run in the opposite direction while watching a race to help you get through your long run. *Caution:* Do not race these races, hold back your competitive nature and run them at a nice and easy conversational long run pace.

2. Practice your race pace. Running a few races from 5 miles to 30K (18.6 miles) at your marathon pace will help you become familiar with that effort. On race day you are likely to be able to continue that pace all the way since you will have rested up and are all pumped up with excitement and confidence.

3. A few hard efforts can be used to measure progress and better select your race time goal. You may wish to compare your times (but be prepared to adjust for hot weather and hills) to previous races of the same distance—or the same race from last year.

Running personal record times at shorter distances rewards you for all the work you have put in. If, for example, you struggled to run a 10-minute-per-mile pace for a 10-mile race you know you are not ready to handle that pace for the marathon distance. On the other hand, if you handled that pace comfortably, you may be able to keep that pace for the marathon. A *rough* rule of thumb for predicting marathon time from half-marathons for experienced marathoners is to double your time and add 10 minutes to approximately predict your marathon fitness. Thus, if you ran a half-marathon in 1:45, you could expect to run a marathon in 3:40—give or take 10 minutes and depending upon comparable weather and course conditions. Often, this guide holds true for beginner marathoners, too, if they have trained properly.

Ideally, you should race at least once a month over the four months going into your marathon. This can give you valuable experience. Do not race more than twice a month. Do not race or do hard speed training for one week after short races (10K and less) or for two weeks after longer races. Do not race on a Saturday and then do a long run on Sunday in an effort to get everything in. You will invite injury if you don't recover from races properly and space them wisely. Your last long race of 10 miles or longer should be no later than three weeks prior to marathon morning; your last short race should be run no later than two weeks before the big one.

Cross-Training
You can minimize the wear and tear on your body by replacing up to 20 percent of your running mileage with biking, swimming, or other aerobic exercise. Do these activities at a pace that will get your heart rate in your training heart rate range.

Injury
Do not attempt to train if you are favoring an injury. Seek advice from a sports medicine expert who is familiar with runners and all their complaints and aches. Replace running with biking or swimming if possible while you recover. If an injury is threatening your health as you approach the marathon, postpone your first marathon until you can safely complete it. Starting a marathon with an injury could result in a serious injury.

The First-Time Marathon Sixteen-Week Training Schedule

Thousands of first-time marathoners have successfully reached the finish line by following my schedule, which is not only printed in this book but is also available in brochure form as the Official New York City Marathon Training Program. That schedule is slightly different from the one here because it is adjusted to fit in official New York Road Runners Club races and long training runs.

Please note that these are *sample* schedules. You can follow them exactly, as many runners around the world do, or you can adapt them to fit your needs. Be compulsive about it, but not *too* compulsive. Follow the theme of the schedules if you make up your own program: progressive increases in weekly mileage with a few plateaus and cutbacks, gradual increases in well-spaced long runs, off days and short runs for recovery to balance long runs and medium runs, a gradual tapering of mileage and long runs over the final three weeks. Long runs are scheduled on Saturdays, but you may wish to change them to Sundays or other days. Carefully adjust your program to fit in a few races—this may mean switching around long runs and making sure to run easy the day before and after the race.

Two sample schedules are included: Figure 14.1 building from a 15-mile-a-week base for at least a month to 35 miles at the peak; and Figure 14.2 starting at a 20-mile-a-week base building to 40 miles a week. The second schedule is my preferred program. If you are not yet at 15 miles per week, you are not ready to build up for a marathon. If you are running more than 20 miles a week when you are ready to start the schedule, just stay where you are until you are on schedule. Those runners who choose to run more than 40 miles a week can just add a few miles to each week on the program. Be careful, however; you can finish the marathon on 35 to 40 miles a week as long as you do your long runs. Too much mileage can lead to failure. It may be wise to save increased mileage for training to improve your marathon time next year.

Mental Preparation: Visualization

Visualization is a mental game used by leading athletes in every sport to enhance performance. But you don't have to be an elite runner to benefit. As long as you have a solid goal and a strong desire to reach it, all you need is a good imagination. Basically, visualization is rehearsing for success. You imagine what you would like to have happen (such as finishing a marathon) and thus

FIGURE 14.1: SAMPLE SIXTEEN-WEEK BEGINNER MARATHONER TRAINING SCHEDULE
(From a 15-mile-a-week base for at least one month)

WEEKS TO GO	MON.	TUES.	WED.	THURS.	FRI.	SAT.	SUN.	TOTAL MILEAGE
Base	Off	3	Off	3	Off	6	3	15
16	Off	3	Off	3	Off	8	3	17
15	Off	3	Off	4	Off	10	3	20
14	Off	3	Off	3	Off	13	3	22
13	Off	4	Off	4	Off	8	4	20
12	Off	3	Off	3	Off	15	3	24
11	Off	4	6	4	Off	10	3	27
10	Off	4	4	3	Off	16	3	30
9	Off	4	4	6	Off	12	4	30
8	Off	4	3	4	Off	18	3	32
7	Off	6	6	6	Off	12	5	35
6	Off	4	4	4	Off	20	3	35
5	Off	5	4	5	Off	12	4	30
4	Off	4	4	4	Off	20	3	35
3	Off	5	5	5	Off	15	3	33
2	Off	4	6	4	Off	6	5	25
1	Off	4	4	4	Off	2	26.2 marathon	14 + race

convince yourself that you can do it. You see and feel success so that when it is actually happening you are not afraid to succeed, but rather embrace it as an old friend. You have to dream that the difficult is not only possible, but that it *will* happen.

Whether your realize it or not, you practice visualization daily. You envision an upcoming event in your life—such as a presentation to your boss or an explanation to your spouse that you must cancel a social engagement to get in a long run—and then play out the scenario in your head.

Visualization trains the athlete to experience mentally the event as if he or she were living it. Dr. Thomas Tutko, author of *Sports Psyching: Playing Your Best Game All of the Time*, tells athletes to "relive" their best performances over and over until they actually can achieve them almost automatically. "It's like putting a tape into your brain, as you would with a computer." Rerun some of your best races and workouts to give you a feel for visualization. Then imagine running an upcoming race. You control the imagery; you should actually imagine your muscles in action as you rehearse

**FIGURE 14.2: SAMPLE SIXTEEN-WEEK BEGINNER MARATHONER
TRAINING SCHEDULE**
(From a 20-mile-a-week base for at least one month)

WEEKS TO GO	MON.	TUES.	WED.	THURS.	FRI.	SAT.	SUN.	TOTAL MILEAGE
Base	Off	3	4	4	Off	6	3	20
16	Off	3	4	4	Off	8	3	22
15	Off	4	4	4	Off	10	3	25
14	Off	4	4	3	Off	13	3	27
13	Off	5	4	5	Off	13	3	30
12	Off	4	5	5	Off	15	3	32
11	Off	6	6	6	Off	12	5	35
10	Off	6	4	4	Off	18	3	35
9	Off	6	6	6	Off	12	5	35
8	Off	5	6	6	Off	20	3	40
7	Off	5	4	5	Off	13	3	30
6	Off	5	6	6	Off	20	3	40
5	Off	6	6	6	Off	13	4	35
4	Off	5	6	6	Off	20	3	40
3	Off	6	6	5	Off	15	3	35
2	Off	5	6	5	Off	5	5	26
1	Off	4	4	4	Off	2	26.2 marathon	14 + race

your race. Neurons will fire just as they do in a race, and muscles contract in minute but detectable amounts.

Kay Porter and Judy Foster, authors of *The Mental Athlete: Inner Training for Peak Performance*, note: "Each time you 'see' yourself performing exactly the same way you want with perfect form, you physically create neural patterns in your brain. These patterns are like small tracks permanently engraved on the brain cells. It is the brain that gives the signal to the muscle to move. It tells each muscle how to move, when to move, and with how much power. . . . Our performance will be tremendously more powerful if we have also trained our minds and created the neural patterns to help our muscles do exactly what we want them to do perfectly."

The technique works because it follows the psychological principle that the closer one comes to simulating an actual situation, the greater one's chances of developing the skill to perform it. By imagining yourself successfully running, you will actually improve your form and racing speed. By training the subconscious mind to perform in the way we want, it will "tell" our conscious mind to perform in that manner. Obviously you can't just dream about a fast time and then do it, but a realistic, challenging goal can be achieved more readily when it has first been "practiced" in your mind.

Visualization is a three-step process: (1) set a goal and create a positive self-image; (2) achieve a state of deep relaxation; and (3) imagine yourself succeeding.

Visualization begins with goal setting and a positive self-image. Write your goal on a piece of paper and tape it to your wall, or take a digital clock and set it for your race time—3:59 for a sub-four-hour marathon, for example—then unplug it and place it in a prominent place so you can see it often. Seeing it often, your mind accepts it as a realistic goal. You then begin to imagine yourself crossing the finish line in that time, making the time seem even more possible. Think about it often, including during your training runs and in the race itself. To help you improve your self-image, place pictures of top runners running with good form where you can see them often. Or place photos of yourself running well in past races in prominent locations to remind you of past successes. Set your goals, believe in them, desire them, expect them, and practice reaching them.

The next step is to achieve a state of deep relaxation as described in Chapter 42. Then focus on your goal. Mentally rehearse the entire race, being as specific and positive as possible. Use all of your senses: "see" the crowd, "hear" the noise, "smell" the air, "feel" your body relax. Visualize the warm-up area, the starting line scene, the course, the spectators, the runners, etcetera. See, feel, hear, and smell the entire experience. Visualize yourself starting your race full of energy, conquering the hills, running with good form, reaching mileage markers at your goal times, and finishing within your time goal. Repeat the whole mental process several times before your key race. You become a movie director and run the movie of your race through your mind.

Visualization can be practiced at quiet times during the days leading into your race, and before your training runs. Some runners continue "visualizing" in brief flashes into their runs and races by "seeing" themselves running up an approaching hill, or finishing the workout or race strongly. It may take a few sessions to get the hang of the technique of visualization. Be patient, be consistent.

Practice it for 5 to 10 minutes several times a week over the last two to four weeks going into the marathon.

Avoid too much mental rehearsing the night before the race. It may leave you emotionally drained. Instead, you may wish to do relaxation exercises to help you get to sleep. On race day, you may benefit from going through your race one more time in your head as a final tune-up. Others find that it leaves them either too hyped up or too relaxed.

When visualizing, you should practice the "perfect" race. But on occasion you should also incorporate some unforeseen problems and see yourself reacting to them calmly. For example: your shoe-lace comes untied, you lose time because of a crowded start. When visualizing, develop a "feeling" for your goals. Concentrate on the actual race itself, one step at a time.

With positive visualization you can be in charge of mental factors, rather than allowing them to be in charge of you. Whether you follow these visualization techniques conscientiously, or merely occasionally daydream about your race, you can see yourself as a confident, successful runner. But remember that you must have a solid training program to back up your visualization. It is not enough just to dream about running fast without putting in the hard training.

Sample Visualization

Here is a visualization program that I use with my New York City Marathon training class. Modify it for your marathon. Remember to first achieve a state of deep relaxation. Choose a slogan (such as "calm," "calm") to repeat on race day to help you stay focused.

You wake up the morning of the New York City Marathon feeling relaxed and refreshed. Feel yourself yawning and stretching like a cat. Taste the cup of orange juice and muffin with jelly that you choose for breakfast. It hits the spot. See yourself putting on your running clothes and pinning on your official number. You look in the mirror and see yourself as being trim and fit. Feel yourself putting on your socks and shoes, which feel very comfortable. See yourself double-checking the bag of race goodies—extra clothing, toilet paper, and so on—that you packed last night. Feel yourself walking toward the buses, your legs stretching out.

You have casual conversations with other runners waiting for the bus. You hear some talking negatively, some positively. Some look very fit and intimidating, others look like they'll never make it. You are prepared for these distractions and calmly take them in. You sit on the crowded bus and smell the various ointments that runners have covered their bodies with. You hear lots of chatter that you can't understand since the bus is full of foreign runners. People ask you what you are aiming for, how you will do. Hear yourself say with both modesty and confidence: "I'm ready to do my best." Hear the bus start up for your journey to the start and feel the nervousness in your stomach. Repeat your slogan: *calm, calm*.

See the bridge you will cross at the start, knowing that you are near the starting area. Hear the voices in the bus become more nervous as you approach the staging area. See yourself calmly getting off the bus and finding a quiet area in which to relax. Every fifteen minutes you get up and walk around, then sit and relax. Feel yourself holding the excitement back, saving energy for the race. You see others wasting energy by getting too involved with prerace nervous talk. You analyze the weather prediction and adjust your race accordingly. If it will be hot or windy, you will start a little more slowly. If it looks like great weather, you will be prepared to go for it.

Hear the announcement to go to the starting line. Feel your heart beating faster and your stomach churning. Feel your positive thoughts emerging. You are not afraid to get started, you welcome the opportunity to unravel your successful race. Feel the runners elbowing each other and hear them chattering as you make your way to the start. See yourself lining up and feel yourself breathing deeply, relaxing as the final minutes are counted down to the start. Repeat your slogan: *calm, calm*. Feel the wind whipped by the loud helicopters overhead, and then hear the cannon explode. Feel your hands touching the runners on each side to protect you from falling, feel your feet making short little strides at the start and then longer ones as you gain room to run. See the time on your watch as you hit the starting line and say to yourself that your race begins now, don't try to make it up all at once.

Feel the powerful vacuum sucking you up the hill and over the bridge. You feel like a powerful horse being reigned in. Repeat your slogan: *calm, calm*. See yourself flowing down the other side of the bridge with proper form. See yourself winding around and then straightening out as you flow in next to the other starting group on Fourth Avenue. You hear the crowds now for the first time, and they are loud and enthusiastic. Feel yourself holding back your energy, not allowing the crowd, the slight downhills, or the overeager runners around you to let yourself go out too fast. See your split at each early mile mark and adjust your pace accordingly—slightly picking it up or slowing down. Hear yourself say that you must subtract the time it took you to reach the starting line from your time to determine how fast you really are moving. Think of how smart you are not to try to make up the time.

See yourself passing runners who started too fast and being passed by others who are full of energy. Feel how your legs are moving smoothly, your breathing is relaxed, you feel in control. Feel the wind. Is it against you, behind you? If it is against you, see yourself tucking in behind others who become shields. See yourself taking water from an aid station; taste the water in your mouth, and feel the second cup you grab as you pour it over your head. Repeat this throughout your visualization.

Concentrate on reaching your next goal—the 5-mile split. You see it up ahead and you reach it feeling real good near your expected goal split. Feel yourself smiling. Hear other runners talking, but you remain quiet, saving energy. See yourself reaching the point where the men and women merge near 7 miles. You welcome the added "scenery." Your next goal is the big clock tower looming ahead at 8 miles. Feel the energy from it pulling you like a magnet. You now aim for the 10-mile mark. Feel your form getting a little ragged and feel yourself picking up the knees, using the arms, breathing comfortably and regaining control of your form. Repeat your slogan: *calm, calm*. See the 10-mile split near your goal time. You feel confidence surging. See a friend jumping out of the crowd and yelling at you.

Your next goal is a big one—the half-way mark at the Pulaski Bridge. See yourself approaching it up a short, but what feels like a steep, hill at this point in the race. Record your split in your mind, multiply it by 2. You will run a great race by keeping the same pace now for the second half of the race. Even if you slow a little, you will do well. Give yourself a mental pep talk. You can do it. You feel happy to have the first half under your belt. You feel full of confidence. Repeat your slogan: *calm, calm*.

The next goal is to get up and over the 59th Street Bridge. You reflect on your hill-training sessions and see yourself changing your form to get up the hill. You see your split at 15 miles near the start of the bridge—again near your goal time. You feel your quads working, your arms pumping, your knees coming up to get over the hill. You see yourself running stronger than those around you who let the hill attack them. You attack the hill with cool confidence. You feel the wind whipping at the top of the bridge, and feel your feet caressing the carpet. You see the majestic New York City skyline and let the power from it pull you like a magnet to the top of the bridge. Repeat your slogan: *calm, calm.*

You feel yourself flowing down the hill now, like a freefalling roller coaster. See yourself holding back slightly, running with good form. Feel the strain on your legs. Hear the loud noise up ahead, and anticipate the surge you will feel as you hit First Avenue. Hear and feel the crowd as you zoom around the corner onto First Avenue. Feel the slight uphill, but feel your form powering you along. Feel the fatigue in your legs, but the confidence in your head allows you to relax and keep moving. See all the struggling runners who are now walking, and you increase in confidence as you power by them—knowing that you paced yourself more wisely, trained yourself better, and have a stronger mind. See friends stationed at this point jump out and encourage you, giving you a rush of new energy. Repeat your slogan: *calm, calm.*

Your next goal is to reach 18 miles—the halfway point between the bridge and "the wall" at 20 miles. See yourself hitting it and talking to yourself—saying, "Okay, wall, you aren't going to get me." See yourself at the end of your long training runs and eating all those carbohydrates. See yourself laughing at "the wall." Yes, it slows you slightly. But as you hit the 20-mile mark you picture yourself smashing through a brick wall and raising your fist in victory. You feel tired, but full of purpose and confidence. A 10K to go. Only a 10K race now. Envision what your finishing time will be by adding a 10K at your goal pace. Sounds good! See yourself patting yourself on the back and saying, "Let's go for it." Repeat your slogan: *calm, calm.*

See yourself shortly after 20 miles, making the turn and heading south toward Central Park. You are on your way home now! Just calm down, concentrate on working the arms and picking up the knees, breathing in a relaxed manner, keeping the neck and shoulders loose. Now you run from mile marker to mile marker, even block to block as you see the street numbers get smaller as you aim for 110th Street—the start of Central Park. Hear the crowds cheering you on, saying, "You're looking good!" Believe them, keep moving. Keep pushing. Don't let up or you will lose time.

Hear yourself talking to yourself. Extolling your body to keep moving. You feel bad off and on but keep moving down the long blue line. See that line. Trust that it will pull you to the finish line. Repeat your slogan: *calm, calm.*

See the trees up ahead—it's Central Park. You hit 110th Street and get a surge of mental toughness. You know you can do it now! Keep the legs moving. Feel the uphill stretch on Fifth Avenue to 102nd Street, and then the short steep hill as you enter the park. Think about how you practiced this hill and just become a robot, running it by memory with good hill-running form. See the 23-mile banner across the road near the top of the hill. Only 3.2 miles to go. Think about how you ran this comfortably two days ago and remember how it felt to run up and down the rolling hills. Remember the joke Glover made: "You only have to run 23 miles on race day, since we're practicing the last 3.2 miles now; you can just become a robot the rest of the way on race day." A friend jumps out of the crowd and yells in your ear. You hear him: "You can do it, go for it." You feel heavy in the legs, but strong in the mind and heart. Think of how tough you are, think about all those long runs you made, all the mileage, all the sacrifice. This is your moment now. This is not the time to give in to fatigue. You concentrate on good form, on feeling relaxed, on being in control. Your body is tired, but it is moving! "I'm going to do it!" Repeat it over and over. Repeat your slogan: *calm, calm.*

The crowd is very excited. They know you will do it. See the 90th Street and Fifth Avenue entrance to the park. A large crowd there gives you a fresh blast of energy. See yourself reaching the 24-mile mark half a mile later. Your next goal is a long, steep downhill at 80th Street. See yourself flowing down the hill. Then look up. You see the New York skyline. Feel the power from the skyscrapers pulling you like a magnet toward them. Repeat your slogan: *calm, calm.* See yourself turning left to leave Central Park as you go under the 25-mile marker. How fast can you run 1.2 miles? Even if you jog it you will have a good time. See what your time will look like at the finish if you finish at goal pace. You are flowing downhill, full of determination. A friend screams at you, you see yourself looking proud in front of him.

Hear the crowd roar as you leave the park and turn onto Central Park South at 59th Street. They become part of you. Their screaming, your willpower, are becoming one powerful machine now. You are too tired to feel graceful. But you do feel powerful. See the quarter-mile-long slight uphill grade ahead, and see the struggling runners you are passing. Feel a few runners who pass you with a finishing rush and see yourself holding on to some of them and going for a ride. See yourself cresting the gradual incline and feel yourself going down now. You are so close! You can hear the announcer at the finish line. Feel the tears welling in your eyes. Feel the anticipation in your heart.

See yourself turning at Columbus Circle. This is it. You are on the last stretch on Central Park Drive. See the crowd up ahead, the balloons, hear the deafening roar of the crowd. You hear them all yelling for you, as you are winning your race. See yourself running under the 26-mile banner. Feel yourself going up the final hill to the finish line. Feel the excitement, feel the pain and the joy of the others around you. You help each other now, push each other toward the moving numbers on the digital clock. See the numbers coming into focus now. See the time—your goal time—and see yourself finishing with great form. See yourself throwing your hands up, your chest out as you cross the finish line. See yourself hugging the runner next to you. You are trembling in fatigue and joy. You did it! See yourself smiling at last. See your family and friends congratulating you. Hear yourself saying to others: "I set a challenging goal, I trained hard, I worked hard during the race, I felt real strong except for a few times, I was determined to do it, I did it! I am so happy and so proud of myself!"

Marathon Countdown

The marathon countdown includes the physical and mental preparation over the last few weeks, days, and hours before your marathon. At this point you start tapering your mileage and get in your last race and long run following the guidelines in this chapter. This is a critical time. If you make mistakes during the marathon countdown you may waste four months or more of carefully planned training. Unlike a 5K or 10K race, you can't do it again in a week or two, so you must be sure to do this part of your marathon training wisely.

This time period is very difficult for many runners, both novice and experienced. As a nervous marathoner hoping for a good race you ask yourself many last-minute questions: Have I trained enough? How fast should I go out? What should I wear? What shoes do I run in? Will I finish last?

To free yourself to focus on your physical tapering and mental preparation, be sure to eliminate prerace details from your concern. Make a checklist of what must be done before the race, and do it. Here are some tips:

▪ Enter the race early. Don't train for it and then find that you missed the entry deadline. If possible, get your race number and information packet in advance so you don't have to stand in line on marathon morning to pick it up.

▪ Use your last long run two or three weeks prior to the marathon as a full-dress rehearsal (just don't go 26.2 miles!). Practice your carbohydrate-loading with the foods you intend to eat for energy and drink the same sports drinks that will be available on the course. Review guidelines in Chapters 19 and 20 for fueling up with carbos and drinking fluids before and during the marathon. Wake up and run at the same time of day you will for the marathon. Wear the same clothes and well-cushioned training shoes you will wear on marathon day. Start the run at your intended marathon starting pace.

▪ Segment the race. Set goals to get to certain mile markers or landmarks and then set out to knock them off one at a time. Know where these key intermediate goals are on the course. If possible, run part of the course (especially the hills and the finish) or drive over it so you can better prepare your mind for the race. Visualize your marathon as detailed in this chapter.

▪ In many ways running your first marathon is like running your first race all over again. Review the guidelines in the previous chapter for prerace tips. This includes setting out the night before the race the clothing (including your race number) and shoes you'll wear and double-checking it in the morning; review how you'll get to the start of the race.

▪ Avoid the premarathon hoopla. Don't spend hours on your feet walking around the prerace clinics, exhibits, and so forth. Attend a few of them for a few minutes to enjoy the atmosphere, but don't spend a lot of time on your feet. Hanging around large crowds of runners at prerace events tends to make you more nervous and drain off energy. Go out to dinner with a few calm, confident, supportive friends and relax. Sight-seeing is a problem for runners who travel to an exciting place, such as New York. Tell your spouse or companions to go ahead and sight-see as you stay behind, except perhaps for a brief bus tour where you can sit down. Don't get caught up going shopping; you'll not only spend a lot of money but a lot of time on your feet. Ideally, if you travel to an event, plan your trip so you can stay for a few days after the race. Use walking tours as part of postrace recovery. You can better enjoy your minivacation once the stress of the marathon is out of the way. Of course, having finished your first marathon, you'll be in a great mood and ready to party!

▪ As you taper, you'll have lots of extra time and energy. Too many runners use it to clean out the garage, wash the floors, or chop wood. Any physical activity that you are not used to could cause injury. Stick to less physical ways to spend your time— read a book or go to the movies—and save your energy for the marathon.

▪ Don't avoid sex the day or night before the marathon. You'll be more relaxed and sleep better. Do avoid staying up all night looking for it.

▪ Get plenty of sleep the week of the marathon. A good night's sleep is most important two nights before the race, so don't fret if your nerves keep you up the night before your first marathon.

▪ Stay off your feet as much as possible the last three days before the race and on marathon morning.

▪ Get the weather report and adjust your clothing and race strategy accordingly. Review Chapters 21–23 for tips on dealing with hot, cold, and other weather conditions.

▪ In hot weather, avoid being out in the sun as much as possible the last few days before the race. Stay in the shade on marathon morning—right up until the start if possible.

▪ Check in with your support crew: this includes family and friends. They can pass you fluids and a change of clothes along the course and cheer you on at strategic spots—such as the top of a big hill, the 20-mile mark, and one mile before the finish line. Also review how you will meet friends and family at the finish area.

■ Wake up at least three hours before starting time to give yourself plenty of time to get dressed, recheck your bag, put on your running shoes and clothing (including your number!).

■ Get to the start area at least an hour (preferably two hours) in advance (earlier if you haven't picked up your number).

■ With 30 minutes to go, take care of all the last-minute essentials:

- Double knot your shoelaces to make sure they don't untie when you're too tired to bend over to retie them.
- Make sure you have money (pinned to your number, or tucked into your shoe) and toilet paper (paper towels work best since they hold up when wet) in case of emergency.
- Make sure emergency contact names and numbers are on the back of your race number or in your shoe pocket.
- Apply sunscreen to protect against sunburn if it's sunny. Also, it might be wise to wear a hat and sunglasses.
- Running for several hours presents added risks of blistering and chaffing due to rubbing. Apply petroleum jelly to your feet (or foot powder), nipples (or try a Band-Aid), and inner thighs.
- Make a final bowel movement and empty your bladder. Don't be modest. Your comfort is at stake, and the bushes may be your only choice.
- At the staging area, turn in whatever clothing you won't be racing in to the baggage claim area or to a friend. If it's cool, wear an old throwaway outfit or a clean plastic bag to keep warm until the race starts. You may choose to start the race with some throwaway clothes. Note: It is better to start the race feeling a little cool since you'll heat up during the race. You will be on the run for a long time, so if the weather looks like it may cool off plan ahead. Tie a jacket around your waist in case you need it later or position your support crew along the course with extra clothing. Weather conditions often change over the course of a four- or five-hour run. It could

get much hotter, or much cooler. It could also rain and then stop, or rain could dampen your spirits late in the run. Try to be prepared as much as possible for changes in the weather.

■ Don't waste energy with a cardiorespiratory warm-up on race morning, especially since you will start slowly anyway. But don't get stiff by standing or sitting too long either. Every fifteen minutes or so move around. Walk, stand, sit. Stretch only after a walking warm-up and make sure not to overstretch while excited and nervous.

■ Throughout the marathon countdown, think calm. Focus as much as possible on staying relaxed. Expect to feel edgy as the big day approaches—this is normal and happens to all marathoners, whether it is their first or hundredth 26.2-mile adventure. Your body has energy to spare, and it misses the hard training. You will have to deal with withdrawal symptoms at the same time you are coping with prerace anxiety. Don't start worrying about losing your fitness and panic. You are not losing fitness, you are ready to run 26.2 miles. Remember this: There is nothing you can do now to improve your fitness, but you can make training errors or mental mistakes that could mess up your race. Concentrate on how confident you are. Keep visualizing yourself crossing the marathon finish line!

Go! Strategy for Finishing Your First Marathon

Goal

Remember your goal: finishing in comfort. A 12-minute-a-mile pace is a five-hour marathon. The first-timer often runs between four and five hours; many finish more slowly than that. Don't be concerned with time goals. Experience your first marathon, don't race it. Run your first marathon, later you can race one. You will be a hero for just finishing—just as you were for finishing your first race—so don't put pressure on yourself by announcing a time goal. Just finishing will give you plenty to brag about. Besides, the slower you finish, the easier it will be to show off by improving your time in the future. Fear not. You won't finish last, and someone will still be at the finish line when you get there. For the New York City Marathon, runners are still coming in after ten hours. You can walk a marathon in that time.

Lining Up

If you intend to start with friends, make very clear plans as to where and when you will meet. Keep a close eye on each other right up until the start. In large marathons it's hard to find someone at the start. Line up according to the pace signs that are posted for most marathons. Be honest—and smart. If you are too far up front when the gun goes off you may get sucked out at too fast a pace; if you start at your pace you'll get in the way of runners starting out too quickly. If you know you'll take five hours or more, then you would be wise to line up way in the back. All those runners that start ahead of you won't be passing you in the race. If you start too far up front, then you'll be passed by hundreds of runners, which isn't good for your confidence. It's better to later pass all those who started too fast.

Due to crowded conditions in most large marathons, it may take several minutes just to reach the starting line and a few miles to settle into your pace. One way to compensate is to deduct, for your personal records, the time it took you to get to the starting line from your finish time. Don't frantically weave in and out of people in an effort to move up: You'll waste energy and risk injury. If you find yourself stuck with the masses, relax and enjoy yourself. After all, it's your first marathon, and without all those other runners, the 26.2-mile run would be much tougher. I assure you, over the last few miles you will be happy to have a lot of company in your struggle.

Start Your Watch and Watch It

You can't always depend on the times given along the course being accurate. Many marathons will have each mile marked but only give times every 5 miles. Wear your runner's watch so you can monitor your pace. (You may also choose to do this with your heart rate monitor—aim to keep within your training heart rate range for your first marathon effort.) Mile markers are sometimes misplaced, and you should be able to quickly detect major errors since you will know approximately what time you should arrive at each mile mark. Be prepared, keep an eye on your watch, and don't panic if mile markers or splits seem to be off occasionally. By regularly consulting a watch, you help yourself concentrate on the race; you keep in tune with your goal and your desire to hold pace. Play a little game: See how close you can come to running mile after mile at the same pace per mile. Be prepared for slower mile splits when running up hills or into head winds as well as faster times with downhills and tailwinds.

Don't forget to stop your watch when you cross the finish line (but try to do it while not looking down or you will ruin any photos taken of you finishing): It may be a long time before you get the official results. Believe it or not, fatigued runners often forget to stop their watch, and then they don't remember the exact time that was on the finish line clock.

Starting Out

Beware, beware, beware! Starting too fast in a short race will mean you'll slow down at the end. Starting too fast in the marathon will either mean a long struggle over the last several miles or a DNF (did not finish). Don't think that you can build a time cushion by starting faster. This strategy will most likely backfire. If you start with a friend or a group of friends, promise each other to keep the starting pace reasonable. Your best bet is to get stuck in the crowd so you have to start with a slow walk progressing to a brisk walk, slow jog, and finally your training pace. Experienced marathoners may race at a pace that is 1–1½ minutes per mile faster than their comfortable long-training run pace. A good bet for novices, however, is to start at the same pace you averaged for your last long run and hold that speed to 20 miles. If you can pick it up a bit from there, go ahead. Or remember this strategy: start slowly and then taper off.

I repeat. Beware of starting too fast. This is the most common error for beginner marathoners. It it's a warm day, be prepared to start slower than your original goal pace.

The First Few Miles: Test the Water

Ease into the race both in terms of your starting pace and your emotional involvement. If you start more than 10 seconds per mile faster than what you plan to average, you are asking for trouble. Slow down gradually and remain calm if you find that your first mile or two are too quick. Emotionally, stay as calm as possible. Treat the first 10 miles like what they are: a controlled run similar to your daily training runs in effort. Try to get in with a pack of runners who are flowing comfortably and help each other.

Adjust for Obstacles: Heat, Cold, Hills, Wind

These factors can play havoc with your marathon effort. Be prepared to adjust your race pace and finishing time goal to safely overcome these obstacles.

Halfway Analysis

This is a critical point psychologically for most runners. If your approximate time goal is four hours and you hit the halfway mark close to that time and feel pretty good, you get a mental lift. If you are a few minutes behind schedule, don't panic. Readjust your time goal by doing away with it. Just concentrate on staying relaxed and making it to the finish line.

The Second Half: Concentration, Form, Relaxation, Mental Toughness

This is where the race begins. In a marathon, fatigue tries to capture you for the last half of the race—that could be for two or three hours. Maintain concentration on pace and the runners around you. Keep relaxed, and remain confident and goal-directed. Maintain good form as detailed in Chapter 34. Occasionally change your form a little to provide relief: drop your arms to your sides for a few yards, thus using muscles differently. When you hit bad patches where you are physically and mentally fatigued—and you will—hang in there.

Think about all that training time and all those long runs that would be wasted if you gave up just because you were uncomfortable. Think about your friends and family waiting for you along the course and at the finish line. Relax, and believe in yourself. Have faith in your training program. Talk tough to yourself: "Come on, let's get going!" Push through periods of self-doubt by internalizing the cheers from the crowd and the fellowship of the runners around you to pull you along. Most likely, if you keep moving, perhaps even take some walk breaks, you will feel better again. If you have to, then alternate running and walking the rest of the way to the finish line, but don't sit down no matter how strong the urge. Accept discomfort. It's real. But use all of your mental resources and your background of solid training to keep it from slowing you down. If you followed my program from this book, don't let me down! Visualize Coach Glover exhorting you toward glory at the finish line.

Bail Out

If you are favoring an injury or bad blister, feeling weak and dizzy because of the heat or illness, or are extremely fatigued—don't be a hero. Bail out at any point and look for medical help. Don't feel that you are a failure if you make an intelligent decision to drop out for reasons of personal safety. You can always try another marathon down the road.

But if you trained properly and do not feel ill or are not hampered by an injury, then you should finish as long as you can handle it mentally. Dig down deep for extra strength and keep going. Everyone feels like quitting many times. You are not alone. But don't unless you need to for health reasons. No one said it would be easy. That's why so many people want to take on the marathon—it's a significant physical and mental challenge.

The Wall

Now comes the real test. But "the wall" is a myth if you are properly prepared following the guidelines in Chapter 19. Most likely you will experience a taste of "the wall" somewhere around 20 miles in your first marathon. But if you trained well, carbo-loaded, and poured in sports drinks since just before the start of the race, you will pass through "the wall" in reasonably good shape.

10K to Go

You will hit two key mile markers in the marathon: the halfway mark and the 20-mile mark. Not only does the 20-mile barrier represent the popular conception of where you will meet "the wall," it also represents the start of a new race. For most beginner marathoners this is the farthest you have ever run. You are entering new and untested territory. From here to the finish you run a 10K race. Of course, it isn't anywhere near the same effort as starting a 6.2-mile run without already logging 20 long miles. But convince your mind that you are familiar with the 10K distance and use that now as your goal distance.

Over the last few miles of the marathon, the mind must take over from the body. You've come this far and your body certainly will feel tired. The willpower that forced you to train through heat, cold, rain, and snow for hour after hour must now be unleashed. Keep pumping the arms and picking up the knees. Somehow you will keep going forward if you can keep the arms and knees in motion.

Break up the course now mile marker by mile marker, landmark by landmark, even block by block—but keep knocking them off, counting down the miles to the mile-to-go marker, then the 26-mile sign, and then the finish line. Work on the runners around you; use them to push or pull you as often and as far as you can. Start thinking in terms of time left until the finish. First get under the 30-minutes-to-go barrier, then 20, then 15, and finally 10: You know you can suffer for these amounts of time, which may seem less threatening than mileage to go.

The Finish

As you cross the 26-mile mark you have only 385 yards—less than a quarter mile—to go. Use the noise of the crowd and the spirit and guts of the runners around you to give you the energy for one more push. As you catch sight of the digital clock over the finish, use it to pull you under to your personal victory. Rejoice, you've conquered! (But please don't drop dead like Pheidippides after his first marathon.)

But you haven't finished yet. You have to stay in line (don't sit down or you might not get back up!) and pass through the chutes in order of finish or you may not get proper credit for your victory.

Fred's Last Marathon

As the director of the New York City Marathon, Fred Lebow had a special place in his heart for first-time marathoners. He loved to go to our marathon buildup and countdown clinics to offer encouragement to the hundreds of beginners on hand and entertain them with stories of what went wrong in his first of nearly seventy marathons.

Battling back from brain cancer at age sixty in 1992, he ran his five-borough New York City Marathon for the first time in a dramatic effort captured on nationwide TV. He finished in 5 hours, 32 minutes. Fred was right where he felt comfortable—running along with back-of-the-packers and novice marathoners. It was Fred's last marathon.

Looking forward to the twenty-fifth anniversary of his event in 1994, Fred struggled one last time with his cancer. In his last days he admitted that he had a few final wishes. One was he wished a member of his family had run his race. His sister Sarah's son, Moshe Katz, volunteered. But Fred had his doubts—after all, it was only five weeks before the event. I didn't have doubts. In fact,

I guaranteed Moshe that if he would follow my emergency plan he would make it to the finish line. Then I told Fred the news. As he laid in his bed, with his running shoes and running hat on, he was barely alive. I said: "Fred, Moshe is going to be the first member of your family to run the New York City Marathon. I guarantee it. I am his coach. I will not only train him, but I will run it with him." Did he hear me? Did he understand? Slowly, but surely, he sat up in bed, looked at me with misty eyes, held my hand, and whispered the words: "Thank you."

But could Moshe do it? This isn't the way I recommend preparing for your first marathon. But Moshe had three things going for him: he was in good shape from playing basketball and had some running experience, he was only twenty-five, and he had the emotional inspiration. Our goal was simple: make good on our promise to Fred. We had another major problem. I was just starting to run again after having been debilitated by a herniated disk. I had been advised not to run marathons any more and hadn't run more than 10 miles in years. But I had made a promise to a dying friend.

So I put Fred's nephew on a training program that involved running every other day for 30 to 45 minutes plus a gradually increasing long run buildup that included plenty of walk breaks. The goal was to be able to at least walk most of the way and please Fred by running across the finish line. Trying to train too much this close to the race would have led to injury and failure. Shelly-lynn Florence Glover helped Moshe with his daily diet, running form, and carbo-loading strategy. She tested him in the physiology lab at Columbia University and was pleased to find that he had a very high aerobic fitness level from his vigorous basketball activity. I ran parts of the course with him a few times while giving him a crash course in mental preparation and racing strategy.

A week after we started training and four weeks before the marathon, Fred left us. Front-page newspaper headlines declared: "Goodbye to Our Marathon Man." But Moshe and I had a sense that Fred was going to run the marathon with us. We committed ourselves to give Fred two of his wishes: to be able to participate in the twenty-fifth anniversary race and to see a family member finish the New York City Marathon.

On race morning we took the bus together to the start of the race. We followed all the marathon countdown tips detailed in this chapter and lined up with the crowd of nearly 30,000 runners. Moshe agreed to a simple strategy. We would start at a pace much slower than his 8-minute-per-mile pace for his shorter runs—we ran about a 10-minute pace. We would stop every mile to walk while drinking fluids. We poured water on us and in us every mile, and drank Gatorade every other mile.

We were inspired over and over again by all the signs and special T-shirts honoring Fred's memory. Whenever I yelled out to the crowd that Fred's nephew was coming through we got huge cheers. Nina Kuscsik, the women's running pioneer and a good friend of Fred's, contributed an important strategy to our effort. At the starting area she penned "Go Mo" across the front of Moshe's shirt. Throughout the race spectators shouted out "Go Mo," which really helped. (You might try that trick! Pen your name to your shirt or have a special shirt made up with your name or town on it: "Go Sally," "I'm from Boston," or "Marathon Grandpa.")

It was a very, very emotional run for the three of us—Moshe, Fred, and I. At 20 miles we sent friends to a phone booth to call the finish line area and deliver a message over the loudspeaker: "Fred, we just crashed through 'the wall.' We are going to make it!" Moshe broke out the bag of candy he carried to treat us when we reached "the wall," but the bag had opened and was now empty. We had looked forward to that moment for 20 miles. No matter, nothing could stop us now!

Each mile Moshe ran faster and faster, passing hundreds of weary marathoners. With less than a mile to go I sent a messenger on ahead—just like Pheidippides—to the finish to announce that we were on the way. But Moshe, who only stopped to drink fluids during the race, was breaking into a sprint and passed him. "Yahoo Fred, look at Moshe go!" He finished his first marathon in 4:22:46. I ran through considerable pain to be there all the way. We embraced and cried, then celebrated with Fred's family and friends. Moshe enjoyed his first marathon so much that he did it again the next year. This time he ran it for himself and broke the four-hour barrier.

If Fred can finish a marathon at age sixty with brain cancer, and if his nephew and I could do it on guts and emotional inspiration, why can't you rise to the challenge, too?

The Aftermarathon

Thousands of runners each year put in hundreds of hours of physical and mental preparation to run the marathon. Very little time or planning, however, is devoted to what happens after the race.

The scene at the finish line of a major marathon resembles a disaster area. The marathon tears down the body, which has been built up for months in anticipation of a strong effort. Injury and illness are frequent not only during and immediately after the marathon, but also in the days and weeks following. The body is weak, and the mind is undisciplined because the immediate goal has been achieved. A postmarathon runner is very vulnerable. How well you recover from a marathon effort and prevent injury from developing depends on how effectively you deal with the three key phases of marathon recovery:

1. your *prerace* preparation

2. *race day* strategy and execution, and environmental influences

3. *postrace* recovery procedures and training for several weeks following the marathon

Immediately after finishing the marathon you must fight the urge to lie down and give up the hope that your pain and fatigue will go away. Force yourself to begin the very important but largely neglected postrace recovery process. If you fail to take care of your aching body properly after the marathon, your legs will soon become very tight and you will be extremely prone to injury over the next few days and weeks of running.

This is the postrace recovery procedure that is most effective in helping runners recover safely and quickly:

The First Hours
Keep moving. When you finish the race, don't lie or sit down for long periods of time. If you do sit down, try to keep your feet elevated. After leaving the chute, drink plenty of fluids, put on warm-ups, walk. Then get off your feet for a few minutes and drink some more fluids. Have any blisters treated immediately by medical personnel at the finish area. Apply ice to any painful areas in the major leg muscle groups, and repeat the process along with taking ibuprofen for the next few days to combat inflammation. It is the swelling around the traumatized muscles that causes soreness and tightness. After you have gained some strength, go for a 10-

to 15-minute walk and eat some food. Do some very light stretching, but don't overstretch fatigued muscles.

Avoid heat treatment of the painful areas for forty-eight hours. However, some people find that a hot bath or whirlpool bath will relax them. If you do take a hot bath, treat the injured area with ice first. After the bath, take a short nap or at least lie down and rest.

Later in the day, go for another walk (15 to 30 minutes), swim, ride a bike, or go dancing. The purpose of this activity is to pump blood into the legs in order to help you recover. Apply more ice and stretch lightly before going to bed.

Fluids. Start replacing fluids as soon as you cross the finish line. Sip fluids if you cannot gulp them. When your stomach settles, pour them in.

You should drink plenty of fluids throughout the day in proportion to the amount of weight you lost. An average runner might lose as much as 8 pounds of water weight running a marathon. Keep drinking until you have clear urine; dark urine is a symptom of dehydration. Force yourself to drink extra fluids. Watch your body weight for the next twenty-four hours. Generally this is enough time to get your fluids—and your weight—back to normal.

Get warm and dry. As soon as possible, get out of your wet clothes, dry off, and put on warm clothes. You'll feel more comfortable and your muscles will not stiffen as much. Your support crew can really help you out here.

Food. Runners who are obsessed with proper diet before a race often ignore it afterward. But what you eat and drink for several days after a marathon will affect your recovery. A balanced diet, with an emphasis on carbohydrates, will replenish all your energy stores of glycogen and allow you to return sooner to a normal training and racing routine.

A marathon will especially deplete your glycogen stores. To recover, and to replace lost glycogen, you should eat plenty of carbohydrates. In effect, this is a carbohydrate reloading to get glycogen back into your muscles and liver. As Chapter 19 details, studies show that your muscles will restore glycogen more quickly during the first hour or two after your marathon effort. So eat soon and continue to fuel yourself often with carbos over the next few days so that you can reload fully. According to Dr. David Costill, director of the Human Performance Laboratory at Ball State University, "Probably the first meal after the marathon should be like the last big meal before. You want to recover as much of that used-up glycogen as possible. It often takes three to five days to recover the glycogen. That's part of the problem of recovering from a marathon. A lot of people don't go after the carbohydrates hard enough, and that is part of the cause for the fatigue and difficulties in getting back into running form again."

The Days Following the Marathon

Joe Henderson commented in his book *Run Farther, Run Faster,* "Recovery seems to go backward at first. You feel worse the morning after the race than you did right after, and worse yet the second day. It takes that long for the 'drunk' to wear off, and the soreness and fatigue to settle in completely. You typically hit bottom about forty-eight hours after racing. You aren't tempted to do much running in this state, and you aren't thinking much about racing again. After another twenty-four or forty-eight hours pass, the worst of the hurts disappear. You think you're ready to start training for another race, but that's where you're wrong—perhaps dangerously wrong. Recovery isn't finished when your legs loosen up; it has only begun.

"Racing tears you down in more ways than one. I see at least three stages of recovery. They are: (1) muscular, (2) chemical, and (3) psychological. Recovery from muscle soreness and fatigue comes quickest. Even marathoners get over it within a few days. But it takes longer to restore body chemistry to its normal balance, and still longer to forget how bad this race felt so you can start looking forward to the next one."

Here are general guidelines to follow for the first week following a marathon.

▪ The morning after the marathon take a bath to relax, but remember to treat injured areas with ice first. Do more gentle stretching, and take a walk. You may be better off forgetting about running for a few days. Stick to non-weight-bearing exercise, such as swimming or biking. The object is to recover by forcing blood into the legs, so why abuse the body by compelling it to run on blistered feet and tired legs?

▪ Treat injured areas with ice for the first forty-eight hours. You may later use heat treatments such as whirlpool baths or ultrasound and massage to promote circulation. Do gentle stretching exercises in the first forty-eight hours, and be cautious—remember, your muscles will be tight.

▪ Get plenty of sleep for several days after your big race. Go to bed early, and take naps if possible. It is extremely important to get much more than the normal amount of sleep. Your immunity is down so rest is important.

▪ Beware of a false high you may experience a few days after a strong marathon effort. Hold back. Even though you feel as if you are very strong, you are not. Also be careful following a disappointing race not to punish yourself by running hard in an effort to improve immediately for your next race.

Rebuilding—Getting Back to Running and Racing

The most common rule of thumb is to take one recovery day for every mile that you race. Thus, you'll need about twenty-six days —a month or so—to rebuild after your marathon effort. Don't rush it. Some runners may recover sooner, but many will need even longer. Recovery deserves as much planning as your premarathon schedule. Besides recovering from muscle soreness (see Chapter 33 for information on delayed-onset muscle soreness or DMSO) and blisters, you need time to restore your body chemistry and glycogen stores to its normal levels and time to regain the desire to train for your next challenge.

Think of it as the pre-marathon taper in reverse—a few off days, then a few short runs, then a gradual increase in weekly mileage until you reach your normal training level. A study at Ball State University in Indiana even indicates that you may be better off not even running a step for the first week after a marathon. Researchers compared a group that did no running at all for a week after their marathon with a group that ran easily for 20 to 40 minutes a day. The result: The nonrunners scored better in tests for muscle strength and endurance three days and a week after the marathon.

Thus, I recommend that you not run for three to seven days after the marathon even if you feel good enough to run. Don't pound away on muscles that need to heal. Non-impact activity such as walking, swimming or biking for 30 to 60 minutes, however, will pump blood to your muscles and help you recover sooner. After three to four days of nonrunning, you may be ready to run easy on soft surfaces for 2 to 4 miles every other day. A good rule of thumb is to increase mileage for the second week to no more than 50 percent of your usual weekly mileage and to no more than 75 percent during the third post-marathon week (but less than this is okay). By the fourth week you may be ready to resume your normal weekly mileage. For the average intermediate runner this may be 15 to 30 miles per week compared to 30 to 40 miles per week when at peak marathon training. If at any point during this four-week buildup or "reverse taper," you feel fatigued or unduely sore, then run less. Remember this rule: Recovery is your priority for at least four weeks after a marathon.

First-time marathoners as well as most intermediate-level runners shouldn't race any distance for five to eight weeks after the marathon. Another marathon shouldn't be considered for at least three to six months, preferably at least a year.

Postmarathon Depression. You put in a lot of time and effort, making many sacrifices along the way, to attempt to race a good marathon. But the marathon is a risky event. If you have a bad day, catch a stitch, develop bad blisters, have problems with your shoes, have an old injury act up, or trip and bang your knee, all your preparation can go down the drain. This is why I encourage you to go for good times for a few shorter races in the last weeks prior to the marathon. You will have something to show for all your training if the marathon race ends up being a disappointment.

Even if you ran a good race, you may feel depressed for the next few weeks. Just as in postpartum depression, your "baby" has reached the finish line and your long-sought-after goal, around which your life revolved for months, has been achieved, leaving you feeling empty. Take some time off from serious running and enjoy activities that you had to give up because you were spending most of your nonworking time running. Maintain minimal mileage levels, however, by doing a few easy runs per week.

Some Concluding Words
You don't ever have to run a marathon. Don't ever let anyone push you into something you don't want to do. The lure of this popular event creates a lot of peer pressure. Desire is the only emotion that will get you through your training and to the finish line. Some

runners never race; some love the 10K races or the half-marathons. Find your desire and follow it.

Also, if you've entered the marathon but your training is not up to the minimum, don't go. Instead, start training for the next marathon. Treat the marathon with respect. Better to postpone than to fail.

Finally, don't take racing, or marathon running, too seriously. Rumor has it that there is life after—or without—marathoning. But there is also nothing like that feeling when you cross the finish line of your first marathon. Here you come—head up, legs tired but still churning, arms pumping. You hug the runner in front of you in the chute. You congratulate each other. You smile, you laugh, you cry. And—damn!—you know you are *good*!

What's Next?

Almost every first-time marathoner says the same thing at the finish line: "Never again." Once you've conquered the marathon and rejoiced, you may indeed be satisfied going back to being a fitness runner, or taking up the challenge of improving times at shorter distances. But many of us catch the marathon bug. We are fascinated with seeing how much faster we can push ourselves over that long road to the marathon finish line.

If you now want to improve your marathon time, you are ready to graduate to *The Competitive Runner's Handbook*, which covers marathon training and racing in great detail.

FIFTEEN

Introduction to Speed Training

I've met few runners who don't want to run faster. And I've met very few beginner and intermediate runners who aren't intimidated by the prospect of speed training.

You shouldn't be. The brutal "no pain, no gain" workouts you hear serious competitors brag about aren't for you. To safely improve, you need only run a little faster than your comfortable everyday training pace and learn to handle a modest amount of discomfort.

Running for health, fitness, and fun is the only goal for many runners. But runners who have reached the fitness stage—running 30 minutes at least three times a week—often want to run faster, whether for self-satisfaction or for performance in races. Most runners run their first few races at a nice easy pace; they are happy just to reach the finish line at any pace. But once that's accomplished, they begin to think beyond "just finishing"—they want to run faster. At this point, you'll still be able to improve your speed somewhat by getting stronger through steady runs, but you'll take a big step forward if you do speed training. Designed properly, speed training will benefit you physiologically, biomechanically, strategically, and psychologically.

Physiological Benefits

When you run aerobically, with your heart rate in its training range and at a conversational pace, there is plenty of oxygen available for energy. But when you start running faster, your heartrate rises and your breathing becomes somewhat labored.

You begin to do much of your running anaerobically, where the body is unable supply oxygen to the working muscles and organs. You may go into "oxygen debt" and lose the ability to converse easily on the run. Eventually, your body rebels and slows down.

This state can't be avoided—by anyone—but it can be postponed. You can condition your body to better tolerate running at fast speeds by practicing anaerobic running in speed workouts.

Biomechanical Benefits

Running form should change somewhat when you speed up. When doing speed workouts, you drive your arms faster, quicken the stride, and really concentrate on relaxed breathing. By practicing running in short segments at race pace or faster, you prepare your body to adjust to the biomechanical differences between training pace and race pace. You'll run more efficiently and faster on race day.

Strategic Benefits

How do you know what pace to start at and hold for your races? One way is by trial and error at races—start too slow and end up wishing you had tried harder, or start too fast and wish you had been more conservative. Either way, you most likely would have run a faster time if you had paced yourself better. Speed training mimics the pacing of races and helps you learn to be aggressive, but sensible, about your starting pace. In speed training you can practice running race pace over and over again to learn what it feels like. On race day you can slip into that gear more easily. By running faster than race pace in speed sessions, you learn to pace hard effort. For example, if, in a workout, you do four half-mile runs spaced by a recovery period in 3:30, 3:40, 4:00, and 4:15, you can see (and feel!) that you started too fast. It is better to learn this in a workout than a race. On the other hand, if you ran them in 4:15, 4:00, 3:40, and 3:30, you know that you could have run them faster. You are better than you thought you were! The best way to run this workout is the same as the best way to run the race—at a reasonably even pace. In this example, that would be half miles run within 5 to 10 seconds of each other: 3:40 to 3:50 for this sample workout.

Psychological Benefits

I've had many students rejoice about running significantly improved race times after only a couple of our speed sessions. I wish I could brag and say it was because of my coaching, but you won't get significant physiological benefits that soon. Rather, these runners improved because they learned there was an athlete hidden within themselves. After learning to push themselves in workouts, they began to feel tougher and faster. Because they *thought* they could run faster in races, they did.

By running controlled segments of the race distance at an effort beyond your perceived limitations, you will gain the confidence to work a little harder in a race. You will find you can run in some discomfort without falling in a heap. Many runners, especially novice racers, underestimate their abilities as athletes; through speed training you can often discover that you are tougher than you had realized. With experience in speed training, your times for workouts improve. You will feel more comfortable starting races at a little faster pace and will know from the feelings you had in speed sessions that you can hang in there to the end.

Generally, you can benefit from speed training if:

▪ It is difficult for you to hold a fast pace during a race, but you finish feeling as though you could have run farther at the same pace: "If only the race had been longer."

▪ You feel uncomfortable with the pace at the start (assuming you didn't start too fast for your fitness) or during the race, or cannot generate a "kick" at the end.

▪ You lack the strength to generate power during a race, especially up hills.

▪ Your running form needs improvement (see Chapter 34).

▪ You need to improve your race pace judgment. This includes learning to start fast enough to do your best, but not too fast to do your worst; and maintaining a reasonably even pace from start to finish.

Easing Into Speed Training

If you are new to racing and speed training, one speed workout per week is plenty unless you are supervised for a second session. You still need to build and maintain enough mileage to get to the finish line in reasonable comfort, and you can't do that safely if you are doing too much speed training. The key is to allow your body and mind to make a safe transition into faster running, not to thrash yourself until running is no longer fun. Speed workouts properly done can be fun, especially if you run them with a group of people. They will especially be enjoyable when they yield tangible results: faster, more comfortable races.

Speed training is quite simple. You run fast (race pace or a little faster) for segments that are much shorter than your race distance, with recovery breaks to minimize the stress on your body. Speed training is based on three variables: quantity, intensity, and recovery.

Quantity. This refers to how many repeat hard runs—popularly termed "intervals"—you do and the distance you cover. Complete enough intervals to give yourself a good workout, but not so many that you can't finish the last run at nearly the same pace as your average interval. Since the first goal is just to acquire a taste for speed training, you should minimize the number of fast runs in a workout. With experience and fitness, you may increase the number of speed runs per workout. For example, to start out, I would recommend doing half-mile runs no more than three or four times. You may build up to six or more later. Generally, the longer the distance and faster the pace the fewer intervals you would attempt. You would not run as many miles as you would halves, and you wouldn't run as many at 5K race pace as you would at marathon race pace.

Intensity. This refers to how fast you run your workouts. The speed will be race pace or faster. The range that I use in classes is from a low-intensity marathon pace to a fairly high intensity of faster than 5K pace. As an introduction to speed training I recommend a pace range between your 5K and 10K race pace except for workouts designed to teach you marathon pace. If you haven't raced enough to know your race pace then just run at an effort that will leave you slightly breathless but not out of breath. Don't sprint—ever. Hard, all-out sprinting will make you more prone to injury. The object is to practice running somewhere near your race effort. You may find that the second time you do the same workout you can run the same pace more comfortably, or you can handle the intervals at a slightly faster pace. This shows that you are progressing with your fitness. However, don't be dismayed if you run more slowly as a result of poor weather, fatigue from increased mileage, or if you just don't feel sharp that day.

Recovery. Recovery is the easy part. It refers to how much rest you take between hard runs. The theory behind intervals is that you can manage a fair amount of hard work in small quantities if the body is rested in between. If you ran very hard with no rest breaks, you would be racing. The body can't handle too many races, but it can handle weekly speed sessions if proper recovery is used between intervals. Basically, you want to recover by allowing the heart rate, breathing, and body temperature to get back down to about the level you would be at for a slow run or brisk walk. For recovery, you can run slowly or walk, or both. Keep moving! Do not sit or lie down—that would place a stress on the cardiorespiratory system. I prefer a walking recovery for all but the faster runners since it allows a more complete recovery and minimizes the pounding on the legs. Don't be shy about pouring fluids on you and in you during rest periods. Make sure you are breathing comfortably before you run fast again. If necessary, rest longer than you had planned or cut short your workout. On the other hand, too long a recovery period will make the workout too easy. The harder you run, and the longer the distance, the more recovery time required. Generally, your recovery period should be 2 to 4 minutes.

These three variables can be juggled in various ways to make the workout more difficult. Adding to the number of intervals run, increasing the pace, or shortening the recovery period makes the workouts harder. I feel that the average runner is best served by keeping the recovery period constant and slightly increasing the number and pace of the intervals. That's the kind of improvement your stopwatch can capture, and it should build your confidence as you approach your races.

A Simplified Ten-Week Speed Training Program
Okay, you've heard enough talk and you want some action. *The Competitive Runner's Handbook* details all the intricacies of speed

training and will guide you beyond the beginner racing stage. But most novices at racing and speed training have modest goals. "Just tell me what workouts to do and I'll do them," you say.

What follows is a sample ten-week speed training program modeled on the typical ten-week program designed by Shelly-lynn for our New York Road Runners Club classes for intermediate-level runners. Hundreds of runners have benefited from these workouts and you will, too. Our program offers a variety of workouts that will allow you to progress in a conservative manner. It is easy to follow, consisting of simple variations on just a few basic themes.

This is a conservative program. Our students know from experience that too little training when it comes to speed work is always better than too much. The key is to run a few high-quality workouts within a limited time period to help you get better without overtraining.

Most runners aim to do well in one or two races each "season." You may wish to train for a very popular 10K or marathon, or just for the local Turkey Trot. The following program assumes that you've developed a reasonable fitness base and are ready to prepare for your races by "sharpening" with a little speed work. To further sharpen for a particular race, you'll benefit from running one or two races during the ten-week buildup program—say a 5K and a 5-miler before a 10K, or a 10K and a half-marathon before your marathon. Try to time your ten weeks so that your last hard speed session is at least ten days before your big race.

The sample ten-week program that follows is just that—a sample. You can use it exactly as explained, or you can adapt it to fit your individual needs and environment. The program is designed to allow average runners to progress in a simple, conservative manner that should lead to improved performances at distances from 5K to the marathon. Just as important, it includes a variety of workouts to keep your training interesting.

Be sure to warm up for your speed runs with easy running for at least 10 minutes and to cool down for the same time period as well. Keep these workouts separated from your long runs by at least two days, and from races by at least four days (both before and after).

Week-by-Week Programs: Ten Sample Workouts

For these introductory speed workouts I'll give you a suggested range for pace: between a little faster than 5K race pace and a little slower than 10K race pace.

Week 1: Mile Intervals

Shelly-lynn often has her intermediates do this workout the first week of class. Why? Many runners have no idea what pace they can run for a mile. This workout will give you a feel for your ability as you get used to running on a track. Note: The best place to run intervals is at your local high school or college track, which is 440 yards (quarter-mile) or the metric equivalent of 400 meters. Four laps equals one mile. If you don't have a track available, just measure off a section on a park road or trail away from car traffic and you'll have your own track.

Shelly-lynn starts off her ten-week program with just two one-mile intervals. Try to run each of the four laps at approximately the same pace—about your race pace for the distance you are training to run. This way you are learning to keep a steady race pace. Hold yourself back the first lap, just as you must at the start of the race. If you feel you can run a little faster on the third or fourth lap, go ahead. How did you feel after your first mile? If you hardly broke a sweat, start a bit faster for your second one after a 3-minute walking recovery period. If you struggled to finish and were slowing down at the end, start the next one at a slower pace. Ideally you ran the whole way at the same pace, finishing tired but not exhausted. Then you should aim to do the same for your second mile interval.

Week 2: Fartlek

What the heck is a fartlek, you ask? The Swedish word "fartlek" means "speed-play" and in its purest form this workout involves spontaneous changes of pace over varying distances. This is a good way to make the transition between easy running and speed training. You do intervals just like you would on the track, but not over an exact, timed distance. Our classes love this workout since it really is play. Shelly-lynn and I always get the most enthusiastic response from our students after these runs, since we take them off the beaten path for a tour of Central Park. If possible, find an interesting park or trail to explore during your fartlek run—ideally over grass or dirt to add even more variety. Don't forget to include some hills!

You can do fartlek two ways. Running fast to a landmark or for a period of time. With our classes, we suddenly announce "pick it up to the top of the hill," or "run fast to the next lightpost." The students never know where we will run next and when we'll start an interval. Fartlek can be fun with a group of people; you can take turns being the leader. Start with a warm-up run of 1 or 2 miles and then pick up the speed to 5K race pace or faster for bursts of 50 yards to a quarter-mile. Pick landmarks to run to, especially the crests of hills. Most people prefer a little structure if they do fartlek on their own. To get you started, I recommend a simple workout. Run four bursts of 2 minutes each with 2 minutes of slow running recovery in between. You might like this workout so much that you'll choose to do it again, replacing one of the following runs. Have fun!

Week 3: Quarters
Back to the track for quarter-mile intervals—one lappers. Now I'll ask you to run a little faster than 5K race pace to improve your speed. Concentrate on pumping your arms, pushing off your feet, and lifting your knees to go faster. This workout will make your starting race pace seem less intimidating and help you get ready for your finishing kick. Run four or five quarters with a 2-minute recovery walk between each one.

Week 4: Long Hills
"Ugh, are you really going to make me run hard up hills," you complain. If you are going to race on them you had better train on them.

Hill repeats are termed "speedwork in disguise." That's because you don't have to run as fast to work hard. It's a good workout to do by yourself since the hill will make sure you get enough of a challenge. I'll introduce you first to long hills. Find one that is about a quarter mile in length and not too steep. It should take you 2 or 3 minutes to run up it. After your warm-up, run the hill at 5K race pace a total of three or four times. Recover by running back down nice and easy. This type of workout will increase your leg strength and bolster your confidence in running hills at or near race pace. If you are bothered by lower leg injuries, skip hill workouts and ease into speed training on the flats.

Week 5: Halves

Back to the track for two-lappers. Now the goal is to hold 5K race pace or faster for a longer distance than for the quarters. Try to run each lap of the track at the same time—this is called running even "splits." You also should try to run each half in about the same time. This is even pacing just like you should run in your races. While doing these intervals, visualize yourself running at the start or midway point of your race. Stay relaxed, stay with good form, stay on pace. Do four intervals with a 2- or 3-minute walking recovery.

Week 6: Tempo Run

"Now what are they throwing at me," you say. Hey, variety will make you a happier, better runner. Tempo runs get you off the track and onto the roads—ideally over part of your race course but not over killer hills. The purpose of this run is to mimic the race itself, but not the whole race. These runs improve racing form and mental concentration while teaching you to stay relaxed and hold a strong pace for several minutes. You want to get into a groove while visualizing yourself cruising along during the middle miles of a race.

After a 1- or 2-mile warm-up run, move into a pace that is comfortably hard. This should be 15 to 20 seconds slower than 10K race pace, or about 30 seconds slower than 5K race pace. This is a continuous speed run. Hold the pace for 20 minutes and then ease into a cool-down run.

Week 7: Mile Intervals

Back to mile intervals, but this time you will not be doing them as an introduction to track training but rather as a peak workout. This one is for the mind. Do three one-mile intervals at 5K race pace or faster with 3-minute recovery walks in between. This is a toughy. Hang tough here and you'll be stronger on race day. For the first interval, hold yourself back just as you will need to for the first mile on race day. For the middle interval, stay calm and concentrate on your pace—again, mimicking your race strategy. The last mile will feel similar to the last mile of your race. Concentrate on good form while remaining mentally tough. Don't give up here or you'll mess up your average time just as letting go toward the end of a race will cost you precious seconds, even minutes.

You can use this workout to test your fitness level and help predict your race-day potential. Ideally, you ran the miles at a faster pace and more comfortably than you did during Week 1 of this program.

Week 8: Short Hills

There's pleasure in them thar hills. Well, at least there is once you've finished your workout. As I tell my students when they groan after finding out that I've scheduled this workout: "I hate hills, too, but they're good for you." Hey, a short hills workout is over quickly and really prepares your body and mind for racing.

Pick a hill that's 100 to 200 yards in length and steep enough to challenge you, but not so steep that it will interfere with good form. You don't have to run these real hard since fighting gravity will take care of the intensity. Charge up the hill as if you are finishing a 5K race. Emphasize good running form—drive your arms, lift your knees. Run all the way through an imagined finish line at the top. It should take about a minute or two for this run. Do four or five hill repeats. Recovery is a very slow run back down.

Week 9: Halves

Here's one last fitness test. You may choose to run one more interval this time—four or five halves with a 2- to 3-minute recovery walk. Compare your times to Week 5 to see how much you have improved! You should now feel much more comfortable at holding a strong pace over distance.

Week 10: Cut-Downs

Cut what? This is just a psychological trick we use to help you peak for your race and practice your finishing kick. It adds variety to your training since you are now getting away from running the same distance for each interval. With cut-downs, each interval is a shorter distance. Here, I recommend a mile, half-mile, and then a quarter-mile. Visualize that each run is your finishing kick. As you get closer and closer to the finish line, pick up the pace. Don't run this workout all-out since you want to finish feeling refreshed, ready for your race later in the week. Run your mile at race pace, your half-mile at faster than race pace, and your finishing quarter quick, but not full steam. Take a 3-minute recovery walk between intervals. As an option, you can do a pyramid workout: you build up in distance and then back down. For example, run a half-mile, mile, and then another half-mile.

Summary
Remember, this is a flexible, *sample* program. Make whatever changes you feel will benefit you and keep your running enjoyable. This simplified ten-week program will help you get as ready as you can get, with a modest amount of work, for a quality race effort. You will learn to run faster. Good luck!

Part V

Equipment

SIXTEEN

Running Shoes

"The worst thing that ever happened to feet was shoes," stated Dr. George Sheehan in the *Encyclopedia of Athletic Injuries*. Or perhaps the second worst, after paved surfaces. These two products of urban civilization—shoes and pavement—have conquered the human foot and created an entire specialty in the field of medicine. Remember, our ancestors crossed continents, pursued wild game, danced for days on end—all without shoes. What about us?

Studies at the University of Leeds, England, by Dr. R. McNeill Alexander, a zoologist, demonstrate that the perfect running shoe may be no shoe at all—that is, perhaps we should be running barefoot. His research shows that ordinary, bare human feet return about 20 percent more useful energy to the legs and body than the best high-tech running shoes. If you have the luxury of running on clean grass surfaces without rocks, glass, or such, then perhaps running barefoot would be ideal for you. But most of us run on hard pavement or over trails that have hidden and sharp obstacles. Running shoes are essential to protect the human skin and provide shock absorption.

Your feet, and those protective running shoes, each strike the ground about 800 times every mile. They hit with the force of approximately three times your body weight. If you run 10 miles a week, then each shoe strikes the ground during your runs more than 400,000 times a year. Your running shoes and your feet absorb the initial impact of running and pass it upward to the ankles, knees, hips, back, neck, and head. Many runners have biomechanically weak feet, which, when pounded on the earth thousands of times a week, incur a wide range of injuries or cause injuries to erupt elsewhere in the body. This alone makes running shoes important.

Today's running revolution has brought the running shoe revolution. When I recall the flimsy items my track coach told me were running shoes back in 1963, my feet ache. They had canvas uppers and gum soles so thin I could feel every stone I stepped on. Well-cushioned running shoes didn't start appearing until the 1970s. My first pair came from a mail-order outfit advertised in *Runner's World*. They didn't fit real well and the leather uppers caused blisters, but they provided some cushioning and I was proud to wear them.

One major innovation in running shoes since we first wrote this *Handbook* back in 1978 is the increasing specialization of shoes. Back then, women most likely bought and wore men's running shoes. Today, a male or female runner can select a shoe to fit his or her special exercise and physical needs and characteristics. As this chapter will detail, there are now shoes for runners who pronate, are heavy, run on trails; or who have high arches, narrow or wide feet, or a particular injury. The list of specialization is almost endless.

But the basic requirements of the shoe remain the same. According to Joe Dula, a footwear buyer writing in *Runner's World*, "A running shoe must cushion the impact of foot strike and it must stabilize the foot and neutralize, as far as possible, a runner's biomechanical imbalances. These are the goals of all running-shoe manufacturers, but they aim to reach these goals in different ways."

This is why one shoe may work well for you and others may cause pain or injury. If you have developed an injury shortly after switching running shoes, suspect the new shoes. Nina Kuscsik, a veteran of more than eighty marathons, suggests minimizing this problem by rotating among different brands of shoes to give your feet different stresses. The same stress repeated over time may cause injury. Still, the best bet may be to find the shoe that fits and works best, and stick with it—and hope the manufacturer doesn't dis-continue the shoe!

Don't think that high-tech or expensive shoes will solve your injury problems. They're likely to be the cause. Over the years, various research reports and shoe surveys have shown that the per-centage of runners who get shoe-related injuries remains about the same despite the many innovations designed to prevent such inju-ries. Why? All that tinkering may solve some problems but it cre-ates others. So don't think that shoes alone will solve your injury problems—or make you a faster or better runner. You will still need to do your preventative exercises and train wisely.

I won't attempt to analyze brands of shoes in this chapter be-cause the shoes change too much from year to year. *Runner's World* and *Running Times* print entire special annual issues that detail the enormous choices we have in running shoes. The best choice for advice on running shoes is your local running shoe store.

Anatomy of the Running Shoe

Running shoes have five major components: last, outer sole, mid-sole, heel, and uppers.

Last

The last is the inside shape of the shoe, which is created from a three-dimensional model. It is an average shape based on the im-pressions of many feet. Nobody has an average foot, yet the shape of the last affects the fit, flexibility, and stability of all running shoes. There are two shapes used in lasting—curved and straight. A curved last turns inward from the heel to the toes. It conforms to an average foot shape that fits about 60 percent of the popu-lation. A straight last has little or no curve from the heel to toe and provides greater support under the medial arch. Variations include slightly curved (closer to straight) and semi-curved (closer to curved).

To determine the shape of your foot, stand on a sheet of paper and have someone trace the outline of each foot. Superimpose this on the soles of your shoes to see if the size and curve are similar. In general, runners with rigid, high arches may feel most comfort-able in curve-lasted shoes. Those with a normal arch may want shoes with a slight curve, while others with a flexible low arch may feel best in straight-lasted shoes.

There are three techniques used to make running shoes: board lasting, slip lasting, and combination lasting. In board lasting, the upper materials of the shoe are pulled over the last and the ends are glued or stitched to a flexible inner-sole board. This shoe will be stiff, requiring a longer break-in period, but is more supportive. With a slip-lasted shoe, the upper material is stitched together on the underside and slipped onto the last. This makes a lighter, more flexible shoe. Combination lasting uses the board method in the heel for stability and the slip method in the forefoot for flexibility. How to tell the difference? Take out the shoe liner and if you see a full-length "board" the shoe is board lasted. If you see stitching, it is a slip-lasted shoe. If you see both, it is a combination.

What should you wear? In general, straight, board-lasted shoes increase stability and are better for runners like myself who wear orthotics or who need shoes that control pronation; this shoe gives us a good running platform. Curved, slip-lasted shoes may feel best on runners who have rigid feet that require as much movement as possible. Slip lasting gives more flexibility and is found in lighter training and racing shoes. If you train in one type of last, you may have difficulty adjusting to racing in another. Many runners prefer the combination-lasted shoes, which provide the benefits of both types.

Outer Sole

This is where the rubber hits the road. The outer sole is the treaded part of the shoe that strikes the ground. It resists wear, provides traction, and absorbs some shock. In general, soles are hard or soft: harder soles are heavier, have less cushion, and wear longer; softer soles are lighter, have less cushion, and wear out faster. The soles of your running shoes should not wear down quickly. The outer sole should also provide good traction, but not too much. There are many sole designs—ripple, waffle, some fancy, some simple. But most get a good grip on things.

Midsole

This is the hidden heart of the running shoe. The midsole, located between the outsole and the foot bed, controls excessive foot motion and provides shock absorption. It is constructed from various types of foam, most often EVA (ethylene vinyl acetate) and PU (polyurethane). Air bags, gel, silicone, and other material may be inserted inside the EVA or PU to increase cushioning. The most important feature of the midsole, however, is its degree of softness or hardness.

The midsole has three functions: to absorb shock from heel and forefoot strike, to flex in the ball of the foot on toe off, and to add stability.

Heels

The heel counter is the firm wrapping around the back of the shoe. It stabilizes the shoe and, therefore, your foot. A rigid heel counter that covers the entire heel is desirable, especially if you pronate. It is usually made from plastic. Squeeze the heel counter to see if it is firm and supportive. A heel wedge, which adds height to the heel, increases shock absorption and reduces strain on the foot and leg. A heel lift of ½ to 1 inch is desirable.

Uppers

On the top part, most running shoes are either nylon, nylon mesh, or a combination. This creates a lightweight, breathable, washable, soft shoe that requires little break-in and dries fast when wet. The mesh uppers do make the shoe somewhat colder during winter weather.

Running shoes have other features such as the ankle collar, which should be padded to cushion the ankle and help prevent Achilles tendinitis.

Lacing

Shoe lacing holds it all together by securing the shoe to the foot. Pull your laces too tight, and you cut off the circulation of blood; too loose, and your shoes flop about. When buying shoes, look for several things. Make sure the tongue is well padded so that the shoe can be laced snuggly against the foot without binding or rubbing. Make sure the eyelets—where the laces pass through the shoes—are strong and will not break. There are three types of eyelets: variable width with staggered eyelets to adjust the width, speed lacing with plastic D-rings substituted for conventional eyelets, and conventional eyelets.

Improper lacing can cause injuries. A common lacing injury is tendinitis on the top of the foot from too tight criss-cross lacing. Other injuries can be eased by using the lacing to draw the shoe tighter, skipping some eyelets to loosen the shoe, drawing the lacing from the eyelets closest to the toe to those farthest to ease pressure on black toenails. Have a shoe salesperson spend some time showing you the variations on lacing.

How to Choose Your Shoes: A Guideline for Beginner Buyers

A good pair of running shoes should provide four basic things: flexibility, cushioning, durability, and motion control. Okay, I'll also add looks. A lot of runners want their shoes to look good. Shepherd got a great pair of running shoes one day after a new runner tossed back a bargain pair with the disdainful whimper: "I don't want white running shoes." After a little dirt-and-grass-staining, Shepherd now runs over the Vermont hills with a good pair of brown-green-and-white shoes. Looks? Pfffffft!

Okay, how a shoe looks may be important to many buyers. But make sure the shoes have the four basics. Same for cost. The most expensive shoes are not always the best for you. The cheapest probably aren't either. I've had the most success with shoes in the mid-price range.

The purchase of a good pair of running shoes is the one critical investment you should make. The best choice for you should come after you check several factors, including your weight, arch type, footstrike pattern, surface you normally run on, how much you run, any injuries, and so on. Watch other runners buying shoes. Talk to them. I go through agony trying to buy the right pair. The store is full of choices and I've had advice from every running magazine (and book!) published. The choice is almost overwhelming. But take your time, and make it as carefully as possible. Most veteran runners, including myself, have a closet where the floor is littered with discarded running shoes.

Invest in a quality pair of running shoes. Too many runners start at either end of the cost line: they buy too cheap or too expensive. You can find a good pair of running shoes that fits your needs, feet, and budget. Remember, the shoes are important and are your only major investment on the road to fitness. The key to finding your running shoes is comfort, not price, looks, or brand name. Also, be sure to try the shoes on in the store. They should feel good there, or don't bring them home.

Here are some tips to help you make better choices:

1. Decide on a budget range, and stick with it. Tell the salesperson your budget.

2. Choose a store that specializes in running shoes and carries a variety in your price range. Before entering the store, narrow your selection. Discuss these choices and your running history with the salesperson. Ask him or her to give you three to five different models to choose from. A good local store will, or should, have experienced salespeople who are also runners and who will know about good running shoes. They should also listen to their customers about what works and doesn't, and the store manager should keep on top of shoe trends and runners' needs. Most good local stores will take your shoes back if you aren't satisfied with them after a run or two. (But don't expect them to take the shoes back after you've logged a lot of mileage, and wear, in them.)

Local stores and salespeople should also know about local races that you may want to enter, or special group runs or classes that may help you in your training. Often these stores also get involved in promoting the sport in your community. You should return the favor when it comes time to buy shoes and other running gear.

3. According to Andy Kimerling, owner of the Westchester Road Runner store in White Plains, New York, where I buy my shoes, a good salesperson will ask about your mileage, how often you run, what surfaces you run on, your immediate running goals. Are you a beginner runner or a runner training for a marathon? You should also describe any tendency to injury or whether you pronate or supinate (as discussed later in this chapter). Bring in your old worn running shoes, if you have them, so the salesperson can see your wear pattern. Kimerling emphasizes that this is very important, "as your old shoes will clearly show the type of shoe you need. The tread wear and stress on the shoe upper will give the shoe salesperson information to guide in his or her advice as to your individual needs." Don't get caught up in the latest popular shoe fad, or ask for the same shoe your friend wears.

4. Now, determine proper shoe size. Have the salesperson measure your foot for length and width. Be sure to measure both feet, since they may differ. Shepherd finds that in some brands the 9½ fits best, but in others he takes a 10 or 10½. Maybe he should run barefoot? Your shoe size will also change—get

bigger—as you run more and grow older. Therefore, have the salesperson measure your feet every time you buy new running shoes.

5. Choose a pair of shoes that fit both feet while you are standing. Try on *both* shoes of the pair; do not assume that since one shoe fits they both will. Always try on the shoes wearing your running socks. Most stores will provide a pair of running socks if you do not have yours with you. Try to shop in the afternoon or evening—or after a run—when your feet are slightly larger due to the natural swelling from normal activity.

6. Allow some room for expansion: feet swell by as much as half a size on long runs in warm weather. Shoes that are too tight in the toe box may cause cramping of the toes, black toenails, or blisters. Shoes that are too long may slide and create blisters, or even curling of the toes, which in turn may cause cramping in the calves or lower back problems.

I need my running shoes to be tight or else I curl my toes, which creates all sorts of painful problems. Most runners need about a thumbnail's width between your longest toe (not necessarily your big toe) and the end of the shoe. You should be able to wiggle your toes freely inside the shoes.

If you are uncertain about which size to go with, take the larger. You can always fill in with padded insoles; your feet will also swell on the run. Shepherd and I also have the problem where one foot is slightly larger than the other. We both fit the larger foot and ask the smaller to work a little harder.

The width should be snug but not pinched. Your foot should not bulge over the midsole material. A shoe too tight in width will not give good support and may cause your feet to numb and cramp due to lack of circulation. On the other hand, a shoe that is too loose will slide and cause blisters and leg problems. Be sure that the heel counter—the cup around the heel—fits firmly but not too tightly. Too loose or too tight, it may cause blisters or Achilles tendinitis. If the shoe is too tight across your instep, start the laces at the second pair of eyelets.

Here's another tip: Once you find a shoe you like, hold onto it but try on one size or a half size larger and smaller for comparison—to be sure.

7. Take your time. Ask more questions. Try on more shoes for comparison (but hold onto the pair you like most). A good running shoe store will even let you take a test run around the block. If they get worried about this, offer to leave your credit card with the manager. (If you do so, be sure to get his or her name.)

8. Check the quality of the pair (or pairs) you select. Place the shoe on a flat surface, such as a countertop. Look at the heel counter to see if it is perpendicular to the sole of the shoe and check for other imbalances. Look for loose threads. Feel the seams inside the shoe to make sure they are uniform, smooth, and well-stitched. Check the quality of the laces and eyelets. Make sure the sole layers are evenly and completely glued to each other and to the upper. Look and feel for lumps and bumps inside the shoe.

9. Check for flexibility. Bend the shoe. Keep in mind that as you break in new running shoes, their flexibility will increase. The shoe may feel stiff when new, but it should flex about 30 to 35 degrees as you bend it with both hands—about the same amount as when you push off your toes. If the shoe is not flexible under the ball of the foot, then the front and back of your leg may get stressed, with resulting injury to your Achilles tendon, calf, or shin muscles.

Seek a balance between flexibility and cushioning under the ball of your foot. The more cushion in the shoe, however, the less flexible it will be. Most quality running shoes are flexible. If in doubt, ask the salesperson for advice.

10. Now check for cushioning. A well-cushioned shoe will minimize road shock to your legs and is recommended for most beginner runners. Cushioning comes from three sources:
- The outersole, which wears out from contact with the ground.
- The insoles, which come with the shoe or can be purchased separately to increase cushioning.
- The midsole, between the other two, which provides the most critical protection.

11. Check out the shoe weight. With the shoe in your hands, feel its weight. The beginner runner, attempting to increase mile-

age, should buy a well-cushioned, supportive shoe that may weigh more than the advanced runner's shoes. Your concern is protection. Most running shoes are made from lightweight materials anyway, and the difference in weight between training shoes will not be important in terms of time or distance to the beginner runner. As you increase your speed and distance, you may want to try lighter weight training shoes or even racing shoes.

Breaking in Shoes

Most running shoes today are easy to break in. The uppers are very soft and, if you follow the guidelines above, you should come home with a flexible pair of shoes. Still, in general try these three steps recommended by Andy Kimerling for breaking in new running shoes:

1. Walk around in your new shoes for a mile or two. Stay alert to any rubbing, poor fit, bumps inside the shoes, or other conditions that might give you difficulty on your runs.

2. Next, try them out on a short run. Again, pay very close attention here to how your shoes fit and wear.

3. If all goes well after a short run, go ahead and run daily in your new shoes. Now pay attention to how your whole body reacts. If you have problems, you might want to run in your old shoes for a while and make the transition more gradual. Run short and medium distances in your new shoes for at least a week before running long distances of over 10 miles, or using them for a race.

Specialized Running Shoes

The Heavy Runner

No two people, and therefore no two runners, are shaped the same. Some runners are large, maybe overweight, but trying to lose with running; some are big-boned but otherwise physically fit; others are simply tall and thus weigh more. Whatever the reason, the more you weigh, the greater the impact force of your body on the ground (and the shock to your feet and legs) when you run. Heavier runners frequently have wide, flat feet and often overpronate.

If you fall within this category, look for shoes with a wide toe box and lots of support for pronation. While elite runners may want a light shoe, the heavier runner should exchange lightness for cushioning, durability, and support. This means a somewhat heavier shoe. Some companies make shoes specifically for larger runners. Ask your running store salesperson to help with recommendations.

Unusual Foot Sizes

Most running shoes come in sizes up to 15 for men and 11 for women. Half sizes are usually not available in shoes larger than 13. Women with large feet may be able to select a men's shoe. This is not ideal, but it's a better choice than not running at all.

New Balance offers most of its shoes in four or more widths to accommodate those runners with wide or narrow feet. Other companies make some models in a variety of widths but may not publicize it. Ask your running store salesperson for assistance with this. You can also make a wide shoe fit better by adding insoles or by using shoes with variable-width lacing systems.

Overpronation and Supination

If your foot rolls inward a great deal when you run, you may be overpronating. Runners with this condition tend to have highly flexible feet and may suffer from runner's knee, shin splints, iliotibial band syndrome, or tendinitis. You can tell because your shoes will be more broken down on the inner border than on the outer. My heel counters slope inward with use in all but my most super-stable training shoes. In general, a straight-lasted shoe with good foot control—a hard heel counter and firm midsoles—is better for the runner who overpronates.

If, however, your foot rolls outward excessively when you run, you may be oversupinating. These runners tend to have rigid feet that cannot absorb shock well and are prone to ankle strains, stress fractures, shin splints, plantar fasciitis, and knee pain. Do not think you have these conditions unless they are chronic and persist over time—say, more than a week. (Obviously, a stress fracture should be checked immediately.) You will notice that your shoes may be compressed on the outside. A slip-lasted shoe or combination-lasted shoe with lots of cushioning, heel support, and a flexible forefoot will serve you best.

If you are experiencing chronic, persistent problems like those mentioned above, check with a podiatrist to determine if you are pronating or supinating. Then, see if your shoe salesperson, working with information from your podiatrist, can find a shoe that benefits you. If the problems continue, you may be a candidate for orthotics to correct the condition (as discussed later in this chapter). Remember, however, that many runners do not pronate or supinate enough to require orthotics; sometimes less expensive inserts will correct, or at least ease the problem.

Motion Control or Cushioning?

Most running shoes emphasize either shock absorption to provide maximum cushioning or motion control for stability. Which should you emphasize? The more cushioning you get, the less motion control. Some shoes try to strike a balance and provide some features of both. You may want to experiment over a year or so to see which you need. Your sports podiatrist and running store shoe salesperson will also help you make this choice.

Does One Size Fit All, or Do Women Need Special Shoes?

For years, women were neglected by the running shoe companies, primarily because they were seen as only a small percentage of the running market (which was predominantly male, like the shoe company executives). At first, women had to get by with men's shoes, then running shoe companies offered scaled-down versions of the men's models in colors that appealed to women.

That compromise was insufficient because the anatomy of a woman's foot is different from, and not simply a smaller version of, a man's foot. For example, in general, a woman's forefoot is wider and her heel is narrower relative to length than a man's. A woman's size 10 shoe is roughly equivalent to a man's size 8½, but a woman's size 10 is ¼- to ½-inch narrower in the heel. (Generally, women's shoes are 1½ sizes larger in number than men's for the same approximate foot size.) Women who bought men's running shoes found that their heels slipped. If they fit the shoes for a snug heel, then the shoes were too tight in the forefoot. Also, women tend to pronate more than men (because they are wider in the hips) and weigh less than men of equal height. Thus they require more motion control and less cushioning in shoes than men do.

Today, large numbers of women are running for fitness, and they make up a significant share of the running shoe market. Not surprisingly, the shoe companies now produce several excellent shoes designed only for women, incorporating technology specific to them. Moreover, in a nice turn of events, women with wide feet also have the choice of buying men's running shoes. Whether you prefer the fit of men's or women's styles, make sure they fit your foot properly. Notes *Runner's World* shoe tester Tom Brunick, "About 90 percent of female runners buy shoes which are actually too small for them."

"To Be Discontinued"

It sure gets annoying when I find the perfect running shoe for me —and then the company discontinues it. Shepherd ran two New York City Marathons in a terrific model of Adidas, but when he went to purchase his third pair—discontinued! After a decade of searching, a running colleague found the perfect New Balance shoe. Then—discontinued! What's going on here? Bob Wischnia, shoe review specialist for *Runner's World*, writes:

> Running shoe companies turn over shoe models for one simple reason: to stimulate sales. Some of the changes in running shoes are purely cosmetic—a new color or a new look for the upper. Many of the changes, however, are in design or materials. The industry has become technology driven, and every running shoe company wants to claim the most advanced design and the latest materials. So the folks in Research and Development fiddle with the shoe, and before you know it, your favorite is gone, replaced by the latest and greatest. Often, it's an improvement. Other times, it's not. Regardless, the replacement doesn't feel exactly like the old shoe.

> If you learn that your favorite running shoe is being phased out, you might want to buy two or three pairs—try each of them on! —and stock up. But sooner or later you will literally run out. What to do? First, don't be influenced by the latest hype over the newest high-tech shoe. Try out other models. Take your old shoe to your running shoe store and ask for help. Beg them to save your feet! This is serious, believe me. You will want to get a shoe with the same or similar last, midsole, cushioning, flexibility, and motion control. You may even find a shoe you like better.

Yikes! As I finish this chapter I've learned that the trusty shoes I've worn during my comeback have been discontinued. I protest!

What About Cross-Trainers?

Beginner runners sometimes ask me, "Can I start running in my tennis shoes?" My answer: "That's better than not starting at all." But running shoes are made specifically for running and offer the best cushioning and protection. Therefore, it is better to start your running program with good running shoes.

But what about cross-trainers? They are advertised as being good for all sports. You could save a bundle that way, right? If you are only running short distances of a mile or two once or twice a week and the shoes give you good cushioning and support, this may be an acceptable compromise. But remember that sports which require lateral motion—tennis, for example—have thinner soles so you won't catch your foot and turn an ankle. Thus, you gain motion but give up the cushioning needed for running. Adds Andy Kimerling, "In general, cross-trainers are not for running."

Street Shoes Are Important, Too

Your feet spend more hours a week inside street shoes than running shoes. Poorly fitting street shoes with little support can also cause problems for your feet and your running. Many runners think they can solve this problem by wearing running shoes most of the day. But wearing the same type of shoe may cause injury from the lack of variety of stress for the foot. On the other hand, wearing street shoes like "loafers" and "wing tips" that have thin and hard soles may hurt your feet. The lack of shock absorption may injure your back or knees. High, loose-fitting heels in boots can irritate the Achilles tendon in your heel and Topsiders, which lack support, may cause heel spurs and can irritate the Achilles tendon, too. The worst shoe is a woman's high heels. Dr. Bill Feigel, a podiatrist writing in *Runner's World*, warns: "Women beware! Look at your feet. If you're wearing high heels, kick them off. Burn them. Use them for kindling."

Any shoe with a heel higher than one inch is detrimental to the health of your feet. A 2-inch heel causes even more harm by lifting the foot into a higher position; 3-inch heels may be lethal. And the damage doesn't stop at your feet. Wearing high heels can result in injuries to your ankles, calves, knees, hips, and back.

The problems start at the tips of your toes. Most high heels stuff the toes into the front of your shoe. They shift your body weight to the forefoot, which places great stress on the metatarsal heads (where the toes connect to the rest of your foot). Your foot screams in agony and produces corns, bunions, ingrown toenails, or heel spurs in rebellion. High heels may also shorten the calf muscles or Achilles tendon. They are flimsy and cause ankle sprains and falls. If you have to wear heels, at least get low ones with a wider heel platform, which will distribute your weight more evenly and make balancing easier.

So what to wear? As with running shoes, make sure the shoes you walk around in all day provide a stable heel, plenty of toe room, support in the arch, and adequate cushioning. Make sure they are replaced if they break down. I found this out the hard way when a pair of running shoes I used just for walking slanted inward and aggravated a hip problem. If you have just started running, or are increasing your mileage, do not be surprised if you need a shoe size up to one and a half your normal shoe size. Feet may swell with running. Remember, any problems with daily street shoes will carry over into your running shoes and your running.

Fortunately, there are excellent brands of health shoes such as Rockport, Clark's, and Easy Spirit that give you good cushioning and support with reasonable fashion. Several running shoe companies like New Balance and Nike make dress shoes for walking. I wear a combination of these types of shoes and cross-training shoes, which feel a bit different on my feet than my usual running shoes. I cannot walk far in thin-soled dress shoes without foot and back pain. To air out my feet and still get good support (instead of slippers or sandals), I wear specially designed sport sandals like those made by Teva or Nike. They provide a foot bed similar to a running shoe and adjustable straps to hold the sandals to your feet instead of flopping around.

Do I Need Special Shoes for Racing?
Racing shoes won't make you faster, but they may allow you to run your best. According to the accepted standard, for every ounce you take off your feet, you will save about a second per mile. The average racing shoe is 3.5 ounces lighter than training shoes; a typical size 9 training shoe weighs 11 ounces and a racing shoe weights 7.5 ounces. Thus, a 40-minute 10K runner wearing the lighter racing shoes could theoretically improve his or her time by 24 seconds and a 3-hour marathoner could improve by 1 minute, 48 seconds. That's the theory.

The fact is that racing shoes are made for speed, not injury prevention. In exchange for lightness and flexibility, the racing shoe takes away cushioning (about 15 percent less), support, durability, and stability. There is less heel lift, which may injure your Achilles tendons, and the curved last may fit much differently from your training shoes. Thus, there is greater risk of injury than in the heavier training shoe. Moreover, if your body is taking more of a beating you may actually run slower in racing shoes despite the advantage of less weight.

A common mistake among runners is to wear racing shoes when they are not necessary. I recommend that beginner racers stick to their heavier training shoes for at least their first several races and their first few marathons. See how it feels. The next step, then, is a lightweight training shoe for races. Who should wear racing shoes? Those runners who are racing at a 7-minute-per-mile pace or faster, and those who are light on their feet and without bio-mechanical problems. Still, I prefer the extra protection of racing in lightweight trainers.

Wear your racing shoes during a few short runs and speed work-outs to break them in before racing. If you have leg or joint pain after training in your racing shoes, you may need to switch back to your training shoes. Start with races of 10K and under. At these distances the benefits of racing shoes may "outweigh" the disad-vantages. Very few runners, however, should wear racing shoes for the pounding that takes place during longer runs, especially the marathon distance. Remember also that racing shoes break down faster than training shoes, so monitor their wear and cushioning properties regularly.

I want to emphasize again that the majority of runners should stick to regular training shoes or lightweight training shoes for racing.

How Long Will My Shoes Last?

Forever, if you don't wear them. More likely, says Dr. Gary Gor-don, a podiatrist at the University of Pennsylvania Sports Medicine Center, running shoes lose significant shock-absorbing character-istics after 200 to 400 miles of running. If you run 25 miles a week, you should change your shoes every three months. If you run 10 miles a week, you should change running shoes after at least six months. Other experts say running shoes should last 500 miles. So I'll give you a range. Most shoes wear out between 300 and 500 miles.

Why worry about this? Well, when your running shoes lose their cushioning and can't absorb the road shocks anymore, that shock has to go somewhere. That's usually through your foot, up your shin, into your knees or hips or back. And that's a pain.

The shock absorbing capacity (SAC) of running shoes has been measured by researchers at the Tulane University School of Medicine. In machine-simulated tests, the midsoles retained 85 percent of SAC for the first 50 miles, 65 percent after 100–150 miles, and about 50 percent after 500 miles. Racing shoes break down much sooner and should be replaced after 300 miles or when they lose their bouncy feeling. Heavy runners and those whose feet strike the ground hard may wear out shoes sooner than this average. Running on soft trails will also extend shoe life. Note that unused shoes sitting around on store shelves or in your closet for a year or longer may lose some cushioning, too.

It used to be easy to tell when to replace your running shoes: when the outsole wore out. But now the outsole is so durable in many models that it often lasts longer than the midsole. If the outer sole is not worn down don't assume that your running shoe is fine. For many runners, by the time wear appears on the outer sole, the midsole—that supportive, cushion area between the outer and inner soles—may be shot. Midsoles break down with use as well as exposure to heat, sunlight, salt, and such.

So the new trick is to watch your midsole. When it starts losing its cushion and support qualities, it's time for a change of shoes. You may be able to determine this by pressing on the midsole with your thumb to check the material's "bounce" or cushion. A good salesperson can also tell you. I can tell that my midsoles have lost bounce because my back and legs start to feel tight after a few miles. Another test is to try on a new pair of the same or similar type of shoe and run in them. If you feel a significant difference in cushioning between the old and the new, you probably should make the switch. Some runners buy two pairs of shoes at the same time. They compare the ones they use daily with the newer ones every month, and they switch to the new ones (and buy another pair) when they notice a significant difference in cushioning.

Here are some more tips on how to know when you need to replace your running shoes:

- If you feel pain in the feet, ankles, shins, knees, and hips. Often your bones will feel the wear before you muscles do.

■ If your feet feel fatigued after running.

■ If the material in the toe box is thin or worn.

■ If the tread pattern is worn down—usually on the ball of the foot or the heel. If you wear down the outersoles unevenly and sooner than 200–300 miles, you might want to consider having them resoled or even use specially made materials to patch them up. But remember, if you've logged more than 300 miles in a pair of running shoes, the midsole is likely to be worn out. Get another pair of shoes.

■ If the heel counter breaks down. Give them this test: Put your shoes on a flat table and look at them from behind. If they roll too much in or out without you in them, throw them out. I used to go through shoes this way after just a few weeks until I started using a very rugged shoe that prevents pronation.

Log in your training diary the miles you have run in each pair of shoes. Number your shoes with an indelible pen to tell them apart and keep track of the mileage. Obviously, if you alternate pairs of shoes each will last a longer period of time, but not more miles. By monitoring the mileage, wear, feel of the cushioning of each pair of running shoes you can avoid or minimize injury by switching to newer shoes.

Care and Repair—How to Make Running Shoes Last Longer

Treat your running shoes like you would treat a new car. The better you take care of them, the longer they will last. Mother Nature can be tough on running shoes. Rain, snow, mud, sweat all contribute to accelerating the breakdown of the materials in the shoes. Here are a few tips to help your shoes last longer:

■ Rotate running shoes. Your shoes should dry for at least twenty-four hours if they get wet from sweat, rain, or snow. Both pairs will wear longer. Further, the midsoles heat up when you run. Alternating shoes allow them to cool, thus the cushioning holds up longer. And if you keep two pairs of shoes going you have a backup if the dog eats a shoe!

■ Store shoes in a cool, dry place where they can air out adequately—not in a locker or sports bag, or a stuffy stairwell.

■ If your shoes become wet, loosen the laces and open the tongue of the shoe. Pull out the insoles and allow them to air dry, or stuff them with newspaper. This will wick out the moisture and help the shoes retain their shape and fit. Studies at Tulane University indicate that shoes which are wet provide significantly less shock protection.

■ Avoid exposing the shoes to direct heat like a radiator or woodstove or hair dryer. Don't leave your shoes out in the direct sunlight or in the hot trunk of your car for a long time. Heat dries out leather and other materials in the shoe and it softens glue, causing it to lose its adhesion. Heat may also damage the midsoles and cause the shoe to curl or twist, thus changing the way it fits your foot.

■ Use foot powder to keep shoes dry, kill fungus and bacteria, control odor, and neutralize the corrosive acids in perspiration. Most shoes can be washed by hand with a soft brush, mild soap, and cold water. Then let them air dry.

As mentioned, if your shoes wear down unevenly you may want to fix them with a commercial shoe repair kit. Do not do this if you have logged more than 300 miles in those shoes. Gary Muhrcke, owner of the Super Runners Shops in New York City, recommends doing the smallest repair possible to preserve the structure of the shoe. "Don't replace the whole sole," he suggests. "The entire shape and structure will be different and that can throw off your stride and possibly cause an injury. It is also important to repair unevenly worn shoes before the wearing-down becomes severe." Many running shoe stores will repair your running shoes.

Running in Snow and Cold
Afraid of slipping and falling in snow and ice? The best bet for "snow tires" are shoes with waffle-type soles that give a strong grip. Or you can go with studded shoes. John Schliffe, an exercise physiologist, trains in the snow in Anchorage, Alaska. He puts ⅜-inch hex-head screws into the outsole of his shoes for his runs

in the snow and ice. He uses pliers to grasp the head of the screw and after a few turns it bites in. When the screw heads wear down, John replaces them. He puts eight to ten screws into each shoe. Let's admit it, this is a screwy idea, but John has never fallen since he studded his shoes. (Does this make John a running stud?)

Another option: snowshoe running. Santa brought me a pair of lightweight aluminum snowshoes that strap on over running shoes. They weigh less than 3 pounds each and come with steel cleats to grip into snow and ice. I'm able to run over packed snow and ice on my wooded trails most of the winter now!

Midsoles can lose up to 25 percent of their cushioning ability on a 20° F. day. This reduction in shock absorption, combined with the stress from the harder cold surface, increases your chance of injury. Sometimes, however, these things even out: Shepherd runs all winter long in Vermont and has logged workouts in weather down to −45°F. (including the windchill). He notices that the colder the temperature, the slower he runs; therefore, the softer his impact on the ground.

Whatever the temperature outside, keep your shoes indoors where it's warm. You might want to add shock-absorbing insoles for cold winter days, or at least run in thick woolen socks (or add a layer of socks). You might want to select a shoe with extra cushioning for cold-weather runs.

Shoe Stuffings

Insoles

One significant and beneficial running shoe innovation during the last two decades has been the addition of removable insoles or sock liners to the running shoe. Removable insoles can be tossed out if you don't like them or need more room. They may be replaced with commercial insoles or orthotics.

The insoles that come with your running shoes are usually constructed of a plastic foam that molds to the shape of your foot. They may provide some extra cushioning and motion control. Some are also treated to reduce friction and thus blisters on your feet caused by rubbing. Obviously, if you are going to insert commercial insoles or orthotics into your running shoes, bring them to the shoe store and insert them into the shoes before you buy them. Do not wait to do this until you bring the shoes home.

Commercial insoles can be purchased at most running shops and drugstores. They are simply inserted into your running shoes in place of the insoles that came with your shoes. These commercial insoles help absorb moisture, reduce blistering, and absorb shock. They can also be used to adjust your shoe size. They may give some support and control to your foot. Sorbothane, Spenco, and Dr. Scholl's are among the more popular insoles available commercially.

Insoles will increase the weight of your running shoes. You may wish to replace them with lighter insoles for speed workouts or races. Or you may add heel pads only, which are shorter and thus lighter. It's a trade off: The insoles add weight, but they also increase protection from injury.

But do they really provide more shock absorption? Dr. Benno M. Nigg and a team of researchers at the Biomechanics Laboratory at the University of Calgary in Canada reported that these special insoles do not provide a more significant amount of additional impact reduction than the insoles that already come with the running shoes. Still, some podiatrists suggest adding both: a light commercial insole over the insole already in the shoe.

It really comes down to personal experience. I've found that special insoles designed to absorb maximum shock really make a difference when I'm doing high mileage on hard surfaces. They leave my legs feeling less fatigued. The best trick I've found for reducing shock and leg fatigue, however, is running on dirt trails rather than harder surfaces. Shepherd suffered from sciatica to the point where he could hardly walk 100 feet, let alone run. After an expensive and fruitless round with podiatrists, he went out and bought a pair of insoles at his favorite running shop, stuck them in his street shoes, and started walking. He was in Kenya at the time, and walked all over Nairobi. The pain disappeared, the insoles next went into his running shoes, and he was off again! You can also add cushioning with thick socks, like those made by Thorlo. Whatever you do, don't overstuff your running shoes. You can lose support at the heel, or cause your toes to jam.

Heel Lifts and Heel Cups

A heel lift may allow you to continue training even when you are troubled by shin splints, Achilles tendinitis, plantar fasciitis, or calf soreness. By raising the heel of the running shoe, you are reducing the strain on the Achilles tendon and the lower leg muscles, thus minimizing the discomfort and helping prevent further strain. A "lift" of ⅛ to ¼ inch will help absorb impact shock and spread your weight over a greater area of the heel. This may ease discomfort from heel bruises or spurs.

Heel lifts or pads may be purchased over-the-counter, or you can cut them out of surgical felt or sponge rubber powder puff pads. Make sure the lift isn't so high that your foot no longer fits the shoe. Wear the lifts in both shoes, or you may cause an injury due to imbalance. Continue wearing the lifts several days after the problem subsides. Build the lifts to a height that gives relief, and then gradually reduce the lift until you no longer need it.

Heel lifts may ease your discomfort and keep you out of a doctor's office. Heel cups are also available in pharmacy and running stores. These devices control movement of the heel, and absorb or distribute impact over a greater surface, thereby relieving pain.

Orthotics

This is a big topic of debate among runners. Orthotics are inserts that you place inside your shoes to change the tilt of your feet as they strike the ground. Podiatrists often compare orthotics to eyeglasses: eyeglasses correct poor eyesight, orthotics correct poor footstrike. In theory, orthotics place the foot in a neutral position and allow it to strike the ground "normally." In addition, they help add more stability to the foot.

More than 500,000 pairs of orthotics are prescribed for sports enthusiasts in the United States every year. Many end up in running shoes. Most are prescribed by podiatrists, but some by orthopedists, chiropractors, and physical therapists. For many runners, including myself, they are saviors.

Back in the 1960s, when orthotics were not available, I suffered from knee pain that ended my collegiate athletic career. I was told that surgery would be necessary and I'd never play sports again. I accepted this condition until 1975 when I met Dr. Richard Schuster, a pioneer in sports podiatry and the crafting of customized orthotics. Dr. Schuster, working over several months, designed and adjusted an orthotic for my shoes. Within three years I was running 100 miles a week pain free and racing marathons. Now, Dr. Schuster and his colleague, Dr. Murray Weisenfeld, periodically upgrade my orthotics to keep me on the run.

Orthotics are not a panacea for all pain or injury from running or exercise. Yet surveys show that about 25 percent of the runners who enter the New York City Marathon wear orthotics and approximately half of the high-mileage runners wear them. Not all these runners need orthotics, although many runners who increase their mileage develop problems that are helped by wearing them.

But they are now also a status symbol: As many as half of all runners wearing orthotics do not need them. Sometimes they are overprescribed by doctors. Sometimes runners insist on them. Dr. Schuster advises: "Unless there are severe imbalances, or pain related to imbalances, the indiscriminate use of orthotic foot devices could stir up a hornet's nest of other problems."

Orthotics, necessary or not, can indeed cause problems. I've seen runners with mild aches and pains that became worse when they inserted prescribed orthotics into their running shoes. (I'm not talking about insoles.) The late Dr. George Sheehan detailed several reasons why orthotics fail to work: they are difficult to fit and mold; they impair the runner's flexibility; rear-foot correction is sometimes excessive; they need adjusting and runners don't bother following up with the adjustments. Badly fitted orthotics, Dr. Sheehan said, "can make you worse as well as better."

Should you buy orthotics? Studies show that between 40 and 75 percent of long-distance runners who wear orthotics report great improvement or complete recovery from a long list of painful conditions. Dr. Mark Caselli, chief of orthopedics at the New York College of Podiatric Medicine, offers this advice: "If you get pain in your feet or legs only during athletic activities, or you have obvious skeletal flaws such as flat feet, orthotics can certainly help." In other words, chronic pain may indicate a biomechanical imbalance that could be corrected with orthotics. The range of possible problems is large: you may pronate or supinate, the front of your foot may need support, you may have one leg shorter than the other, your feet may be too flexible or not flexible enough, and so on. To determine if you are a candidate, Dr. Caselli suggests looking at your sports shoes. If the soles wear out unevenly or too fast, or if the upper part of the shoe deteriorates very quickly, your feet may be unstable in the shoe.

But orthotics are expensive. Before going to custom-made orthotics and the agony of adjustments, first try commercial over-the-counter orthotics. Available at most running stores, they are contoured to the shape of the average foot, and modified to reduce excessive pronation. Runners who think they need professionally fitted orthotics may wish to use one of these devices first. They may help with mild pronation problems or cushioning. Shepherd, for example, developed a slight knee problem, and acting on my free advice he purchased a pair of over-the-counter orthotics, wore them until the pain went away, tossed them in the back of his closet, and never needed them again.

If your running pain lessens using commercial orthotics, but doesn't go away, or if your symptoms return with an increase in mileage, you may wish to consult a sports podiatrist to see if you need custom-made orthotics. Commercial orthotics are sold by shoe size, and may produce results if your foot size is close to the model used. But many runners have slight differences in arch height, leg length, and range of motion not adequately corrected by these standard devices. Most over-the-counter orthotics wear out at about the same rate as your shoes, so be prepared to replace them when you buy new shoes.

If you do need custom-made supports, a podiatrist trained in the craft is your best bet. The podiatrist will perform a series of tests to check biomechanical weaknesses. She or he will also ask you questions about your training and injury patterns, and examine your shoe wear. An early first step may be for the podiatrist to try out some shaped, leather pads with special felt panels glued underneath to lift them in areas specific to your complaint and foot problems. These may be worn for several weeks to determine their effect on your pain.

The next step may be prescribed orthotics. Most orthotics are fashioned in a lab from a plaster or foam mold of your foot. They are corrected over several weeks by your podiatrist and the lab to adjust to the structural weaknesses of your feet. Breaking them in may also take time.

In general, orthotics fall into three groups: rigid, semi-rigid (the most common), and soft (for people with minor problems). The material needs to be rigid enough to control pronation, but malleable enough to facilitate natural movement. The orthotic can be made from a variety of substances, but most are now constructed from strong, light, and relatively flexible polypropylene. A more temporary orthotic is constructed from plastizote, a Styrofoam-like material used to help in overcoming specific injuries.

When breaking in orthotics, first wear them while walking and then gradually increase their use when running. If they do not feel right, have them adjusted. (Follow your podiatrist's advice about this.) Most runners only need minor adjustments. My feet are fussy and my orthotics required several adjustments. You may need to have your orthotics readjusted every few years as they wear and your needs change. If you wear orthotics, remove the insole that came with the shoe, or at least cut out the arch support like I do, to help make the shoe fit your foot and to avoid interference with the orthotic's function.

What Shoe Should I Use with Orthotics?

Ask your podiatrist and shoe salesperson about the best running shoes for people wearing orthotics. The shoes should be straight lasted or slightly curved, and have removable sock liners. Shoe charts will assist you on this choice, too.

When trying on running shoes, be certain to bring your orthotics and insert them into every pair. Do both feet. Remove the shoe insoles so they won't interfere with fit and feel.

Should I Race with Orthotics?

According to a study at Arizona State University's Department of Health and Physical Education, orthotics increase, not decrease, the energy cost of running—that is, you'll run slower wearing orthotics. Actually, in the Arizona tests by Drs. Lee Burkett, Wendy Kohrt, and Richard Buchbinder, running barefoot turned out to be the best way to go, followed by running in regular shoes, with running in shoes with orthotics coming in last. For the fitness runner, the extra energy used due to the added weight is probably offset by the absence of pain and the need to prevent injury. According to the Arizona study, orthotics increased the energy cost by about 1.7 percent—that might reduce running speed by as much as 5 meters per minute.

And as is so often the case, another study shows different results. Researchers at the Spaulding Rehabilitation Hospital in Spaulding, New Hampshire, tested runners with and without their orthotics on a treadmill for oxygen consumption. Despite the extra weight, there was no difference in the results. They theorized that the orthotics make up for the extra weight by allowing the runners to run more economically due to the correction of biomechanical problems. The lesson of all these studies is really simple: Don't fear losing precious seconds off your race times at the risk of injury and discomfort.

We are talking about a very fine edge in running here. Standard orthotics add just 2 ounces to your training shoes. You can compromise. Wear lighter, soft orthotics made of material like plastizote for races. Or have your doctor tape your feet for extra support. But what are we aiming for? Unless a few seconds in short races and a minute or two in marathons are very, very important to you, then I suggest you will be better off in your orthotics. My choice is to wear orthotics for racing—it is more important to me to keep from getting injured than to run perhaps a bit faster. Believe me, I have known the joy of personal victory after years of agony from de-feet.

SEVENTEEN

Apparel and Accessories

Picture this:

Me, Bob Glover, running in Central Park in skintight tights.

Check it out. Just look at the photo on the cover of this book.

That's not all. I can now wear sleek sunglasses that adjust to solar brightness, or run in the rain and not get soaking wet. I can run with a wristwatch that not only tells time but also lights in the dark, acts like a stopwatch, checks my pulse, and records and computes my pace and time per mile. Hey, I used to turn my wristwatch to twelve noon and count from there to time my runs and races.

I used to run in an old T-shirt and plain shorts, not in matching multicolored singlets and shorts. Where's my old faithful gray sweatshirt and red nylon windbreaker?

Gone forever? For better or worse, running clothes and accessories are now high tech and high fashion—and a multimillion-dollar industry. And this doesn't count running shoes! Old or young, slim or pudgy, you can look fast and slick in stylish running gear.

Because these advancements are changing so rapidly, this chapter can only give you an overview. We'll talk about the new fabrics, clothes, and equipment. But a more comprehensive report would be too long and soon out of date. Review this chapter and then head for your favorite running store and have fun exploring the new styles. But bring along several credit cards!

Also, keep one important thing in mind. You may look terrific and feel fast in these new high-tech, high-priced duds, but a runner's clothing has only two major purposes: warm weather clothes keep you cool and dry; cold weather clothes keep you warm and dry.

Fabrics

It used to be so simple. Runners wore cotton or wool socks, cotton T-shirts, and cotton or nylon shorts. Over that you wore a cotton sweatshirt and sweatpants, or maybe a nylon jacket. That was the good news. But the fabrics were often abrasive and caused chafing. The clothing stuck to you as you sweated. When it rained or snowed everything wicked up the water and drooped with the extra weight. You could get quite cold and uncomfortable. The nylon jacket let heat build up and sometimes caused overheating. Keeping dry and warm without overheating was always a problem on cold or rainy days.

Now the choice of fabrics changes almost weekly. Fiber technology has revolutionized the clothing industry. My old gray sweats ain't what they used to be: Today I can dress to prevent moisture and wind from getting in while allowing body heat and moisture from sweat to get out. And the changes and improvements keep coming. In fact, the apparel included as we write this section may well have changed by the time you read this. Only the principles of the clothing combinations remain.

The Old Fabrics

Cotton. This standby remains popular because it is cool and soft. But 100 percent cotton T-shirts are also expensive. Try a cotton blend, which is cheaper, doesn't shrink, and lasts longer. Cotton gets wet and clingy on hot sweaty runs. Also, when cotton gets wet it tends to dry slowly and promote heat loss from the body, thus it is not a good fabric for cold weather if you sweat heavily. Nor is it a good material for socks because wet socks can cause blisters.

Wool. The old-time, cold-weather favorite because it keeps you warm even when wet. But wool is itchy against the skin and is bulky.

Nylon. This fabric is lightweight, dries fast, holds body heat, washes easily, protects against the wind, and repels some rain. What's the problem? Nylon is a hot fabric and can allow heat to build up against your body. It doesn't "breathe" like the new fabrics, and thus prevents body heat from escaping. Moisture trapped inside your windbreaker may also cool you on cold winter days.

These old fabrics—cotton, wool, and nylon—are not as effective in keeping you warm and dry in cold weather and cool and dry in warm weather as the newer high-tech fabrics.

The New Fabrics

New innovations in warm-dry and cold-dry fabrics continue to improve comfort for runners each season. It is impossible to keep up with all the high-tech improvements, but I will list some of the most popular fabrics at the time we went to press.

Fabrics to Be Worn Against the Skin in Cold Weather

Polypropylene. Nicknamed "polypro," this old-new fabric was first popular with cross-country skiers. It is now found in outer and innerware, thermal underwear, socks, gloves, hats, and jacket linings—from head to toe you can be outfitted in polypro. Why is polypro so popular? It offers excellent insulation, lightweight protection, and "breathes" well. It traps warm air next to the skin while also "wicking" or removing moisture from it. As a result, your skin maintains a constant balance of heat and humidity without the dampness of other thermal fabrics like cotton. To be effective, polypro must be the first layer next to the skin and should fit snug so moisture passes through to the next layer.

On mild days, you need no fabric over polypro. On cold and wet days, a loose-fitting cotton or wool layer over it will keep you warm and absorb moisture. Polypro is not waterproof or windproof. It should be worn under a protective outer garment to keep you warm and dry. It will not work alone to keep heat next to your body. There are many other fabrics with similar properties. A common layering scheme for a cold day is a polypro shirt next to the skin covered by a short-sleeved or long-sleeve shirt and then a Gore-Tex jacket.

DryLete. This is one of my favorites. It was developed by Hind. Besides wicking moisture away it also keeps you warm and dry through a unique push/pull mechanism. The inner layer pushes moisture away from the body; the outer layer pulls the moisture to the surface to provide for quicker evaporation. This fabric doesn't require a second layer to absorb the wicked away moisture. DryLete can be worn in a wide range of weather to keep you warm but not too warm. On very cold days adding a windproof jacket will keep you dry and warm.

Fabrics for Outerwear Protection
Gore-Tex. This fabric is used in running suits and foul-weather gear. It lets body moisture out but won't let wind, rain, or snow in. It is almost completely waterproof. It insulates your body without letting you overheat, or get cold or wet. Gore-Tex works by allowing water and vapor to escape, but keeping wind and larger water drops out. It is especially effective on cold or rainy/snowy days over a fabric like polypro. There are other fabrics on the market with similar properties.

Windproof outerwear. Waterproof outerwear is fine for cold, wet days. However, the technology that keeps out rain doesn't let heat out as efficiently as windproof, water-repellent outerwear.

Other New Fabric Clothing
Coolmax. This stuff is real cool! Coolmax is made up of channeled polyester fibers, grooved to pull moisture away from your skin and allow for quick evaporation. It is ideal next to the skin on hot weather days to keep you from getting soaking wet. The fabric is lightweight and soft. It is used in shirts, singlets, shorts, and as liners in jackets. It is amazing to run without your sweaty clothes sticking to your sweaty body. Coolmax retains eight times less moisture than nylon, and fourteen times less moisture than cotton.

Fleece. Polyester fleece (such as Polartec) is warmer than wool and quicker drying, easier to care for and more durable. It is a great outer layer or, on very cold days, middle layer since fleece retains heat even when wet.

Lycra spandex. This is a form-fitting, stretchy material made by Du Pont that is used in tights and other clothing in combination with other fabrics to provide maximum comfort, mobility, and sleek good looks. It has the ability to stretch as much as 500 times its length, then return to its original shape.

Supplex. Supplex nylon is a popular outerwear used in shorts, windshells, etcetera. It feels like soft cotton and is lightweight, wind resistant, flexible, quick-drying, and tough. It also "breathes" and is water-repellent. Supplex is often blended with Lycra spandex.

ProCore. A soft material that wicks well. Composed of rayon, Du Pont polyester, and Lycra spandex, it is used in sport tops and tights.

Clothes

Okay, so I admit that one purpose of running clothes is looking good. But beyond high fashion we need clothing that protects us from the elements—cold, rain, heat, sun. There is a far wider choice of quality running clothing than when I started running more than thirty years ago.

What you wear can help you run your fastest. Looking and feeling great is important—it will help you get out the door and off running more often. Clothes, however, can make you run slower. The heavier the clothing and the more you wear, the slower you will run.

In this chapter we review various clothing choices. Specific guidelines for clothing for hot and cold weather (layering) running are detailed in Chapters 21 and 22.

Shirts/Singlets

Many runners prefer cotton blend T-shirts or singlets on hot days because they are comfortable and cool. The new singlets and shirts made with fabrics like Coolmax stay dry and are comfortable on hot, sweaty days. Their moisture transfer and evaporation properties will help keep you dry. Many runners are switching to these and saving the T-shirts they get at races for after the run. Test the differences with the new fabrics. Go for a run on a hot day in a cotton T-shirt. On a similar day try one of the new fabrics. You may be amazed. The T-shirt will be wet and heavy, but not the high-tech top.

In hot weather the key is coolness and comfort. Your shirts or singlets should have excellent ventilation, dry quickly, and feel

smooth against your skin. Soft fabrics and loose cuts are important. When trying on the clothes in the store, check for labels and
seams that might rub your skin.

Cotton and other materials may, when wet, cause chafing of the
nipples in men and women. To prevent this try applying petroleum
jelly to the area before you run. Or, select shirts or singlets that
have a panel of material such as nylon across the chest. Women's
singlets include a higher fit under the arms and wider shoulder
strap to cover their bra straps.

In cold weather a short- or long-sleeved polypro, Thermax, or
similar shirt should be worn against the skin, perhaps covered by
a fleece shirt. Shepherd adds an old cotton turtleneck on top with
an extra-long necksleeve that he can pull up over his mouth and
nose as needed.

Running Suits

Are those fancy running suits worth the cost? In a word, maybe.
The new fabrics solve the problems of repelling water, letting out
body moisture and warmth. But if you run for 30 minutes a day
or less, you probably don't need an expensive running outfit. A
nylon shell will hold the hot air in and keep the cold air out. Beyond 30 minutes of running, however, you might appreciate a
breathable windproof or waterproof suit. My waterproof suits tend
to overheat on mild days, so I go with the cooler, lighter windproof
suits and save my waterproof suit for those cold, rainy runs. But
if you have one running gift request from Santa, I'd definitely recommend a high-tech waterproof suit.

What are we looking for here? Waterproof, breathable fabrics
are great in bad weather, but in cold without rain or snow a soft
fleece jacket is fine. Shepherd even runs in an old turtle neck and
a light down vest. The shell should have a ventilated mesh lining
and a front or back vent. Zippered jackets (zip up and down to
adjust for warmth), with pockets and reflective stripes for running
in low visibility are also important.

What not to buy? Don't even think about running in rubberized
suits. Many years ago coaches and trainers thought that by sweating more you would melt fat. This is not true, although you will
lose some temporary water weight. Moreover, plastic or rubberized
clothing is dangerous: It prevents evaporation of perspiration,
which cools your body.

Shorts

As we write this, the most popular fabric for running shorts is a Supplex nylon short with a Coolmax liner. The liners should let your body "breathe" and wick moisture from the skin to keep you dry. Who knows what the fabric will be when you read this? Whatever the material, your running shorts should be comfortable, soft, loose, light, and fast drying. And they should fit you. The slits on the side should allow for a full stride. Some runners prefer shorts with Lycra/nylon, which are somewhat longer, like biker's shorts, and hug the body. There is a difference between women's and men's shorts: They are made to fit their specific body builds.

Tights

Running tights are usually made from Lycra combined with a soft fabric like Supplex. Tights come in all sorts of colors and styles, and you wear nothing under them but a brief or support. Tights made from materials such as polypropylene, or ProCore are heavier and add warmth in cold weather. Running tights are excellent for cold weather because they keep the legs warm and minimize the chance of muscle tightness. In most cold weather conditions you may find that your running tights will replace the need for pants. In very cold weather, I wear tights under my running pants for extra warmth.

If you want something a little more loose-fitting than the stylish tights, try a cotton-Lycra combination like SportHills or Hind's Munich Tight. These offer many of the advantages of running tights without making you feel naked. Tights are available with reflector stripes for running at dusk or in the dark.

Men's Supporters

The bulky cotton jockstrap is dead. It has been replaced by high technology. Most men prefer to wear running shorts with built-in briefs. Others like a separate sports brief made from a soft, seamless, absorbent stretch fabric. MAX produces a variety of supports for men including cotton blend/Lycra clothing that are a cross between underpants and the old jock. Coolmax briefs are extra cool. MAX's "CoolJock" has thin straps and offers support and comfort as does the jockstrap from Le Jacques and Sportjock.

The new support waist bands hold their shape and stretch much longer than the old jocks. They also provide some protection against cold. And getting those private parts wet and cold on a winter's day can be very uncomfortable, as well as dangerous. Special windbriefs, some with a nylon panel in front, made of polypro provide extra protection. One style affectionately called the Aussie—because it keeps you warm "Down Under."

Sports Bras

One of the most welcomed improvements in running clothes has been the sports bra for women. It used to be that women runners struggled with flimsy bras that were uncomfortable when running. Most major bra manufacturers now make at least one type of sports bra. But it didn't used to be that way. How was the running bra discovered?

In 1977, Lisa Lindahl and Hinda Miller, cofounders of Jogbra, Inc., were runners who couldn't find a bra that gave them support during their exercise. Fed up, says Lisa, "Hinda bought and sewed two jockstraps together, and when I wore it for running, it worked."

Today, women are even wearing sports bras as outerwear. What would my grandma have thought of that? Look around. You'll see women in sports bras of all colors and styles. "We always maintained that the proper sports bra is an essential piece of sports equipment," Lisa told *Runner's World*. "And now, women recognize that they need and will perform better with the right equipment. In some cases, a good sports bra actually empowers a woman to be athletic."

Not only do sports bras come in all sizes and colors, but they are also specialized to your activity: running, tennis, aerobics, basketball, and so forth. Sports bras are primarily designed to minimize breast discomfort that may occur during exercise. The support also helps to minimize breast discomfort just prior to a woman's monthly period.

Sports bras utilize one of two basic support systems: compression or encapsulation. Women with small breasts often favor the compression style, which presses both breasts against the chest wall in a single mass. Most women with large breasts prefer the encapsulation style in which each breast is held separately in a sturdy cup. Breast size is based on heredity and body fat, and since breasts are composed mostly of fat, breast size often decreases with an increase in running. Thus, your sports bra size need may change as you increase or decrease the amount of your exercise.

The most important thing—as with all sports clothing—is that

the sports bra fits you comfortably. A good sports bra should minimize breast motion but not be constricting. It should stretch horizontally, to allow you to pull it on and off, but not much vertically
(which would minimize support).

A sports bra is made from a nonabrasive, breathable material.
The bra should be comfortable and reduce the risk of chafing and
irritation by using seamless cups. It should have wide, nonslip
straps, roomy armholes, and a back design that spreads the weight
of your breasts. Finally, it should provide for a full range of arm
motion and prevent slippage. Some manufacturers use Coolmax
fabric inside the cups to help make them "breathe" and make them
cooler. Others also place mesh in the bottom of the cups and under
the armpits. To keep you dry in the winter, some sports bras come
in fabrics such as DryLete that wick away moisture.

Always try on the sports bra in the store before you buy. Run
in place or do some jumping jacks to get a feel for the bra and
check its support. Swing your arms in a running motion and raise
them over your head and take several deep breaths, expanding
your rib cage. The bra should not interfere with your movement
or breathing. Popular manufacturers include Jogbra, Jembra, Dan-
skin, and Olga.

There is some controversy concerning whether or not running
contributes to sagging breasts. Dr. Joan Ullyot, in her book *Wom-
en's Running*, argues that sagging breasts are not the result of
bouncing while running and that the only reason for wearing a bra
is comfort. Still, many women develop soreness after running without a bra. Some studies, for example one conducted at Oregon
State University by LaJean Lawson, an exercise physiologist, indicate that exercises like running may cause the breasts to bounce
and stretch with each footstrike. If the breasts are not supported,
the repeated stretching and rebounding may lead to permanent
stretching of the skin and to sagging breasts. Other experts maintain that the main factors that contribute to sagging breasts are
breast size, body weight, genetic makeup, and pregnancy. To be
more comfortable, most women will want to wear a sports bra
while running.

Gloves/Mittens
Should you wear gloves or mittens in cold weather? Being a Glover,
I prefer gloves, but I'll go to mittens on extremely cold days. Mit-
tens are warmer because the fingers are together and warm each

other. I also like polypro DryLete or Thermax gloves because they are very light, keep the moisture away, and don't let my hands overheat. Cotton gloves retain moisture when wet, which will make your hands cold. Gloves need to stay dry so you can stay warm.

Many runners prefer mittens to gloves. Shepherd is a mitten man and wears them throughout the winter in Vermont and England. His hands get so warm that he often removes the mittens during his runs and tucks them into the pouch of his sweatshirt. On bitter cold days, you might try a polypro or similar fabric glove as a liner with a mitten made of Gore-Tex, or other windproof, waterproof, breathable fabric. Can't make up your mind? Manzella produces a convertible glove/mitten with a flip top to set your fingers free.

Never throw your gloves or mittens away during a race or run. Tuck them into your shorts, stuff them into a pouch or pocket somewhere. If your hands get wet, or you turn back and face a head wind, you'll want those gloves to protect against frostbite.

Some runners prefer to run with their hands in their sleeves rather than wear gloves or mittens. Your hands should be kept free for balance.

Head Gear/Face Gear

To stay warm, keep your head covered. As much as 50 percent of your body heat escapes through the top of your head. A cap or hat traps that heat.

On cool days I like to wear a bike cap. Actually, this is one of those official New York City Marathon caps. It keeps me warm without overheating and protects my head from sunlight. On cold days, some runners prefer the old wool or wool blend hats, but polypro, Thermax, and other such fabrics are less bulky. Runners with enough hair (unlike me or Shepherd) to trap heat may prefer not to wear a hat but only a headband to protect their ears from frostbite. These also come in polypro, fleece, and other fabrics. On extremely cold days and nights you may combine the headband with one of those high-tech hats. You may unzip the hood from your jacket and pull it over your hat for extra protection and warmth. Your jacket should zip to make a high collar that protects your neck. Scarfs, turtlenecks, or neck gators can also be used to keep out the wind.

To protect their faces, some runners wear face masks that have openings cut out for the eyes and mouth. Many runners find these masks too restrictive. I prefer the polypro or balaclava (or head-gator), which serves as a hat and can be pulled down to fit over my mouth and nose for protection; there is a slit for the eyes. I can just pull it down over my chin if I get too hot around the mouth. Breathing through this in cold weather minimizes my asthma, which gets worse when I run in the cold. Face masks also come with extended necks.

Socks

Just reach in the drawer, pull out that pair of favorite running socks, and off you go, right? Not so fast. Even selecting socks is a high-tech choice now. Most running socks in the 1960s and 1970s were cotton with some acrylic; you wore wool socks in winter. Your only other choice was size and length. Now, most socks are 80 to 100 percent acrylic; the most popular acrylic fabrics are polypropylene, Coolmax, and Orlon sometimes blended with cotton, nylon, or other fabrics. Wool or a wool-polypropylene blend will keep your feet warm in winter and dry faster if you do get wet. You can also choose tube, regular, three-quarter length, or anklet styles.

Socks do more than keep your feet warm and dry. They also prevent blisters and protect your feet and shoes. Some runners try to run without socks, but this may cause blisters, abrasions, excessive foot odor as well as premature deterioration of the shoe. Blisters are a major concern. Dr. Douglas Richie, a podiatrist, and students at the California College of Podiatric Medicine conducted a study of 400 runners in the Long Beach Marathon to find out how socks affect blisters. They distributed among the runners commercially available socks made from cotton, wool, polypropylene, and acrylic; these included thin and thick socks, and double or single layer socks. Here's what they found:

1. Keep your feet dry. If your feet do get wet, it doesn't matter what kind of sock you're wearing. Blistering risk increases dramatically. Wet skin produces more friction and thus more blisters.

2. Cotton makes a great sock—when dry. But cotton absorbs moisture and wet cotton socks lose their shape and cushioning, and create blisters. Wool holds its shape a little better and dries faster. Synthetics like acrylic or Orlon don't absorb water into

the fibers but wick it away from the skin. The water can evaporate and your feet stay drier. In the California College study, acrylic socks had the lowest incident of blistering. Cotton had the highest. In fact, cotton socks resulted in twice as many blisters as acrylic socks—and the blisters were three times larger.

3. Thicker and more heavily cushioned socks caused fewer and less severe blisters than thinner socks.

Dirty socks also create blisters. Don't try to get an extra run out of your socks to save on laundry like some runners I know (admit it Shepherd!). Make sure your socks fit. If they are too loose they may bunch and cause blistering.

Equipment
Here are some of the newer equipment items that might tempt you. Even adults can have fun with toys!

Headsets
A little music may go a long way if you're running. But then why do they call it a Walkman? Running with a headset can be dangerous, as I detail in Chapter 24.

Heart Rate Monitors
These are wonderful gadgets that are fully explained in Chapter 8. They are helpful if you want to be sure you are running within your training heart rate range.

ID Tags
The safety value of these items, which are carried in most running stores, is detailed in Chapter 24. They may be bracelets, small cards for your shoes or running shorts pocket, little pouches, or other types of ID. Along with your name, they should include blood type, medication, home and work phone number, and other vital information.

Night Running Apparel
It is critical to your safety to be seen when running. This is true any time of day or night, but especially important after dark. Shepherd likes his bright orange reflective vest, the type used by high-

way crews—probably because it's inexpensive and he's a thrifty New Englander. He wears it during day or evening runs, in rain and snow, year-round.

There are all kinds of ways you can signal your presence on the road. You can buy jackets, tights, hats, even shoelaces that reflect light. You can get reflective tape to put on your favorite old gray sweats. A special blinking red light (Jogalite) powered by batteries can be attached to your body, usually your arm or waistband. This creates an unusual effect as you run: a blinking light that moves horizontally (your running path) and vertically (the motion of your arms, legs, or feet). Whichever reflective device you like, get one. And use it.

Runner's Watches

Computerized watches time your runs, give you split times for each mile of a race, and much more. Sports watches include alarms and pacing beepers (which may annoy other runners who are keeping track of their own pace). An inexpensive watch with a chronometer is a good investment since I believe it is better to run for a set period of time (say 30 minutes) than for distance. Watches with lights are great so you can check your times in the dark.

The price on these watches continues to fall so much that you can afford a high-priced watch for work and partying, then switch to the handy and inexpensive runner's watch when you lace up your shoes. I wear mine all the time and so does President Bill Clinton. That way when I decide to take off for a run I don't have to remember where I put it. Top manufacturers include Casio and Timex, and the watches are sold everywhere including large mall stores.

Sunglasses

Another trendy result of the running revolution. The Sunglass Association of America claims that sales of shades have tripled; more than one-third of those sales were in running, biking, and skiing sunglasses. Sporty sunglasses may protect your eyes from the sun's rays and make running more comfortable. They will definitely make you look cool.

But do you need them? Running in sunlight exposes you to the sun's ultraviolet (UV) rays. Extended UV exposure triples your risk of eye cataracts and increases your chances of developing keratitis from inflammation of the cornea. The sun's heat can also dry out the eyes and cause eye fatigue and other ailments. Exposure to sunlight causes eyestrain from constant squinting. Extended UV exposure has also been linked to noncancerous eye growths; it may also cause damage to the retina. Water, snow, and ice reflect additional UV radiation back at your eyes and there's more UV at higher altitudes. So if you do a lot of running at the beach, over snow or ice, or at altitude, you have an increased risk and may want to spend the money for sunglasses. Or you can alter the time of day you run to lessen the impact of sunlight on you.

The choice is yours. Most quality sports sunglasses come in a wraparound style to ensure maximum UV blockage; good sports sunglasses should offer 100 percent UV protection. The glasses should have a lightweight, durable frame and lenses that are shatterproof. Many come with adjustable ear stems and frame angles. You can get them with interchangeable lens tinting that adjusts to variations in sunlight. Each lens tint provides a different balance of light transmission, color, absorption, and light reflection.

Ask a salesperson to help you select the glasses that best meet the conditions you will be running in. A good pair should feel snug yet comfortable on your nose. They shouldn't bounce as you run. A removable strip of foam across the top of the frame in some glasses may help soak up sweat and keep the glasses from slipping. Leading manufacturers include Oakley, Bollé, Gargoyles, Vuarnet, Smith, and Revot. Look for glasses with the ANSI (American National Standard Institute) seal.

Sunglasses can make your run more comfortable by reducing eyestrain and shielding your eyes from wind (and sun) and airborne objects. I admit that I resisted until I got a pair for a present; they really do help me stay relaxed when running in the sun. They will also protect your eyes from bugs (now if I can just remember to keep my mouth shut, too).

Where to Find Apparel and Accessories

Check to see if there is a well-stocked store in your area that specializes in running shoes and apparel. This is your best bet, since its manager and salespeople are likely to keep up with what runners need. If not, many general athletic stores have a good selection. You might also want to check the articles on apparel and ads in running magazines like *Runner's World* and *Running Times*.

Mail-order houses that specialize in running equipment also have catalogs filled with pages of exciting things to wear and use. Still, I recommend that most of your running equipment be purchased from your local running store, since they should give you the best personalized service.

Part VI

Food and Drink for Health and Energy

EIGHTEEN

Nutrition for Health

Runners understand the old saw: You are what you eat. We are forever in search of food, drink, and vitamins that will increase our stamina, energy, strength, performance, and recovery.

Proper nutrition means a balanced diet that includes six essential nutrients—carbohydrates, fats, proteins, vitamins, minerals, and even water—that are consumed and used for optimal health. Runners don't need a special diet, just a healthy one based on sound nutrition. What we eat can make us sick as well as strong. In fact, five of the leading causes of death in the United States—heart disease, cancer, stroke, diabetes, and atherosclerosis—are exacerbated by poor diet. What you eat or don't eat may also cause obesity, high blood pressure, osteoporosis, and dental diseases. Dr. C. Everett Koop wrote in the groundbreaking *Surgeon General's Report on Nutrition and Health*: "If you are among the two out of three Americans who do not smoke or drink excessively, your choice of diet can influence your long-term health prospects more than any other action you might take." Exercise, of course, is important, too.

Those of us who are interested in fitness tend to be people who like to take care of ourselves and control our lives. Managing our diet and exercise can have big payoffs. To maintain a healthy diet means carefully selecting what you eat, and understanding the basic value of each of the essential nutrients. They provide the body with fuel and the materials for growth and repair of body tissues. They assist with the normal body processes. Each nutrient is independent of one another. We all need them, but the amounts we need vary according to age, gender, body size, environment, and exercise level.

The majority of Americans know about the link between high-fat diets, cholesterol, and coronary artery disease. Six out of ten Americans reported to the surgeon general that they had changed their diets to prevent chronic diseases. Unfortunately, surveys to determine what we actually eat—not what we *say* we eat—show a disturbing contradiction. Few Americans pay much attention to what they eat. Dr. Koop's study found that we consume too much fat, usually in the form of meat, dairy products, cooking and table fats, and too few carbohydrates and fibers.

Dietary Guidelines for Americans

The "Dietary Guidelines for Americans," first released in 1980, provide the basis for federal nutrition policy and nutrition education activities. The guidelines are updated every five years by a joint committee of the Agriculture Department and the Department of Health and Human Services. Its seven key recommendations for eating right include:

▪ *Eat a variety of foods.* To obtain the nutrients and other substances needed for good health, vary the foods you eat. Foods contain combinations of nutrients and other healthful substances. No single food can supply all nutrients in the amounts you need.

▪ *Balance the food you eat with physical acitivity; maintain or improve your weight.* For the first time in 1995, the federal nutrition guidelines added this important emphasis about exercise. In order to stay at the same body weight, people must balance the amount of energy in food with the amount of energy the body uses. Exercise is an important way to use up food energy.

▪ *Choose a diet with plenty of grain products, vegetables, and fruits.* These foods provide vitamins, minerals, complex carbohydrates (starch and dietary fiber), and other substances that are important for good health. They are also generally low in fat, depending upon how they are prepared and what is added to them at the table. Most Americans of all ages eat fewer than the recommended servings of these foods, even though their consumption is associated with a substantially lower risk for many chronic diseases, including certain types of cancer. Most of the calories in your diet should come from these foods. Eat more grain products (breads, cereals, pasta, and rice), vegetables, and fruits. Increase your fiber intake by eating more of a variety of whole grains, whole-grain products, dry beans, and fiber-rich vegetables and fruits such as carrots, corn, peas, pears, and berries.

▪ *Choose a diet low in fat, saturated fat, and cholesterol.* A diet with less total fat, saturated fat, and cholesterol is important to good health. Foods high in fat and cholesterol should be used sparingly. Choose lowfat milk products, lean meats, fish, poultry, beans, and peas to get essential nutrients without substantially increasing calorie and saturated fat intakes.

▪ *Choose a diet moderate in sugars.* Limit sugar in your diet. Americans consume far too much.

▪ *Choose a diet moderate in salt and sodium.* You should reduce salt intake and choose foods low in sodium. Take the salt shaker off your table or use a salt substitute.

▪ *If you drink alcoholic beverages, do so in moderation.* Alcohol intake of one drink a day for women and two for men is acceptable according to the guidelines. Avoid drinking alcohol if you are pregnant, driving, operating machinery, or taking medication.

The Food Guide Pyramid
The United States Department of Agriculture (USDA) published a new food guide that replaced the "basic four" food groups that most of us runners were raised on. The new guide included changes in the number and sizes of servings. In a major change, the four key food groups was expanded to five by breaking the important fruit and vegetable group into separate classifications. It also lists

a sixth group—fats, oils, and sweets—as a category to use minimally. The new recommendations tell us that a nutritious diet should consist mainly of foods high in complex carbohydrates and low in fats. They dropped the foods from animal sources—milk and meat—from one-third in the old plan to as low as one-fifth in the new guide. The new food groups and recommendations for daily servings are listed in Figure 18.1. The number of servings recommended are expressed as ranges—individuals should eat at least the lowest number of servings from each of the five major food groups. Age, sex, and activity level will determine the number of calories and servings needed each day.

It should be emphasized that the guide recommends that some food from each of the five major food groups should be eaten every day and that no one food group is more or less important than another. However, some foods or food groups should be eaten more often than others.

What counts as one serving according to the USDA? For example:

Milk, yogurt, and cheese: 1 cup of milk or yogurt; 1½ ounces of natural cheese; or 2 ounces of processed cheese

Meat, poultry, fish, dry beans, eggs, and nuts: 2–3 ounces of cooked lean meat, poultry, or fish; ½ cup of cooked dry beans (1 egg or 2 tablespoons of peanut butter count as 1 ounce of lean meat).

Vegetable: 1 cup of raw leafy vegetables; ½ cup of other vegetables, cooked or chopped raw; or ¾ cup of vegetable juice.

Fruit: 1 medium apple, banana, orange; ½ cup of chopped, cooked, or canned fruit; or ¾ cup of fruit juice.

Bread, cereal, rice, and pasta: 1 slice of bread; 1 ounce of ready-to-eat cereal; or ½ cup of cooked cereal, rice, or pasta.

If you eat a larger portion, count it as more than one serving. Again, eat at least the lowest number of servings from the five major food groups listed. No specific serving sizes are given for the fats, oils, and sweets group because the message is to use them sparingly.

The pyramid graphic (figure 18.1) visually shows which foods should comprise the bulk of the diet according to the new guidelines for daily servings. Bread and grains make up the foundation of the diet. Fruits and vegetables share the next layer, topped by the narrower layer shared by the milk and meat groups. Symbols for fats, oils, and sweets, with instructions to use sparingly, cap off the pyramid. The Food Guide Pyramid thus visually prioritizes the foods we should eat by volume with the foods we should eat most at the broad-based bottom and those we should minimize at the narrow top. Those who exercise at high levels, such as when marathon training, need to increase the servings from carbohydrate sources—the three base categories of the pyramid.

For further details on the Food Guide Pyramid, contact the Superintendent of Documents, Consumer Information Center, Department 159-4, Pueblo, CO 81009.

FIGURE 18.1: FOOD GUIDE PYRAMID
A Guide to Daily Food Choices

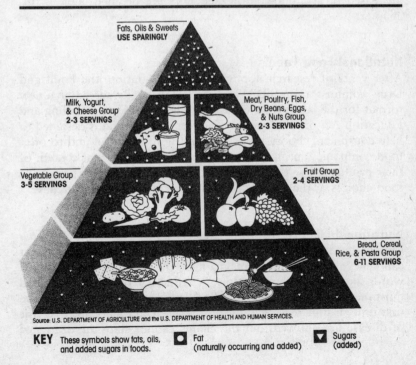

Fats, Oils & Sweets
USE SPARINGLY

Milk, Yogurt,
& Cheese Group
2-3 SERVINGS

Meat, Poultry, Fish,
Dry Beans, Eggs,
& Nuts Group
2-3 SERVINGS

Vegetable Group
3-5 SERVINGS

Fruit Group
2-4 SERVINGS

Bread, Cereal,
Rice, & Pasta Group
6-11 SERVINGS

Source: U.S. DEPARTMENT OF AGRICULTURE and the U.S. DEPARTMENT OF HEALTH AND HUMAN SERVICES.

KEY These symbols show fats, oils,
and added sugars in foods.

■ Fat
(naturally occurring and added)

▼ Sugars
(added)

Recommended Daily Allowances (RDAs)

The National Research Council, a government committee, meets every five years or so to review the most current scientific research on the nutritional needs of the body. They develop standards for optimal nutrient intake that are called Recommended Daily Allowances (RDAs). The RDA of a nutrient is an estimate of how much is needed for an individual to maintain good health. These are only recommendations because factors such as age, sex, height, weight, and activity level will result in varying nutritional needs. They are based upon "average" people: females age 23 to 50, 5 feet 4 inches tall, and 120 pounds; males age 23 to 50, 5 feet 10 inches tall, 154 pounds. The figures are also based on adults who only perform light physical activity. Many nutrition experts believe that the recommended RDAs for many nutrients are too low, especially for physically active individuals.

The RDA used to be listed on food labels (listing the percentage of the vitamins and minerals in each food item). They were replaced on the new food labels by the Daily Values (DVs), which are based on a 2,000-calorie diet. DVs are detailed later in this chapter.

Nutritional Food Labels

After years of research, lobbying, and negotiation, the Food and Drug Administration (FDA) and the USDA finally agreed on a new format for the labels on most foods. The Nutritional Labeling and Education Act of 1990 went into effect in 1994 and is designed to help consumers choose foods that are more healthful and to offer food companies an incentive to improve the nutritional content of their products. Use the guidelines on the labels to help make your food choices at the grocery store and for the meals you prepare.

Nutritional Claims

One of the key results of the government regulation is that you can believe most of the claims made on the package. If a label uses words like "less," "light," "low," "reduced," or "free," the food must meet strict standards—by law—such as those below. For the first time, claims of a relationship between nutrients and the risk of disease are allowed, but the claims cannot state the degree of risk reduction and can use only "may" or "might" in discussing the connection.

When a label makes the following claims, the product must contain the following:

- Low calorie: 40 calories or less per serving
- Reduced calorie: At least 25 percent fewer calories compared to the standard product
- Light or Lite: A third fewer calories, or 50 percent less fat or sodium than the standard product
- Low-fat: 3 grams of fat or less per serving
- Fat-free: Less than 0.5 grams of fat per serving
- Low saturated fat: 1 gram or less per serving
- Low sodium: Less than 140 milligrams per serving
- Very low sodium: Less than 35 milligrams per serving
- Low cholesterol: Less than 20 milligrams per serving
- Cholesterol free: Less than 2 milligrams of cholesterol and 2 grams or less of saturated fat per serving
- Lean (meats, poultry, fish): Less than 10 grams fat, less than 5 grams saturated fat, and less than 95 milligrams cholesterol per 3½ ounce serving
- Sugar free: Fewer than 0.5 grams of sugar per serving
- Good source of a nutrient: At least 10 percent of the daily value for that nutrient
- High in a nutrient: At least 20 percent of the daily value
- More in a nutrient: At least 10 percent more of the daily value

When a label makes the claim:	*The product must be:*
• "Foods low in saturated fat and cholesterol may reduce risk of heart disease"	Low-fat, low saturated fat and low cholesterol, or extra lean
• "Foods low in fat may protect against certain types of cancer"	Low-fat, fat free, or extra lean
• "Fruits and vegetables may protect against cancer"	Fruits and vegetables must be low-fat and a good source of dietary fiber, vitamin A, or vitamin C

Nutrition Facts

According to the new government regulations, most packaged foods are required to carry an up-to-date, easy-to-use nutrition information guide on the back or side panel to help consumers plan a healthy diet. It is titled "Nutrition Facts" and provides information on serving size, numbers of servings per container, the number of calories, calories from fat, and the amount and percent of Daily Value of total fat, saturated fat, cholesterol, sodium, total carbohydrates, fiber, sugar, protein, vitamins, and minerals. Figure 18.2 is a sample.

Serving sizes are standardized to reflect the amounts that people actually eat, and they are expressed in household and metric units to allow for easy comparison between products. For example, on the enclosed sample label, the typical serving size is ½ package or 21 grams and there are two servings in each container.

Calories for one serving are listed along with how many of those calories come from fat. Calories from fat are shown to help consumers follow recommended guidelines to get no more than 30 percent (runners should strive for less than 25 percent) of their calories from fat. In our sample, 20 of the 70 calories come from fat, or 29 percent of total calories. Thus this food source is a bit on the high side for fat content.

The labels replace the Recommended Daily Allowances—which had been used for vitamins, minerals, and proteins on food containers since 1973—with Daily Values (DVs) and set official recommendations for total fat, saturated fat, cholesterol, sodium, carbohydrate, and fiber. DVs are based on a 2,000-calorie-per-day reference diet consisting of 30 percent calories from fat, 60 percent from carbohydrates, and 10 percent from protein. By consulting the Daily Values, you can determine how much or how little of the major nutrients you are eating on a daily basis. For example, health experts state that a 2,000-calorie daily diet should contain no more than 65 grams of fat, so 65 is the DV for fat. Our sample food contains 2.5 grams which is 4 percent of this figure. This percentage is called the "% Daily Value." For fat, cholesterol, and sodium, choose foods with a low % Daily Value; for total carbohydrate, dietary fiber, vitamins, and minerals the goal is to reach 100 percent of each from combined food sources each day on the average.

The % Daily Value column can quickly tell you if a product is high or low in a nutrient and how a food fits into the overall daily diet. Less than 5 percent is considered low. The column shows the percentage of a person's daily diet that each serving of a food contains (the actual amount in grams per serving is also listed). These percentages, as noted, are based on a 2,000-calorie-a-day diet, which may be low for some exercisers. Some marathon runners for example may need 3,500 or more calories per day. You need to adjust these guidelines for total fat, saturated fat, carbohydrate, fiber, and protein if you consume more or less than 2,000 calories per day on the average. The DVs for cholesterol, sodium, vitamins, and minerals are the same for all calorie levels. Nutrients listed—fat, sodium, carbohydrate, and protein—are those considered by the government to be the most important to your health. Except for carbohydrates, these nutrients are consumed at levels higher than recommended for good health in the average diet.

The label not only lists the food's total fat, but it also lists the amount of saturated fat per serving. These bad guys as well as potential dietary hazards sodium and cholesterol are listed both in total quantity and as the % Daily Value they supply per serving. For example, the sample food in Figure 18.2 supplies a whopping 39 percent of the Daily Value for sodium. Too high! Minimize this food, especially if prone to high blood pressure. DVs for the bad guys: 20 grams of saturated fat, 300 milligrams of cholesterol, 2,400 milligrams of sodium.

Total carbohydrates (DV of 300 grams) includes the amounts of complex carbohydrates and simple carbohydrates (sugar) combined. Sugar is listed separately, thus in our example the total carbohydrate makeup is 4 grams of sugar and 8 grams of complex carbohydrates. No recommended limit is set for sugar, but a good guide is to keep it under 10 percent of total calories—or under 50 grams in a 2,000-calorie diet. The amount and % Daily Value for dietary fiber is also listed. The DV for fiber is 25 grams and our sample includes 1 gram, or 1 percent of the % Daily Value. Thus, this food isn't a good source for important fiber in the diet. Protein is listed just by grams (DV = 50); % Daily Value is an optional listing for food manufacturers.

Only A and C among the vitamins, iron and calcium among the minerals (other than sodium as discussed) are listed, since they are most often deficient in the average diet, and the food label includes the % Daily Value for these important nutrients. For example the DV for iron is 18 milligrams and our sample food contains 2 percent of this amount. If a claim is made about other vitamins or

FIGURE 18.2: SAMPLE FOOD LABEL

Nutrition Facts

Serving Size 1/2 of packaged (21g)

Servings Per Container 2

Amount Per Serving

Calories 70   Calories from Fat 20

	% Daily Value*
Total Fat 2.5g	**4%**
Saturated Fat 1.5g	**6%**
Cholesterol Less than 5mg	**1%**
Sodium 940mg	**39%**
Total Carbohydrate 12g	**4%**
Dietary Fiber 1g	**6%**
Sugars 4g	
Protein 2g	

Vitamin A 0%   •   Vitamin C 0%

Calcium 6%   •   Iron 2%

* Percent Daily Values are based on 2,000 calorie diet. Your daily values may be higher or lower depending on your calorie needs:

	Calories:	2,000	2,500
Total Fat	Less than	65g	80g
Sat Fat	Less than	20g	25g
Cholesterol	Less than	300mg	300mg
Sodium	Less than	2,400mg	2,400mg
Total Carbohydrate		300g	375g
Dietary Fiber		25g	30g

Calories per gram:
Fat 9 • Carbohydrate 4 • Protein 4

minerals, then information about it is mandatory and would be listed here. An orange juice carton, for example, may list % Daily Value of thiamine, Niacin, Folate, and Vitamin B_6. Fortified cereals will list its % Daily Value for all vitamins and minerals added to the food.

The lower portion of the label may not be listed on smaller packages. This section is the same on all food labels and gives the Daily

FIGURE 18.3: PERSONALIZED NUTRITION AMOUNTS FOR SIX DIFFERENT CALORIE LEVELS

Food Component	1,600	2,000	2,200	2,500	2,800	3,200
Total fat (g)	53	65	73	80	93	107
Saturated Fat (g)	18	20	24	25	31	36
Total Carbohydrate (g)	240	300	375	375	420	480
Dietary Fiber (g)	20*	25	25	30	32	37
Protein (g)	46**	50	55	65	70	80

* 20g is the minimum amount of fiber recommended for all calorie levels below 2,000.
** 46g is the minimum amount of protein recommended for all calorie levels below 1,800.

Values for diets of 2,000 and 2,500 calories. Amounts listed for fat, saturated fats, cholesterol, and sodium are recommended maximums; amounts listed for carbohydrates and fiber are recommended minimums. The 2,000 level was designed to apply to most women, children, and older men. The 2,500 level was designed for very active women, teens, and younger men. Most regular exercisers will be at least at the 2,500 level. Athletes in heavy training, such as when preparing for a marathon, may require 3,500 calories or more. Use Figure 18.3 to adjust your nutrient amounts for six sample calorie levels from 1,600 to 3,200 calories.

The calories per gram noted at the bottom of the label is a reminder to consumers that each gram of fat contains 9 calories compared to 4 for carbohydrates and protein.

In addition, the ingredients of the food is listed on all packages (but not within the "Nutrition Facts" chart) and must be more specific than previously.

Nutrients

The body requires at least forty nutrients that are classified into six groups: water, carbohydrates, fat, protein, vitamins, and minerals. All of these nutrients are essential, but some are more important to exercisers than others. Nutrition experts consider the four "primary" nutrients to be water, carbohydrates, fat, and protein since these substances are required in large quantities in order for the body to function properly.

Carbohydrates, fat, and protein are the energy nutrients—they contain energy that is measured in units called calories (water, vitamins, and minerals do not contain calories). When we exercise, we burn these energy nutrients to fuel our bodies. An excess of calories results in a gain in body weight. Chapter 41 details weight management and the calorie-balancing game, and Chapter 19 discusses how foods fuel our exercise.

The recommended diet would include 60 to 70 percent of calories from carbohydrates, 20 to 25 percent from fat, and 10 to 15 percent from protein. However, dietary surveys show that most exercisers don't meet these standards for carbohydrates, but exceed the recommended percentage in protein and, especially, in fat.

Linda Houtkooper of the University of Arizona College of Agriculture summed up the needs of endurance athletes in *Medicine and Science in Sports and Exercise*: "Foods in endurance sports training programs should provide adequate fluids to prevent dehydration; energy intake that is high in carbohydrate, low in fat, adequate in protein, and that maintains desirable body weight and desirable proportions of fat and lean weight; and sufficient amounts of vitamins and minerals."

Water

Despite containing no calories, water is the most important nutrient. It is the most important environmental substance to human life except for oxygen. Water makes up approximately 50 to 60 percent of your body weight. It provides the medium in which most of the body processes occur. As the main component of sweat, it stabilizes body temperature by acting as a coolant. Water is a major component of blood and thus helps transport nutrients to the cells and fuel to the exercising muscles. As the main component of urine, it helps to dissolve waste products and carry them away. Water lubricates your joints and softens food for digestion. It is critical to the healthy functioning of your body.

About 60 percent of our daily requirements for fluids come from drinking; 30 percent comes from the water in foods we eat, and 10 percent is produced in our cells during the metabolism of carbohydrates, protein, and fat. How do we lose water? Sixty percent is lost through urine, 5 percent through fecal loss, 15 percent is evaporated from the skin, 15 percent is lost as we humidify air taken in through respiration, and 5 percent is lost through normal sweating (more through sweat with exercise). The amount of fluids we take in and lose each day is surprisingly constant: about 2½ quarts. But we may require twice that amount or more if we exercise, and at least half of that should be water. As we will learn in Chapter 20, approximately 90 percent of water loss during exercise is caused by sweating, and when the total water output exceeds input, the result is the threat of dehydration.

We can get our water from a variety of sources, including watery fruits and vegetables, juices, milk, and soups. High sugar choices such as sodas contain lots of calories. Coffee and other caffeinated drinks as well as alcoholic beverages provide fluids, but they also increase fluid loss through urination. Sports drinks are a good source, especially while on the run.

What is the best source of drinking water? From the tap, or bottled? The United States has one of the cleanest water supplies in the world. When traveling to foreign countries, it may be wise to stick to bottled water. Our water sources are monitored for relative purity and our water is purified to meet federal standards. Yet pollutants still find their way into your town's water system or well. The Environmental Protection Agency (EPA) establishes standards for the maximum acceptable amount of various contaminants in our water, which include toxic metals, such as lead; pathogens, including bacteria and viruses; radioactive gases, including radon; and organic chemicals, such as nitrate. Federal law requires your supplier of water to make public their test results of its water's purity. It may also be a good idea to have your water tested from your own faucet since impurities such as lead can come from household plumbing as well as from water-company pipes. Use a state-certified independent laboratory. Contact your town or county health department for information.

Water quality and taste can vary from town to town, home to home, and tap to tap. You may choose to invest in a commercial water-filtering or water-purifying device. Besides removing potential contaminents, they may improve the taste of your water.

Many runners don't trust the local water and don't like its taste. The chlorine used to treat local water (to kill bacteria) may leave a bad aftertaste. Bottled water, which is disinfected with ozone, may be a good alternative. But it will be a much more costly source of fluids than the relatively cheap local water supply. Bottled water used to be a simple alternative to tap water. But over the last few years it has been marketed heavily with fancy names and bottles as a chic (and expensive) alternative to soda and alcohol. Your many choices of bottled water include spring water (natural sources with no added minerals or carbonation), sparkling water (carbon dioxide added naturally or artificially), mineral water (contains minerals naturally present at source and may or may not be carbonated), club soda (artificially carbonated tap water with added minerals and salts), and seltzer (carbonation added to tap water but no minerals). Some seltzer water may be sweetened to add taste and thus will add calories.

What's best for you? If your tap water tastes good and is safe why spend the money on fancy water? On the other hand, if you enjoy the bottled sources, drink up. The more fluids you drink as a runner the better.

Carbohydrates

As the most important food source for long-distance running, carbohydrates have basked in the glory since researchers proved conclusively during the running revolution of the 1970s that carbos, not proteins, are the key to running fast and long. Pasta dethroned steak as the meal of champions. Whenever your runs increase to an intense pace, or whenever your runs extend beyond one and a half hours, you may deplete carbohydrates stored in the body as glycogen. This is the primary energy source for vigorous exercise as detailed in the following chapter. As a runner, 60 percent or more of the calories in your diet should come from this highly efficient energy source. Besides fueling our exercising muscles, carbos are essential as the fuel for the central nervous system. They also assist in the digestion and assimilation of proteins and fats, which are needed as additional energy sources. There are two classifications of carbohydrates: simple (sugar) and complex (starches).

Simple carbohydrates are one-molecule sugars (monosaccharides such as glucose; fructose or fruit sugar; and galactose) and two-molecule sugars (disaccharides such as sucrose, or table sugar; and lactose, or milk sugar), which are quickly converted to glucose and rapidly absorbed into the bloodstream, providing you with quick energy. Sounds like a great system. This process, however, also causes a response in which insulin, a hormone produced by the pancreas, removes sugar from the bloodstream and places it in the cells. The result is that after a quick blood sugar high comes a blood sugar low accompanied by decreased energy and performance. Sugar is found in two forms—refined and natural. Many concentrated sweets such as cookies, cakes, doughnuts, candy, soda, and other refined-sugar sources are "empty calories." They contain plenty of calories, and often contain plenty of fat, but they don't contain essential vitamins, minerals, and fiber.

No other food has been so overemphasized in our diets as sugar.

The average American consumes 125 pounds of sugar a year. That's half a cup every day, and sugar makes up 18 percent of the average daily caloric intake. Health authorities suggest cutting our sugar intake to 10 percent or less. Excess sugar in the diet has been linked to obesity, diabetes, heart disease, stomach and bowel disorders, some forms of cancer, mood swings, hyperactivity in children, dental cavities, premenstrual syndrome, and more.

But, like me, you love sweets anyway, you say? It is possible to fit a few sugary treats into a well-balanced diet. A candy bar once in a while or a cookie for dessert are fine. Just don't eat the whole bag of cookies or skip lunch and eat candy instead, like many of us did as kids when Mom wasn't looking. If we aren't careful with our diets the urge for sugar can take over. Nancy Clark warns in her *Sports Nutrition Guidebook*: "If you find yourself craving sweets, determine whether you've eaten adequate calories to support your activities. The chances are that you've let yourself get too hungry. Sweet cravings are simply a sign that you're physiologically ravenous. To prevent this craving, eat more calories at breakfast and lunch (and snack in the afternoon if you eat a late dinner), so that you curb the cookie monster that tends to arise in the later afternoon and evening." Eating (or nutritious snacking) every three to five hours will help you avoid periods when you might feel low because of declining blood sugar.

If you feel you crave sugar, try substituting a high-carbohydrate snack like fruit, low-fat and dry low-sugar cereal, a sports bar, or a sports drink. I've found that the secret is to keep good snack sources handy and to keep poor nutritional sources out of sight.

Natural simple sugars are good for you in moderation and have an important place in our diets. They are found in fruits, juices, and vegetables and include valuable vitamins, minerals, and fiber. An apple, orange, or banana can meet your needs for a sweet treat and are nutritionally valuable.

Complex carbohydrates are composed of a chain of sugar molecules and in most cases (potatoes, rice, and white bread are among the exceptions) take longer to convert to glucose. Thus they are absorbed more slowly into the bloodstream, resulting in a slower, more steady energy supply. Good complex carbohydrate sources include pasta, cereal, bread, and vegetables. The majority of the carbohydrates we consume in our diet should be of the complex variety. Many of these foods are also high in fiber, which the surgeon general promoted as an important element of a healthy diet.

Fiber is a natural "broom" that sweeps through our intestines and moves food along quickly and easily. It softens waste, adds bulk, and attracts water to the stool. It thus prevents constipation and eases hemorrhoidal conditions. The American Health Foundation states that reducing fats and increasing fiber in the diet will reduce our chances of getting cancer of the colon. The recommended diet for good health and good performance thus should emphasize bread, grains, vegetables, and fruits.

Fats

Not to be confused with body fat, which is discussed in Chapter 41, dietary fat is an important nutrient found in the food we eat. It serves several major functions. It is a source of energy, and it transports fat-soluble vitamins A, D, E, and K. Fats also add flavor and palatability to foods, and it prolongs digestion by slowing down the stomach's secretions of hydrochloric acid.

Consumed fats may end up stored as body fat, but so will excess calories from carbohydrates and proteins. The problem with dietary fat is that most of us consume much more than we need. The average American consumes approximately 35 percent of his or her calories as fat. The federal government, American Heart Association, and other major organizations now recommend that no more than 30 percent of our daily calories come from fat. Many experts suggest that we—especially runners and other aerobic exercisers—cut back our intake of fats to only 20 to 25 percent of our total diet and replace them with carbohydrates. Don't panic here. These recommended percentages of dietary fat intake don't apply to each and every meal or snack. It's the recommended amount for the average diet over time, not individual items or meals, that is important. In other words, you can enjoy your steaks periodically and even your favorite ice cream (but not the whole carton).

Fats contain more than twice as many calories per gram as carbohydrates and protein; thus, a high-fat diet will add plenty of excess weight. Foods that contain lots of fats include ice cream, butter, mayonnaise, salad dressing, red meat, egg yolks, whole milk, cheeses, and chocolate.

Fats in the diet come in two basic forms: saturated (the bad guys) and unsaturated (the good guys). Foods don't necessarily consist of one type of fat, so you can choose foods that have a high ratio of unsaturated to saturated fats. Saturated fats come primarily from animal sources—red meat, milk, and butter—but also from coconut, palm, and hydrogenated vegetable oils. Saturated fats raise LDL cholesterol (the bad guys) and total cholesterol. Despite being the least healthy type of fat, saturated fat is still required by the body in small amounts. Unsaturated fats, which are usually liquid at room temperature, are divided into monounsaturated and polyunsaturated categories. Monounsaturated fats are the healthiest of the fats and can actually lower blood cholesterol. Sources include most natural oils including olive, peanut, and avocado oils. Polyunsaturated fats are found in corn, soy, sunflower, safflower, and fish oils and many margarines and butter alternatives. These fats tend to reduce total cholesterol, but they also cause HDL levels (the good guys) to fall some. Beware of hydrogenated fats, which are made by adding hydrogen molecules to mono- and polyunsaturated fats in order to make it easier for cooking and eating. This process negates many of the benefits of these fats and may raise blood cholesterol. Check food labels to see if this process was used on your peanut butter and other foods. Nutritionists recommend that one-third of fat calories ingested should come from each type of fat—saturated, polyunsaturated, and monounsaturated.

Most people should strive to control their total fat intake—saturated and unsaturated—since both types are bursting with calories. But saturated fats should be particularly minimized since they are closely linked with coronary heart disease and other chronic illnesses, including obesity, diabetes, and some cancers. According to the *Surgeon General's Report*, the average American gets 14 percent of the calories in his or her diet from saturated fat high in cholesterol. The recommended limit is 10 percent. Chapter 39 details the relationship between cholesterol, heart disease, and exercise.

How can we cut back on fats in our diet? First, practice healthful shopping. Choose leaner cuts of meat, switch to reduced-fat and nonfat dairy products such as skim or 1 percent milk and low-fat cheeses and yogurts, and replace ice cream with frozen ices and frozen yogurt. Buy more poultry and fish and less red meat. Load up your shopping cart with fresh fruits, vegetables, grain foods, and meat substitutes such as dried beans and lentils. Read labels on all processed foods and don't choose those that contain more than 3 grams of fat per 100 calories. Cut back on those products that contain highly saturated oils or lard. Labels proclaiming food to be "cholesterol free" don't mean the food is necessarily free of fat, and they could be full of excess calories. Also beware of labels bragging about snacks that are "low in fat." They usually replace those fats with sugars and what remains is still high in calories. If they have to brag about it chances are that something isn't right nutritionally.

Next, keep a low-fat kitchen. Trim all visible fat from meat and remove the skin from poultry parts. How you cook your food affects fat intake. Frying and sauteing foods are added-fat methods. Instead, use lower-fat cooking methods such as broiling, steaming, and poaching. Last but not least, control the size of your servings. A beef serving, for example, should be 3 to 4 ounces—or about the size of the palm of your hand. More than that and you are loading up way too much on saturated fats and calories.

In summary, the message is clear to runners: cut down on fats in the diet and increase carbohydrates. Especially avoid fats prior to running or racing since they are slow to digest.

Protein

Although it only makes up 10 to 15 percent of the recommended diet, protein is still essential to life and to athletic performance. Proteins are best known among exercisers for their role in building muscles. They are natural body builders that help bone and tissue grow, maintain, and repair. With exercise, our muscles and tendons may experience small tears or traumas that are repaired by the protein in our diet. Thus, protein is especially important to runners who are recovering from intense workouts or long runs such as in marathon training. Proteins are also a major building material for blood, skin, hair, nails, and the internal organs.

Proteins are the major structural component of our body's cells. They aid in the formation of hormones that control growth, sexual development, and the rate of metabolism; proteins control the balance of acids and alkalines in the blood and regulate the body's water balance. They also fight off disease by helping to form antibodies that ward off infection. Proteins make up part of the important hemoglobins that carry oxygen and carbon dioxide in the red blood cells. Last but not least, protein provides a small but significant source of energy for exercising muscles.

Protein is found primarily in muscle and it makes up approximately 15 percent of our body weight. Protein is made up of twenty types of small units called amino acids—the "building blocks" of the human body. Eleven of these amino acids are referred to as "nonessential amino acids" because they can be synthesized by the body. The nine "essential amino acids" can only be obtained from our diet. It is these amino acids in our food then that are critical to meeting our protein needs. Animal protein—including meat, fish, poultry, eggs, and milk—are called complete proteins because they contain all of the essential amino acids. Proteins from vegetables, grains, and other sources are incomplete proteins; they do not supply all of the essential amino acids. If you are on a vegetarian diet, you need to plan your daily diet by eating a variety of foods that will give you all the essential amino acids.

The theory that huge amounts of protein are needed to build muscles is a myth. When I competed in college, all athletes—from the beefy football players to the skinny cross-country runners (that's me!)—were told to eat plenty of meat, including the pre-event training meal. Some athletes and coaches swore by protein supplements. Many athletes, coaches, even nutritionists thought that extra protein contributed to extra strength and better performances. Little attention was paid to—indeed, little was known about—the value of carbohydrates and their role in sports and exercise. Now, of course, endurance athletes emphasize carbohydrates, not protein, in their diet and pre-event meals.

So don't pay attention to those glitzy adds promoting amino acids and protein supplements. There is no evidence to support the claims that these expensive supplements promote exercise performance. In fact, excessive protein will be stored in your body as fat. Too much protein—we are talking here about excessive amounts of supplements that many body-builders and football players ingest in an effort to build bigger muscles—may damage your kidneys or liver. Exercise, particularly resistance work such as weight training, and a healthy diet including sufficient protein are the keys to developing bigger muscles (unless you cheat and take anabolic steroids—another health hazard).

Okay, so we know now that athletes don't benefit from excessive amounts of protein, but do runners and other serious exercisers still need more protein than the average nonexercising person? Peter Lemon, Ph.D., of Kent State University in Ohio has done studies that show that protein needs increase with exercise. In looking at the protein balance of highly trained distance runners, Dr. Lemon found that a diet based on the Recommended Daily Allowance for protein was too low. Runners who consumed only the RDA (0.4 grams per pound of body weight) showed a loss of body protein.

"Don't pay attention to the RDA for protein," says William Evans, Ph.D., of the USDA Human Nutrition Research Center on Aging at Tufts University in Boston. "It was worked out for sedentary people who don't use protein for exercise. Runners burn 5 to 6 percent of their fuel as protein so a lack of this nutrient could result in an energy drain."

According to nutritionist Maureen Smith Plombon, an adviser to the American Running & Fitness Association, "Athletes participating in certain events may need more protein than the RDA, but should not exceed a level of two to two-and-a-half times as much. This may also be estimated as 12% to 15% of total daily calories." The fitness runner fits somewhere between the RDA and the needs of serious runners. Nutritionist Nancy Clark recommends that endurance athletes consume 0.5 to .75 grams of protein per pound of body weight.

Most athletes who are low on protein, and thus risk health and performance, do so for one of three reasons. First, they may be starving themselves in an effort to lose weight. Second, vegetarians have a limited source of proteins in their food and thus need to pay attention to balancing their diet. Third, runners, especially when training for marathons, may pay so much attention to stuffing in the carbohydrates that they don't eat enough protein. Increase carbos at the expense of fat, not protein, which is needed to help muscles recover from training.

Most of us can easily meet our protein needs by eating a balanced diet. In fact, dietary analyses show endurance athletes average one and a half to two times the RDA for protein. Good sources of protein include lean meat, fish, poultry, legumes, nuts, beans, whole grains and cereals, egg whites, low-fat milk, low-fat cheese, and some vegetables. Peanut butter is a fun source—but watch the fat.

In sum, too much protein in your diet will not help you gain strength and is harmful to your health. However, restricting your protein intake will also be harmful, since the exerciser needs more protein than the sedentary individual, and more than the RDA.

The word "protein" comes from ancient Greece and means "of prime importance." So don't forget that it is important to include enough protein from healthy, low-fat sources in your diet.

Vitamins

Vitamins are not a direct source of energy (and thus contain no calories), but they aid or initiate the conversion of carbohydrates, fat, and protein into energy. We need them in only small quantities, yet they are essential to growth and good health. Vitamins primarily serve as catalysts that regulate our bodies' chemical reactions and allow us to utilize the other nutrients in our diet. Vitamins help regulate the metabolism of our bodies and form bones and tissues.

Natural vitamins are found in plants and animals as organic food substances. Because our bodies cannot synthesize most vitamins, we must get them in our diet or with supplements. As runners strive for a low-fat, high-carbohydrate diet, they need to be sure to get enough of the thirteen essential vitamins, each of which has a specific function. Vitamins are grouped into two types: fat soluble or water soluble. Vitamins A, D, E, and K are fat-soluble vitamins—they are absorbed during digestion bound to fats. Any excess of these vitamins is stored in the body causing toxic buildup. Water-soluble vitamins include the B-complex and vitamin C and are absorbed during digestion along with water. Most excess is excreted in urine, thus toxic buildup is rarely a problem.

Antioxidants. This is perhaps the most controversial nutritional topic of recent years. Antioxidants are substances that neutralize toxic compounds, called free radicals, that damage cells. Free radicals are produced when the body burns fuel for energy. A small amount of the oxygen we inhale is metabolized into free radicals that career through the body, mutating and killing healthy cells. When you are under a lot of stress or when you exercise very intensely, you produce lots of these dangerous free radicals. These chemicals are also produced when you are exposed to cigarette smoke, exhaust fumes, radiation, and excessive sunlight.

Antioxidants act like fire extinguishers, counteracting those nasty free radicals. Antioxidants are manufactured by the cells of our body and are found in our diet. Research indicates that aerobic training increases the amount of these enzymes produced by the body. Studies indicate that by increasing your intake of certain vitamins (C, E, and A—in the form of beta-carotene), you'll be better armed to fight off the attacking free radicals. Antioxidants may protect your health from the effects of pollution, stress, and ultraviolet light, and from the damaging effects of strenuous exercise. Since free radicals are believed to contribute to the development of cancer, cataracts, and heart disease—and even to the signs of aging—antioxidants serve as important disease fighters.

But is there really sound evidence that antioxidants reduce disease? According to Dr. Jeffrey Blumberg, associate director of the USDA Human Nutrition Center on Aging, and chief of the Antioxidants Research Laboratory at Tufts University in Boston, "The scientific basis is really quite substantial. Epidemiological studies have shown repeatedly that people with the highest intakes of antioxidants are at the lowest risk for heart disease and cancer, the two leading killers of Americans. I'm talking about prevention—not treatment. Antioxidants can also reduce the incidence of cataracts and infectious diseases." But the Food and Drug Administration and many other experts want to wait for more scientific proof before recommending increasing the RDA for these antioxidants. And some studies even seem to prove that the antioxidant theory is wrong.

Dr. Blumberg, and many leading authorities, think that enough evidence exists, and that since we are faced with a public health crisis in chronic diseases we should act now. He told *American Health* magazine his reason for taking antioxidant supplements: "There is very likely a significant health benefit without risk of toxicity. . . . But even a 10% reduction in heart disease, which kills more than 800,000 Americans and costs over $110 billion a year, would be a tremendous benefit. I'm not suggesting that antioxidants are magic bullets. You can't eat a high-fat, low-fiber diet, smoke cigarettes, drink alcohol excessively, not wear seat belts, skip exercise and practice unsafe sex and say, 'It's OK, I take Vitamin E.' Nutrient supplements are not substitutes for a healthy diet."

But how much antioxidants are needed? Dr. Blumberg's answer: "That's highly controversial. Recent research suggest that the optimal amounts are much greater than we can get readily from our diet. The ranges that look optimal now—total intakes from diet and supplements—are between 250 and 1,000 milligrams a day of vitamin C, between 100 and 400 international units of vitamin E and between 6 milligrams and 30 milligrams of beta-carotene." Dr. Kenneth Cooper, the "father of aerobics," recommends taking even larger dosages in his book *Dr. Kenneth H. Cooper's Antioxidant Revolution*. The RDA for vitamin C is 60 milligrams, and for vitamin E it's 30 international units; there is no RDA for beta-carotene. If you were to eat three to five servings of vegetables a day and two to four servings of fruit you would come close to meeting Blumberg's recommended ranges for vitamin C and beta-carotene. But 90 percent of the population probably doesn't meet this standard in the diet, so supplements may be necessary. Reaching the recommended antioxidant dosage for vitamin E is difficult through the diet because most sources contain more fat than is wise to eat, thus supplements become even more valuable.

Vitamin A (Retinol). This vitamin is critical to the development of strong bones and teeth, and helps to maintain eyes, skin, lining of the nose, mouth, and digestive and urinary tracts. It also enhances the immune system and helps to prevent red blood cell damage. Deficiencies contribute to skin disorders, increased risk of infection, retarded growth, and night blindness. Healthy sources include dark green leafy vegetables, yellow-orange vegetables and fruits, liver, milk, butter, and egg yolk.

Beta-carotene is an important form of vitamin A. It is a plant pigment that may be converted to vitamin A if needed. What isn't converted is available as an antioxidant, and studies indicate that beta-carotene fights heart disease, cataracts, and certain cancers. Good sources of beta-carotene include carrots, pumpkin, sweet potatoes, butternut squash, spinach, broccoli, apricots, cantaloupe.

Vitamin B-complex. The B-complex vitamins help provide the body with energy by converting carbohydrates into glucose. They are also essential to the metabolism of fats and proteins, assist in growth, and contribute to appetite. They may be the single most important factor in the health and normal functioning of our nervous system. B-complex vitamins include: B_1 (thiamine), B_2 (riboflavin), B_3 (niacin), B_6 (pyridoxine), B_{12} (cyanocobalamin), folic acid, pantothenic acid, and biotin. A deficiency in one of the complex vitamins may impair use of the others. Folic acid, found in liver, lentils, and many beans and leafy green vegetables, is of particular concern to runners since it aids in the formation of blood cells. If you don't take in enough of this vitamin, you may be prone to anemia and fatigue. In addition, folic acid is necessary for normal fetal growth and development. Healthy sources of B-complex vitamins include whole grain cereals, green vegetables, nuts, beans, poultry, fish, liver, and some dairy products.

Vitamin C (ascorbic acid). Made famous by Dr. Linus Pauling's promotion as the cure for the common cold, vitamin C is one of the most controversial vitamins. It facilitates the formation of connective scar tissue, helping to heal wounds and burns; it promotes iron absorption from the intestines and aids in the forming of red blood cells. It prevents and relieves scurvy. Some studies indicate that vitamin C fights bacterial infection, fever, and reduces the impact on the body of some allergy-producing substances. Studies show that it may not prevent the common cold, but taking plenty of vitamin C on a regular basis and even more when you have a cold will help alleviate the symptoms. As an antioxidant, it fights cancer, cataracts, and heart disease.

Studies at the University of Birmingham in England show that vitamin C supplements more than six times in excess of the RDA resulted in improved muscle recovery from hard workouts. Research at the University of the Witwatersrand in Johannesburg, South Africa, found that vitamin C supplementation in amounts ten times the RDA may cut endurance athlete's risk of upper-respiratory infection by 50 percent. Most nutritionists agree that the RDA (60 milligrams) for this beneficial vitamin is too low and that taking in more (about one gram a day) is of little risk since it is water-soluble. However, excessive intake of vitamin C over an extended period may interfere with the absorption of vitamin B_{12} and promote the formation of kidney stones. Good natural sources include most fruits and vegetables including broccoli, tomatoes, brussels sprouts, oranges, strawberries, cantaloupe, and grapefruit.

Vitamin D (cholecalciferol). Essential in the absorption of calcium from the intestinal tract and in the breakdown and assimilation of phosphorous, vitamin D is thus critical for bone development and strength. Without it, bones and teeth will not calcify properly. It is also valuable in maintaining a stable nervous system, a normal and strong heartbeat, and normal blood clotting. Good sources include fish-liver oils, fortified milk, egg yolks, and tuna fish. Sunlight on the skin also produces vitamin D.

Vitamin E (tocopherol). This is another of the antioxidants that particularly seems to protect against heart disease. Some studies indicate that vitamin E helps to slow the aging of cells, lessens oxidative damage after hard training, and prevents lung damage from many of the pollutants we inhale. Vitamin E minimizes red blood cell damage, is vital to the immune system, and promotes aerobic energy production. This vitamin protects and maintains cellular membranes. Good sources include vegetable oils, wheat germ, whole grains, leafy vegetables, rice, liver, and peanut butter.

Vitamin K. Essential to blood clotting, this vitamin is found in green leafy vegetables, liver, soybeans, vegetable oils, fishmeat, oats, rye, and alfalfa.

Should you take vitamin supplements? If vitamins are good for you then more will make you even stronger and faster, right? Wrong! Anita Singh, Ph.D., and colleagues at the Uniformed Services University of the Health Sciences in Bethesda, Maryland, tested trained exercisers for performance in aerobic capacity, aerobic endurance, muscular strength, and muscular endurance. Half of the subjects took megadoses of vitamin and mineral supplements twice a day for ninety days; the other half took a placebo. The result: no significant differences in their performance tests. A study performed by researchers at the Sport Science Center in Cape Town, South Africa, on thirty distance runners came to the same conclusion. However, subjects in these studies had no preexisting vitamin or mineral deficiencies prior to testing. Other studies indicate that if you have a vitamin or mineral deficiency, then supplements can help you improve performance. The Bethesda study concluded, in *Medicine and Science in Sports and Exercise*, "If you have a vitamin or mineral deficiency, supplements will help bring your levels up to par, but once you've repleted your stores you're better off meeting your needs with a balanced, varied diet than with expensive supplements. Once back on track with a good diet, there's no reason to think that supplements will give you an edge."

Okay, vitamins won't help you run faster or get stronger, but what about the claims from the billion-dollar vitamin industry that supplements fight off everything from colds to cancer? Liz Applegate, Ph.D., wrote in her nutrition column in *Runner's World*:

Scientists have assured consumers for years that a balanced diet provides plenty of vitamins and minerals—a surplus even. Recently, however, these same scientists seem to be eating their advice—and their supplements, too. The word out now is that additional vitamins provided through supplements may improve health; ward off cancer, heart disease, and cataract formation; and even hasten recovery from athletic injury.

Although many scientists are uncertain whether taking vitamins in supplement form is as healthful as eating them in food, most agree that taking a supplement that provides 100 percent of the RDA is safe, even though it will send your vitamin and mineral intake above the RDA.

Why? Many agree that the RDAs are too low for some vitamins and that modern health stressors including poor air quality require additional vitamins.

Running and other forms of exercise do not increase your need for vitamins. But runners may be vitamin deficient due to a poor diet. If your diet isn't well balanced because of poor planning or a hectic lifestyle, then vitamin supplements may help you keep healthy and prevent a loss of performance. Many experts state that natural and synthetic vitamins are equally beneficial, and tests have shown that most cheap vitamins are as good as the expensive ones. A "one-a-day" vitamin and mineral supplement that provides no more than one to two times the RDA for any one vitamin is recommended. You may choose to take even more if you agree with the antioxidant theory. But remember: Large doses of these supplements will not improve performance and may be poisonous, especially the fat-soluble vitamins.

Confused? So are most Americans. That's because studies come out every year that contradict previous recommendations, and what our government recommends isn't always in step with the recommendations of leading experts in nutrition. The best bet is to discuss your diet and your potential need for vitamin and mineral supplements with your sports doctor and/or sports nutritionist. They should be able to advise you according to the latest findings, which may even differ from what we are discussing here in this book.

Minerals

Minerals are inorganic substances found in the soil and picked up by plants. We get our minerals by eating plants, or animals that have eaten plants. Minerals, therefore, exist in most foods and in the body.

Minerals make up approximately 4 percent of your body weight and are essential for normal cellular functions. Like vitamins, they are not used for fuel but work with other nutrients to ensure a smoothly functioning body. They are essential for the functioning of the heart and the contraction of muscles; they are constituents of the bones, teeth, soft tissues, muscles, blood, and nerve cells; they are essential to maintaining the body processes, strengthening skeletal structures, and the vigor of the heart, brain, and nervous system. Minerals aid in warding off fatigue and cramps, maintain the body's delicate water balance, and aid in the transportation of oxygen.

Each mineral has a unique function. There are seventeen essential minerals that are divided into two categories. Macrominerals are those which are needed in large amounts (over 100 milligrams per day). These include calcium, chloride, magnesium, phosphorus, potassium, sulfur, and sodium. Microminerals (or trace elements) are needed in smaller amounts. These include chromium, cobalt, copper, fluoride, iodine, iron, manganese, molybdenum, selenium, and zinc.

Some minerals, called electrolytes, produce ions that can then be involved with chemical reactions. Electrolytes are lost with sweat during exercise. Sodium and chloride are lost in the greatest amounts; calcium, copper, magnesium, potassium, and zinc are lost in lesser amounts. The electrolytes lost with sweating can be easily replaced with a well-balanced diet. In fact, a well-balanced diet will provide you with all the minerals your body requires. However, iron and zinc may be hard to obtain if you don't eat red meat, and calcium levels may be low if you don't eat dairy products. Supplements of minerals aren't as popular as vitamins, which have more magical, as well as some proven, claims. Calcium and iron are generally the minerals that may require supplementation. If you take a one-a-day multivitamin, it should include mineral supplementation in small quantities as well. Many minerals, as with vitamins, may cause health problems if taken in excess.

Although each mineral has an important, essential function, the following are of particular importance to runners.

Calcium. Your body needs more of this mineral than any other— 40 percent of the mineral content of the body comes from calcium. It is best known for building and maintaining bones and this is where most of it is needed. Remember how many times your mom told you to drink your milk so you would grow up with strong bones? Well, we also need calcium as adults to maintain those strong bones and to prevent stress fractures to runners. Most people stop growing by the end of their teens, but peak density for bones isn't reached until your early thirties. After about age thirty-five your bones start to thin with the aging process. If we don't consume enough calcium in our diet, then the bones weaken, leading to osteoporosis (see Chapter 28)—a brittle bone condition that affects mostly women, especially after menopause. Men are mostly affected in their seventh and eighth decade of life.

A regular program of weight-bearing exercise such as running and weight training combined with a calcium-rich diet will slow this process. And this plan should start in childhood and continue throughout our lives. The earlier we build and maintain strong bones the better. Said Sandra Raymond, executive director of the National Osteoporosis Foundation in Washington, D.C., "Achieving maximum peak bone mass in youth may be the most critical factor in preventing osteoporosis later in life." Yet studies show that most Americans—men and women of all ages, kids through senior citizens—do not consume enough calcium and do not get enough exercise. This is a concern particularly among adolescent girls who, studies show, don't come close to consuming the recommended amount of calcium. Too much calcium with excessive supplementation can cause constipation or decrease iron absorption.

Calcium also helps build and maintain teeth, helps regulate heart function, is important to coagulation and acid-base balance, assists muscle growth and contraction, and the passage of nutrients through cell walls. It is also essential for nerve impulse transmission. In addition, research indicates that calcium-rich diets may help control high blood pressure and reduce the risk of colon cancer.

Extended emotional stress and lack of exercise increase the need for calcium. Good sources include low-fat milk and dairy products, calcium-fortified fruit juices, beans, cauliflower, oranges, eggs, and dark leafy vegetables like broccoli and spinach. Lactose-intolerant runners should drink lactose-reduced milk.

Plenty of vitamin D helps to increase the absorption of calcium. Since milk is a great source of calcium in the diet, it is fortified with vitamin D. Sunshine also contributes to vitamin D supplies and thus calcium absorption. Alcohol decreases calcium absorption and increases calcium losses. Consumption of protein and sodium in excess, as do most Americans, increases the amount of calcium lost in urine. Too much phosphorous or zinc can also lower calcium levels as does cigarette smoking. Caffeine or high-fiber foods eaten at the same meal with high-calcium foods or supplements may interfere with calcium absorption. Calcium supplementation may be recommended by your sports doctor or sports nutritionist, but they are not absorbed as well as milk sources. Besides, the ads are true—milk is good for you, in many ways. How much milk should we drink? The National Institutes of Health recommends five glasses a day for a teenager or an older woman and at least two for everyone else. They recommend taking far more calcium than the outdated RDA set in 1989.

Chloride. Chloride, potassium, and sodium allow for the nerve impulses that control muscular activity. They also maintain water balance and distribution, blood-acid balance (pH), and normal cardiac rhythm. Chloride is also needed for hydrochloric acid production in the stomach. It is consumed as table salt (sodium chloride).

Iron Although this is a micromineral and is present in the body in very small amounts, it is important to good health and running performance. This is because it is critical to oxygen transportation. Iron is required in combination with protein for the formation of hemoglobin, which is found in red blood cells and carries oxygen from the lungs through the bloodstream to the body tissues, including the working muscles. It is also required in the formation of myoglobin, which transports oxygen into the cells.

As much as one-quarter of the world's population is iron-deficient. This results in anemia—a condition in which the blood's oxygen-carrying capacity is decreased. Fatigue, loss of energy, headaches, behavior change, and impaired intellectual performance may result from iron deficiency anemia. Iron also aids in resistance to disease and stress, and benefits muscle contraction. Women are more prone to anemia than men because they lose iron in blood during menstruation. Pregnancy also contributes to iron losses. Women of menstruating age need approximately twice as much iron as men. It is estimated that 30 to 50 percent of all women of childbearing age have iron-poor blood. Studies show that as many as 10 percent of male athletes may be iron deficient, too.

Iron deficient anemia occurs more frequently in runners than in the general population. "Runner's anemia" may result in high-mileage runners, men or women. According to the U.S. Olympic Committee Sports Medicine and Science Division, training affects iron status in many ways, including losses through sweating, decreased iron absorption, and the impact of hard footstrikes that may destroy normal red blood cells. But this type of anemia usually doesn't occur until runners reach at least the 40- to 50-mile-per-week level.

Some iron shortages occur in the blood, others in the body's stored sources. Iron levels can be low for many reasons, including an inadequate diet or physiological problems in absorbing iron from food.

A sports doctor or sports nutritionist can best help you determine if you are iron deficient and what the causes are with blood tests. Be aware that standard tests (hemoglobin and hematocrit) may not detect the problem as they test only for anemia, the final stage of iron deficiency. The hematocrit test compares the ratio of fluid in the blood—plasma—to the number of red blood cells as well as the amount of oxygen carried by each. Depleted iron stores in the bone marrow, liver, and spleen could occur for months prior to the onset of anemia and these shortages may not be detected with these tests despite the symptoms of fatigue, irritability, and so on. Thus, it may be a good idea to have a complete blood count and iron profile. This will measure other factors including ferritin, a marker of stored iron.

If you are feeling tired and sluggish, the cause may very well be iron deficiency. Studies show that aerobic performance improves significantly within a few weeks with iron supplementation, but only to the extent that a deficiency exists—that is, iron supplements do not allow you to process more oxygen and thus run farther and faster if you are not iron deficient.

Natural sources include lean beef, lamb and pork, liver, dark meat poultry, leafy green vegetables, nuts, lentils, dried fruits, blackstrap molasses, shrimp, scallops, iron-fortified cereals, and breads. Cooking in a cast-iron skillet also contributes needed iron. Those who do not eat meat and those who train intensely or at high mileage seem to be particularly prone to iron deficiency. Temporary shortages may occur with surgery or blood donation. Supplementation may be advised by your sports doctor or sports nutritionist, but for many it may cause intestinal discomfort, and high levels of iron have been linked in some studies to increased risk of cancer and heart disease.

Normally, only about 10 to 15 percent of the iron ingested is absorbed by the body, although this varies widely from person to person and from time to time. Vegetable sources of iron (nonheme iron) are not absorbed as well as animal sources (heme iron). Only about half of the iron in vegetables is assimilated. Vitamin C–rich foods enhance iron uptake so eat these foods when you are ingesting iron-fortified foods and supplements. The vitamin C in a glass of orange juice, for example, stimulates a threefold increase in the amount of nonheme iron absorbed from a breakfast cereal. But coffee and tea inhibit iron absorption, so don't drink them with your iron sources if you are prone to anemia.

Magnesium. This mineral aids the body's energy production and regulation of body temperature, combats stress, assists in bone growth, and muscle and nerve function. Of importance to runners, it helps maintain muscle contraction. Prolonged diarrhea, large amounts of alcohol, and profuse sweating will contribute to lower levels of this mineral. A Gallup survey found that two-thirds of regular aerobic exercisers were not obtaining the RDA for magnesium in their diet. Natural food sources include fresh green vegetables, wheat germ, soybeans, figs, corn, apples, nuts, whole wheat bread, and tofu. The most popular choice for distance runners: bananas.

Phosphorous. This mineral plays a role in almost every chemical reaction in the body, helping it use carbohydrates, fats, and proteins for growth, cell repair, and energy. It also stimulates heart and muscle contractions, helps prevent tooth decay, and maintains kidney function. It is closely linked to calcium (forming calcium phosphate) providing strength to bones. A shortage may result in loss of energy and cellular function. Good sources include lean meats, fish, chicken, eggs, whole grains, seeds, nuts—and, surprise, chocolate.

Potassium. This mineral assists sodium and chloride in functions listed above, but also aids in the conversion of glucose to glycogen, helps with cell metabolism, stimulates the kidneys to eliminate body wastes, and nourishes the muscles. A potassium-rich diet strengthens arteries and protects against high blood pressure. Good sources include green leafy vegetables, bananas, oranges, whole grains, potatoes, raisins, tuna, tomatoes, dried fruits, prunes, watermelon, molasses, and sunflower seeds.

Sodium. This mineral assists potassium and chloride in functions listed above. We lose electrolytes (sodium, potassium, and chloride) with sweat, so hard exercise in hot weather could cause some deficiencies. Sodium ingested with water after exercising helps retain fluids needed to counteract dehydration. Sodium in sports drinks helps improve taste, absorption and retention of fluids, and stimulates the thirst mechanism so we'll drink more fluids. Good food sources include seafood, poultry, carrots, and beets.

Sodium and chloride combine to form the salt compound (table salt is called sodium chloride). Forty percent of it is sodium, but this is the mineral that relates to high blood pressure for some individuals. Sodium is a critical mineral, but since the average American diet contains at least three times what is needed, deficiencies aren't common. Table salt is widely used in the preservation, processing, and preparation of foods. Salty foods to avoid include table salt, potato chips and other junk foods, salted crackers, smoked and cured meats and fish, pickles, processed cheeses, and commercial salad dressings. According to the *Surgeon General's Report* we should "reduce intake of sodium by choosing foods relatively low in sodium and limiting the amount of salt added in food preparation and at the table." Look for foods labeled "low sodium."

Do runners who sweat heavily in hot weather need to replace all the salt that is lost? Susan Kleiner, Ph.D., wrote, in *The Physician and Sports Medicine*, "As a rule of thumb, if you exercise intensely in hot conditions, let your taste buds guide you. If you find yourself craving salty foods, that may be your body's way of telling you to consume more sodium." When this happens to me I munch on a *few* potato chips, crackers, or pretzels and wash them down with a sports drink.

Zinc. This micromineral is necessary for protein metabolism and contributes to carbon dioxide transport and metabolism. This is important to runners since it helps to remove carbon dioxide from your working muscles during exercise. It also aids in healing, boosts the immune system, and, working as an antioxidant, protects against pollution. Good sources include organ meats, lean beef, lamb, chicken, sunflower seeds. As with iron, vegetarians may be deficient in zinc since animal sources of this mineral are absorbed better. Zinc is lost through sweat, which may be why some studies show lower blood levels of zinc in runners.

Caffeine

Caffeine has no nutritional value and can become toxic if taken in excess. Despite this, it is one of the most widely consumed drugs in the world. According to the International Food Information Council, 80 percent of Americans regularly consume caffeine, which is found in coffee, tea, cocoa, soft drinks, chocolate, and other foods. It is also found in many over-the-counter medications such as Anacin, Excedrin, and Dexatrim. Caffeine affects people in different ways—some more positively or negatively than others.

Many people intentionally consume lots of caffeine. Why? They love the way a cup of coffee perks them up in the morning and how coffee, tea, or cola picks them up during the day when they need to feel more alert, such as when studying, driving, or working. Caffeine increases the body's production of adrenaline, which causes a big "rush." But many people who drink caffeine regularly don't notice the increase in adrenaline after a while—they build up a tolerance. It is those who don't drink it often who are more susceptible to its stimulating effects. I'll admit that I sometimes drank cola to help me keep alert while working the many long hours involved in writing this book. But if I drank cola too late in the day it kept me from getting to sleep at night. What's a safer way to get a quick pickup when feeling drowsy? An exercise break. A short run or walk in the fresh air will invigorate you without the need for drugs. My two dogs appreciated my breaks during the writing of this book because it meant several extra walks for them. Another great pickup technique: a 15- to 30-minute nap!

Similar to but weaker than amphetamines, caffeine stimulates the central nervous system thereby increasing mental alertness and concentration, elevates mood, decreases fatigue and delays its onset.

Caffeine may also improve performance in some athletes. For one thing, drinking caffeine prior to exercise may improve mood and thus make the exercise seem easier. Indeed, I find that a glass of cola prior to a run seems to help me. It may just be a psychological boost, but I'll take all the help I can get! Some runners find that preexercise caffeine drinks help them, others find that it causes them to be too jittery or causes stomach distress. Chapter 19 examines the mixed reviews of whether caffeine can help improve running performance (some studies prove it helps some runners, others prove it doesn't). The International Olympic Committee bans large amounts of caffeine for competitive athletes (equivalent to about five or six strong cups of coffee in one to two hours) since it has physiological affects on the body that may improve performance. The message seems to be that a little caffeine to make you feel a little more perky is one thing, but to take it to gain an unfair competitive advantage isn't ethical.

On the negative side, caffeine can cause irregular heartbeats (and increase resting heart rates), hyperactivity, anxiety, sleeplessness, headaches, and intestinal discomfort. It may aggravate conditions like ulcers, gout, or high blood pressure. Pregnant and nursing women should avoid caffeine since it may stimulate the unborn infant and make its way into breast milk, which could stimulate babies, interfering with sleep for both the baby and the parents. Caffeine works as a diuretic, promoting urination and body water loss, thus increasing susceptibility to dehydration and heat illness. This is a good reason for runners to eliminate or minimize caffeine when training during hot weather or the day before and morning of races. Caffeine may also interfere with the absorption of calcium (and thus contribute to osteoporosis) and iron (and thus contribute to anemia) if taken with the sources for these minerals or within an hour after.

Studies have shown that some, but not all, individuals can become caffeine dependent, and when trying to give it up can suffer powerful withdrawal symptoms—headaches, irritability, dizziness, and in some cases vomiting and diarrhea. Doctors advise patients to cut out caffeine gradually to minimize withdrawal symptoms. Try switching gradually to decaffeinated coffee or tea or herbal teas.

Doctors generally recommend that caffeine lovers limit their intake to 50 to 200 milligrams per day, which is equal to one to three cups of coffee, two to five cups of tea, or one to four 12-ounce colas. The average caffeine consumer drinks about 280 milligrams daily or about four to five cups of coffee a day; at this level, adverse affects take place. According to the American Council on Science and Health, some 11 million Americans consume this much caffeine daily.

How much caffeine is in your favorite drinks? A 6-ounce cup of coffee has 110–150 milligrams; 25 milligrams for decaffeinated coffee. A 5-ounce cup of tea has 20–46 milligrams; a 12-ounce cola has 30–60 milligrams.

Alcohol

The Departments of Health and Human Services and Agriculture has issued guidelines for the consumption of alcohol. They recommend a maximum consumption of about one drink a day for women and two drinks a day for men, who break down alcohol faster than women. The guidelines define one drink as 12 ounces of regular beer, 5 ounces of wine, or 1.5 ounces of distilled spirits, 80 proof.

According to the *Surgeon General's Report*, "Alcohol is a drug that can produce addiction in susceptible individuals, birth defects in some children born to mothers who drink alcohol during pregnancy, impaired judgment, impaired ability to drive automobiles or operate machinery, and adverse reactions in people taking various medications. Excessive use of alcohol is also associated with liver disease, some types of cancer, high blood pressure, stroke, and disorders of the heart muscle."

Although a cold beer may seem refreshing after a run on a hot day, it is a poor choice as a sports drink. Some think that it is a good source of carbohydrates and fluids and thus is an excellent postrace choice. This isn't true. A can of beer contains only about 10 grams of carbohydrate compared to 30 grams in a bagel. Before you could get nearly enough carbohydrates from beer after a race you would get loaded, not carbo-loaded. It isn't a good fluid replacement either. In fact, it's the opposite—it works as a diuretic causing an increase in urination and thus contributes to dehydration. You may think you are drinking in plenty of fluids with beer, but you'll end up losing more in your trips to the bathroom than you can consume. Beer "passes through" me at a very fast rate! Don't drink alcohol for a few days before a big race (especially in hot weather). Limit yourself to one beer after runs or races. Be sure to have something to eat and drink some water first, to counteract the fluid loss it will cause. Beware that you can get drunk on very little alcohol when dehydrated and hungry after a run. If you run and drink, don't drive.

Drinking alcohol prior to a sports event will impair performance because the brain will not function as quickly, the muscles won't

as quickly, and you will be prone to dehydration. This
ly includes the day of the run, but the night before, too. A
t of heavy drinking will not only leave you with a hangover
e next morning, but with less stored energy. The liver stores carbohydrate as glycogen for energy. If the liver is busy processing
alcohol, then carbohydrate metabolism is affected. The result is
that liver glycogen isn't readily available to supply adequate blood
sugar to the brain and you feel fatigued and irritable. Drinking
thus interferes with two critical substances that runners need plenty
of for good performances—water and glycogen.

Alcohol contains 7 calories per gram—almost as high as fat.
These are "empty" calories that provide no appreciable amounts
of vitamins or minerals and most often end up stored as unwanted
fat. Drinking alcohol is a good way to gain weight since not only
is it high in calories but drinkers often consume it with high-calorie
snacks. It also inhibits the absorption of calcium.

Before you call me a party pooper, let me say that a cold beer
or two still has a place in the life of runners who enjoy it. A beer
or two with a meal or with popcorn while watching TV a few
times a week is fine as long as you're not pregnant, on medications,
or will be driving. Just don't drink too close to races. Drinking red
wine may even be good for you. Studies have demonstrated that
moderate consumption of red wine raises HDL cholesterol (the
good guys) and lowers LDL cholesterol (the bad guys), which results in a lower risk for heart disease and stroke.

Even the feds are willing to party—in moderation. For the first
time, in 1995, the "Dietary Guidelines for Americans" acknowledged that consuming some alcohol can be healthful. They even
went so far as to recognize that "alcoholic beverages have been
used to enhance the enjoyment of meals by many societies throughout human history."

Vegetarianism

Many runners choose to become vegetarians. Their reasons range
from religious beliefs to moral beliefs to concern about their health.
There are many degrees of vegetarianism. Pure vegetarians are
called vegans and they eat only food from plant sources. Those
whose diet comes from plants as well as dairy products are called
lactovegetarians. Ovovegetarians eat plant foods and eggs; lacto-
ovovegetarians eat plant foods, dairy products, and eggs. Dieticians

now recognize a new category, called "alternivores"; these are people who choose to eliminate meat, or at least red meat, on a part-time basis for health reasons. It is important to point out that if you don't eat meat but do consume dairy products, you may not be following a low-fat diet unless you choose low-fat dairy sources.

There is indeed lots of evidence for becoming vegetarians, particularly as increased water pollution makes more seafood unsafe, weight enhancers contaminate poultry and beef, researchers link red meat with colon cancer, and physicians tell us to lower our cholesterol and fat to fight heart disease. Plant foods generally contain more fiber, less fat, and less cholesterol than meat besides offering antioxidants to fight various diseases.

For the first time, the 1995 "Dietary Guidelines for Americans" endorsed the healthfulness of a vegetarian diet. There is a wealth of studies backing the health benefits of such a diet. In one research project in Great Britain, 6,115 vegetarians were compared to 5,015 meat eaters over a twelve-year period. The vegetarians had a 40 percent lower risk of dying from some forms of cancer and a 20 percent lower risk of dying from any cause. Other studies have demonstrated that vegetarianism lowers the risk of obesity, diabetes, high blood pressure, and heart disease. Studies by Dr. Dean Ornish of the University of California at San Francisco have presented evidence that narrowing in coronary arteries can actually be reversed through a vegetarian diet, exercise, and stress reduction. But can athletes remain healthy on a vegetarian diet? According to a position statement by the American Dietetic Association, "Vegetarian diets are healthful and nutritionally adequate when appropriately planned." The key is in eating a variety of foods and proper meal planning to compensate for those nutrients you do not consume from animal sources. Meatless diets need alternate sources of iron and zinc; dairyless diets need alternate sources of calcium. Since there are no plant sources of vitamin B_{12}, supplements may be necessary. Plant sources aren't complete proteins so no one source will supply all your protein needs. Thus you need to combine a variety of plant foods.

Fatigue and poor performances have been a result of switching to a vegetarian diet for some athletes. This is most likely due to poor food selection. If you are considering switching to a vegetarian diet, make your dietary adjustments gradually so both your mind and your body can get used to it. Consulting a sports nutritionist for help in making the changes is recommended.

Here's a good daily food guide from the American Dietetic Association's booklet *Eating Well—The Vegetarian Way*, which is an adaptation of the Food Pyramid:

- Breads, cereals, rice, and pasta: six or more servings

- Vegetables: four or more servings

- Legumes or meat substitutes: two or three servings

- Fruits: three or more servings

- Dairy products (optional): three or more servings

- Eggs (optional): limit to three or four yolks per week

- Fats, sweets, and alcohol: use sparingly

Those who exercise at high levels, such as when marathon training, need to increase the servings that contribute carbohydrates: the first four categories on the above list.

Meals

Eating regular meals and eating breakfast regularly, as mentioned in the introduction to the wellness section, are two of the seven good health practices linked to living longer, not to mention living better. Eating three meals every day combined with healthy snacking prevents a wide change in your blood sugar, which in turn affects your appetite, energy level, and ability to handle stress. That is why some people sometimes feel "on edge" when they skip a meal or have a meal out of schedule. If you have to skip a meal, skip lunch; never skip breakfast—unless you choose to skip it or minimize it prior to exercising. Many nutritionists advise eating smaller meals every four hours. The next chapter includes guidelines for eating prior to running or racing.

Dinner traditionally is the time when the family gathers at the end of the day and eats together. But its value as quality family time has dwindled as more members of the family have busy schedules—including running—that interfere with this time of togetherness. Set a daily family goal: eat together for breakfast or dinner—or perhaps a combination. Breakfast may be the best time to gather during the week.

Breakfast

Breakfast is considered the most important meal, primarily because it provides the fuel needed to get our engines going for the rest of the day. We should provide that engine with premium fuel: complex carbohydrates, protein, fiber, vitamin C, calcium, iron, and potassium. The National Cancer Institute reports that most Americans eat no high-fiber cereals or whole-grain breads at all.

Why bother with breakfast? Studies show that people who eat breakfast tend to be more alert, productive, and efficient than those who skip this meal. They are also more likely to perform well at sports, including running. There are four major dietary ingredients to athletic success, says sports nutritionist Nancy Clark. These are iron, calcium, carbohydrates—and breakfast. Clark wrote in *Runner's World*:

A substantial breakfast sets the stage for a productive, high-energy day. And when you eat healthfully (a wholesome breakfast rather than the 10 o'clock binge), you feel not only better, but also better about yourself. . . . If you skip breakfast, your ability to concentrate is likely to be diminished later in the morning, and you will work or study less efficiently. You may feel irritable and short-tempered. You may fall short of energy for your afternoon run. And worst of all, you may gain weight rather than lose weight.

Calories consumed at breakfast are more likely to be burned during the day than those eaten late in the day. A good choice is to eat a solid breakfast and then diet during the rest of the day if your goal is to lose weight. You may not be hungry after your early morning run, so drinking orange juice and milk may hold you off until you are hungry for a nutritious breakfast by mid-morning.

Nutrition experts rank cereal at the top of the list for good breakfast choices. Many cereals are rich in carbohydrates, the best source of energy for your muscles, and loaded with fiber and iron, but low in calories, fat, and cholesterol. Cereal can in fact form the center of a convenient, balanced breakfast that starts you on your full and active day. But I also recommend that you read the nutrition labels on the side of the cereal boxes. You will be surprised to find that many cereals are high in salt, fat, or sugar.

Breakfast should provide one-quarter to one-third of your daily calories as well as many essential vitamins and minerals. A cereal breakfast does that and best of all it's a quick and easy meal. Start your day like I do, with a high-fiber, vitamin- and iron-enriched cereal topped with a banana with one percent (or skim or nonfat) milk, and one or two glasses of orange juice. Sometimes I'll add a slice of bread or a bagel or muffin topped with jam as well as a glass of low-fat milk.

You don't have to eat cereal every day. When you have the time, perhaps on weekends, you may want to cook eggs (poached or boiled not fried) or good healthy carbohydrate foods such as pancakes or waffles, or other traditional breakfast foods (but beware of the fat in bacon and sausages). But breakfast should never be a cup of coffee and a doughnut on the way to the office or school —a typical breakfast for thousands of Americans.

Teenagers need special attention to make sure they eat a good breakfast. According to the National Adolescent Student Health Survey (NASHS), half of our teenage girls and one-third of our teenage boys reported eating breakfast on only two days or less during the previous week. Many of them skip lunch as well.

Lunch

Lunch is a time to recharge, but always recharge with nutritious foods, not junk. If you can't get a healthy meal at lunchtime because you're at work or at school, a "brown-bag" lunch can provide what is needed for a healthy and light meal. Beware of consistently rushing to a fast-food store for a quick, nutrition-poor lunch. Many adults either eat too much—the proverbial business lunch—or skip this meal. Some good choices for quick lunches: pizza (without extra cheese and meat toppings), turkey or chicken sandwiches (with mustard instead of mayonnaise), a peanut butter and jelly sandwich.

How does exercise fit with lunch? Exercise done at lunchtime suppresses appetite. Instead of using your lunch hour to go out to eat, you can exercise (even a 15- to 30-minute walk will help) and eat a light, nutritious lunch at your desk, such as low-fat yogurt and fruit.

Dinner

Traditionally, dinner is the main meal of the day for the American family. But it also tends to be the largest meal, and that adds calories. Research shows that when people slant their food consumption toward the evening and nighttime hours, they gain more weight than those who consume most of their foods in the morning and early afternoon. But not Shepherd. He practices the old English adage: Eat breakfast like a king, lunch like a prince, and dinner like a pauper—that is, he has his largest meal in the morning and the smallest (in terms of calories) in the evening. Besides helping to control weight, this system helps to fuel you up for your runs, which most often come prior to nightfall.

You should exercise little after dinner, although evening walks are recommended to help you relax and burn off a few additional calories. A full stomach does not promote sound sleep. Research by Dr. Kenneth Cooper indicates that exercising vigorously about two hours before the evening meal is more likely to cause a loss of body fat than exercising at other times of the day. Why? His theory is that exercise depresses your appetite just before what is typically the heaviest meal of the day.

Snacks

Snacking is permissible as long as you don't add too many extra calories to your daily diet or load up on foods full of fat and sugar. "Grazing" during the day, in fact, may be good for athletes since it serves to keep blood sugar more level—resulting in more energy for performance and mental alertness. It will also keep you from getting too hungry and overeating later, or from craving sweets. When I'm exercising a lot, I usually need a snack mid-morning, mid-afternoon, and two hours before bedtime. But I combine these with light meals rather than heavy meals so I don't take in too many calories.

Good healthy snacks would include pretzels, low-fat popcorn, raisins, fresh or dried fruits, juice, sports drinks and sports bars, low-fat granola bars, low-salt crackers, low-fat yogurt, baked potatoes, nuts, seeds, bagels, fig bars, and carrots. Another good choice—here it is again: cereal either dry or with low-fat milk. Please notice this list does not include potato chips, candy, soda, ice cream, doughnuts, and other favorite junk foods.

Nutrition Hotline

If you need a quick answer to a nutrition question, the National Center for Nutrition and Dietetics, a branch of the American Dietetic Association, offers a nutritional hot line. Call 1-800-366-1655 to talk to a registered dietitian or listen to recorded messages on nutrition.

NINETEEN

Fuel for Running

We should all concentrate on a well-balanced diet high in carbo-hydrates and low in fats. But how do we adjust what we eat and drink prior to our runs and races? Do we need to eat on the run? Is it important what we eat after we run? How do our energy needs change if we move beyond training runs at a relaxed pace and begin to run and race longer distances, even train for the marathon?

Where Do We Get Our Energy for Running?

As discussed in the previous chapter, carbohydrates, protein, and fat provide us with energy. At any level of activity, a mixture of fuels is generally being used. The intensity and duration of exercise will affect the proportion of the fuels that are used.

Your body actually prefers fat for energy since it releases 9 calories per gram when burned compared to only 4 for carbohydrates and protein. But fat, unlike carbos, isn't an efficient fuel for vig-orous exercise. Carbohydrates are the preferred foods for exercis-ers. It is the nutrient most important to endurance athletes.

During the digestion process, carbos are broken down into sim-ple sugars like glucose, which is used by the body in three ways:

Blood glucose. A small, but significant amount of glucose circulates in the blood to keep us exercising and to feed the brain to prevent mental fatigue.

Liver glycogen. Some of the glucose that is converted to glycogen is stored in the liver where it can be reconverted to glucose and quickly released into the blood to meet the energy needs of the body.

Muscle glycogen. The majority of the glucose is converted to glycogen and stored in our working muscles. Glycogen stored in muscle fiber is directly available only to that fiber. It is this muscle glycogen that is the key to vigorous exercise, not fat.

According to Nancy Clark in her *Sports Nutrition Guidebook*: "The average 150-pound active male has about 1,800 calories of carbohydrates stored in his liver, muscles, and blood in approximately the following distribution:

Muscle glycogen	1,400 calories
Liver glycogen	320 calories
Blood glucose	80 calories

"In comparison, the average *lean* 150-pound man also has about 60,000 to 100,000 calories of stored fat—enough to run hundreds of miles!"

Your body burns both carbohydrates and fats—along with some amounts of protein—at the same time to produce energy. You don't just run out of one fuel source and switch to the other. The percent of each used at any time is determined by the amount of oxygen needed (intensity of exercise) and by how quickly fuel is needed. At low intensities, oxygen is readily available to burn fat for fuel. But it takes approximately three times as much oxygen to burn a gram of fat as it does a gram of carbohydrate. Thus, at higher levels of exercise intensity, with increased oxygen demands, a higher percentage of energy comes from carbohydrates. Carbos can be delivered quickly. Most of it is stored as glycogen in your muscles right where it's needed. Glycogen converts to glucose and is burned by the muscles for energy. Fat, however, is stored in large complex molecules all over your body. It takes a much longer time for fat to break down and make its way to your working muscles to supply energy.

You don't need a lot of energy to read this page; so fats supply most of your needs. You are burning approximately two-thirds fat and one-third carbohydrates. But start to run and this mix changes. You need more oxygen, more fuel, and you need it faster. To meet this need, your body increases the amount of carbohydrates it burns. During the first few minutes of exercise, you burn about 80 percent carbohydrates and 20 percent fats. Once you have settled into your pace during light to moderate aerobic exercise, and your heart and lungs are efficiently supplying enough oxygen to the working muscles, you use fat and carbohydrates about equally. Thus, most of your easy-paced runs will be supplied with approximately 50 percent of energy from carbohydrates and 50 percent from fats. The longer or more intense the activity, the greater the use of carbohydrates. With high-intensity running, such as in racing or speed training, 70 to 80 percent of your energy needs come from carbohydrate sources. Your glycogen stores determine how long you can exercise at your desired pace.

Marathon running demands a lot of carbohydrates: for the average runner, up to 70 percent (up to 80 percent for elite runners) of the total energy used in a marathon will come from carbohydrates compared to 30 percent from fats. In the late miles of a marathon, as carbo stores deplete, fat becomes valuable as an energy source and protein is also used more.

All runners should concentrate on including plenty of carbohydrates in their diet. According to Dr. David Costill, Ph.D., director of the Human Performance Laboratory at Ball State University, the best diet for most runners—indeed, for most healthy people—contains at least 50 percent, but ideally 60 percent or more, carbohydrates, less than 20 to 30 percent fat, and 10 to 15 percent protein. The runner who puts in 50 miles a week or more, such as in marathon training, probably needs to consume about 700 additional calories a day, and that diet should include up to 70 percent carbohydrates. Most of these should be in the form of complex carbohydrates.

As a beginner or intermediate runner, your 20- to 30-minute runs will be fueled almost equally by stored fat and stored carbohydrates (glycogen). Your body has plenty of fat stores—enough to run for many hours—unfortunately, glycogen stores are much more limited. Glycogen stores will be diminished after intense exercise, such as racing or repeated sprints, or after long runs of one and a half hours or more. You will still have enough fat to offset the lack of glycogen, but since it doesn't burn as efficiently as glycogen, your performance will suffer. When you run low of glycogen, you will not be able to exercise intensely and may experience significant fatigue. You may "hit the wall," which we detail below.

Further, glycogen depletion can be caused by chronic heavy training. During successive days of high mileage or intense running—such as marathon training—glycogen stores can become progressively lower, resulting in fatigue. To keep muscle glycogen at high levels you need to eat a diet high in carbohydrates and follow a sensible training program that provides for rest days. Overtraining and not eating enough carbos will lead to poor health and mediocre runs and races. Proper training will help here: A study by Dr. Costill demonstrated that well-trained muscles develop the ability to store 20 to 50 percent more glycogen than untrained muscles.

Hitting "the Wall"

Hitting "the wall" refers to that point when you run short of glycogen. This is an experience that every runner should try—once. After you've survived it, you will respect the need to prepare better for your next marathon.

If you have never hit "the wall," let me describe it to you. In my early days of marathoning I learned the hard way about the values of long training runs, tapering, eating plenty of carbos, and not starting too fast. Ignoring these factors all contribute to hitting "the wall." I remember my first marathon. I was running well for 15 miles, and then I started to feel leg fatigue. By Mile 20, I felt as if I were sleepwalking. I was very tired and had an overwhelming urge to quit and find a good place to take a long nap. My pace quickly dropped by a minute per mile and then 2 minutes per mile. It got so bad that runners twice my age who were walking passed me as I ran. Yet I struggled to the finish line of my first marathon.

Hitting "the wall" is most often associated with the marathon event, but you may experience it even in half-marathons if you haven't properly prepared. After an hour and a half or so of running, you begin to run low on glycogen. For most runners that will be 10 to 13 miles into a run. The average well-trained runner may store enough glycogen to last 15 to 20 miles, depending upon such factors as pace, body weight, fitness level, and how well they loaded up on carbohydrates going into the race.

When you run low on glycogen, your body attempts to conserve what remains by burning more fat for energy. But since fat is 15 percent less efficient than carbohydrates as an energy source, you are unable to hold your pace and have to slow dramatically. Long training runs develop mechanisms for your body to utilize fat more efficiently throughout your race, thus "sparing" some glycogen for use later. Workouts at marathon pace and faster will also train your muscles to utilize carbohydrates more efficiently at these paces. In addition, starting your race at a conservative pace will help conserve glycogen for later in the run. Tapering for a marathon (see Chapter 14) combined with carbohydrate-loading (detailed later in this chapter) is the key to surviving "the wall."

Liquid Carbohydrates: Sports Drinks

Most sports drinks fall into one of two categories: fluid replacements and carbohydrate-loaders. Fluid replacement drinks like Gatorade not only help you hydrate, but they also supply some additional energy for exercise. Typically, they will have a carbohydrate concentration of 6 to 8 percent. These drinks may improve performance by helping runners maintain blood glucose levels that otherwise would fall and cause fatigue in runs of an hour or longer. These sports drinks can be used before, during, and after running to energize your body. These types of drinks are usually available at liquid stations during most major marathons. Fluid replacement sports drinks are discussed in more detail in the next chapter.

Carbohydrate-loading sports drinks such as GatorLode, Carboplex, Ultra Fuel, and Exceed High Carbohydrate aren't meant to replenish fluids. They are primarily used to help build energy stores. They typically contain a carbohydrate concentration of 20 to 25 percent (three to four times the typical concentration of regular sports drinks). Basically, these are not drinks; rather, they are liquid meals that are to be ingested an hour or two before running, or after. Don't drink liquid carbos during your runs—they are not intended for that purpose. (A lower concentration of carbohydrates as provided in regular sports drinks is needed to allow for fast and efficient absorption of fluids on the run.)

Liquid carbohydrate drinks provide a mix of complex and simple carbohydrates, and they normally contain no fat or proteins.

These drinks leave the stomach faster than solid foods and allow you to pack in carbos easier and faster.

You should consume 60 to 70 percent of your daily calories as carbohydrates. If you are not able to meet this standard, these high carbohydrate drinks may be used to supplement your diet. It may also be difficult to eat enough carbos without feeling too full during periods of heavy training. Again, liquid carbos may come to your rescue. An 8-ounce glass of one of these drinks may provide as many carbohydrates as two cups of pasta. If you don't have time to cook a high-carbo meal, you can load up with fluids. But don't look to these liquid meals as a replacement of your steady diet— they don't contain all the essential nutrients you need for good health. Stick to a balanced diet and use these drinks as a supplement to pack in more energy.

These drinks are most effective to ensure prerun loading and postrun replenishment for runs of one and a half hours or longer. Liquid carbos will be of minimal benefit to beginner and intermediate runners, but they may be of help if you move up to marathon training. If you try them, experiment with liquid carbo boosts one or two hours before your training runs. Some runners find that these drinks do not agree with their stomachs.

Sports Bars

One dietary supplement that gained popularity among exercisers in the 1980s and 1990s was the "sports bar." When Shepherd first heard about them way up there in Vermont, he thought they were something with a curved oak railing, brass footrest, and Monday night football on a big screen. On the contrary, ol' Shep, a sports bar is an energy bar that is ideal for a quick snack, light meal, preexercise fuel boost, energy pickup during a long run, or a post-exercise recovery food. Instead of grabbing that candy bar or box of cookies when you're hungry and have a workout coming up, grab a sports bar instead. They are designed for active people who need nourishment in a hurry that won't bog them down.

You should choose a bar with less than 30 percent fat and more than 60 percent carbohydrates. In comparison, candy bars will have 60 percent fat with few carbohydrates and will contain two or three times as many calories per ounce. Most sports bars provide lots of carbohydrates to energize your run as well as some amounts of protein, vitamins, minerals, and fiber. The composition of the carbos packed into sports bars is important, too. Most sports nutritionists recommend a fifty-fifty mix of simple carbohydrates (sugars) and complex carbohydrates (starches). The simple carbohydrates give immediate results: They replenish blood glucose and so are quickly used as a source of energy. The complex carbohydrates take longer to break down and so provide a steady stream of energy later in the run.

Beware: Some sports bars are ripoffs and are high in fat or contain substances such as bee pollen accompanied by unproven claims of high performance. Read the nutrition labels carefully. A pioneer and leader in the field is PowerBar, founded by former Canadian Olympic marathoner Brian Maxwell. This sports bar provides a mix of simple and complex carbohydrates, soluble fiber, protein, and branched-chain amino acids (which delay the breakdown of protein in the muscle tissue). They are fortified with several vitamins and minerals and each bar provides 225 calories of which 75 percent is from carbohydrates and less than 10 percent is fat. Other popular sports bars include Exceed Sports Bar, PR Bar, GatorBar, and Edgebar.

A relatively new option as an energy food source are concentrated carbohydrate gels. ReLoad, a gel developed by Gatorade scientists, packs 20 grams of carbohydrates into a small, easy-to-open packet. Just tear it open and squeeze out the carbos for an easy-to-chew (or slurp), easy-to-digest energy boost. Use one or two packets one or two hours prior to running in a marathon, or within 30 minutes after finishing a long run or race.

If you want to supplement your diet with a sports bar (or gel), experiment before, during, and after training runs until you find one you like. Don't eat them for the first time before a race since they may upset your stomach. You should drink plenty of water or nonalcoholic fluids (8 to 16 ounces) when you eat the bar or gel to aid in digestion, especially in hot weather when you will need to combat dehydration as well.

The earlier sports bars tasted like mud, but many of them are now quite tasty and come in all kinds of flavors. However, don't chow down a bunch of them during the day, because they each contain approximately 200 calories. Save them for when you really need them—to help you perform better for a workout or race. I'll eat a sports bar an hour before a hard workout or race (along with plenty of water to increase absorption), but not on the run (my stomach doesn't agree with them while running). I also enjoy chewing on them afterward, when I need to restock my energy stores but have a limited appetite.

Caffeine

Will caffeine improve your runs and races? Depends on who you ask. Some runners swear it helps, others swear at it. For every runner that feels he must have that cup of coffee to pick him up before exercising, there is another who finds that caffeine prior to exercise makes her too jittery and causes untimely bathroom stops. Some runners even seem to benefit from drinking defizzed cola during races—as Frank Shorter did on the way to winning the 1972 Olympic Marathon in Munich. I know runners who mix water and defizzed cola fifty-fifty and have friends hand them their magic drink at key spots along the marathon course. The sugar helps reenergize them and the caffeine perks them up. I find that a quick drink of cola late in a long training run helps me regain alertness and gives me a perception of feeling stronger.

How much of this is physiological and how much is psychological? If it works, who cares? Researchers have proven that caffeine enhances performance, particularly for events of one mile to 5K. Other researchers have proven that it doesn't, and that it may contribute to dehydration—particularly for runs of one hour or more in hot weather.

What should you do? Dan Becque, Ph.D., and colleagues at Southern Illinois University in Carbondale reviewed all the caffeine studies, including some of their own, and reported on their findings to the annual meeting of the American College of Sports Medicine. Their conclusion was that caffeine can improve performance under some conditions, but considering the potential performance-impeding and health-risk side effects (remember this is a drug), why bother? They suggested that the better way to go is to boost performance with carbohydrates. They added that if you usually enjoy one or two cups of coffee, or colas, prior to running, there's no reason to change, but if you don't normally consume caffeine-containing drinks, there's no reason to start.

Besides, caffeine probably does not enhance athletic performance in beginner and intermediate runners: Studies show the greatest measurable performance enhancement benefits are with well-trained elite runners. Beginner and intermediate runners may benefit from some caffeine to perk them up enough to get them out the door.

Fasting

Some feel that the best way to eat to improve performance is to not eat at all—that is, fast to run fast. This was one of the more controversial myths of the 1980s. Some 13 percent of the distance runners surveyed back then by *Runner's World* said that they fasted regularly for one to three days at a time, consuming only water and juices. Others fasted for up to two weeks. Some runners believe that fasting cleanses and "detoxifies" the body, and prepares its metabolism for the stress of long-distance racing after its glycogen supplies are low. But there are many potential side effects to fasting that are not good for your health. I experimented with fasting for a few days at a time back in those serious running days. The result for me was that I ran poorly.

Indeed, for regular exercisers, fasting appears to have the opposite effect of carbohydrate-loading—it "unloads" the runner. A study of marathon runners by Dr. David Nieman and researchers at the Human Performance Laboratory of Loma Linda University in California showed that those runners who fasted, compared to those tested who were fed, had a 45 percent decrease in endurance. The fasting runners also had a hard time going faster—they reported difficulty in holding their pace. Prior to the run, the fasting runners had leg muscle glycogen levels 17 percent lower than the fed runners. The study's researchers made an interesting summary of their results: "Fasting for 24 hours prior to a competition is like running for 90 minutes prior to the competitive event."

Fasting appears to offer no endurance bonuses. Fortunately, very few runners today fast. If you need to fast for religious or other reasons, be sure to cut back on your training until you can get back on the recommended high-carbohydrate, low-fat balanced diet that we recommend for good health and optimal performance.

Should You Eat Before Your Run or Race?

According to Nancy Clark, in her *Sports Nutrition Guidebook*, any preexercise or prerace meal has four functions:

1. To help prevent hypoglycemia (low blood sugar), with its symptoms of lightheadedness, needless fatigue, blurred vision,

and indecisiveness—all of which can interfere with top performance.

If you run low of blood sugar, your brain doesn't receive enough fuel. This can happen during a 30-minute run for beginner runners or during a marathon for highly trained athletes. It can affect your mental stamina to perform up to your abilities. It may cause you to want to just quit, give up. When your blood sugar is low, your liver breaks down glycogen to glucose and releases it into the bloodstream to maintain a normal sugar level. If your muscle glycogen depletes, you hit "the wall." But if your liver glycogen depletes, you get brain drain.

How do you prevent this? By timing your meals properly. It is several hours between dinner and a race the next morning. You may be fully loaded with glycogen in your muscles, but you may have burned off much of the limited glycogen stored in the liver just from normal bodily functions. Your body will be ready to run but you may lack fuel for the brain. This could cause you to have a lousy run or a poor race. Liver glycogen can be topped off by eating a small carbohydrate meal two or three hours before running. This small meal will prevent mental fatigue caused by low blood sugar. Easy-to-digest carbohydrate drinks or sports bars may be taken an hour before the run to combat this problem.

2. To help settle your stomach, absorb some of the gastric juices, and abate hunger feelings.

Many runners can't run on an empty stomach for these reasons. For others, this isn't as much of a problem as dealing with food that may irritate the digestive system while under stress. Much more than half a bagel or a slice of toast and I'm in trouble.

3. To fuel your muscles, particularly with food eaten far enough in advance to be digested and stored as glycogen.

4. To pacify your mind with the knowledge that your body is well-fueled.

If you are worried that you don't have enough food in you for your run, you won't perform with confidence.

We need to find out for ourselves what are the best foods for us to eat before exercising and racing—and whether to eat at all. And your body's reaction to eating may change. It used to be that I couldn't eat anything for several hours before running. That was when I was younger and faster. Now I find that if I don't eat in the morning before running I feel very weak. On the other hand, if I eat too much or the wrong foods, I have to make a few pit stops.

I've known runners who could wolf down a full dinner, lace up the shoes, and go out for a run. No simple habit or food will bring a great run for everyone. You've got to find what is best for you.

Preexercise Eating Tips

Here are a few suggestions that may help you with your prerun meals:

- Avoid foods with a high sugar content, especially in the hour before running. These include soft drinks and candies. They will give you a quick "sugar boost," and then turn around and give you a "sugar low" during your workout. Suggests Clark: "If you simply must have a little bit of something sweet, eat it within 5 to 10 minutes of exercise. This short time span is too brief for the body to secrete insulin, the hormone that causes low blood sugar. Because the body stops secreting insulin when you start to exercise, you should be able to handle this sugar fix safely *if* the food settles comfortably."

  Also avoid high-fat proteins like cheese and red meat that take a long time to digest. Milk causes problems for many runners, so be careful about having it prior to running (including with your cereal). Fructose (the sugar in fruit and honey), unlike glucose, will not contribute to performance and it may cause stomach distress. The best bet is to choose high-starch, low-fat foods—trusty carbohydrates such as breads, bagels, pasta. The key here is to select easily digestible, quick-energy foods. These are the foods that you should eat daily for good health and for good running performance.

- Prior to racing, don't eat anything you haven't previously eaten. Experiment before your regular workouts, not your races. Don't be unpleasantly surprised by trying something new on race day—or the night before for that matter.

▪ Allow plenty of time for digestion. This may vary from an hour or two for a small snack, sports energy bar, or a liquid carbohydrate meal to two to four hours (or even more) after a meal. Your last meal before exercising should be a light one, not a heavy feast.

Allow more time for digestion before intense exercise than before light or moderate exercise. What works well before training runs doesn't always hold up—or stay down—during races. I can eat a bagel and wash it down with a sports drink an hour before an easy half-hour run, but I can't eat even a small meal for at least three hours before a race. During an intense workout your muscles require more blood so your stomach may get only 20 percent or so of its normal blood flow, which slows digestion. During an easy run at your conversational pace, your stomach will still get about two-thirds of normal blood flow, which will still allow near-normal digestion to take place.

▪ If you can't handle food in the morning prior to your runs or races, even a liquid meal, make sure to eat well the day before. Try a bedtime snack instead of breakfast. But beware that overnight fasting reduces liver glycogen stores that, if not replaced in the morning prior to exercise, may result in a poor performance due to a shortage of available blood glucose.

▪ What works well for you before nonimpact activities such as biking or swimming may differ from what works with running. The up and down movement associated with running may contribute to abdominal stress.

▪ Drink plenty of water and other nonalcoholic and noncaffeinated fluids with your meals to aid digestion and to prevent dehydration.

Carbohydrate-Loading

You "carbo-load" to improve your performance for long races lasting more than one and a half hours. The goal is to avoid hitting "the wall." You may carbo-load for a 10-mile or half-marathon race, but for most runners this ritual comes into play mainly for marathoning. Packing in the carbohydrates seems to work as well for the average runner as for the faster runner. In fact, the back-of-the-packers may benefit the most from it.

Dr. Costill, coauthor of *Physiology of Sports and Exercise*, notes,

> The difference between elite and average marathoners is that even if both started out with the same amount of glycogen, the elite marathoner would spare it by burning a higher ratio of fat. Although more oxygen is required to burn fat, the highly developed oxygen transport system of the elite runner allows this. Furthermore, he moves more economically, which means that he uses less oxygen to accomplish the same task. The average runner, on the other hand, depletes his glycogen supply sooner and doesn't have as efficient an oxygen transport system to burn fat. That's why hitting the wall is so devastating and why carbohydrate loading is more important for the average runner than for the elite runner.

Not only that, the average four- or five-hour marathoner has to keep running much longer than those sub-three-hour runners after becoming glycogen depleted.

The key to carbo-loading is to rest the muscles going into the race, thus hoarding glycogen in the rested muscles, while at the same time increasing the carbohydrates in your diet, thus adding to your glycogen stores. This combination allows your body to "load up" on glycogen, which should give you an increased energy supply for long-distance running.

Here are the basic ingredients for carbo-loading:

▪ Start cutting back on your training two or three weeks before a long race or marathon. Especially minimize your running the last three days. If you are running less, you'll be burning less glycogen for fuel and can store more for the marathon race. See Chapter 14 for more information on marathon tapering.

▪ Stick to your normal diet, which should consist of approximately 60 percent carbohydrates until three days before the event.

▪ With three days to go, increase your carbohydrates to 70 percent of your diet. Really pack in the carbohydrates. The key is to increase the percentage of carbohydrates in your diet, not the calories. This may be a good time to use liquid carbohydrates to supplement your meals.

■ Don't eliminate protein from your diet as you get close to the marathon. Your body still needs protein on a daily basis. But stick to small servings of low-fat protein such as chicken.

■ Drink plenty of water as you are loading. Water is stored in muscle tissue along with glycogen, and your muscles will take from other organs if enough isn't supplied from the outside, which could lead to dehydration. You may find that you'll gain a few pounds (2 to 4) and feel bloated while loading, but don't worry about it. This is to be expected since your body stores 2.6 grams of water for every gram of glycogen that you load. Most of that is water weight, and you'll lose that and more during your run as you start to sweat. You should pack in about 3 ounces of water for each ounce of carbohydrate stored.

■ Beware of fats hidden in your high-carbohydrate diet. This includes ice cream, cookies, extra cheese on pizza. Skip the butter on your toast, pancakes, and baked potatoes; cream cheese on your bagel; and rich sauces on pasta.

■ Eat a high-carbohydrate meal that will agree with your stomach the night before your marathon or long race. Years ago coaches used to promote a big steak to build muscle as the preevent meal. Indeed, my college cross-country team used to go out for a steak dinner the night before our races. Now the meal of choice is pasta! Don't eat too late at night and don't eat too much for dinner or you may not fully digest it prior to a morning race. Spaghetti, macaroni, and noodles are popular choices. Steamed or boiled rice is fine (fried rice contains too much oil), and potatoes. Good carbohydrate sources are fruits, starchy vegetables, and breads. Some runners, myself included, like to load up on pancakes or waffles. Drink plenty of water or other nonalcoholic and noncaffeinated fluids to help you pack in the carbos and hydrate for the race.

This "last supper" is an important meal. You should eat about 6:00 P.M. when preparing for a morning race the next day. A light snack, such as an apple or banana or sports bar, around 10:00 P.M. may help you feel more prepared. Select carefully where you eat the night before. Make reservations, or if dining out at the prerace feed, get there early. Don't upset your stomach by standing in line, and don't attend that spaghetti feast for the masses if the scene is too exciting for you. Don't eat anything that is unfamiliar to you. The best option may be the dullest and safest one: a quiet meal at home or in your hotel room.

■ Eat a light, high-carbohydrate breakfast two or three hours prior to running your race if you have found doing so before a long run and race works for you. Good choices: bagels, toast, bananas, raisins, rice, liquid carbohydrates. You may wish to eat a sports bar an hour before to give you an extra energy boost.

■ Drink 8–16 ounces of a sports drink (with 6 to 8 percent carbohydrates levels) 5 to 15 minutes before the start of the race. And you can keep loading during your run by drinking 4–8 ounces of sports drink every 10 to 20 minutes (or every 2 miles).

Food for 5Ks and 10Ks

Shorter races of less than 90 minutes, particularly less than an hour, don't diminish glycogen stores nearly as much as marathons. Thus, carbohydrate intake isn't as critical. Nevertheless, muscle glycogen still plays an important role since you need to burn plenty of carbos to fuel an effort that will most likely be much harder than your training pace and much faster than your marathon pace. If you follow a recommended daily high carbohydrate diet of at least 60 percent carbohydrates and taper your mileage three to seven days before your race, you shouldn't need to be concerned about a prerace meal to pack in more fuel. Eat what makes you comfortable and eat it two or three hours prior to the race. This will ward off hypoglycemia and brain fatigue. If you choose not to eat, it may be helpful to take in some sports drink or sports bar an hour before. Be aware that the amount and types of foods you can eat the morning of a slower-paced marathon may not work for you at the more intense pace of a short race. I may eat a small meal three or four hours before a marathon, but never before a shorter race.

In research at Texas Christian University, runners were tested in 10K races after trying out different types of carbohydrate foods an hour before each event. They also raced after drinking water with no carbohydrates included. Average race times were the same for all concoctions, including the one with no carbos. They concluded that a carbohydrate snack or drink an hour before a short race didn't harm performance, but neither did it help it. These runners, however, sped through the 10K in 40 minutes. In races over an hour (including 10K runners racing at 10 minutes per mile and slower), certainly over an hour and a half, you may benefit from prerace carbohydrate intake.

Fueling Up During Exercise

Adding fuel on the run isn't that critical for shorter runs. You should have enough glycogen stored in your muscles to meet your needs. For workouts lasting an hour or more, however, added fuel during the run will boost performance. In the early stages of a long race most of your energy will come from stored muscle glycogen. Later, the sugar in your blood (blood glucose) and your liver glycogen becomes more significant as you start to deplete stored muscle glycogen. Carbohydrate intake before and during your run will help you meet this energy need. But how do you eat while running? One simple way is to drink in the fuels with a sports drink that has a 6 to 8 percent carbohydrate solution. Not only do such drinks as Gatorade help keep you hydrated, they boost performance by sustaining blood glucose levels and sparing muscle glycogen, allowing you to work out longer and harder.

A study directed by Clyde Williams, Ph.D., at the Loughborough University of Technology in England compared the effect of fueling up for races to just drinking water. Four men and three women raced each other over a 30K (18.6-mile) distance. Before the events they stuck to their normal daily diet. On race day they drank 8.5 ounces of a 5 percent carbohydrate drink before starting, and they drank another 5 ounces every 5K of the race. Before another 30K race, they drank the same amount of fluids, but this time it was water. On the average, the runners ran 3 minutes better with the carbohydrate drink for an improvement of 2.3 percent. For a marathon that would equate to a difference of approximately 5 minutes for the average four- or five-hour performer. The runners ran the same pace with both types of fluids, but without carbos the runners slowed significantly over the last 5K. They hit "the wall."

Research at Florida State University in Tallahassee has documented, as have many other studies, that carbohydrate drinks taken just before and during exercise improves performance. Highly trained runners were given either a 7 percent carbohydrate drink or a placebo—both right before running as well as every 15 minutes during a run. They ran until exhausted. The result: On the average, those that drank carbos lasted 29 percent longer and they reported their effort to be easier during the run.

What about eating solid foods? University of North Carolina at Greensboro researchers found that solid bananas were as helpful as liquid carbohydrates when fed during exercise—and both improved performance compared to just drinking water. Studies at the University of Texas at Austin and at the University of New Mexico in Albuquerque also found that solid carbohydrates were as effective as liquid carbos. Their conclusion was it may be helpful to eat small pieces of bananas or sports bars during long, hard workouts since they pack in more carbos than liquids do. However, you need to drink plenty of water with them to facilitate absorption. This works for some. Others find that anything solid eaten on the run causes stomach distress.

What should you do? Again, experiment in your long runs and practice races, not during an important race like a marathon. I consume a sports drink every 2 miles in long races and will eat small pieces of bananas a few times during the race as well. In between, I drink water. For example, at the New York City Marathon, they give Gatorade every 2 miles and water every mile. I'll drink water at the odd miles and Gatorade at the even miles. Indeed, University of Texas research backs that strategy. They found that drinking only water or only liquid carbos would result in a smaller performance gain than if you drank both.

The best strategy appears to be to drink 8–16 ounces of a sports drink 5 to 15 minutes before a long, hard effort and then, every 10 to 20 minutes, take in more carbos either in liquid (about six swallows) or solid form. Continue to drink plenty of water, especially on a hot day. About 30–60 grams of carbohydrate per hour is recommended to keep blood glucose levels high. This strategy will work to fight off the effects of dehydration, hypoglycemia, and glycogen depletion resulting in a more comfortable, improved performance. It is important to point out that fatigue during your runs cannot be prevented by fueling up on carbohydrates on the run. It can, however, be delayed.

Fueling Up After Exercise

Runners have two replacement priorities after exercising. First, as discussed in the next chapter, you need to drink plenty of fluids to replace what you've lost with sweating. You also need to replace the stored carbohydrates that you depleted during your run. Carbohydrate "reloading" is as important as carbohydrate-loading before your run.

Beginner and intermediate runners completing workouts of 20 to 60 minutes do not need to be concerned about reloading muscles with glycogen after their runs. As long as they follow a high-carbohydrate daily diet the body will easily replenish what is used within a day. But if you run one and a half hours and longer— such as in marathon training and racing—then you should pay attention to the "carbohydrate window" theory. This is even more important to those high-mileage runners who may run over an hour and a half several days in a row, or run twice a day.

According to research by John Ivy, Ph.D., at the University of Texas, muscles are most receptive to glycogen replacement if you eat within the first two hours following long or intense runs. Subsequent research by Ivy and also by W. Michael Sherman, Ph.D., at Ohio State University, further refined that theory: The sooner you can ingest carbohydrates after running the better. According to Ivy, "The longer you wait before consuming carbohydrates, the less 'hungry' your muscles become. If you wait longer than 15 minutes, the rate of absorption is decreased by roughly 50 percent." Eating while this "window" is open will help you recover sooner, allowing you to maintain a higher energy level throughout the day and be better prepared for your next run.

But what should you eat after running? Carbos, again. You need to reload. But it isn't practical to sit down to a big dish of pasta right after you've finished a long training run, certainly not as soon as you've finished a marathon. A quick way to get large amounts of these carbos into your system when you have a reduced appetite is to consume high-carbohydrate drinks and energy bars (taken with large amounts of water). Low-carbohydrate sports drinks that you consume during your runs will help you replenish fluids and give you a start on your carbohydrate needs until you feel ready to consume foods or drinks high in carbohydrates.

Liz Applegate, Ph.D., wrote in her nutrition column in *Runner's World*,

Postrace refueling is essential for quick recovery. . . . Take in about 50 to 100 grams of carbohydrates within the first 15 minutes after your race. Go for liquids first, until you have an appetite for bulkier items; then stay with foods such as bread, bagels and raisins, which all get into your system quickly. Following a long race, your goal should be to consume 600 grams (or 2,400 calories) of carbohydrates in the next 24 hours. So pace yourself at about 50 grams every 2 hours, on the average (dependent on body size). A recent study showed that including protein with carbohydrates in those first meals after racing replenishes glycogen faster.

Still more studies by Dr. Sherman at Ohio State suggest you can load even more glycogen into the muscles by eating smaller amounts of 25–60 grams of carbohydrates over the next four hours at more frequent intervals—every 15 to 45 minutes. Most of you don't train at high mileage and race at very intense paces, so if this is too much for you to bother with I suggest the following: reload within 15 minutes of running with at least 50 grams of carbohydrates and then another 50 grams or more within two hours, then eat every two hours until you eat a regular meal.

FIGURE 19.1: SUMMARY OF FOOD INTAKE FOR RUNNERS

Daily	Low-fat, high-carbohydrate (60 percent of calories or more) diet
Before running	Eat a small high-carbohydrate meal two to three hours prior to running, or a liquid carbo meal or sports bar one to two hours prior. Drink 8–16 ounces of a sports drink 5 to 15 minutes prior to long runs or races.
During running	Drink 4–8 ounces of a sports drink every 10 to 20 minutes during long races. Banana pieces also help. Also, 30–60 grams of carbos per hour is recommended.
After running	After long runs and races, consume 50–100 grams of carbos within 15 minutes, another 50 grams every two hours until you eat a regular meal.

TWENTY

Hydration for Running

Everyone who exercises must drink, drink, drink—before, during, and after your runs and throughout the day. Hydration is important no matter what the weather, but you should be especially attentive to your fluid needs in warm weather (further guidelines for coping with hot weather running are detailed in the next chapter). The closer you can come to replacing all the fluids that you lose during running, the better off you will be both performance-wise and health-wise. Prevention of dehydration and heat illness is even more important than carbohydrate replacement. If you are low on carbos, you just slow down. But you can die from dehydration.

According to exercise physiologists David Costill, Ph.D., and Jack Wilmore, Ph.D., in their book *Physiology of Sports and Exercise*, "It has been estimated that we can survive losses of up to 40 percent of our body weight in fat, carbohydrate and protein. But a water loss of 9 percent to 12 percent of body weight can be fatal."

Here is how your body reacts to exercise. Heat is produced in the exercising muscles as calories are burned for energy. Your body produces fifteen to twenty times more heat during exercise than it does at rest. As your body temperature rises, your brain signals for sweat production. So when we run, we sweat. This is both good and bad. Sweating cools the body—4 ounces of sweat prevents a one-degree rise in body temperature. When body fluid is lost through sweat and not replaced, you may dehydrate. The result: reduced performance and an increased risk of the heat illness as described in the next chapter.

Exercise and Water Loss

Approximately 90 percent of water lost during exercise is by sweating. Most of the rest is lost through respiration. The average sweat rate during running is about 1 to 1.5 quarts per hour. Since you will lose about 2 pounds of body weight per quart of sweat produced, you would lose 2 or 3 pounds per hour for most runs. You will lose even more when running at a faster pace and in hot weather. Runners exercising vigorously have been measured with losses of over 2 quarts of sweat (4 pounds of body weight) per hour.

The combination of dehydration, heat buildup generated by the workout, and warm air temperatures can dramatically increase your body temperature. Your normal body temperature is 98.6° F. If you run on a hot day it will rise to over 100° F., making you vulnerable to heat-related illnesses. Life-threatening heatstroke occurs when your body temperature rises above 104° F. It is critical to hold down your body temperature by replacing lost fluids. Studies by Dr. Costill have shown that rectal temperatures in runners are two degrees (F.) cooler when the runner drank fluids during a two-hour run than when they did not.

An adequate water supply allows your body fluids to accomplish several tasks that are essential to exercise. When you are dehydrated, your cells malfunction and work inefficiently, sweating decreases, heart rate and body temperature increase, blood volume decreases, and you have less blood to transport oxygen and glucose through your body.

Besides the risk of a heat-related illness, performance is also affected by water loss. According to Costill and Wilmore, "Even minimal changes in your body's water content can impair endurance performance. Without adequate fluid replacement, a subject's exercise tolerance shows a pronounced decrease during long-term activity because of water loss through sweating. Studies have shown that dehydrated people are intolerant of prolonged exercise and heat stress."

Studies conducted by Dr. Costill show a steady decline in exercise performance (as measured by aerobic capacity) with dehydration: a 1 percent loss of body weight yields nearly a 5 percent loss in aerobic capacity; a 2 percent loss of body weight results in a nearly 10 percent decline in exercise performance; a 4 percent loss of body weight results in a nearly 25 percent loss in the capacity for prolonged aerobic effort. Performance can be affected in as little as 30 minutes of running; the longer you run the more you dehydrate and the more your pace will decline.

How much we sweat on the run depends upon several factors:

- Temperature: The hotter it is, the more we sweat.

- Humidity: High levels increase sweating but interfere with the evaporation of sweat.

- Wind: Head winds help cool the body thus reducing the need for sweat production.

- Body size: Bigger people will sweat more.

- Fitness level: A well-conditioned person will have more and enlarged sweat glands producing more sweat to cool the body. They also perspire sooner into a run.

- Exercise intensity: The harder you run, the more you will sweat.

- Genetics: How much you sweat is also in part determined by genetics. Some people, like myself, sweat more than others and have more trouble coping with the heat.

- Gender: Women tend to sweat less and more efficiently than men.

You also need to be concerned with chronic dehydration, which can affect you later in the day or even several days later. Dehydration can be a result of a single run, or from running several days in a row without proper rehydration. Warning: Dehydration can occur even in cold weather if you don't drink enough fluids.

How Do We Know If We Are Dehydrating?

Thirst is not an early sign of dehydration. Runners, especially those over age sixty-five and kids, need to drink more fluids than thirst demands. Any one of us can lose as much as 2 quarts of fluids before getting thirsty. The easiest way to know if you have sufficiently replaced lost fluids is to check the color and frequency of your urine. A good flow of clear or pale yellow urine indicates that your body has good normal fluid balance. Dark and little urine may indicate, among other things, the need to replace lost fluids. If you need to urinate frequently over the next few hours after your run then most likely you're getting enough fluid.

I remember many years ago getting the scare of my life. After running 20 miles on a hot day and drinking very little fluids on the run, my urine turned purple! Then I remembered drinking two bottles of grape soda after I finished my run. My body was so dehydrated that the fluids went right through me faster than the body could filter out the food coloring in the sodas.

Another good monitor is to weigh yourself before and after exercise. If your weight in the morning is 2 pounds or more below that of the previous morning, your sudden weight loss is most likely due to too much water weight loss. Don't celebrate yet. Drink up! Besides checking your urine and weight loss, also pay attention to how you feel. If you feel tired several days in a row, especially when training a lot in hot weather, suspect that you may be chronically dehydrated.

What to Drink in Your Daily Diet

Your body is 50 to 60 percent water and it needs a good fresh supply every day to function normally. There is little danger of consuming too much water; any excess is flushed away by your kidneys. On the other hand, not drinking enough fluids when you are running a lot can place a strain on the kidneys, as I found out the hard way after developing a painful case of kidney stones.

A general guideline for everyone is to drink at least eight 8-ounce glasses of fluids daily. Half of these 2 quarts should be water. But how much fluid your body needs depends upon several factors:

- Size: The bigger you are, the more you need.

- Caffeine and alcohol consumption: These are diuretics that increase the amount of fluids you lose through urination. Drinking lots of coffee, cola, and beer will not rehydrate you—in fact, it dehydrates.

- Exercise: The more you run, especially in hot weather, the more fluids you will need in your daily diet. In order to compensate for fluid lost while exercising, runners need at least an additional 2–3 quarts of fluid daily, and half of this should be water. Try to set a goal of drinking a glass or two of fluids with each meal as well as at least a glass of fluids mid-morning, mid-afternoon, and in the evening. This is in addition to fluids that you will drink right before, during, and right after running. Make sure during hot weather that you drink more than your thirst dictates.

You will get some of the fluids you need from food (approximately 30 percent). Excellent sources include bananas, oranges, tomatos, cucumbers, and lettuce. Almost any drink that doesn't contain caffeine or alcohol is a good source of fluids as part of your daily intake. Sports drinks and water, however, are your best bets while on the run.

Another factor to remember when pouring in fluids is that you are also pouring in calories. In my comeback to racing, I upped my mileage and cut back on extra calories—even my favorite desserts! But I couldn't shake those extra 10 pounds. The more I ran, the more fluids I drank, including lots of juices, sodas, and sports drinks. I was downing more than 4 quarts a day of these drinks to satisfy my thirst and keep me hydrated. Then I looked on the labels to see how many calories were in these drinks. Yikes! Each glass of soda, milk, or juice was worth about a mile of running (about 100 calories per 8 ounces depending on the type of drink and pace of my runs). At least the Gatorade was a better deal—at about 50 calories per serving, I could burn off the calories of two glasses in a mile. But the beer I liked to drink with my unbuttered popcorn in the evening is worth 150 calories per 12-ounce bottle! Do you remember how many calories I said are in a glass of water? Yep, zero.

I had to make some changes to get my weight down so I could run faster. The problem was drinking, not eating. To just cut back on fluids would cut calories, but then I would be prone to dehydration. I realized that I seldom drank just plain old water. Why? It just isn't that glamorous. I like the taste of juices and sodas, not to mention my Sam Adams brew. I added up how many calories I would save by replacing these drinks with water. Would you believe 500 calories a day, 3,500 for the week—which equals one pound! Not to mention enough money to buy a few pair of running shoes each year.

I literally replaced my high-calorie drinks with no-calorie drinks by filling an empty soda bottle with tap water and putting it in the refrigerator outside my office. I put another one in the fridge in the kitchen. By keeping cold water handy, I pass on the urge to grab something else. For me, the key was in keeping the water very cold. In most parts of the country, ice-cold tap water tastes great. If yours doesn't, try filtering it or buy bottled water. Water bores you? Spice it up with a slice of lime or lemon and a few ice cubes like that high-living Shepherd, or drink seltzer water, which is full of sparkles but has no calories or added sodium.

Each type of drink has its place and time. Fruit juices are a good choice and they provide plenty of vitamins and minerals. Milk supplies some important calcium to your diet. Minimize the drinking of soda, beer, and coffee. Sports drinks aren't needed during the day as much as they might be needed before, during, and after running long distances.

Sports Drinks

Plain water was the main choice for fluid on the run until the high-tech sports drinks started to become popular during the running boom in the late 1970s. Prior to then, a few wily runners concocted their own drinks or downed juices or sodas on the run. I even competed against old-timers who drank brandy during races—and beat me!

Sports drinks are now a billion-dollar industry. Available at first only at selected races and running stores, they now fill the shelves at supermarkets and delis. Gatorade was the first sports drink and remains the industry leader. It actually was formulated in 1965 by medical researchers at the University of Florida, where it was first tested on the Florida Gators football team, hence the name. Many runners prefer other choices, such as All Sport, Exceed, PowerAde, and 10K.

Sports drinks are valuable for several reasons:

1. Sports drinks containing a 6 to 8 percent carbohydrate concentration do two things that are important to runners. First, they are absorbed into the body up to 30 percent faster than water and much faster than drinks such as soda and juices with higher concentrations. This means they are an excellent fluid replacement. If the carbohydrate concentration of a drink is too high, the fluids will not be absorbed as well as water and thus will affect rehydration. Second, they improve performance and fight off fatigue during runs by quickly supplying glucose.

2. Many sports drinks contain small amounts of electrolytes. Since these electrolytes are lost with sweat, sports drinks help to replace them. Sodium is especially valuable because it helps increase absorption, improves taste, and stimulates the thirst mechanism, encouraging you to drink more. A study directed by Ronald Maughan, Ph.D., at the University of Aberdeen in Scotland found exercisers who worked out in the heat retained more of the fluids they drank from electrolyte-replacement drinks than plain water. This was because water lacks the salt that aids fluid retention. Much of the plain water was lost in the urine over the next two hours.

Some claim that electrolytes such as potassium lost while sweating might cause cramping and impair your body's normal functioning. Studies by Dr. Costill and others, however, indicate that electrolyte loss is very small during running and that a balanced diet supplies enough replacement electrolytes.

3. Most runners find that sports drinks are easier on their stomachs than fruit juices and sugared drinks because sports drinks have a lower concentration of carbohydrates. Drinks that have a concentration of more than 8 percent are more likely to cause stomach distress because they are absorbed too slowly. Experiment with sports drinks in your training runs and buildup races.

If you are running an important marathon, find out what type of sports drinks will be offered and get used to drinking it prior to the race.

4. Studies show that runners choose to drink more when offered lightly flavored, moderately sweet sports drinks than when offered plain water. This is important when you really need to take in plenty of fluids before, during, and after running and racing.

5. Sports drinks can be used to replace soda and other high-calorie sugar drinks with your meals and snacks.

Thus, I recommend the use of sports drinks. They'll supply fluids faster than water along with needed carbohydrates for energy. But water lovers take heart. Good old-fashioned H_2O is still of great value to the running community. Drink plenty of it during the day to supply needed body fluids without extra calories, during your training runs when sports drinks aren't available, and along with sports drinks during your races. During runs and races of less than an hour it makes little difference whether you drink water or sports drinks.

Drinking Before Running or Racing

It is important to prepare for exercise by drinking before your workout. You especially want to drink extra fluids in the days before a warm-weather race. Also, if you are carbohydrate-loading for a long race, you will require additional fluids. Stay away from alcoholic and caffeinated drinks the day before a race, especially a long one on a hot day. On the day of your run, drink up to two hours before exercising. At least two 8-ounce glasses of fluids about two hours before running is recommended, especially on a hot day if you are running long. But stop drinking two hours before running. Your body needs 60 to 90 minutes to eliminate excess fluids through urination. Avoid sugared drinks within two hours of running (it's okay within 5–10 minutes, however). You may have an insulin reaction that will temporarily lower your blood sugar, leaving you prematurely exhausted.

Drink one or two cups (8–16 ounces) of fluids 5 to 15 minutes prior to running, especially before races and long runs. If you don't know exactly how much you're drinking, a good estimate is one big swallow equals an ounce. Your kidneys shut down when you start running, so last-minute fluid intake will remain in your body. These fluids will be absorbed within 20 minutes of drinking to help replace fluid loss from sweating. If you will be running for less than an hour, this drink can be water or a sports drink. Beyond that time it is recommended that you choose a sports drink that will provide additional carbohydrates for energy. Look for fluid stations at the starting area of races. Most good races offer a choice between water and sports drinks. Again the warning: Don't drink something before or during running your big race that you haven't tested before training runs and buildup races.

Drinking on the Run

In warm weather, you should drink 4–8 ounces (or four to eight big swallows) of fluid every 10 to 20 minutes during your run. This is as much as your body can absorb in that amount of time. In races, this would be about every 1 or 2 miles. For training runs, you should drink at least every 2 or 3 miles on hot days. Studies show that cold fluids are absorbed more quickly. However, studies at the University of Aberdeen have shown that warm fluids are absorbed a little more quickly than cold ones, so it may be best to drink room temperature or cool (but not ice-cold) drinks on the run. Don't wait until late in the run or until you feel hot and thirsty to start drinking; it takes up to 20 minutes for the fluid to be absorbed. Drink right before you start and then start drinking again 10 to 20 minutes into the run. What you drink in the last 2 or 3 miles of your run won't help you then, but it will aid in your postrun fluid recovery.

Even beginners only out for a 20-minute run-walk on a hot day should drink before running and again after 10 minutes. You may lose a pound of sweat in as little as 2 miles. Fast runners don't gain much by drinking fluids before short races, such as a 5K (3.1 miles). They will be finished before any fluids taken are absorbed. Prerace and postrace fluid intake for short distances is still recommended for all runners, however. As a rule of thumb, if you run for more than 30 minutes during a race, drink fluids during the race as well as before and after.

Do you need to drink on the run even in cold weather? You may drink somewhat less on cooler days. For training runs of less than an hour, a glass of water or sports drink prior to running will probably be enough unless you are overdressed and thus overheat.

You still should drink on long runs—at least every 3 to 5 miles—despite the temperature. You'll benefit from drinking during races of 30 minutes or longer on cold days—running will raise your body temperature and deplete fluids even when the spectators are wearing winter coats. Be careful, however, not to overdrink on cold days and cause stomach distress.

Where can you find fluids during your training runs? Plan ahead. Know where you can find water. Most parks have plenty of water fountains. If there aren't any water fountains along your route, scout out a friendly gas station, school, or home along the way. Look for water faucets or hoses. As a backup, bring money with you like I do. If I've run for too long without finding water, I'll look for a place where I can buy some bottled water or sports drinks.

Plan your course to make sure you can get fluids. On long runs, I'll loop back to my house at least once to get cold sports drinks. You can also plant sealed bottles of drinks along your route ahead of time. Some runners prefer to carry their drinks with them. A bottle can be attached to a belt around your waist or just held in your hand. A variety of water-carrying systems have been designed. Some of the fancier models have insulated pouches to keep drinks cool and you can drink on the run through a plastic tube that extends around your waist or over your shoulder. I can't stand to carry drinks with me, but I know many runners who don't mind it at all. They *do* mind not having enough to drink. When they run low, they just find a place to refill.

The best solution is to have family members or friends provide support. They can take the car and meet you along the way or they can accompany you on a bike. This, by the way, is a good way to involve your spouse or kids in your training. Don't worry that you are cheating when you take a break from running to get a drink. You will enhance the quality of your run and protect your health if you take frequent fluid stops. Never think that not drinking during training runs will toughen you for hot weather races. The body can't be trained to adapt to running without fluids. You can condition yourself to tolerate heat better by training in it, but you always need to replace lost fluids. So go ahead and stop halfway through your 20-minute run and drink from a water fountain, or every 2 or 3 miles for longer runs. I'll stop two or three times on hot days at water fountains for each 6-mile loop of New York's

Central Park. It takes just a few seconds. You don't need to jog in place while waiting behind someone at the fountain, but try to get moving as soon as possible after drinking or your muscles will get stiff.

How to Drink During a Race

Drinking during a race can be tricky. What's more important, getting in plenty of fluid or keeping moving? Studies have shown that time lost drinking is more than recovered down the road. Remember: Your pace will slow by 2 percent for every 1 percent of body weight lost through sweat.

All races should provide fluid stations at least every 2 or 3 miles. If they don't, don't run them, especially in hot weather. Race directors should tell you before the race starts where the fluid stations are located. Most long races offer a choice between water and a sports drink. The New York City Marathon, for example, offers water every mile and Gatorade every 2 miles. I try to pour some of each in me during long races, but I try to remember to only pour water over me. (Once, in the heat of competition, I poured a sports drink over me and I felt quite sticky by the time I finished!)

You have three choices on how to take in fluids during a race:

1. Completely stop and drink a full cup of fluid.

2. Grab the fluid and keep taking swallows while walking with it. When finished, ease back into your run.

3. Grab it and do your best to keep running while drinking.

The first option could present problems. The tendency is to gulp the drink down too fast, which would cause stomach distress. And suddenly coming to a stop could cause muscle cramps. I recommend the second option for beginner runners and beginner marathoners. Taking a few walk breaks while making sure you take in enough fluids will give your muscles a break from the pounding of the running while allowing your body to cool off a bit. Look at it as a good excuse to rest. If you are holding a cup of water while walking doesn't it seem justified to take a break? Your goal is to finish, and by making sure you get plenty of fluids you increase your chances of reaching your goal. So go ahead, walk, drink, and then run. I give you permission. Besides, you may find that you'll lose less time and take in more fluid that way than if you tried to clumsily drink while on the run.

If you are an experienced racer and want to minimize time lost while drinking in order to run a good time, you'll need to master the art of drinking on the run. Here are some tips to help speed you on your way:

- Be on the lookout for fluid stations. As you get close to one, maneuver to that side of the road. If you suddenly cut to a water table you may cut off another runner.

- Plan ahead, look for your best shot at getting fluids quickly. Sometimes you may be able to choose from volunteers handing out cups at the tables or grabbing a cup off the table yourself. Usually, it is more crowded at the beginning of the stations, so take a quick glance to see if fluid is available a few feet farther along. I try to grab a cup at the beginning and another at the end of each fluid station. Try to thank the volunteers if you have the energy. Without their often thankless efforts you'd be in trouble.

- Run defensively. Runners of all sizes, shapes, and speeds converge at fluid stations. Some will be running full speed and will be in a hurry, others will be staggering and fuzzy-brained. I've been both. You and the other runners need to be aware of the traffic heading into and out of the water stations. It isn't unusual to see runners cut off or knocked down. Also be aware that the footing may be slippery around the water stations—the roadway will be wet and strewn with cups that have been tossed away.

- When grabbing a cup on the run, keep your eye on the cup and watch as your hand reaches for the cup. It is easy to miss if you don't pay attention. If you are grabbing a cup from a volunteer, yell out or point to them and make eye contact so they can be prepared to assist you in the transfer. If you need to grab a cup from a table, slow down slightly and move your arm back as you make contact with the cup. This way you won't hit it at full running speed and it will be easier to pick it up without spillage. If you fail to grab a cup on the run, stop and make sure to get the fluids. Especially in hot weather or in long races it is important to consume fluids despite losing a few seconds in attaining it.

■ Try to take in at least four big swallows (4 ounces) of each cup. You should be able to take in that much even if you spill some. Many races hand out 8- to 10-ounce-size cups so you have room for error. You will need to slow the pace at least slightly to be able to drink on the run. Experiment with the best way to hold the cup. Some runners pinch the top of the cup together as soon as they get it to prevent too much of the fluid from splashing out. Then they'll sip it a little at a time. I just hold it in one hand and take a mouthful, swallowing it a little at a time before taking another mouthful. I try to stay relaxed, breathe normally between swallows, and take my time finishing the cup while maintaining a relaxed pace. Others try to gulp it down quickly in one or two big swallows and off they go again. Budd "Rookie" Coates, fitness director for Rodale Press, passed on this tip in *Runner's World*: "Grab a cup, using your fingers as pincers. Place one or more fingers inside the cup and your thumb on the outside, and squeeze the wall of the cup between them. Then, with your free hand press the side rims of the cup together, and drink from one end of the slit." I call him rookie because he went out too fast on a hot, humid day in his first marathon and I passed him late in the race. He went on to become a national class runner with a best of 2:13.

If you are concerned about your drinking technique make sure to run a few practice races that have fluid stations. If not, set up a table along your route and every 5 to 15 minutes loop by it and practice your drinking form.

You don't have to wait until you reach fluid stations before you drink. By supplementing the official fluid stations, you don't need to down as much fluid each time—downing 4 to 8 ounces during a race without spilling it isn't easy. Some races don't supply fluids often enough to meet your demands. Also, in some big races, it is very hard to get fluids without literally standing in line and fighting for them. And sometimes they run out for those folks in the back of the pack. So it is helpful to have a backup fluid-supply system.

A good, safer way to make sure you consume enough fluids is to form a support team—friends, relatives, kids—and make them a part of your racing success. Position them along the course with cups of fluids or small plastic squeeze bottles filled with water or your favorite road-tested sports drink or concoction. You can run along with the bottle and spray the fluids into your mouth. This way you know what you are getting, and you're getting it from encouraging supporters. Just be sure to be precise as to where they will meet you. Be prepared to yell out their names so they can find you—it's hard to pick out runners as they run by.

Sometimes, in an effort to break away from competitors or save precious seconds, a runner will skip a few fluid stations. Some races and personal records have been won this way. But others have been lost by competitors who suddenly fell apart from lack of fluids. When in doubt, be cautious. Drink.

Pour It On You, Too

Besides pouring fluids in you, pour them on you. Douse yourself with water during races and long runs on hot days to help you at least temporarily feel cooler. During training runs I'll cup my hands under water fountains and splash my head and chest with water. On my hot weather runs out in the woods I'll stop and splash myself with *cold* spring water, which really helps revive me when I'm struggling with the heat. During races, I take two cups of water at each station. I drink one and pour the other over my head. Between stations on hot days I'll grab water whenever I can to keep myself watered down. Many races provide sprinklers or hoses to run through to help cool runners. When dousing yourself, be careful to minimize getting your shoes and socks soaked, which could result in blisters.

If you have to choose, pour it in you, not on you to fight the heat. Research at the University of Wisconsin shows that skin-wetting doesn't lower body temperature and doesn't help keep you cool. But it sure seems to work for me. If nothing else, it provides a great psychological boost when you need plenty of help coping with the mental stress of running on a hot day.

Drinking After Running

After your run or race, you must replace lost fluids. If you have been sweating a lot, you have lost salt during your run. Be sure to eat some salty foods (a small bag of salty pretzels) and take sports drinks (which contain sodium) to assist in the retention of the fluids you consume. You should drink two cups of fluids (16 ounces) for every pound of body weight lost during your run. A good choice after hot weather runs is to drink at least twice as much as you feel is necessary. A good rule: Drink, drink, and drink until you have a good flow of clear or pale yellow urine. Even if the scale doesn't show that you've lost any weight after a 30-minute run on a cool day, you should still drink at least a cup of fluids after your run. Marathoners often lose 6–12 pounds, or the equivalent of as much as 1–1.5 gallons of fluids. This is not weight loss; it's fluid loss, and it's not permanent. But the sooner you get that fluid level back to normal the better.

To rehydrate adequately following a long hard run may take one or two days. So continue drinking heavily for a day or two after these longer sessions of an hour or more. Weigh yourself before and after every long workout and race to see how much fluid weight you are losing. And then keep drinking. How much you drink before and during your run will minimize how dehydrated you will be after your run. Start replacing fluids immediately after you finish running to help bring down your body temperature as well as replace lost fluids.

If you want to enjoy a postrun cold beer, first drink plenty of water and eat some food. If you are dehydrated and don't have food in your stomach, the alcohol will hit you much harder. Drink plenty of water to go along with the beer, since alcohol causes you to urinate more and thus adds to dehydration, not hydration. Remember: Don't run, drink alcohol, and then drive. Caffeinated drinks should also be minimized while you are rehydrating since they are also diuretics. In cold weather, drink cold fluids first to replace lost fluids, and then add something warm if you like—hot chocolate or soup. But after long runs or races, always start with water and sports drinks to get fluids in you, and don't forget that within 15 minutes you need to eat or drink at least 50 grams of carbohydrates to replenish lost muscle glycogen. Here's where those high-carbohydrate sports drinks come in handy.

Don't risk chronic dehydration by consuming too little fluid after running. This will lower your tolerance to fatigue, reduce your ability to sweat properly, elevate your rectal temperature, and increase the stress on your circulatory system.

FIGURE 20.1: SUMMARY OF FLUID INTAKE FOR RUNNERS

Daily	3–4 quarts or more, at least half of it calorie-free water
Before running	Drink 16 ounces of water two hours before running, particularly long runs in hot weather. Then, stop drinking until just prior to running. Drink 8–16 ounces 5 to 15 minutes prior to running. A sports drink is recommended for races longer than one hour.
During running	4–8 ounces (four to eight large swallows) every 10 to 20 minutes. A sports drink is recommended for runs and races over an hour.
After running	At least 8–16 ounces. Drink 16 ounces for each pound of body weight loss from sweat. Continue drinking more for several hours after long runs on hot days. Drink until urine is clear or pale yellow.

Part VII

The Running Environment

TWENTY-ONE

Hot Weather Running

Most runners hit the roads and trails more often in the warmth and extra daylight hours of spring and summer. Some runners love the heat. They cannot wait to get outdoors in hot weather. Shepherd's good friend Bowden Quinn is a lawyer-runner in Chicago. Bowden started running during his years working in Zimbabwe and now loves the summer heat of Illinois. He thinks running in the heat and humidity is as close to heaven as we come. Shepherd, who enjoys running in the winters of Vermont, thinks it's certain hell. I love to train in the heat, but I hate to race in it.

I know many runners who insist that they can't cope with the heat. They'll just stop running until it cools off. But by following the guidelines in this chapter and using common sense, you can learn to cope better with hot weather running. If you prefer to take off when the going gets hot, go ahead. But at least keep exercising by working out indoors where it is air-conditioned, or go swimming. Beginners can beat the heat by switching to walking, which generates less heat than running, on those miserable, muggy days.

Running in hot, humid weather and direct sunlight carries risks. Racing in it can be dangerous. Heat and humidity may cause muscle cramps, fatigue, heat exhaustion, or heatstroke. Combined with air pollutants and sun exposure, heat can cause many problems for careless runners.

Heat threatens everyone who exercises, no matter how well-conditioned—although the more fit you are, the better you are able to cope with heat. Running in hot weather, your body initially produces more heat than it can give up into the environment. You sweat. The moisture is evaporated, which cools you. But if your cooling system cannot keep up, your internal temperature will rise. A significant increase in body temperature may cause your body to malfunction. As you sweat, you lose fluids and this in itself may interfere with your body's ability to regulate heat. Too much fluid loss combined with heat can lead to serious problems.

Some heat factors you can control, and some you can't. Heat affects some runners more than others and even the same runners differently on different days. Heat also affects heavier runners more than lighter ones; older runners as well as children may have more trouble running in the heat. Alert runners understand head and tailwinds and use them to advantage. In any weather, hot or cold, a head wind is cooler and a tailwind is warmer—that is, a head wind (blowing toward you) evaporates sweat and carries body heat away from you, but a tailwind (blowing against your back) wraps body heat around you like a blanket and therefore reduces heat evaporation and heat loss. The position of the sun and any cloud cover are also factors. Direct sunlight at high noon will result in more body heat; clouds, of course, shield the runner.

One of the key factors in coping with hot weather running is replacing fluids by drinking before, during, and after your runs. This important topic was discussed in detail in the previous chapter. Here, I'll present guidelines for other key factors for running in the heat, including humidity, sun, clothing, and adjusting training runs and race strategy.

Humidity

Air temperature is a major factor to consider when starting on your run. Humidity is another. The key to regulating body temperature in hot weather is sweat evaporation. This accounts for as much as 90 percent of heat removal. Under very humid conditions, little sweat can evaporate, and it becomes difficult for the body to lose heat.

The National Weather Service uses a Heat Index to measure discomfort and the potential danger of heat-related illnesses. The

Heat Index (Figure 21.1) is expressed as an "apparent temperature." It is basically the summertime equivalent of winter's wind-chill factor. It expresses what a combination of temperature and relative humidity feels like.

How bad can it get? It is not unusual in the United States for summer weather to reach 95°F. with 75 percent humidity. That combination creates an oppressive 130°F. in "apparent temperature." (Ugh! That's the time I head indoors for an air-conditioned workout on my exercise bike.)

The basic premise of the Heat Index is simple: The higher the temperature and the higher the humidity, the higher the Heat Index. An actual air temperature of 85°F. combined with 95 percent humidity is more dangerous than an air temperature of 100°F. in a dry climate.

When the Heat Index goes above 90°F., the possibility of heat-related illnesses increases sharply. The National Weather Service issues a heat advisory when the Heat Index exceeds 105°F. At that point you should exercise outdoors only with extreme caution—better yet, head inside for your workout. *When the Heat Index exceeds 130°F., do not exercise outdoors!*

Adjust to the Weather

You can and should adjust to the weather. Prepare yourself for the heat. You cannot run faster in the heat, so the next choice is to prepare yourself to run in it more safely. Follow these guidelines for running in the heat whether you are a beginner runner or a competitive racer.

Wear light-colored, loose clothing. Choose a lightweight, breathable fabric, such as Coolmax, that wicks away the sweat. Minimize clothing to maximize skin surface from which perspiration can evaporate. A loose, light-colored (to reflect the sun's rays) singlet and shorts are best. If running for a long time in the sun, protect your body with a loose shirt that covers your shoulders and upper arms, and a hat that shades your head. You might even add cool sunglasses to protect your eyes and help you stay relaxed in the bright sunshine.

Pour water in you and on you. As detailed in Chapter 20, drink before, during, and after your runs. You may also benefit from pouring it on you. Shepherd even soaks his favorite old floppy

FIGURE 21.1: HEAT INDEX

	AIR TEMPERATURE (F°)										
	70°	75°	80°	85°	90°	95°	100°	105°	110°	115°	120°
	Apparent Temperature (what it feels like)										
0%	64°	69°	73°	78°	83°	87°	91°	95°	99°	103°	107°
10%	65°	70°	75°	80°	85°	90°	95°	100°	105°	111°	116°
20%	66°	72°	77°	82°	87°	93°	99°	105°	112°	120°	130°
30%	67°	73°	78°	84°	90°	96°	104°	113°	123°	135°	148°
40%	68°	74°	79°	86°	93°	101°	110°	123°	137°	151°	
50%	69°	75°	81°	88°	96°	107°	120°	135°	150°		
60%	70°	76°	82°	90°	100°	114°	132°	149°			
70%	70°	77°	85°	93°	106°	124°	144°				
80%	71°	78°	86°	97°	113°	136°					
90%	71°	79°	88°	102°	122°						
100%	72°	80°	91°	108°							

RELATIVE HUMIDITY (left axis)

Apparent Temperature	Heat Stress Risk with Physical Activity and/or Prolonged Exposure
90°–105°	Heat cramps or heat exhaustion *possible*
105°–130°	Heat cramps or heat exhaustion *likely*
	Heatstroke *possible*
130°+	Heatstroke *highly likely*

running hat in water before he runs. (I suppose he chews it if he can't find a drinking fountain!) I pour water over my head and chest at every opportunity on hot days. Despite the fact that some studies show this doesn't lower your body temperature, it sure helps me psychologically and I feel cooler.

Avoid the heat. This sounds sensible, but you'd be surprised how many runners ignore this simple advice. As Noel Coward said, only "mad dogs and Englishmen go out in the midday sun"—and that was composed when the British Empire controlled some rather hot parts of the earth!

If you don't plan to race in the heat, don't train in it. Run during the cool of early morning or late evening. Or just stay indoors and exercise where it's air-conditioned.

Adjust your pace. Start slow and run a steady slower pace in both training runs and races. You can't hold the same pace with the same effort in the heat anyway, since blood diverted to get rid of body heat isn't available to carry oxygen to your exercising muscles. You may need to slow down by as much as a minute per mile or more and make further reductions along the way. Take walk breaks if needed to keep your temperature down. Take heart rate checks to monitor the effect of the heat on your heart.

Adjust your distance. When the weather is hot, shorten your running distance. Postpone a long run for a cooler day or shift your long run to a cooler time of day.

Give yourself time to acclimatize. If the weather suddenly turns hot, or you have traveled to a hot climate, pull back. Ease into running in the heat—slow down your pace, shorten your runs. During your first workout in the heat, cut your intensity by a minute or more per mile. Give yourself seven to ten days to slowly adjust to the heat.

Heat train for races. This advice will seem counter to everything I've just said, but if you plan to run a race in hot weather, train in hot weather. Give yourself ten to fourteen days of progressive heat training. A few times a week, run at the hottest time of day. But go easy. Remember to adjust your time goals—no matter how well you heat train, you can't run as fast on a hot day as you can on a cool day.

Replenish your body's minerals. Your body loses fluids, vitamins, and minerals during hot weather workouts. You need to be conscientious about replacing them. Magnesium, salt, and potassium in particular are lost through sweat. Fresh fruits and vegetables, especially bananas, watermelons, cantaloupes, carrots, and tomatoes are rich in minerals. So are their juices. Or you might want to try some of the commercial electrolyte-replacement sports drinks.

Be in shape. An unconditioned runner places an extra burden on his or her body by running in the heat. So does an overweight runner. If you insist on running in the heat, follow all of these rules and be sure you're in good shape first. Running in the heat to *get* into shape is a bad and perhaps dangerous idea.

Run in the shade. Select tree-lined paths to protect you from the hot sun. Or run from shady spot to shady spot. Shepherd switches from one side of the road to the other when running in the heat in Vermont. (Watch for cars and bicycles!) In the shade, he also removes his hat to let his body ventilate through the top of his head. (Maybe *that's* when he chews his hat?) Also, if you are running a race in hot weather, stay in the shade prior to the start to avoid raising your body temperature.

Run on cool surfaces. Pavement burns your feet. Heat reflected up from the road warms your body. Try running on the dirt shoulders or on grass. A light gravel or woodchip path may be best.

Remember to warm up and cool down. You still need to prepare your body for a run with a cardiorespiratory warm-up even in hot weather. To adjust to the heat, after a few minutes of limbering exercises, start your workout with a walk and then a slow jog. Then bring the pace up to a comfortable level—a pace that is slower than usual. After running in the heat, your body temperature will remain high. The blood vessels in your skin and arm and leg muscles are dilated. Stopping suddenly may stress your heart as it continues to pump blood through these dilated vessels. Cool down by walking slowly for 5 to 10 minutes to bring down both your heart rate and body temperature. Then drink plenty of fluids and stretch thoroughly.

Use common sense. If you feel dizzy, overheated, or cold, stop and walk. Get out of the sun and get fluids into and on you. Do not race or train hard in very hot or humid weather. Heat-related disorders (detailed below) can affect any level of runner, seasoned competitor or novice alike.

Heat-related Illnesses

Even if you follow all of the advice above, you may still run into trouble. The four stages of heat-related illnesses are listed here in progressive order of seriousness:

Heat stress. Thirst, fatigue, and dizziness are early warning signs that your body is becoming heat stressed. Stop running immediately. Walk. Drink fluids.

Heat cramps. The next step may include sudden, painful, involuntary contractions of your muscles, most often in the calves, arms, or abdomen. To treat these cramps, massage them with your hands and cool the body with cold water and wet towels. Drink fluids immediately; you should include electrolyte-replacement fluids since loss of electrolytes may have caused the cramping.

Heat exhaustion. This occurs when your cardiorespiratory system is overworked, and while rarely life-threatening it may precede heatstroke. It may appear after vigorous exercise or come on gradually over several days or weeks as a result of dehydration. Symptoms include headache, dizziness, nausea, a weak but rapid pulse, weakness in the legs, cramping, profuse sweating, dilated pupils, and vomiting. You may feel a flushed, hot sensation around your head and shoulders. The skin may become moist, pale, and cold. Body temperature will be elevated.

If you experience any of these symptoms, stop running immediately. Seek help and medical attention. Find a cool, shaded spot and lie down with your feet elevated. Loosen or remove excess clothing. Drink fluids as soon as possible and continue doing so until you feel better.

Heatstroke. This is an extreme emergency situation and can be fatal. Symptoms include not sweating although it is very hot, a chilling sensation, flushed and red skin, a burning sensation in the legs and/or chest, difficulty breathing, rapid heart rate, a feeling of dizziness, an inability to think clearly or run a straight line, and suddenly finding yourself on the ground. Heatstroke occurs when the body's thermoregulatory mechanism fails and the body temperature rises above 104°F. The skin is hot and dry. The runner may develop convulsions, suddenly collapse, or go into a coma.

Too often, runners ignore the warning signs of heat exhaustion and run themselves into heatstroke. By then the runner may not be able to understand the warning signs; others will have to help. You may have to physically pull this runner off the road, since he may not understand how serious his condition is.

Get the runner out of the sun immediately. Find a way to lower his or her body temperature immediately. If fluids are in short supply, pour them on the body rather than force them into the person. Seek medical help immediately even if the person claims to feel

better. The runner will need fluid replacement, probably intrave-
nously.

Caution: Studies show that the severity of heat-related disorders
increases with age. Conditions that cause heat cramps in a seven-
teen-year-old may promote heat exhaustion in someone forty and
heatstroke in a person over sixty.

Sun

I used to run shirtless at high noon to get a good tan along with
a solid workout. No more! Now we know that too much exposure
to the sun both in summer and winter increases the risk of skin
cancer and eye damage. More than 750,000 new cases of skin
cancer and one million cataracts are reported each year in the
United States. Why? Because people are spending more time outdoors and the ozone layer in the atmosphere that screens the sun's
rays is deteriorating. Skin damage is now a year-round threat.

"All sunburn and suntans are visible evidence of injury to the
skin," writes Dr. David Bickers, a dermatologist and director of
the Skin Diseases Research Center at Case Western Reserve University in Cleveland, Ohio. "And while a tan will help prevent
further injury, repeated exposure leads to premature aging of the
skin and accelerates the development of nonmalignant skin
cancers."

Runners should protect themselves. A well-tanned body is no
longer an image of fitness. Keep in mind the following tips:

- Avoid exercising between 10:00 A.M. and 3:00 P.M., the peak
period for ultraviolet B radiation from sunlight.

- Be aware that sand, concrete, water, and snow reflect the sun's
rays and increase your exposure to harmful UV rays. You are
also more vulnerable at high altitudes.

- Avoid tanning salons and sunlamps.

- Apply sunblock liberally on all exposed areas. Choose a sweat-
proof sunscreen with a sun protection factor of at least 15. Studies at the University of Melbourne in Australia showed that not
only did those who use sunscreen exhibit 30 percent fewer new
precancerous spots, but some of their existing spots disappeared.
Spread the sunscreen over all exposed areas of the face, neck,

and body. The areas most commonly neglected: ears, the area between the mouth and nose, the nose, and the hairline.

- Wear a loose-fitting shirt that covers at least your shoulders.

- Wear tightly woven clothing when exposed to the sun for long periods of time.

- Wear sunglasses and a hat or visor to protect your eyes, face, and head.

To publicize the danger of sun exposure, the National Weather Service and the Environmental Protection Agency (EPA) developed an experimental daily UV Index. This daily index forecasts the amount of ultraviolet light that will hit the earth's surface at noon the next day in most American cities. The index uses five exposure levels: minimal (0–2), low (3–4), moderate (5–6), high (7–9), and very high (10–15). The scale is based on upper-atmosphere ozone levels and cloud cover. Ozone blocks ultraviolet radiation, that part of solar energy that causes sunburn and is blamed for skin cancer and eye cataracts. Clouds may help block out UV rays, but you will still be exposed. According to Drusilla Hufford of the EPA: "I think one of the most important messages we're going to get out is: Know your skin type." The lighter your skin, the more the danger.

The EPA has divided skin phototypes into four categories and calculated the minimum time it takes for each type to burn, given various UV exposure levels—see Figure 21.2.

1. Never tans; always burns; pale, alabaster-colored.

2. Sometimes tans; usually burns; sometimes freckles.

3. Usually tans; sometimes burns; light tan, brown, or olive.

4. Always tans; rarely burns; brown, dark brown, or black.

In addition to checking your weather report for the Heat Index, also check out the UV Index. Combined, they will give you good guidelines for how to dress and train in the sun and heat.

FIGURE 21.2

EXPERIMENTAL UV INDEX		MINUTES TO BURN SKIN TYPE 1	MINUTES TO BURN SKIN TYPE 4
Minimal	0–2	30 minutes	more than 120 minutes
Low	3	20	90
	4	15	75
Moderate	5	12	60
	6	10	50
High	7	8.5	40
	8	7.5	35
	9	7	33
Very High	10	6	30
	11	5.5	27
	12	5	25
	13	less than 5	23
	14	4	21
	15	less than 4	20

Note: Times do not factor in a person's base tan and the amount of sunscreen used.

TWENTY-TWO

Cold Weather Running

Some runners stop running when the weather turns cold, dark, or blustery. Like cats, they prefer the warm and sunny spots. I know plenty of runners—especially at the beginner and intermediate levels—who just refuse to run on cold days. Some even hang up their running shoes until spring arrives. But for every runner who loves hot weather, there is another like Shepherd who can't wait to see the snow swirl. Out they go, like little kids, into the elements.

With proper adjustments in clothing and training, cold weather running can be a safe and enjoyable change of pace from warm weather running. The biggest obstacle in cold weather running is just getting out the door. Although it may sometimes seem unpleasant—in thought, if not actual deed—even running in extreme cold isn't much of a problem once you learn to dress and prepare for it. And you get the added bonus of being in much better shape when the warm weather returns. But, like hot weather, cold weather can have a significant affect on your body's physiological responses to exercise resulting in an increased health risk.

Freezing Lungs

Let's start right at the heart of the argument. You've already heard this, first from your mother, then from your significant other, and always from those runners who curl up by the fire for the winter: "You go out there and you'll freeze your lungs."

Wrong.

And tell 'em Bob Glover said so.

Freezing of the lungs is a myth. The air we inhale while running in the cold is warmed by the air passages. Runners like me with sensitive bronchials and asthma, however, will find that cold air irritates these conditions. Wearing a face mask, like I do, or a scarf will help alleviate that condition. It helps to warm the air you inhale before it even reaches your air passages.

Frostbite

Frostbite is a real danger to the fingers, toes, ears, face, and other exposed (and in men, as we shall see, not so exposed) parts. One cold and windy day I stopped running because of an asthma attack brought on by exercising too hard in the cold. I walked home through the snow. But by the time I got to my front door I had no feeling in my toes. The first stage of frostbite had set in. To this day, those toes bother me when I stand around in the cold. If I keep running they're fine.

The danger of frostbite increases with wind. If you run in cold weather, you should understand the windchill factor and know what it is as you start out the door. The windchill factor is the air temperature plus the effect of any wind. Figure 22.1 is a chart to help you. Remember that running into the wind cools you further, thus increasing the effect of the windchill factor. On a 10°F. day, for example, a 10-mile-an-hour wind results in a windchill factor of −9°F.

Frostbitten skin is usually cold, pale, and firm-to-hard to the touch. The first step in treatment is to warm up rapidly without excessive heat. Use warm water. Do not massage or, in the case of the toes, walk on the injured area. Do not rub with snow (another old myth). Drink warm fluids. Take the frostbitten runner immediately to receive medical attention.

To prevent frostbite, keep your exposed skin to a minimum. Cover your hands and face. Keep dry. Keep moving. Avoid running into strong head winds, especially if you have been perspiring greatly or you are otherwise wet. A mild form of cold injury called

FIGURE 22.1: WINDCHILL FACTOR CHART

	ACTUAL THERMOMETER READING (F°)											
	50	40	30	20	10	0	−10	−20	−30	−40	−50	−60
EST. WIND SPEED (MPH)	EQUIVALENT TEMPERATURE (°F.)											
calm	50	40	30	20	10	0	−10	−20	−30	−40	−50	−60
5	48	37	27	16	6	−5	−15	−26	−36	−47	−57	−68
10	40	28	16	4	−9	−24	−33	−46	−58	−70	−83	−95
15	36	22	9	−5	−18	−32	−45	−58	−72	−85	−99	−112
20	32	18	4	−10	−25	−39	−53	−67	−82	−96	−110	−124
25	30	16	0	−15	−29	−44	−59	−74	−88	−104	−118	−133
30	28	13	−2	−18	−33	−48	−63	−79	−94	−109	−125	−140
35	27	11	−4	−20	−35	−51	−67	−82	−98	−113	−129	−145
40	26	10	−6	−21	−37	−53	−69	−85	−100	−116	−132	−148

(Wind speeds greater than 40 mph have little additional effect.)	LITTLE DANGER (for properly clothed person). Maximum danger of false sense of security.	INCREASING DANGER Danger from freezing of exposed flesh.	GREAT DANGER

frostnip precedes frostbite. Be aware of warning signals: numbness, tingling, burning sensations, or whitening of the skin. Do not ignore these early signs.

Hypothermia

Hypothermia occurs when the core temperature of the body falls well below normal—under 90°F. compared to an average body temperature of 98.6°F. This generally happens when you are outside in extremely cold weather and get wet. The most common occurrence is when someone falls into icy water during very cold weather. But it may also occur when you are exercising in the cold and get wet from sweating.

As your body temperature falls, the body responds with shivering, which is the muscles' attempt to produce heat. If ignored, the runner could next become incoherent, lapse into a coma, even die.

If, on a very cold day, you get wet from sweat or other sources, such as getting splashed with slush, keep moving and get inside quickly. Take off your wet clothing immediately. Take a hot bath and drink warm fluids. Hypothermia almost got me. After finishing a 20-mile race in good shape, I hung around talking to friends; I still had my wet running clothes on under my warmups. Before I knew it, I was feeling very disoriented. I quickly took a taxi home and got warm and dry.

If you see a runner developing hypothermia, remove all wet clothing and warm his or her body with blankets or your own body heat. Get medical help quickly—but do not stop your efforts to warm the runner.

Cold Weather Clothing

The key to running in the cold is wearing the right clothes in the right combination. Here are some basic rules:

- Dress to keep warm and dry.

- Dress to stay warm, but also to let heat escape as you exercise. This will keep sweating to a minimum and help you stay drier and warm. Choose fabrics that let out any excessive heat that builds up.

- Dress to protect your extremities—toes, fingers, ears, as well as your face. Keep your ears covered with a pull-down hat, head-band, or earmuffs. Try to cover your face with a pull-up turtle-neck, pull-down hat, mask, or some other protection. Some runners slather the exposed portions of their face with petroleum jelly for protection.

How to dress? In Chapter 17 we discuss the various fabrics important to cold weather running. Here are some suggestions about how to use those fabrics in layering.

Layering

The secret to maximum comfort during cold weather running is layering: an inner wicking layer, an insulating middle layer, and an outer windbreaking layer. You may not always need three layers, and some of the functions may be combined. Sometimes conditions will be so fierce that you may need four layers.

An efficient layering system traps body heat between layers of clothing and keeps you warm. You adjust your temperature by unzipping or even removing the outer layer, or more (see below). If you cool off, you merely zip up or put the layer back on. Not only do layers of clothes effectively trap and allow you to regulate your body heat, but they also allow perspiration to move readily through the thin layers of clothing. Moisture is wicked away from your skin by the inner layer and transferred to the second or third layer for evaporation. If one piece of clothing in the system fails in this function, you will not keep as dry and thus as warm. Wet clothing can't keep you warm.

The inner (wicking) layer. This is the one against your skin. It should consist of fabrics like polypropylene, Coolmax, DryLete, or Thermax, which are "breathable" and thus allow water vapor to pass through. This "wicks" perspiration away from the skin and helps keep you dry. This layer should be lightweight and fit fairly snugly to your skin. Women will find sports bras available in wicking fabrics, too. You should not wear an absorbent fabric like cotton next to your skin: It will get wet and make you feel uncomfortable and cold.

I heat up pretty quickly, so I usually wear a very lightweight DryLete or Coolmax long- or short-sleeved shirt against my skin, but then go to a heavier DryLete or polypro long-sleeve shirt in colder weather. Shepherd still prefers lightweight short-sleeved undershirts.

The middle (insulating) layer. This layer is generally used only on really cold days. It is essential for adding additional space to trap heat—just like the insulation in your attic at home. This layer is usually heavier than the inner layer, but it also needs to be breathable and to wick moisture away from the skin. The middle layer has two functions: It traps heat to keep you warm, and it passes moisture to the outer layer to keep you dry.

This layer should fit more loosely and should be easy to open or to remove so you can make adjustments if you get too warm. Runners like Shepherd who don't sweat too much may prefer a long-sleeved cotton shirt or turtleneck for this layer. But if you sweat a lot like I do, this won't work. Go with fabrics that will keep you dry: fleece, wool, Thermax, Polartec, and so on. According to Andy Kimerling at the Westchester Road Runner, "Many runners will wear a cotton T-shirt as the middle layer because it will act like a diaper and soak up the moisture coming through an inner polypro shirt."

The outer (windbreaking) layer. This one protects you from the wind; it should also be of a fabric that will repel rain and wet snow. It must be "breathable" to allow perspiration moisture and excessive body heat, passed from the inner wicking layer to the middle insulating layer, to continue their journey and escape into the environment.

Your biggest enemy in keeping warm is not the air temperature but strong winds that can blow away your body heat. This outer layer, therefore, should fit loosely and be zippered so you can make easy temperature adjustments. An additional plus comes if the outer layer is waterproof, or at least water repellent. Waterproof layers tend to be too warm if you are running hard or long. Outer layers may consist of windproof, water-repellent clothing like Windkiller and Windstopper, and waterproof fabrics like Gore-Tex. Nylon windbreakers—the old standby—will protect you against the wind, but since nylon is not "breathable" you may find it too warm. My recommendation is to wear waterproof clothes only in cold, wet weather; use water repellent outerwear on windy days or in mild temperatures.

Winter Clothing

How should you combine fabrics and layering?

Upper body. In the coldest weather wear a long-sleeved wicking fabric against your skin. Cover this with an insulating layer like fleece. As mentioned, a long-sleeved cotton T-shirt works for most runners if you don't sweat a lot. Add a windproof jacket or shell. Ideally, your jacket will have covered zippers, a hood, and pockets for storing your mittens and hat (if you remove them). It should be cut long enough to cover you below the waist and should also have drawstrings and a high collar you can close. In very cold weather you will want to add an additional middle layer of clothing.

Shepherd thinks your outer shell should also have a Velcro cuff—rather than elastic—to allow you to open the cuff to cool off. An elastic cuff will trap heat and cause moisture to build up around your wrists, which may make you very cold. The best outer shell Shepherd ever bought was on sale not in a runners' shop but in a backpacking store. It had all of the above plus a nylon mesh overlap across the upper back and large Velcro cuffs that he could easily tear open while running. He also favors turtlenecks to keep cold away from his neck. Others may protect this area with a scarf or gator.

Legs. Your legs generate a lot of heat and need less protection than your upper body and head. One layer is usually enough. The most common choices are tights or a pair of nylon, Coolmax, or Gore-Tex pants over a pair of shorts. Lycra spandex tights are warm enough in most weather. For colder runs try heavier tights made of wicking fabrics like DryLete. On really bitter cold days, wear tights covered with windproof pants. These two layers are the most any runner will need.

Private parts. If you get wet and then catch a strong head wind, your private parts may get uncomfortably cold—or worse (see the story at end of the chapter). One choice is a special moisture-wicking windbrief with a nylon panel in the front. The combination keeps you dry and holds the wind at bay. A good pair of long windproof pants usually provide more than enough outer coverage.

Women should also take precautions to keep warm. Running briefs, tights and special sports bras that wick moisture and keep out the wind are recommended.

Feet. Wear socks that are warm and stay dry to protect your feet. Remember: Most running shoes are nylon with a mesh across the top. They will let in a lot of cold air and water. So you need to make sure that your socks stay dry and provide insulation for heat. Your feet will probably not get cold while you are running and dry.

One layer of wicking socks made of acrylic or polypropylene or that old standby wool is usually enough. In very cold weather you may choose to go with a thin inner sock made of a wicking fabric such as polypropylene and an insulating outer sock made of an acrylic. Be careful about the socks rubbing together and bunching up, which may cause discomfort or blisters. Some veterans of the cold and wet wear biker's booties or plastic bags over their socks to stay warm and dry in nasty weather.

If your feet get wet on a cold day, stop the run and get indoors immediately. Get your wet socks and shoes off, and warm your feet quickly.

Head. Always wear a hat for cold weather running. More than 40 percent of your body heat is lost through your head. You can also remove the hat when you get too hot, then put it back on to warm up. It is also important to protect the ears from frostbite; you might select a hat that covers them.

Runners with plenty of hair may get by with just a headband over their ears or earmuffs. In very cold weather, I wear a headband covered by a fleece, DryLete, or polypro hat. Still colder and windier weather brings out my hood over the hat. On those days, I may add a face mask.

You wouldn't recognize me out on my runs in bitter winter weather. Sometimes I have to say a secret code to get back into my own house! I wear my DryLete face mask covered by a fleece hat. The face mask covers my mouth. This warms the air and assists runners like me who have bronchial problems in the cold. If it isn't real cold, I may wear my lightweight bikers cap and carry a polypro hat in my pocket. I might trade back and forth a few times during a run to keep comfortable.

Some runners slather petroleum jelly on exposed portions of their face to fight off the biting cold wind. Others use an all-purpose balaclava worn as a watch cap or pulled down over their ears and neck to protect against the cold.

Whatever you choose, just be sure to cover your head and help your body store heat.

Hands. Fingers and hands need protection in very cold weather. Mittens, or even socks worn as mittens, keep your hands warmer than gloves because of the warmth shared by your fingers. I like light breathable gloves for most cold days since I tend to get warm quickly. DryLete or polypro liners don't get too hot and can be covered by mittens on cold days. Thermax gloves in heavier weights add a little more warmth. I prefer windproof, waterproof ones that I slip on and off depending on rain and wind. Shepherd prefers mittens to gloves for his hands while running in Vermont winters. (He claims he has run at −45°F. with windchill!) Avoid collecting moisture in your hands. Don't be afraid to take your gloves or mittens off if your hands get wet. Carry one in each hand or tuck them in your jacket or pants and put them back on when you get cold.

Plan Your Runs in the Cold

Here are some winter running tips to make your cold weather runs more pleasurable and safer:

- Carefully plan all workouts, whatever the weather. Warm up properly—good advice even if you are planning to shovel snow, which may be far more dangerous to your heart. Start with some gentle stretching exercises and then go out with a brisk walk. Move into a slow jog and gradually find your normal pace.

- When running an out-and-back course, always begin by running into the wind. Otherwise you'll build up a good sweat with the wind at your back, and then turn into the biting wind for your return. This may cause extreme discomfort, cold, perhaps even frostbite or hypothermia.

- Peel off layers. As you run and begin to warm up, the first item to remove is your hat. Tuck it into your pants or carry it in one hand. Next, take off your mittens. Unzip your outer shell if you start to overheat and get wet. If you continue to be hot, remove the shell, hold a cuff in each hand and twirl it in front of you a few times. This will make it tight and it will tie easily around your waist.

  As you cool, replace the clothing in reverse order, the outer shell going back on first.

- Be alert to conditions. During a single cold weather run, the conditions may change several times. You may get very warm (even hot) if the sun and wind are at your back, and then turn around and run against the wind and get chilled. Or you may suddenly encounter cold rain or wet snow. *Never* toss away any articles of clothing when you are out running in cold weather. Don't even leave them along the road to be picked up on your return loop. Tuck, tie, fold, squeeze them into your pockets and around your body. Shepherd knows New England runners who carry a little mesh bag on an outer belt and tuck their hat, mittens, and shell into the bag, spin the bag around to their fanny —and never miss a step. All that warm, dry clothing is hanging there when the sun goes down and the north wind howls.

▪ Don't forget that UV rays reflect off the snow. On bright sunny days with snow on the ground, it is wise to wear sunscreen and sunglasses.

▪ Underdress or overdress? There is far more danger in underdressing than in overdressing. Figure it out. You leave that warm hat and those mittens at home, you don't have them when you need them. You wear them, or tuck them into a pocket or waistband, and they're there when you start feeling cold.

Beginner runners are more likely to overdress. This could lead to dehydration or even a heat-related illness. More advanced runners have been out in almost every condition; they know what to wear, how to shed it, store it on their bodies, and retrieve it. Ask me or Shepherd what we wear in any given condition and we can tell you right down to the type of socks we'll wear.

The key, however, is knowing what to wear *and* wearing as little as possible. A good rule of thumb is to dress as though it were twenty degrees warmer out there than it really is. You should feel a little chilly when you first go outside. Your body will soon warm up. If you are racing, you may want to wear "throwaway" clothes at the start or leave your extra clothes with a friend down the road. Just remember that you can't go back and get them. Also, you'll need something to keep you warm once you cross the finish line.

▪ Walk briskly for at least 5 minutes after your run. After removing wet clothing and toweling off, stretch thoroughly. Drink fluids and take a warm shower.

▪ Drink plenty of fluids before and after your runs—and along the course if you are running more than an hour. You don't need as much fluids as in hot weather, when you perspire more, but you can still dehydrate in cold weather due to sweating.

▪ If traveling to a race or for a training run, be prepared with warm dry clothing to put on as soon as you finish. Don't wait until you get home—it may be too late.

Winter runs may be shorter and slower because of the cold and the difficult footing. But they are important in continuing to build endurance to stay in shape or for racing in warmer weather.

Alternative Training

You don't have to run every day during the winter. But you also shouldn't quit running when the cold weather sets in. Instead, you might cut back your mileage and do something else as an alternative or cross-training. See Chapter 35 for guidelines. The most likely exercise when it snows is to cross-country ski. Try it! It's great! Use the same clothing and warm-up guidelines as for running. I not only enjoy this sport but also enjoy running in the lightweight snowshoes Santa brought me.

Keep Winter Running Fun

Here are some tips to help get you through the doldrums of a long, dark winter.

- Run during the daytime rather than after dark, if possible. Daylight running is more cheerful in winter, and it's warmer when the sun is out.

- Make a date a few times a week to work out with other runners to keep winter running from being too lonely.

- Don't pay as much attention to your pace. With all the clothing you're wearing you have an excuse to run slower. Just run fast enough to keep warm and within your training heart range. Don't run too far at once if the weather is too cold or the footing bad.

- Take a runner's vacation. A week, or even a long weekend, in a warm-weather spot like Florida, Arizona, or the Bahamas will give you a real boost and a break from battling the snow and cold. Many resort areas offer weekend packages to attract runners who may need only the slightest excuse to escape for a few days. Be careful to gradually acclimate to hot weather running.

Running in Snow, Slush, Ice

Running during a light snowstorm or on newly fallen snow can be a joy. The silence is broken only by your breathing and the sound of your footsteps. It's also fun to watch your footprints break a path in the snowy wilderness. I'm like a kid: I can't wait to go out for a run in the new snowfall. In fact, more than once I've left my house to run at midnight in a snowstorm. With the white snow on the ground, you can see quite well. A light layer of snow also provides some cushion. But you do need some precautions.

Footing. Slow your pace when it snows. Watch your footing, especially where the newly fallen snow may have covered ice. When the snow gets packed down, you may want to search for dry areas to run. Waffle or ripple soles seem to grip best.

Walk around the icy areas. I know too many runners who have slipped on ice and broken an arm or leg. If you find yourself on ice, do not try to stop suddenly. You'll slide. Try to slow down, run flat-footed, stay relaxed and flexible. Be especially careful of downhills. Walk if necessary. When my dirt trails are covered with slippery stuff I prefer strapping on my cleated runner's snowshoes. The pace is slower but still vigorous, and safer.

Vision. If it's snowing, try wearing goggles or sunglasses to protect your eyes. Sounds will also be muffled, so be alert to vehicles, other runners, cross-country skiers, and the like. Motorists will also have poor visibility, so stay off roadways. Run defensively.

Stride. Shorten your stride to prevent slipping. Since your muscles are working differently, don't overdo it and risk muscle fatigue or injury.

Injuries. The most common winter running injuries come from slipping and sliding in the ice and snow. Poor footing causes you to tighten muscles to guard against this. A runner may alter his or her running form, which can lead to further problems. Lateral foot slippage often occurs on icy spots and may cause a pulled muscle or tendon. Running in snow forces you to work muscles normally not used as much. Limit your running in snow and slippery conditions and be alert to stresses and strains on new muscle groups.

Warm up carefully and well. Stretch before and after your run, as always. Start with brisk walking or a slow jog; this will also let you test the surface conditions. Try to run relaxed. Adjust your pace to the conditions.

The Final Cold-War Story

A good cold-war story comes from Dr. Melvin Herskowitz of Jersey City, New Jersey, who wrote the following tongue-in-cheek account, warning about the danger of frostbite for the inadequately dressed male runner. It appeared in the *New England Journal of Medicine* (January 20, 1977):

To the Editor: A fifty-three-year-old circumcised physician, non-smoker, light drinker (one highball before dinner), 1.78 meters tall, weighing 70 kg with no illnesses, performing strenuous physical exercise for many years, began a customary 30-minute jog in a local park at 7:00 P.M. on December 3, 1976. He wore flare-bottom double-knit polyester trousers, Dacron-cotton boxer-style undershorts, a cotton T-shirt and cotton dress shirt, a light wool sweater, an outer nylon shell jacket over the sweater, gloves, and low-cut Pro Ked sneakers. The nylon shell jacket extended slightly below the belt line.

Local radio weather reports gave the outside air temperature as −8°C, with a severe windchill factor.

From 7:00 to 7:25 P.M. the jog was routine. At 7:25 P.M. jogger noted an unpleasant painful burning sensation at the penile tip. From 7:25 to 7:30 P.M. this discomfort became more intense, the pain increasing with each stride as the exercise neared its end. At 7:30 P.M. the jog ended, and the patient returned home.

Physical examination at 7:40 P.M. in his apartment at comfortable room temperature revealed early frostbite of the penis. The glans was frigid, red, tender upon manipulation, and anesthetic to light touch. Immediate therapy was begun. The polyester double-knit trousers and the Dacron-cotton undershorts were removed. In a straddled standing position, the patient created a cradle for rapid rewarming by covering the penile tip with one cupped palm. Response was rapid and complete. Symptoms subsided 15 minutes after onset of treatment, and physical findings returned to normal.

Side effects: at 7:50 P.M. the patient's wife returned from a local shopping trip and observed him during the treatment procedure. She saw him standing, legs apart, in the bedroom, nude below the waist, holding the tip of his penis in his right hand, turning the pages of the *New England Journal of Medicine* with his left. Spouse's observation of therapy produced rapid onset of numerous, varied, and severe side effects (personal communication).

Pathogenesis of the syndrome was assessed as tissue response to high air velocity at −8°C, penetrating the interstices of polyester double-knit trouser fabric and continuing through anterior opening of Dacron-cotton undershorts, impacting upon receptor site of target organ to produce the changes described.

The patient continues to jog, wearing an athletic supporter and old light cotton warm-up pants used in college cross-country races in 1939. No recurrences are expected.

Apocryphal? I'd hate to be the one to test it.

I know of runners who work out in a windchill temperature of −125°F. Now that's cold enough to frostbite any appendage! The coldest I've ever run in was −19°F. during the 1976 Jersey Shore Marathon. Three months later I was in Boston running when it was 99°F. Mother Nature is an extremist.

TWENTY-THREE

Running with Mother Nature

Mother Nature provides us with seasons for running—from the snap and color of autumn to winter's windless mornings with fresh snow, to summer's mugginess, to spring's flowers, blossoms, and hope. Mother Nature gives us sunshine and darkness, heat and cold, snow and rain, steep uphills and downhills, wind and calm, and woodland perils when we venture off the beaten path. With perhaps too much help from humans, she also provides a variety of surfaces to pound and pollutants to breathe.

Runners go out in every season. As we expose ourselves more and more to running, we also expose ourselves to the vagaries of the environment. We still have a lot to learn about running with Mother Nature. We need to know the challenges and prepare for them. You've read my detailed guidelines for hot and cold weather running; now I'll guide you through still more environmental obstacles.

Running in Rain, Sleet, Hail, Lightning

I ran my first marathon during a tornado warning in Kansas. First came rain, then sleet, and then hail. I thought maybe Mother Nature didn't want me to run the race, but I soon felt like a kid running under the sprinkler.

I can't believe how many runners won't set foot outdoors for a run if it's raining. I get calls all the time from runners wanting to know if their running class will be canceled because of rain. My answer is that only lightning stops us from going out. After all, what do you do when you return from a run? Get wet in the shower.

During warm weather, once you're wet running in the rain is fun! A cold rain, though, is something else—you may want to get some of those fancy foul weather outfits discussed in Chapter 16. As with all runs, take off your wet clothing as soon as you get home. Never, under any circumstances, stand around wet.

Treat running in the rain like running in snow. You will be more tense because you are afraid of slipping. This may cause some muscle tightness. Stretch well before and after your run. Shorten your stride. Stay relaxed on the run and under control. Slow your pace. Beware of wet, slippery leaves.

Lightning is serious. My best friend and his eight-year-old son were both hit by lightning while exercising. The boy was killed.

Watch for lightning. "Sheet" lightning at some distance should make you very alert. Bolts of lightning should send you into a building or vehicle. Do not seek shelter under a tree. If there is no shelter, lie flat on the ground away from tall objects. Do not stand upright in an open area. Stay away from water or high, exposed land; do not touch metal.

Wind

I've already said a lot about head winds and tailwinds in terms of heating or cooling. But wind will also affect your speed. A 10-mile-per-hour head wind will slow your forward progress by about 8 percent. A 10-mile-per-hour tailwind will push you along by about 5 percent faster. You read that right: Mother Nature doesn't play fair! A head wind slows you more than a tailwind helps you. According to studies at Penn State University, you may expend as much as 8 percent of your energy to overcome a head wind. And the stronger the wind, the greater the effort.

Moreover, the slower the runner, the more he or she will be affected by a head wind in terms of time loss. Again, unfair. Jack Daniels, Ph.D., an exercise physiologist, has determined that a three-hour marathon runner will lose 11 seconds per mile when running into a 5-mile-per-hour head wind and 25 seconds per mile when facing a 10-mile-per-hour head wind. That's more than 4 minutes every 10 miles! The four-hour marathoner will lose between 15 and 32 minutes over the marathon distance!

Now the good news: A tailwind will help the slower runner more. The three-hour marathon runner may run 8 seconds per mile faster with a 5-mile-per-hour tailwind and 18 seconds faster with a 10-mile-per-hour tailwind. The four-hour marathoner, however, gets pushed along at between 10 and 24 seconds per mile.

You can control this somewhat. Run into a head wind by leaning into it a little to decrease resistance. Stay as relaxed as possible to minimize the loss of good running form and thus conserve energy. If you're in a race, duck behind other runners and use them as windbreaks. If you're running with friends, take turns serving as the windbreak. You might also use this technique during training runs.

According to Chester Kyle, a professor of mechanics at California State University in Long Beach, you can cut your wind resistance by 31 percent if you stay about 10 feet behind another runner. Move up to 5 feet and you cut the wind resistance by about 50 percent! What else are friends for?

If you are racing, take advantage of a tailwind and fly. You may never get an opportunity to race this fast again!

Running Surfaces

God gave our ancestors the soft earth to cushion their feet. Then along came pavement to mess up the system. Hard surfaces and slanted roads contribute to injury in runners. A well-cushioned shoe will help minimize this problem, but will not eliminate it.

Sand, beaches. If life is a beach, then running on it can be hell. I don't recommend it. The beach is soft and, closer to the water, slanted. The footing is uncertain and there are hidden objects, from shells to such refuse as glass and even needles. Your heel will sink into the sand causing strain on your Achilles tendon. Then there is the problem of heat and too much sunshine and not enough shade. You get the idea.

Sure, it may be fun to run on the beach. But run out and back to compensate for the slant and always wear shoes for protection. I'd limit beach running to 10 minutes for starters and build to no more than 30 minutes. The best advice is to use the beach to relax, not train. Look for a boardwalk to run on.

Grass and dirt. I run on grass and dirt as much as I can as an alternative to running on pavement. This type of running provides constant changes in surface, so you don't have the same chronic repetitive stress that you get with road running. It results in less impact shock than road running and forces your muscles to work harder (and thus strengthens them) at pushoff.

This is good for your body, but ease into it. It is also real tough on your ankles and feet. Some runners don't like the uneven character of grass and dirt. I do, but I also recommend that you get accustomed to it.

Trails. If you are lucky like me, you can find trails and dirt roads in the country or in city parks. City trails are generally well maintained, safe, well lighted, and fun. Some cities have well-marked wood-chip trails. New York City's Central Park has a 1.55-mile cinder path around the reservoir that is maintained by the New York Road Runners Club.

Gravel, concrete, asphalt. Gravel can be rough, especially if the stones are too large, and unstable. Concrete is the worst surface in terms of shock absorption; if your choice is between asphalt and concrete, take asphalt. Many runners prefer asphalt to grass or dirt. The surface is at least dependable.

Roads. When you run facing traffic in the United States, which is the safest way to run, the road surface slants upwards on your right leg. Your right foot, therefore, will turn in more (pronate) and your left foot will turn out more (supinate). Run on the opposite slant and, of course, the opposite feet and legs are affected. Whichever side of the road you choose, the effect is the same: excessive movement all the way up to the knee and hip, which can cause injury. It also results in your right leg being, in effect, shorter than your left—another source of injury.

What to do? Stay off slanted roads as much as possible. Or try to run on roads with less slant. If possible, run on park roads that ban car traffic. Then you can safely run on the crown of the road where there is little slant, or alternate your direction every few miles.

Tracks. The same problem is true when you run on slanted indoor tracks. One leg is "higher" and therefore "shorter" than the other. Usually you cannot reverse direction; to keep the flow steady everyone must run the same way. Some clubs change the direction on alternate days to cut back on the risk of injury.

Flat indoor tracks are even worse to run on; slanted banks at least help to minimize the stress of tight turns. Stay away from indoor tracks that don't have high-quality cushioned surfaces. Indoors or outdoors, you are better off on a slower, more cushioned and bouncy track in terms of injury prevention.

What is the safest surface for a runner? Arkady Voloshin, associate professor of mechanical engineering and biomechanics at Lehigh University in Pennsylvania, studied runners on asphalt, grass, and an artificial track of polyurethane. Voloshin's conclusion is not surprising: "The polyurethane surface produced about 20 percent less shock than did grass or asphalt. Over time, that means a lot less wear and tear and fewer injuries."

So where to run? If your local high school or university has an indoor or outdoor polyurethane track, check it out. Runs up to 30 minutes won't be too boring. After that, you'll feel like a gerbil.

The next best surface is a well-maintained dirt or cinder trail. Only run on grass and rugged trails if you are in real good shape and have strong, flexible ankles and feet. Stay off concrete and minimize your beach running. If you intend to race on paved surfaces, you should do some training there.

Variety is best. But beware of sudden changes in your running surfaces. Start cautiously. Try your new surface just for short runs at first. Don't run on it two days in a row until you have adjusted, perhaps after a week or more.

Altitude
Above 3,000 feet, you will notice the altitude as you run. Since you have less oxygen at high altitude, you will tire more quickly. The higher the altitude above sea level, the greater the effect. With each 1,000-foot increase in altitude above 5,000 feet, your aerobic capacity drops 3 to 4 percent. Your maximal heart rate decreases, lactic acid levels increase, and the amount of oxygen passing through your lungs into the bloodstream also decreases.

As I have found out the hard way, air at higher altitudes is cooler and drier, which is tough on the respiratory system. You also dehydrate quicker, overheat more readily, and may be exposed to greater amounts of sunshine and therefore sunburn. Keep this in mind if you move to a higher altitude or travel to, say, Denver, Colorado. Your running will be affected.

Elite runners go to higher altitudes to train because they believe this helps them improve their performances. Research, however, shows otherwise. Because you can't train as fast as you can at sea level, high-altitude training will not benefit you much. On the other hand, if you live at a high altitude and train or race at a low altitude, you might have an advantage.

If you are a reasonably fit runner visiting at high altitudes, you should start with shorter runs at a slower pace. Within a week, you may be able to gradually increase the intensity and duration of your running. The higher the altitude, of course, the longer the period of acclimatization. At 3,000 feet you may adjust in about a week. At 6,500 feet—Denver's altitude—it will take you two weeks; at 8,000 feet, take four weeks.

Hills

The way I see it, you have three options when it comes to running hills:

1. You can run the other way whenever you see one.

2. You can struggle up hills, cursing Bob Glover with every step.

3. You can outsmart the hills by preparing to meet their challenge.

I heartily recommend options 1 and 3.

All runners talk about hills. They brag about conquering them. Then they complain about how hills slow us down. Our coaches get cussed every time we introduce our beginner runners to the hills. But hills condition you for running and for life. They tire your legs and leave you winded, but they also hone your running form and speed, strengthen your body and mind, and add fun and variety to your running routine. If you are going to race on hills, you'd better train on them. Besides, without hills life would be all flat; there would be nothing to train for and conquer, no wonderful rewarding view from the top.

To win this struggle, repeat and practice the runner's credo: Attack the hill before it attacks you.

Beginner runners, especially if they are overweight, should keep it flat at first. Hill running dramatically increases your heart rate, tires your legs, and makes you feel—let's be blunt about this— awful. Because the beginner's goal is to run easily for 20 minutes, you should avoid hills.

Eventually you will become fit and strong enough to start exploring hilly terrain. You'll know when. Listen to your body. If you've been running the flats and now find them boring, lift your eyes to the gentle hills. Don't suddenly shift to hill running. At first, run hills only once or twice a week. Later, as you gain strength, be sure to include days of flatter, easier running. The ideal is every other day. Minimize the amount of downhill running you do. Downhill running causes more injuries than uphill running. If you face a very steep descent, do the Bob Glover Chicken Walk down it.

Prepare mentally when running hills. Concentrate on good form. Beginner runners should run up as far as they can while running comfortably, then alternate running with walking. But keep going. Pick a spot 50 yards ahead and run to it, then another, and another. (Shepherd runs the Vermont hills from farmhouse to farmhouse.)

Don't start or end your workout on a steep uphill or downhill, if possible. Starting uphill will raise your heart rate quickly at a time when you want to ease into your run. It will stress muscles that haven't yet warmed up. My runs in the country often begin with a large hill, so I walk up it and start my run. When I return, I finish my run at the top and then walk down. If you must finish on an uphill run, make sure you walk around until your heart rate comes back down below 100 beats per minute.

See Chapter 34 for guidelines on running form when going up and down hills. Chapter 15 discusses tips for using hills to train for races. Running uphill will take more out of you than you will gain from running back down it. If you are nursing lower leg injuries, such as shinsplints or Achilles tendinitis, running hills will aggravate your problem.

My favorite training routine is to run to the top of the nearest big hill. I don't race it. I take it as a tourist would—casually, watching the surroundings change as I ascend. At the top of the hill I'm rewarded with a lovely view. The best view I ever earned —and believe me, I worked hard for this one—came at the peak of Mount Washington in northern New Hampshire. There is actually a race to the 6,288-foot summit of that mountain, the tallest on the East Coast. The good news is that there is only one hill. The bad news is that the road up the hill is 8 miles long.

The day I ran Mount Washington the temperature was 90°F. at the bottom and 52°F. at the top, with high winds above the tree line. It was torture all the way, and at times I found the grade enough to make walking faster than running—I found this out when a pair of old geezers passed me with a brisk walk. At the top I looked out across miles of New England; I could even see the little red barn in the valley where we had started.

You, too, can be rewarded with a justly earned "view from the top" if you include hills in your training. Making it up the hills on your runs brings you strength and confidence. In races, outperforming others on the tough hills adds to your personal victory. But the key to being "king of the hills" is to conquer them in practice.

Woodland Perils

I moved to Westchester County to get away from the foul air of New York City and to enjoy running on miles of trails through woods with deer, geese, ducks, wild turkeys, coyotes, and more. But I found that running in the woods comes with its own dangers: poison ivy, mother goose protecting her goslings, Lyme disease, flies, and other biting and stinging things. Most of these can be avoided by staying on the paths, bringing your own toilet paper on your runs, and using insect repellent.

Lyme Disease

Over the last few years, Lyme disease has become an increasing problem for runners. One of the fastest-growing diseases in the United States, it is spread to humans by a common deer tick. If you run through tick-infested areas and you later experience fever, aches, or pains or develop a rash that resembles a bull's eye, see your doctor. Lyme disease can be treated very effectively and cured if diagnosed early.

The first rule is: Stay on the path. I restrict my running to wide trails and avoid running in any area where my body can easily come in contact with grass or brush. If you must relieve yourself, stay on the trail (if you can). (If you use leaves as toilet paper, please learn what poison ivy looks like!) Dress in light colors and wear high white socks so that you can see any ticks that may hitch a ride on you. Use insect repellent with 30 percent DEET.

It takes twenty-four hours for a tick to fully attach itself to a host. You can prevent this by removing ticks without delay. After running, shower immediately and inspect yourself and your clothes for ticks. These may appear as small, pin-head-size dots. (If you've run with a *very close* friend, you might do this for each other; ticks have been known to scamper into those hard-to-see places on the human body!) Your dog can pick up ticks, too. Handling ol' Bowser after you both return from a run in tick country can transfer ticks to you.

If you find a tick on your skin, remove it with tweezers pulling straight out with gentle traction. (If the tick is enlarged with your blood, Shepherd suggests heating up a paper clip and holding it against the tick, which will then dislodge itself.) Apply antiseptic to the area.

Getting Lost or Hurt
Another problem for the runner in the woods is getting lost or hurt, especially those city slickers who go out to the country for a weekend. I got lost once, and then darkness set in. Fortunately, I was able to locate car lights and found my way to the road. The key is to keep some significant object in mind—a river, a highway—and to orient yourself to that object. (For example, keep it always on your left or right; run toward it or along it.) I've also known runners who have turned an ankle while running in rugged terrain. In both cases, the best thing is to have someone with you. If this is not possible, let someone know your running course and the approximate time you will return.

Allergies
Forty million Americans suffer from allergies. Unfortunately, running outdoors gives allergy sufferers added trouble because it exposes them to annoying allergens. You can be exposed to these substances by contact or by inhaling airborne allergens. These substances, which are harmless to many people, can cause physical reactions in allergy sufferers—sneezing, a runny nose, itchy and watery eyes, difficulty breathing and sleeping, fatigue. Needless to say, it's hard to get in a good run with these symptoms.

Some people battle allergies year-round, but most people suffer only seasonally—their symptoms appear at about the same time every year. You may be allergy-free for most of your life, like me, and then gradually find yourself more and more allergic to more and more allergens. You may move your home or office, as I did, to eliminate many of the allergens that were causing you problems only to discover different, more irritating ones to battle.

Mother Nature challenges us with three types of allergens:

- Pollen from weeds, grasses, and trees

- Mold spores

- Dust mites

It is hard to avoid these irritants because they are so small you can't see them. What can you do to minimize the problem of allergies?

Here are some recommended steps that I have learned to take in fighting allergies:

Determine What Is the Cause of Your Allergies
You may be able to figure this out yourself by judging how your body reacts when exposed to different irritants. An allergist can test you to determine what allergens you are most sensitive to and recommend a program to minimize your suffering. If possible, go to an allergist that is familiar with a runner's needs.

Limit Your Exposure
Fight humidity. Mold spores and dust mites are year-round threats that thrive in moist conditions. Use a dehumidifier (clean them regularly) to keep humidity at about 45 percent in your house and basement. Place a few humidity gauges around the house to monitor moisture.

Clean regularly. Eliminate any mold or mildew you find with a strong cleanser such as chlorine. Have a contractor clean your heating system annually to prevent it from becoming a source for spreading allergens throughout the house. Encase your mattress and pillows in a washable cover designed to contain dust mites. Wash your sheets, pillowcases, bedspreads, and blankets in hot water regularly to eliminate dust mites. Clean the house often to eliminate dust and mold buildup. Vacuum rugs regularly or eliminate them. While you are at it, clean your pets and their bedding frequently since pets can carry allergens (you can also be allergic to your pets).

Run away from your problems. If you know which pollens cause your allergies then you can attempt to eliminate them from your property and avoid them on your running courses. This may mean you have to change your favorite routes during allergy season. Trees that cause the most problems include ash, birch, cedar, elm, maple, and oak. (Yikes, I've got most of them in my yard!) Grasses that do the most damage include Kentucky bluegrass, timothy, ryegrass, Bermuda, and Johnsongrass. (Got some of them in my lawn, too.) Major weed allergens include ragweed (the major cause of hay fever), pigweed, English plantain, and sagebrush. I can't cut down all the trees on my property and dig up the lawn, so the best I can do is keep my windows closed and run the air cleaner and/ or air conditioner during allergy season. When is that?

Since most allergens are seasonal, you can find out what time of year you need to avoid which pollens. For example, in the Northeast, allergy season is at its peak for trees from March to June, for grasses from May to August, and for weeds from August to October. Many newspapers print a daily "allergy watch." My local paper lists the previous day's total pollen count, predominant pollens, and a ranking from "absent" (no symptoms) to "very high" (almost all people with any sensitivity will have symptoms) for each of the three major categories of pollens—trees, grasses, and weeds.

Adjust your runs to minimize the problem. Run later in the day, when pollen levels are lower. Plants produce the most pollen between 5:00 and 10:00 A.M. Also, pollens will be spread around more on windy days, so you may choose to wait for the wind to die down before starting your run if your allergies are bothering you. A good time to run is after a rain since it clears pollens from the air and washes it away.

Protect yourself from pollens. You may choose to wear a face mask that filters out pollen. Glasses or sunglasses will provide some protection from eye irritants. As soon as you finish your run, shower and rinse your eyes to eliminate allergens that have attached to you. If pollen counts are very high and you are very sensitive to them, work out in your home or at your gym with aerobic exercise equipment. Air-conditioning cleans pollens from the air.

Consider Medications
Try an over-the-counter antihistamine tablet a half hour before running. Choose one that doesn't cause drowsiness. If that doesn't work, your doctor may prescribe inhalants or sprays such as those described for asthmatics (see Chapter 30). Allergies often contribute to asthma attacks, so your doctor may need to treat you—as mine does—for both conditions. Some allergy sufferers find success with immunotherapy—a series of monthly shots that combat specific allergens.

Learn to Be Flexible
You may need to adjust your training and racing schedule according to your allergy symptoms. I find that I can continue to run for fun and fitness despite my allergies, but need to cut back on hard running—speed training, long runs, and races—when my allergies are bothering me. When I challenge Mother Nature here, I often lose. For me, the result is usually a severe bronchial infection that weakens me for a week or two.

Not from Mother Nature
Not all of the obstacles runners face come from Mother Nature. Some of the worst are man-made, like concrete or slanted roadways. Here are a few more.

Air Pollution
More than 150 million Americans now live in areas where air pollution reaches harmful levels. Air pollution levels can get so high that public health warnings are issued. People are told to stay indoors, to not exercise. Some of the most beautiful areas in America, from southern California to Vermont, are now blighted by air pollution. People living in cities with the dirtiest air had a 15 percent higher mortality rate during a seven-year period than those living in the least polluted cities, according to a Harvard School of Public Health study of 552,138 people in 151 cities.

If you run on hot, hazy days, you may have had an experience similar to mine. One summer day, I took a break from writing this chapter. New York City was in the middle of a terrible heat wave: three straight days with temperatures higher than 100°F. Warnings were issued against exercising strenuously due to high ozone levels. Having just lost six months of running because of a back injury, I was trying to get back into shape. When fit, I could handle the heat. So I didn't think much about going out and running for an hour at a fairly brisk pace. Off I went, but near the end of the run I felt like I hit "the wall." I slowed and finished, but I felt lightheaded and then nauseous. Later came a headache and diarrhea. That was one more reason for me to move my running gear to the country.

Owen Anderson, the exercise physiologist, writes in his *Running Research News*:

> Unfortunately, one of the most common myths of running is that runners don't need to worry about air pollution because their lungs are in "better shape" than those of sedentary persons. Although runners' respiratory systems are usually functionally superior to the lungs and airways of more vegetative folks, that superiority does not include protection from cankerous air. In fact, runners are quite vulnerable to the effects of air pollution, and the risk of damage rises during the act of running.

Our respiratory systems are exposed to greater amounts of pollution when we run compared to those people breathing at rest. The difference is 6 quarts of air per minute at rest compared to 80 to 100 quarts while running briskly. Another problem, Anderson adds, is that while we runners mostly breathe through our mouths; nonrunning people mostly breathe through their noses. The nasal passages remove many pollutants from the air, while breathing through the mouth bypasses this natural filtration system.

The two major enemies of runners today are ozone and carbon monoxide, which come from internal-combustion vehicles and industry. Other air contaminants include sulfur dioxide, lead, and nitrogen dioxide. Not only can short-term exposure to these irritants affect your running, but it can also cause coughing, wheezing, headaches, nausea, and other problems. Chronic exposure may cause more serious pulmonary problems such as bronchitis, emphysema, and even pneumonia.

Ozone
Ground-level ozone is a colorless, toxic gas produced by sunlight reacting with vehicle exhaust and industry emissions. At high con-

centrations, ozone causes irritation to the eyes, nose, and throat and loss of proper functioning of the lungs. Chest tightness, headaches, coughing, and wheezing are other symptoms. Exercise physiologists at the University of California at Davis found, not surprisingly, that people riding exercise bikes who breathed high levels of ozone could not complete their workouts. Another study, reported in the *Journal of Applied Physiology*, noted a 10 percent drop in aerobic capacity among exercisers breathing ozone at peak levels in smog-prone cities. That means you run 10 percent slower with the same effort.

Ozone levels peak on hot, sunny, windless afternoons. Urban areas in valleys and basins tend to trap the highest level of these pollutants.

Carbon Monoxide

Studies show that the worst place to run (or walk) is along a highway or busy street. That's because of the carbon monoxide spewing from the exhaust pipes of internal-combustion vehicles like cars, trucks, and buses. This very toxic pollutant is quickly absorbed by the body and attaches itself to the blood's hemoglobin. This reduces the capacity of red blood cells to carry oxygen. Thus the heart must work harder to meet the demands of exercise. A study at New York Hospital–Cornell University Medical Center shows that runners working out for 30 minutes in heavy New York City traffic increased the level of carbon monoxide in their bloodstreams by as much as tenfold. This is the equivalent of smoking a pack of cigarettes. Symptoms from overexposure to carbon monoxide are similar to ozone: headache, watery eyes, tightness in the chest.

The only good news is that pollutants from vehicles dissipate quickly beyond 50 feet from roadways. If you must run along a road, keep your distance!

Living with Pollution

What should serious runners do?

First, keep track of the ozone and carbon monoxide levels through news reports. If the air quality in your region becomes "unacceptable," postpone your outdoor run to another day. Men and women with a medical history of lung or heart problems should not run during air pollution warnings.

On days when the pollution is high but not high enough to trigger an air pollution alert, I follow the advice of the late Dr. George Sheehan. The scale tips in favor of running. As Dr. Sheehan said: "People who worry more about air pollution than about attending to their physical condition are deluding themselves. They would feel much better running in the city and becoming fit than they would sitting around all day doing nothing in the pure air of the country."

Still, a little pollution is one thing; a lot of pollution is another. When the level is at the warning stage, adjust your workouts. Run shorter and slower. Be aware of the symptoms of pollution. If you are a beginner runner, you may be better off skipping the challenge of the heat and pollution and working out indoors where the air-conditioning screens most of the pollutants. Go for a swim, ride an indoor bike, or run on a treadmill.

Pollution is at its worst in the United States from May to September. In warm weather areas like southern California, it lasts almost year-round. The highest levels of ozone occur in the afternoon. Therefore, the best time to run in hot weather is in the morning or late in the evening. Avoid exercising at midday to avoid high ozone levels.

Ozone is less a factor in cold weather, but carbon monoxide still is. The highest levels of vehicle exhaust are rush hours: from 6:30 to 9:30 A.M. and from 3:30 to 6:30 P.M. So the time to run in cooler weather is non–rush hours and midday when there is less traffic. Run in open spaces where wind currents will help dissipate the exhausts.

Some runners wear filter masks to protect them against air pollution and pollen. This may be useful for those runners whose lungs are irritated by the air.

Country Training, City Racing

If you live in the country but plan to race in the city, you may want to spend a few days getting acclimated. Shepherd, the Vermont runner, finds it takes at least two running days in New York City before he can run there without thinking his arms and legs have turned to concrete. Studies show that exposure to ozone will allow you to adapt to it over a period of days. It may take four or five days for your lungs to become desensitized to the ozone and for your bronchial passages to adjust.

So, to run or not to run? Does running in air pollution increase your health risk?

Once again, ol' George Sheehan was right. Dr. William Adams of the Human Performance Laboratory at the University of California at Davis is a world-renowned expert on the effects of ozone on the human body. His research shows that the lung's ability to repair itself after ozone injury is remarkable. Although a runner may experience a lot of discomfort after exposure to high levels of ozone and other pollutants, studies indicate that most frequently the lungs are completely normal again within twenty-four hours of the end of exposure. Since the long-term effects of such exposure are unknown, however, Dr. Adams does not recommend running regularly during high levels of air pollution.

Running during low levels may be okay. The trade-offs are clearer. Running during air-quality alerts is not recommended, however. If you must run under these conditions, first look for an air-conditioned, indoor track. If you go outdoors, make the run short and slow. Better yet, wait for the air pollution alert to pass. Give Mother Nature a chance to bounce back.

Part VIII

Running Lifestyle

TWENTY-FOUR

Safety

Most runners are confident people. After all, we are fit and conditioned, we can run for long periods of time, and we feel good about ourselves. Running regularly gives us this confidence and it increases as we become better runners. We carry this attitude over into the rest of our lives.

But this confidence can betray us. We may think we can take chances out on the road, like running alone at night or in an unsafe area or not turning back when an unfriendly group appears ahead. We think our strong legs can outrun all danger. This is an unsafe, foolish attitude. Increasingly in the last several years, runners have been attacked in all sorts of settings: city parks, suburban streets, and along country roads. Their attackers have been alone or in groups; on foot, bicycles, cars, even running; they have often carried weapons. We must also face the danger of sharing the road with vehicles.

What should you do? Most important of all, don't let overconfidence make you foolish. Use common sense. Dress to be seen. Run defensively. Run in groups. Run in familiar places. Choose a safe alternative. Be very alert at all times. Watch and know your surroundings. Project self-confidence—a runner who appears hesitant or fearful is more likely to be attacked.

Here are some tips to follow.

Use a Buddy System

Most running clubs offer group runs. Use them. The New York Road Runners Club, for example, has a regular group run in the evenings and on weekends. It also puts together a "buddy board"—a bulletin board listing runners willing to team up with others—and its volunteers have formed a safety patrol that runs in Central Park watching for safety problems. If you are traveling, ask about local running clubs and join their group runs. There is safety in numbers.

Consider Running with Your Dog

I've never heard of a runner getting mugged while running with a dog, though that doesn't mean it hasn't happened. But if you must run alone, take Rover with you. Just be sure to ease your dog into training—dogs get out of shape, too. Keep it hydrated along with you, and keep it on a leash so it won't be a hazard to other runners. Remember: Having the dog along doesn't guarantee your safety, so don't be overconfident.

Plan Ahead

Whether you run alone or in a group, plan your route in advance. Avoid poorly lighted areas, alleys, deep brush; you should also avoid running alone at night. Rapes in New York's Central Park, for example, have taken place when a lone female runner ran near a remote and densely wooded area. The rapists grabbed the victims and dragged them into the brush where they couldn't be seen. Don't stretch your luck, or invite trouble, by running in areas or at times that are obviously dangerous. Few incidents in city parks occur during the prime running hours before and after the normal workday or during the weekend daylight hours. Most problems occur late at night, or during mid-morning or afternoon workdays.

Practice in your head what escape routes you would use at various points along your regular running route. If you see something different or dangerous ahead of you on your run, do something radical. Run into a store, a building with a doorman, a police or fire station, or, as a last resort, a well-lighted home. Scout these along your route beforehand. If you are visiting a new place, ask your hosts (friends, hotel manager, innkeeper) what they might do in case of sudden danger on a run. (Other safety tips for traveling runners are discussed in the next chapter.)

Tell someone where you will be running and when you'll be back. Then, if something happens and you don't return on time, the police can be notified sooner and have a better chance of finding you and/or the person who hurt you.

Also, when you return to your car or home after running, have your key in your hand. Do not fumble around for it in front of your door—this gives a mugger an opportunity to grab you. And don't wear jewelry that may attract attention.

Act Defensively

If someone harasses you verbally during your run, do the only sensible thing: Ignore it. But if this escalates, be prepared to move away from the trouble. Reverse direction. Change your route. Make lots of noise. Carry a whistle and blow it loudly and repeatedly.

If in doubt, play it safe. Always know who is ahead of you— including who has just passed you and where he or she has gone —and have in mind the nearest safety choice. Be alert to drivers who stop to ask directions. Do not approach the car; instead, answer at a distance. If you think a car is trailing you, turn and run in the other direction. Follow the same strategy if you encounter someone in or on other vehicles, including bicycles.

If you are attacked by someone who is unarmed, try to escape. Again, make a lot of noise. Scream, yell, blow a whistle. Let others near you know clearly that you are being attacked. As a last resort, fight back. But: If your attacker is armed, don't resist. Your life is too valuable to risk. Concentrate on being able to give the police a good description of your attacker—but don't tell the attacker you are doing this! People have been killed during robberies because they told the robbers they would identify them to the police.

Do not show fear or plead. This may intensify the aggression. Talk to the aggressor while watching for an opportunity to escape. Look for a moment of indecision or distraction.

If you are out running and someone calls for help, go to their assistance. *But be careful!* If you think a call to the police may prevent an incident, get to a phone! (Tuck phone change—a quarter usually works—into that little pocket of your running shorts. What else do you think it's for?)

Shepherd had just returned from a run in New Hampshire one day and was entering a pizza parlor—to carbo-load, he claims—when he thought he saw a large young male college student punch a woman student several times. He had actually walked by them on the sidewalk and into the pizza parlor when he suddenly realized what he had witnessed. The woman had not made a sound—nothing, not even a brief outcry. Shepherd looked out the window just in time to see the young man push the woman to the sidewalk. He and a friend were on the student immediately and yelled for help. The police came and an arrest was made. But Shepherd couldn't get over this simple fact: The assaulted woman never uttered a sound.

Act defensively. And make a lot of noise if something happens that you don't want to happen.

Choose a Safe Alternative

If you are unsure whether it is safe to run in a certain area, or you lack a running partner, or the weather is bad, or it's dark—*don't run*. A home exercise bike or rowing machine is great for these occasions.

Watch Out for Cars: Run Defensively

Cars weigh more than you and move faster. You won't win in a collision with a car. I know too many runners who were killed or injured by cars while running.

Bill Coughlin, a good friend and running partner from my days in Rome, New York, was killed by a car while running in Jackson, Michigan. Kathy Damon, one of the sub-three-hour marathoners I coached, was knocked off the road and hospitalized by a hit-and-run driver on Long Island. She was lucky: She got out of the hospital and ran her marathon anyway.

Since Bill's funeral, I refuse to run on roads shared by cars. I stick to trails or run in parks closed to traffic. But many runners have limited choices. And cars are a constant danger. What should you do? Here are some tips:

- Don't run on high-speed roads. Why take the risk?

- Always run facing traffic. Most incidents of cars hitting runners occur when the runner is overtaken from behind. Pedestrians are twice as likely to be killed when moving with traffic as when facing traffic, according to data from the National Safety Council. Facing the traffic allows you to see every vehicle coming your way and to make eye contact with drivers at corners or in moments of confrontation or decision. You can convey your moves and the driver can respond.

An exception is when you must run around a blind curve. Then you should run in such a way that cars from both directions can see you at the earliest possible moment. Shepherd runs on a narrow, winding Vermont road that has seven sharp curves within a half mile. He alternates the side he's on in order to give drivers the longest possible view of him.

▪ Stay as far from the traffic as possible. Along a busy highway, run on the outside of a wide shoulder.

▪ Pay special attention when crossing roads. Don't think you can dart across and beat an oncoming car. If you are tired, or your judgment is blurred, you're gonna become roadkill. Wait.

▪ When in doubt, step off the road and stop. Face the approaching vehicle.

▪ Wear bright and reflective clothing at all times—day *and* night. It helps drivers see you.

▪ If possible, avoid running after dark anywhere, but especially on roads. It is much safer and more interesting to run along sidewalks in residential areas than on roads after dark. Or run around a large, well-lighted, well-populated parking lot.

▪ Do not look directly at headlights. This may temporarily blind you.

▪ On country roads, do not simply listen to cars as they pass and then step out onto the road without glancing back.

▪ Avoid the road on snowy, icy, or rainy days. The harder it is for a driver to see, the greater the danger for a runner.

▪ If you are running in a group, run single file. Don't fill the road and think you own it. The road belongs to vehicles, not you.

▪ Stay alert. Don't allow yourself to fall into a trancelike state. Hey, I've almost run out in front of cars while deep in thought. I've actually seen runners run right into the sides of cars.

▪ Don't challenge any vehicle. They always have the right of way in terms of your safety.

▪ Finally, if you plan a fast or long run, confine it to traffic-free routes. If you can't think of any, call your local runners' club. Runners training for a marathon are especially prone to carelessness during their long runs.

Remember to avoid overconfidence. The only study I've seen on the subject of runners and vehicles—a survey by the U.S. Insurance Institute for Highway Safety—found that in 31 percent of accidents involving runners, the runners were at fault. That's almost one out of three! In another 28 percent of cases, the runners were equally at fault with the motorists. So, in almost 60 percent of all accidents involving runners and vehicles, the runner is at least partly at fault.

Watch Out for Bikes: Run Defensively

Be alert to bikes. I would also add in-line skaters. Anything on wheels should be considered a vehicle moving your way at high speed.

I know from experience that runners and bicyclists don't mix. I was clobbered by a bicyclist only two weeks before a major marathon attempt. That wiped out twelve straight 100-mile weeks of training. So treat bikes like cars. Be careful when running in crowded parks or streets even when they are closed to vehicular traffic. Cyclists often weave in and out to avoid runners and walkers. On the other hand, avoid weaving all over a crowded road yourself. As the study above points out, runners themselves cause many accidents. Respect the pace and rights of others on the road. Run defensively.

Dress Defensively

Shepherd wears his bright orange reflector vest whether he runs day or night. Even his shoes have reflectors on them.

Take Off Your Headphones

I get complaints from runners every time I tell them this. So, you don't want to hear it from me? How about Capt. Joe Raguso? Captain Raguso is a veteran runner and a New York police officer who at one point in his career was in charge of safety in Central Park. Headphones on runners are his "number one complaint," he says. "I love the things myself and enjoy them at home, but not while running. They are dangerous because they cause a loss of perception. Runners, especially women, must constantly monitor what's going on around them—speeding cars, a suspicious man behind bushes, etc. Since headphones have become popular, crime involving runners has dramatically increased. Muggers love them —the majority of muggings and many rape attempts we see happen to runners wearing headphones."

Headphones encourage crime for several reasons. They are attractive targets themselves because they can be snatched and then quickly resold. They also impair your sense of what is happening around you. I've seen a biker wearing headphones ride smack into the side of a truck, and a runner, bopping to music, run into a stop sign. If you are focusing on the music, you are less aware of what is happening around you. If you aren't aware of the music, why wear the headphones? Even when the music is turned low, your sense of danger is still impaired. For example, in Brooklyn's Prospect Park, women runners were attacked in a series of rapes or attempted rapes in broad daylight. In at least three cases, the women were running alone and wearing headphones.

Playing loud music can also cause hearing damage. A study conducted at the University of Nevada at Reno found that the cardiovascular system is stressed during exercise, diverting blood and oxygen from the ear, making it more sensitive to sound. Playing headphones at a comfortable level will not cause hearing loss. A good rule is don't play them louder than a loud conversational speech. If, when you take them off, you have ringing in your ears or speech sounds muffled, consider this a warning sign. Turn it down to 85 decibels or less.

Still, many people find that their workouts are more enjoyable with music, and studies at Springfield College in Massachusetts show that people who listen to music can exercise longer. If you insist on running with headphones, here is my safety rule: Run only in an area free from car and bike traffic with plenty of other people around. This might be your local track, a wooded trail frequented by other runners and hikers, or along a busy path. Otherwise, save the headphones for working out on your stationary bike or treadmill at home or at your gym.

Shepherd used to wear a headset attached to a tape recorder in a small fanny pack. Then one day while listening to Fauré's "Requiem" during a run, he started to cross a winding country road and a car passed so close it actually tore his running shorts. He never heard it. But he learned a lesson.

Respect Other Runners

A collision between runners is considerably less dangerous than a collision between a runner and a vehicle. Either way, you're still going to be black and blue, at the least. In most U.S. cities, the parks and trails are crowded with runners, cyclists, rollerbladers, race walkers, and all manner of strollers and gawkers.

Collisions seem to be the norm and on the increase. To avoid them, stay alert. Keep to the right when facing and running by another runner and always pass other runners on your right. Crowded tracks may have posted rules. Note which way the runners are going—clockwise or counterclockwise—and do the same. You'll also notice that there is always one runner who can't figure this out and insists on running against the flow. Keep your eye on him. He hasn't read this book!

Be polite. Notify other runners when you are about to overtake them from behind: "Excuse me. Coming through on your right. Thank you." Shepherd wants me to add this note: When you are passing someone older than you, add a little lift for their ego. Tell them that they are "looking good" or "really taking that hill." Give your fellow runners a boost.

Identify Yourself

For several hours after my friend Bill Coughlin was killed in Michigan no one knew who he was. Like too many runners, Bill didn't carry identification. Hey, he was just going for a run. What could happen? He had run for decades with no problem.

If you are involved in an accident, ambulance EMTs and hospital emergency room staff will need to know your blood type, name, medications, and so on. Your loved ones will also want to know if you've been hurt, so they can come to your side. I usually stick a business card in that little pocket in my shorts or under the laces of my shoes (or even under my orthotics). You should list your name, address, an emergency contact person, and any important information such as blood type, medications, and allergies. When you travel, add the name of your hotel (but not your room number) or where you are staying.

Dogs

I've stepped on snakes in Vietnam, tripped over rats along the Hudson River, been stung by bees, swallowed bugs, and a bear narrowly missed me in Yosemite Park. But dogs are the worst.

Some wary runners plan routes to avoid passing the houses of certain dogs. Others, in their anger at being chased and snapped at, have almost fulfilled that great journalistic definition of what constitutes news: Man bites dog.

Not all dogs are interested in runners, but any dog that comes out to check on you as you run by is a potential danger. Keep your eyes on him, especially as you pass. Dogs often bite from behind. Shepherd was jogging in New York City's Riverside Park when he passed two well-dressed ladies talking and letting their little poodles sniff and scratch. Just as he went by, Shepherd heard the growl and snap. One poodle had lunged at him and missed only because it was on a leash. The owner said, "My, my, Tootsie, it's only a silly man."

You can lower the risk of provoking trouble from a dog. Many dogs protect their territory and will defend it if they feel threatened. Keep in mind that as a runner you approach their territory faster than they are used to; this may excite even docile dogs. Do not come up quickly and unexpectedly on a dog. Always speak to any dog you approach. Talk to dogs in a firm but soft voice. Say things like "good doggie" over and over (most owners address their dogs in this tone). Tell the dog to "stay home, stay, stay," or just say "no"—firmly.

Try to anticipate a dog's intentions. If the tail is erect, ears straight up, lips curled, hair raised on the back of its neck, he means business. If you find yourself confronted with such a dog, there are four techniques you may want to use to deal with it:

1. You can run. This works only if you are challenged by a dachshund or a dog on a leash (do not trust a rope). Dogs are animals with hunting instincts. If you run, the dog will sense your fear and chase you. A better bet: Imitate the fleet Masai of

East Africa, who know that if they encounter a lion in their path they must stop and face him and stand still. To run is to die.

2. You can try to make friends. This also contains risk. Some dogs are trained guard dogs. Others consider the world their territory. That hand offered for a sniff may appear to be a threat. If this tactic doesn't work, at least your arm gets the bite, not your legs. You will still be able to go out for a run.

3. You can threaten the dog. Shouting or growling—I know some runners who are splendid growlers—sometimes works. Clap your hands loudly. Shout "No!" or "Sit!" or "Bad dog!" Waving your arms or shooing the dog away, however, may be considered menacing. Sometimes, dogs will retreat if you bend down and pick up a stone or stick. (Be sure not to let the dog come too close before you bend; in that position you are vulnerable to a fatal bite.) If you grab a stone and the dog halts, *slowly* raise your arm to throw it. He may get the message and retreat. If he doesn't, then you retreat: back off slowly. Keep your arm raised with the stone in it. You may need to throw it at the dog if it continues to come forward.

4. Spray the dog. Some runners clip a can of Halt! or other spray to their shorts. Others carry small water pistols with a half-and-half mixture of ammonia and water. That's also effective, although water pistols often leak. Shepherd always carries Halt! when he runs in the country. But there are risks here. Owners can become irrational if you threaten to spray their dogs. Also, the one time I tried out my trusty dog spray I was downwind of the dog. I cried all the way home; the dog ran off laughing.

As a last resort, you might try my father's trick. He was out for his morning walk when a dog that had been bothering him for weeks came up. My father knelt down quietly and when the mutt came within range, he punched him in the nose. He wasn't bothered again.

Be especially wary of any dog whose owner proclaims, "Oh, he won't bite." He will, you can be sure. If you are bitten, do not fight back. This may cause the attack to continue. If the dog runs off, try to remember what it looked like and where it lived. Go immediately to the hospital and also report your injuries to the police, even if you don't think you are hurt. If there are bites that break the skin, the dog will have to be tested for rabies and you may have to go through a series of rabies injections.

Owners of dogs can be nuts. Most communities now have strict leash laws, primarily to protect dogs from vehicles and animals that might be carrying rabies. But owners, especially those in the country, often ignore the laws and let their dogs run free. So the sweet little things, obeying that hunting instinct, chase deer and runners. When two large German shepherds attacked and bit me, the owner said I had provoked the attack by throwing rocks at his dogs as they slept innocently on the front porch. Jack Cohen, a New York Road Runner, ran a favorite course in upstate New York where he was continuously harassed by the same dog. He began telephoning the owner in advance so she could tie up the dog until he had passed. But when ole poochie howled, the lady got tired of tying him up. One day she suggested that Jack change his route. "After all," she told him, "the dog was here before you were."

TWENTY-FIVE

Travel

I often hear runners complain: "I was keeping up with my exercise program until I had to travel on business. I got so far behind that I quit." I always tell them: "You can find the time to exercise (it may not be running). Be flexible."

All of us are very busy. We carefully schedule our lives—and that includes our runs on certain days, at certain times, and even along certain training routes. Such planning is the heart of our personal fitness programs. But no matter how carefully we schedule our exercise, business trips and vacations can disrupt this routine. With proper planning, a flexible attitude, and an inquisitive spirit, you can continue to exercise when your routine is broken. Approach running in new locations as an adventure—and add a dash of caution.

Shepherd and I are, in the words of his Vermont neighbor, "comin' and goin' cats." I've traveled on business to Europe, Southeast Asia, and China, while he is always off and running in England, Eastern Europe, and sub-Saharan Africa. Believe me, we know how hard it is to stay in shape while traveling. This chapter is what we've learned (so far).

First, some general suggestions.

Attitude. Think of your trips as exercise opportunity gained, not lost. If you are convinced that your trip will destroy your fitness base, you might very well let that happen. Open yourself to new adventures and different forms of exercise. Sightsee on the run.

Sure, we all lose a little training edge when we travel. But take what you get and don't stop your exercise routine.

Flexibility. As a runner who also travels, you need to be very adaptable. You have to fit your exercise in with your business, travel, and leisure plans. You must also respect the fatigue that is part of travel: jet lag, increased emotional stress, lost sleep.

What do I mean by being flexible? Simply this: Take your exercise when, and in whatever form, you can. Don't expect to be able to run at your usual time, pace, or distance. Find opportunities whenever your schedule and your body allow. You may skip a day, but that's all right—but try not to miss two days in a row.

Don't force yourself to work out if you're tired. Try a short walk or swim instead. Catch up on your sleep and get ready for a good run the next day. Strive for high-quality runs that enhance your vacation (or your relaxation), not for lots of miles to enter in your training diary.

How's this for being "flexible"? A millionaire executive I coached carried an exercise bicycle on his private jet so he could workout while traveling around the country. That's really taking altitude training to new heights!

Or, there's the story a running friend told me about his traveling companion who was very upset because his flight was delayed. He was going to miss an entire day of running. Then the plane finally left and about two hours into the overnight flight, the captain announced to the passengers that they might have to make an emergency landing. There was a strange, unidentifiable noise coming from the rear of the plane. One of the attendants saved the flight by discovering the cause of the noise: the compulsive runner was jogging in place in one of the toilets!

You can even run while on safari. Dr. Chris Mupimpila, an economist from Zambia and a friend of Shepherd's, runs six out of seven days every week. Nothing stops him! During a conference at Italia Game Reserve in South Africa (home of white and black rhinos), Chris logged his miles every morning by running back and forth across the fence-enclosed compound—200 yards each way-

—for five miles! Chris ran on the inside, the lions and rhinos ran on the outside!

The first day I arrived in China, I was worn out from the long flight in a plane that seemed to be filled with smokers. I took it easy the first day, and then had a great run on the second. In fact, my sight-seeing runs in the countryside showed me a China I could never have seen from a tour bus. I only ran six out of the ten days on that trip, and my mileage was lower than I had hoped, but I was able to enjoy what running I did and returned to the States full of enthusiasm about China, its people, and my running routine there.

Commitment. To exercise when traveling you simply need commitment. Try to schedule exercise during the business day by writing it into your calendar. Don't be shy about offending someone more senior than you. They will generally understand. Shepherd remembers standing in a formal English garden at Emmanuel College, Cambridge University, while a young Swedish-American woman, Dr. Cecilia Albin, looked through her pocket calendar to make an appointment with a very senior faculty member.

"I'm free," she told him, "until noon, when I run, and I'll be free again after two." That was fine with her English host.

- Try to block out time in your pocket calendar every day for exercise. Most people, like the British professor at Cambridge, understand the importance of exercise. (If not, you have an excellent topic for discussion.) Your best bet when traveling may be to work out first thing in the morning before your day fills with appointments or tours. Otherwise, you may end up running out of time or energy for your exercise.

- Be a little selfish when you travel. Don't hesitate to ask your clients (or family) to shift reservations an hour later so you can enjoy a brief exercise break.

- Be creative. If you cannot exercise even when you've scheduled it, or you can't find a good place to run in a strange city, try the fitness center at your hotel, the local sports club, or YMCA. This may also be safer in a new city than running outside in unfamiliar territory. A half hour or more of vigorous exercise in the pool or on the exercise machines is as good for your heart and muscles as running.

Shepherd, one of the oldest little kids I know, loves the new computerized rowing machines you find in most hotel fitness centers.

For a change of pace, you might want to exercise with your business clients or with local runners. I've played soccer in China with a bunch of giggling kids. And I'll never forget the most unusual "workout" I ever enjoyed at a sauna in Germany. Hundreds of nude men and women of all ages packed the huge facility for a series of co-ed rituals followed by an invigorating sprint across the snow in subzero weather, then a jump into hot tubs. Who said exercise was boring?

▪ Try contacting local running clubs to see if there are any group runs. The New York Road Runners Club, for example, has regular evening and weekend runs that welcome visitors to the city. In Nairobi, Kenya, the Hash House Harriers run every Wednesday evening; don't worry about lions.

These clubs can be found through phone books, running stores, or the concierge at your hotel. Just ask at the desk when you check in for admission to the hotel's fitness center for the names of any running clubs. Some hotels post notices from such organizations. They are a great way to work out in a strange place and to make new friends.

Don't overdo it, however. I've found that, when traveling, it is always better to do a little less; you'll enjoy it more. Better to coast through a 3-mile run and leave time for an unrushed shower than to squeeze in an hour of running and arrive late for a meeting or dinner frazzled rather than relaxed.

Always leave time for proper warm-up and cool-down. I once rushed back from a long morning run on a hot day, jumped into a hot shower, and zoomed without eating or drinking to a presentation I was making before a large group of doctors. As I was giving my slide show I remember yelling at the projectionist several times to focus the slides. But I was the one out of focus; a few seconds later I collapsed. There was a mad rush of doctors to see who would be the first to attend me. I finished the talk, but I was really embarrassed.

Finally, be adventuresome, but also be wary. In China, I decided to explore along a river and ran right by a sign in Chinese that I didn't understand. Soon I was facing two young Chinese soldiers who pointed the barrels of their rifles in my face. I have no idea what I did, but after a lot of hand waving and smiling, I was out of there in a sprint!

Now, let's discuss some more specific ideas.

Packing

If you're going to travel, you're going to get good at packing. I have three rules:

1. In terms of weather, pack for where you're going, not for where you are.

2. Take the least amount of clothing you can. Actually, Shepherd and I pack our running gear first. Whatever fits in after that, we also take along.

3. Always take your running shoes, shorts, shirts, and orthotics (if you wear them) on the plane with you. The airline can lose your regular clothes for a few days and you'll survive. But the loss of your favorite shoes and running gear would be traumatic.

Here are some other tips:

▪ Most running clothes wash easily and dry overnight. (You might also pack a small plastic bag half full of your favorite laundry soap; double bag it and tuck it into the toe of one of your shoes.)

▪ Pack your running gear in a separate bag that you can easily carry on board with you. You can also find your gear quickly should you need it for a workout.

▪ Make a list of the things you use at home for your workouts. Put it with your running bag. Remember the little things: Vaseline, sunblock, and so on.

▪ Pack a large plastic bag—a supermarket bag is fine—for your dirty and wet clothes. Some hotels provide plastic laundry bags; look in the closet or the desk drawer—or ask the maid.

▪ Don't forget a few extra new T-shirts, if you have room. They are great to trade with other runners, especially in a foreign country, or to give as gifts. Anything with the name of your running club and its logo, a U.S. city or college (you don't actually have to be associated with the college!), or the word "marathon" on it is a terrific gift.

Remember to pack light. Also, if you're traveling to a race and have been mailed your number *don't forget to pack it!* The best bet is to pin it to your running shirt and pack them together with all your other race information and directions. Also, carry this gear on the plane with you. Don't check it!

Accommodations

In a study conducted by the American Hotel & Motel Association, 25 percent of travelers said that their decision about a place to stay was based on the type of recreational or sports facilities available. Many hotels and motels also have "no smoking" rooms. Fitness facilities are also becoming common hotel amenities.

When making reservations, ask about the hotel's fitness center. When checking in, ask again and get a special key, if needed. Most hotels with computer-programmed keys can make them fit both your room and the fitness center.

If the hotel you are staying in does not have a fitness center, ask if they have arrangements for guests to work out in a nearby club—most do, and be sure to inquire if there's any additional cost.

Most large urban hotels have fitness centers; some also have small exercise swimming pools. The fitness centers are usually open twenty-four hours a day—you'll have no excuse not to exercise! —and along with the weight, rowing, and running machines they will have stacks of clean towels and even a television set. You can lift, row, or run and watch your favorite show.

But be careful: Most hotel fitness centers have no employee in attendance. Many do not even have a closed-circuit TV monitor so that the front desk can at least watch who comes and goes in the fitness center. Therefore, take no valuables to your workout. Both men and women should enter the fitness center cautiously and check out anyone else in the room. Before you start working out, see if the phone is working and learn the emergency number. If you sense something wrong, leave or call the security desk.

Shepherd has used hotel fitness centers from Amman, Jordan, to Portland, Oregon. He's never had a bad incident in any of them. Moreover, he has found that most hotel employees can also direct you to excellent running trails and other workout amenities. So, ask and enjoy!

Jet Lag

This is the bane of all runners—and all travelers. In theory, traveling east (when you "lose time") across several time zones is harder on you than traveling west (when you "gain time"). North-south travel is not as much of a problem, although some trips are long in duration. Either way, your internal clock is thrown off and you'll need time to adjust. There are several things you can do to minimize the impact of travel even before you step on the airplane.

Before You Fly

Three or four days before your flight, try to change your schedule to coincide more closely with the time at your destination. This is tough to do, but try to prepare beforehand by changing your schedule—getting up or going to bed an hour or two earlier— especially if you are traveling a long distance. Go into the trip with as much sleep as possible.

Set your watch at the local time of your destination and eat and sleep (as much as possible) by that schedule for a few days before you fly. Run the day before you fly.

Flying

During your flight, eat lightly and forgo caffeine and alcohol. The combination of alcohol and low cabin pressure may disturb your adaptation process. Drink plenty of water. Dehydration, caused by low cabin humidity, adds to your fatigue. You may want to bring a large bottle of water on board with you. During the flight, get up and walk around every 30 minutes or so. Try some gentle stretching and relaxation exercises. Wear loose clothes and remove your shoes. Your feet (and hands) may swell considerably due to the pressure in the cabin.

Shepherd has an in-flight routine that is truly bizarre, but it works for him. His advice:

■ No partying! Follow the above diet rules, especially when ordering beverages from the cart. Eat lightly.

■ On flights longer than two hours, put in ear plugs, remove your shoes and put on light slippers, cover your eyes with an eye shade. Forget the in-flight movie. Have you ever seen one you'd recommend to a friend?

■ On overnight flights, do all of the above plus your usual bedtime ritual: brush your teeth, etcetera. (Okay, you can skip reading *Goodnight, Moon.*) Shepherd even takes half an over-the-counter sleeping pill to help him get about four hours or more of sleep.

If you do this, try a pill at home at least a week before your flight to see what effect the sleeping tablet will have on you the next day. You want to be able to wake up suddenly—in case of an emergency on the plane—and move around easily the next morning. After all, you will have to get your bags and take some form of transportation to your final destination.

■ Ask the flight attendant to wake you about an hour from your destination. Get up, stretch, eat any breakfast served, do your morning ritual (teeth, hair, face, shaving, etc.). On long flights, Shepherd even changes into a fresh set of underwear (running shorts) and a clean shirt. Feels terrific.

Can you imagine flying with Shepherd? No booze, no partying, no in-flight movies; slipper socks, ear plugs, eye shades, and a little over-the-counter numb-numb! This guy is definitely not Charlie Party, but, hey, when he arrives he's ready for work and exercise.

Arriving

After a long flight, it is best not to run as soon as you arrive. You'll be tight and prone to injury. Get to your destination, settle in, check out the exercise opportunities, plan your schedule. Then, stretch and go for a walk or a swim to loosen up and relax. Don't expect to feel real peppy on your first few runs after a long trip.

Pay attention to things you might take for granted at home: altitude, climate, road surface, road safety. Dr. William Haskell of the Division of Cardiology at the Stanford University School of Medicine suggests some cautions to the traveling runner: "It's wise to back off a bit from your usual running schedule. If you've gone suddenly from a moderate climate to a hot and humid one, the demand on your cardiovascular system, of course, is going to be greater. The same is true when going to a cold climate. Or to high altitudes."

Get into a regular sleeping pattern as soon as possible. Most travelers have a rule of thumb about recovering from jet lag: One day recovery for every hour in time zone change. If you fly to Europe (say Paris) from the east coast of the United States, there's a six-hour time-zone change. Expect to take six days to get yourself feeling normal again. Prior to that, adjust the distance and pace of your runs according to your level of travel fatigue.

Athletes in competition try to lessen the impact of jet lag by arriving those time-zone days before a competition. Or, they fly in right before the competition and hope that the jet lag doesn't kick in until they've finished competing. Professional sports teams generally have a much worse record on the road than at home. Why? In part because they know their home field and draw in the energy of their home crowd. But much of it comes from travel-related fatigue. A good rule of thumb: Arrive one day before your race for each time zone you cross.

By car. If you are traveling long distances by car—and you may do this every day in your work—try to get out every two hours or so, walk around, and stretch your legs and back. If possible, take turns driving with others.

Where to Run on the Road

I make arrangements to stay at hotels near my favorite running trails. For example, near the lakefront trails in Chicago, the Charles River in Boston, Fairmount Park in Philadelphia, the Mall in Washington, D.C., the routes to Golden Gate Park in San Francisco. For me, of course, the most convenient and most exciting place to run is in New York's Central Park. This park is only a few blocks from many fine hotels.

Most hotels provide maps of running trails. If information isn't available from the hotel, call the local YMCA, running club, or a running store for help.

One of the best services available for the traveling runner is the Running Trails Network provided by the American Running and Fitness Association (1-800-776-ARFA). They have maps for more than 250 North American cities showing the best places to run. ARFA also invites runners to send them maps of their favorite running places so they can add them to their data base—big cities as well as routes from smaller towns and suburban areas. As an incentive, if you contribute a map to the Network you will receive, in return, a different map free. Handmade maps are welcome.

Adventure Runs

Some runners like to follow a map and a route. This is also safer. I prefer to get lost.

I really love the adventure of running in new territory. Put me in a new city and the first thing I need to do is go for a run to scout my way around. I'll scale the highest hill for a view and search for routes along the local river or lake. I'll run until I find the Washington Monument or the steps to the art museum in Philadelphia that Sylvester Stallone made famous in the film *Rocky*.

While all of this is adventuresome and fun, there's a price. Here are some things I learned the hard way:

- Bring with you the name, address, and phone number of the hotel you are staying in.

- Before running too far, note a landmark—tall building, lake, mountain—to serve as a guide during your exploration.

- Carry some bills for a taxi in case you get hopelessly lost.

- Learn to overcome male conditioning—ask for help before you get too desperately lost.

When Carl Eilenberg was working as the radio announcer for Syracuse University football games and the team played away, he loved to explore on the run. One weekend before the Syracuse-Navy game, Eilenberg trotted out of the Holiday Inn near Bowie, Maryland, where he and the Syracuse team and coaches were staying, and took off. It was a magnificent autumn day and he felt as though he could run forever. He soon forgot how to get back.

"I got lost," he admits. He stopped to ask a man sleeping in a car: "I'm lost. Where am I?"

The man eyed his fancy running outfit and replied: "You're in the United States of America, son."

Eilenberg told him he wanted to get back to the Holiday Inn. The man asked: "Holiday Inn One, Two, or Three?" Eilenberg didn't know.

Running out of energy and time, Eilenberg hailed a taxi. When he got back, the entire Syracuse football team, coaches, and press corps were standing at the entrance to the hotel. "The boos, jeers, and catcalls persisted for weeks."

Not only that, he had to borrow $20 for the taxi fare.

■ Run in a large loop where you can keep your return point to your left or right at all times. Or, run in one direction, keeping track of the time, and turn around at the halfway point (say, after 20 minutes). Be sure to run straight back! I learned a lesson in San Francisco when I went sight-seeing on a long downhill stretch and then had to return up those hills!

■ Run for time. When you travel, don't count on trails or roads being marked for distance. Take a break from logging miles and just run for time. If you run for 30 minutes at a pace that feels like a 10-minute-per-mile pace then give yourself credit for a nice 3-miler.

Safety, Local Laws, and Customs

I've been stopped by the police three times while running. The first time I was running after dark in a ritzy residential section of Beverly Hills. The second time I was running shirtless (Hey, it was 95°!) in a fancy little town near the beaches of Long Island. In both cases, the local police regarded me as intruding riffraff. My third "offense" was "jayrunning" in Minneapolis—crossing the street between the crosswalks. I plea-bargained that one: Jayrunning is a way of life in New York City, where I lived at the time.

Having a police record like that has made me create some basic rules for running (or even walking) in a new place:

■ Be conservative and cautious. Learn the customs. Women need to be especially wary: In some parts of the world customs frown upon, or outright forbid, women to show their legs (or arms) while on the street. Be especially careful about this and ask before you go out. Women runners, especially those running alone, may also attract other equally unpleasant kinds of attention.

▪ Always carry an ID or at least a business card tucked into the tongue or under the inner soles of your running shoes. How else are they going to notify next of kin? You're in a strange city where no one knows you. How do you convince anyone, from cop to morgue officer, that you are you. ("That's Glover." "Nah, don't look like him from TV.") You can also write your hotel, address, and phone number on the back of your business card before you tuck it into your shoe.

▪ Be alert to traffic. I know, I sound like your father. But in some places in this world drivers come at you from the opposite direction. On her first day in Nairobi, Shepherd's wife stepped off the curb and looked left. Trouble was, they drive on the "wrong" side and traffic came from the right. A taxi passing at high speed actually caught her skirt and turned her around. In a couple of countries I've been to they drive all over the road—at full speed.

Best bet: Stay off the roads in a strange country.

Food and Drink

Go ahead: taste the local menu. Try the salad. Drink the water. But you will pay for that genuine native dinner at that quaint little out-of-the-way spot during your run the next day. There are two dangers to travel, even within the United States (or your home country): food and drink.

It's easy to overeat, starting with the airplane meals. Moderation and caution are the order of the day. Your digestive system takes no holiday. Here are some guidelines:

▪ If you are uncertain about the water, buy bottled water. Use it for brushing your teeth or to hydrate yourself just before a run. In restaurants, drink only from bottles that are opened at your table. If an opened bottle is brought to the table send it back. It may be a refill.

▪ Eat only cooked food, fruits that you peel yourself, and only well-cooked vegetables (although these are risky). Avoid salads since they are washed in the local water.

- If you are afraid of not eating a balanced diet, bring a supply of vitamin pills.

Drinking fluids while you run can be a problem anywhere. In the United States and some developed countries (Western Europe, Japan) you might be okay drinking from the fountains in a park. Here the local running club people can be helpful.

In the United States, because of federal and local water laws, your only worry is likely to be finding where the drinking fountains are located. If need be, loop back to your hotel every few miles to get water. Or bring money to buy bottled water.

If you like long runs, you'll need to replace lost fluids. In that case, you'd be wise to invest in one or two small plastic water bottles that you could carry in either hand. Overseas, fill them with bottled (or boiled) water. In the United States, draw water from a tap after letting it run for about a minute.

Nothing is a sure thing, however. Take the race I helped organize in China. I strongly told the local officials that they must carefully boil the water that the runners would drink during the race to prevent them from getting sick. Race day came, we all started out, and as the temperature reached 90°F. I got hot and thirsty. I hit the first water table 2 miles into the race. I gulped the water—and quickly spit it out. It was hot! Indeed, the race officials had carefully prepared boiled water for the runners, and then kept it boiling!

None of this should make you stay home. Travel! Explore! Be adventuresome! And remember to exercise on the run.

TWENTY-SIX

Time Management

"I don't have time to run."

I hear this a lot! It's the number one excuse people have for putting off an exercise program. And you know what? They're right. Running and exercise do take time and time is a priceless part of our hectic lives. But invest time in a running and fitness program and you'll save time in the end. How? You are likely to live a better quality of life and thus get more done. You are also likely to live longer. You can even work on the run.

In this chapter, I detail guidelines for managing your running and fitness time. In the next chapter, I discuss how to manage your life so that you keep running and fitness in proper balance.

Let's start with the example of Tom Monaghan, a very busy man who doesn't seem to have time to run. Tom is founder and president of an empire of Domino's Pizza stores and the former owner of the Detroit Tigers baseball team. Monaghan says there are five priorities that he always makes time for in his life: spiritual, social, mental, physical, and financial. But at one point, he didn't include the physical part and he soon found himself overweight and flabby, not to mention unhealthy. He started to exercise and diet. The challenge of completing a marathon pulled him into running. He enrolled in a special program I developed for young corporate presidents. Following the marathon training schedule from *The Runner's Handbook*, Tom Monaghan completed his first New York Marathon in 4:19:16.

How does this busy executive find the time to exercise? For one thing, he runs to work almost every morning, a distance of about 6 miles. This gets him started and generally does not cut into his workday. For another, he schedules workouts in his daily routine. "I've been called a fitness fanatic," he says. "But to me it's a matter of sticking to habits that I know make me feel and function better all day along. If I run for an hour, I can get along on an hour less sleep. So it really takes zero time out of my day."

Many runners with busy schedules, and perhaps families to raise, can structure their time to allow them to train enough to reach realistic exercise goals. True, the elite runner training twice a day and running more than 100 miles a week has little time for anything else. As Bill Rodgers warned when he was a top marathoner in the 1970s: "No one who works a forty-hour week will ever beat me." Maybe not, but those of us who work at least forty hours a week can indeed fit exercise training into our routines at some level.

When Should I Run?

First, select a time of day when it's best for you to exercise—morning, noon, or night. Most runners I know do the bulk of their training after work on weekday evenings and on weekend mornings. But there are also plenty of runners who, like Tom Monaghan, prefer early morning runs; others like to break up the day with a run at noon or in the afternoon.

When to run depends on the time of day you enjoy running and how easily you can fit running into your schedule. Your schedule should be flexible, but you should also stick to it. Be firm. Set a priority.

I usually run at noon two days a week, then in the evening twice a week with our class workout, and again late on a Saturday or Sunday morning, if not both. Most of my business meetings and social outings are scheduled around these times (or rather around my son's schedule and then my running preferences). Shepherd, running in New England where the light changes by as much as four hours during the year, runs in the late afternoons and evenings in summer and gradually switches back toward noon for the winter. That way, he gets the cool summer evenings and the warmest part of the days in winter. And he runs in about the same amount of daylight.

Most important, make a schedule and then follow it. For example, Monday, Wednesday, Friday, and Sunday; early morning, noon, afternoon, or evening. Put it in your appointment book. Bill Horowitz, my running dentist, says, "I schedule an appointment for myself each day just as patients schedule themselves to see me. I run when scheduled, 'Come hell or high water.' "

Morning Runs

Morning is Shelly's favorite time to run, but not with me. My morning runs start at noon. Other runners are getting into the habit of working out early in the morning before going to work. They tend to be more consistent runners. Makes sense. By running first thing in the morning, you don't have the risk of last-minute business or personal demands stealing or cutting short your runs. Morning runs in hot weather also avoid the heat and, in some regions, the air pollution.

Some runners say that running in the morning clears their head and leaves them full of energy for the rest of the day. If you are a morning runner—and I'll cheer you on (from my bedroom window, that is)—here are some tips:

- Get to sleep early if you intend to run early the next morning. Some of the most restful sleep comes during the last two hours. To wake up to go for a run before your body is ready may leave you fatigued rather than refreshed. Don't cut an hour of sleep out of your schedule to run early. Go to bed an hour earlier. (Try watching the ten o'clock news rather than the eleven!) Most exercisers need at least seven to eight hours of sleep every night. If you cut into that, you may pay for it with lousy running and sluggishness at work.

- Warm up properly. Don't attempt vigorous stretching exercises—your muscles are too "cold" to stretch properly. When you wake up in the morning your muscles will be stiff. According to our circadian rhythms, body temperature is lowest between 4:00 and 6:00 A.M. So, before about 6:00 A.M. and for the next few hours your muscles are going to be stiff and cold (Is this why I feel like dead meat in the morning?) and much more prone to injury. A study by Dr. John Pagliano, a California podiatrist, indicates that morning runners indeed get injured more often than noontime or evening runners. Avoid hard running, speed workouts, or races until you have been up and about for at least two hours. Start slowly. Too many early morning runners are in a hurry and skip the warm-ups. This gives them a higher risk of injury. Better to skip a few minutes of running than to risk injury.

■ Start with easy limbering up exercises and go for a brisk walk for 5 to 10 minutes. Then, ease into a slow run for a mile or two before you settle into your normal pace. An early morning normal pace may be slower than a pace you run later in the day. That's okay as long as you are within your training range. Be sure to stretch slowly and carefully when you return.

■ You don't need to eat before your early morning runs. This might cause stomach cramps. If you feel that you need something to settle your stomach, or give you a little energy, try dry toast or a glass of cool water, juice, or even coffee or tea. You should drink something, even if you run before the sun comes up or after it goes down.

Midday Runs
This is my time to run. If you have flexible hours (like me), a midday run is a great option. There are a lot of pluses: You don't have to worry about darkness and it generally isn't as cold during the winter. You also aren't as stiff as you are in the morning. A run will lessen your appetite; a light lunch at your desk afterward will help you maintain weight control. A midday run helps clear the mind and provides a break from the stresses of your workday. A midday run, like one in the early morning before the family gets

up, may eliminate hassles at home when your spouse or children
want and need your attention after work.

The midday run is becoming so popular that workers have
negotiated for company showers and lockers. I think the midday
run can be a working runner's dream. By starting work a little
earlier or finishing a little later to make up for the long lunch
break, you can easily schedule a midday run into your workday.
Of course, you may pass on the midday run during the summer
heat; or you may substitute a swim, bike ride, or treadmill
workout.

Evening Runs

This is Shepherd's time of day. The cool of evening, the beauty of
the slanting sun, the pressures of the workday behind you. This is
also the easiest time to find running partners. (Maybe this is why
most evening runners are single. In fact, in the evening, the scene
at the main entrance to the reservoir running trail in New York's
Central Park often resembles the runner's version of a singles bar!)
Another plus: According to a study at the Cooper Clinic Research
Institute in Dallas, exercising in the evening was most effective in
controlling weight in runners.

Some people find that the evening run interferes with their social
life; dinners and evenings out often have to be rescheduled to accommodate the evening runner. Others use the excuse that they're
too tired to run after work. But those of us who do it know that
the evening run energizes you: Shepherd always feels more alert
and wide awake after his evening run.

Running too hard late in the day may make it difficult to relax
and go to sleep. If this is true for you, try taking a little extra time
to stretch and cool down, maybe even do some yoga. Take a warm
bath instead of a shower. Drink a glass of warmed milk.

Run to Work

Some runners find that running to and/or from work saves time,
adds to their workday, and invigorates them. Other runners commute longer distances. They may keep a change of clothes in the
office, and either shower there or clean up with a wash cloth
and towel. A little splash of deodorant or aftershave, and they're
ready.

Race Time and Race Times

I'm a night owl. Much of this book was written well past midnight. Little of it was written before noon. I perform better at the computer and on the road later in the day. As I said, I'm worthless in the early morning. So what do I do if I have to run a race at 9:00 A.M.—the time many races are held? Am I at such a disadvantage against early morning runners?

In a study reported in the *Journal of Applied Science*, Penny Burgoon and colleagues from California State University at Northridge tested runners who had identified themselves as morning, midday, or evening runners. The subjects were tested using a maximal exercise test at three set times: early morning (defined as between 7:30 and 8:30 A.M.), noon, and evening (7:30 to 8:30 P.M.). The results? Runners don't gain an advantage by racing at the same hours they train; nor do they lose anything by racing at hours other than when they train. In short, the morning runners didn't outperform the evening runners on early morning exercise tests, and the evening runners didn't outperform the morning runners on the evening tests.

The only noteworthy outcome was that all runners, regardless of when they trained or preferred to run, performed best in the evening. In a University of Texas study, subjects did all-out tests on a bike between 7:30 and 9:00 A.M. and again between 4:00 and 5:30 P.M. They performed nearly 10 percent better in the afternoon than in the morning. Several such studies have indicated that aerobic capacity peaks in the late afternoon and early evening. If you can find a few evening races, you may find it easier to turn in a good race time. In fact, several world track records have been set at night.

Working on the Run

Don't look at running as a waste of time or only as exercise. Running does make us more fit, but it is also a time to think of little else, to clear the mind for work to come. Sometimes I just relax and keep my mind blank. Other times I work on the run. I've spent many runs by myself sorting out my thoughts and coming up with great ideas. Often I dash for pen and paper when I return and get the ideas down before they are washed away in the shower. Much of this book was developed on the run. And when I have a business or personal problem that I find difficult to deal with, I focus on it during a solitary run and often come up with ideas on how to solve it.

I even have meetings on the run. They save time and often result in great ideas. I invite my staff or potential business partners for a run to discuss both business and pleasure. It beats those stuffy big lunch meetings that are so much a part of business—and leave you feeling sleepy and physically drained.

You, too, can save time by working on the run. But don't carry this to the extremes that some New Yorkers do. I once saw a man running in Central Park and talking on a cellular phone! That's ridiculous: For me, one of the attractions of running is that it takes me away from the phone.

Running Partners

One of the best ways to manage your time and make sure you get your exercise in is to run with others. You might make an appointment to run with a friend or business partner three times a week. This will guarantee that you exercise at least three times a week and allow you to do some business on the run.

Bill Clinton takes his running seriously—he calls it "my thinking time"—and tries not to miss a day. As president, he could have his pick of running partners and he often runs along with chosen individuals, seldom in a crowd. His fellow runners have included a few members of Congress, mayors, governors, members of his cabinet, and even the president of South Korea. "Running with the president," said a White House aide, "is bigger than an audience in the Oval Office." But—embarrassingly—most can't keep up with his steady 8-minute mile pace.

Clinton is also known to do business on the run. When the first Clinton budget vote was in the Senate, the president summoned Senator Bob Kerrey (D.-Neb.) for a run and a chat. Kerrey, who has an artificial right leg, pounded along wearing a "Hillary Knows Best" T-shirt and later said they talked "a great deal after the run about policy, about trade, about Vietnam." Clinton got Kerrey's pivotal vote and the budget passed—by a tiebreaking vote from Vice President Al Gore (another avid runner).

If you can't manage an invitation to run with Bill, another running partner is your dog. (If you don't have one, get one!) It eats up an hour or more each day to take ol' Fido out for his walk. Why not turn this chore into a part of your run—get that mutt in shape and save time while both of you get fit.

You can put the baby into a running stroller and take kiddo along with Fido. When my son, Christopher, was old enough to talk, he would chatter away enjoying the scenery and motion and being happy with his dad. I was doubly happy: I was out running and I was spending time with my son while showing him off to other runners in the park.

TWENTY-SEVEN

The Runner's Triangle

Now you are up and running, and filled with the excitement that comes from regular exercise and being fit. But we are going to turn around and tell you something you may not want to hear: Take it easy. Do not make running the central focus of your life. Balance it with other things that are important to you: friends, loved ones, family, work.

When running as an everyman's sport took off across America in the mid-1970s, everyone started talking about running as the "positive addiction." Runners became "addicted" to their exercise, and it was good for them. I even discuss "positive addiction" in this book. Running is, in fact, an excellent way to overcome the stress in our lives and to add purpose and direction. We set running goals and achieve them. Some of us experience the release of endorphins, which give us pleasurable feelings while running. Many of us find running to be a positive force in our lives. We run on a regular basis because along with fitness it gives us a sense of achievement, well-being, and control.

In the late 1970s, running was the central focus of my life. I was single, working for other people, and could devote much of my life and energy to training and racing. Then, several things happened.

Seeing the wreckage of bodies and hopes after the hot 1978 New York City Marathon, I was distressed that so many men and women had put so much of their emotional, as well as physical, selves into that race only to lose it to the heat and sun. Not long afterward, I married and became the father of a very energetic son. I saw the demands that running, family, and work put on a person. And I saw how some men and women, especially in the high-stepping 1980s, became obsessed with running and excluded the other parts of their lives. But running cannot be the focus of one's life; it carries pain and disappointment, and, most important, it is no replacement for family, friends, career, religion. So I coined the phrase "the runner's triangle." I saw this as the need to balance the triangle of life: the physical side of running (body), the intellectual and career side (mind), and the spiritual and emotional side (soul).

Most of us run a moderate amount to keep us fit. But others cross over the imaginary line, a line as measurable as "the wall" in a marathon. While the professional runner can accept a life of commitment to running, those of us who run for fitness and maybe enter a few races, also have lives away from running. When we get too immersed in our running, our lives become unbalanced. We lose sight of, or ignore, the other things and we have a serious problem. This may be termed "exercise addiction" or "exercise dependency." Runners who become dependent on exercise make it, like someone hooked on drugs, the central focus of their lives. They may treat running the way some workaholics treat work: running for up to two hours a day may be as much a behavior disorder as working twelve or more hours every day. Make them stop running and these men and women have actual withdrawal symptoms.

Studies by Dr. William P. Morgan at the Sports Psychology Laboratory at the University of Wisconsin at Madison show two very interesting—and opposite—results: Vigorous exercise within the ranges discussed in this book can decrease anxiety and increase a sense of well-being. But, when Dr. Morgan and his lab studied Wisconsin varsity men and women swimmers, he found that as training becomes more intense, it actually causes significant emotional and psychological problems. This created a paradox: While moderate amounts of exercise can reduce it, he found, "depression also seems to be a product of overtraining," and includes chronic fatigue, insomnia, increased emotional tension, and decreased li-

bido. Overtraining may also lead to significant metabolic, hormonal, and cardiovascular changes. Most of us are not part of a
university team. Our overexercising is self-inflicted.

Many running-related injuries are due to overexercise. Running
addiction cannot be gauged by mileage. Some runners who run
100 miles per week know exactly when they should ease back or
stop their training. Some runners who run as little as twenty miles
per week may be strongly addicted.

Runners believe that if they exercise they automatically gain positive mental health. As we have seen, running does help improve
one's self-image and this carries over into daily life. But no amount
of running by itself will make us happy, healthy, successful in our
relationships, or emotionally balanced. One of the better New
York City runners jumped out a window to his death; running
hadn't saved him from the deeper stresses in his life. A forty-five-
year-old British executive died from an overdose of aspirin and in
his suicide note he said that life was no longer worth living: He
couldn't run because of a knee injury. That man had lost his perspective on life: Running had become an obsession.

We need to balance career, family/loved ones, and running—the
three points of "the runner's triangle." All of us, every runner,
encounters the struggle. On the one hand, we want to run because
we know it makes us physically healthier, emotionally more balanced, eager to tackle the challenges of everyday life, more relaxed,
and ready to enjoy the simple pleasures of family and friends. This
is what makes running a positive addiction.

On the other hand, the very things regular running prepares us
for—a better business and social life—often infringes on our running schedules. How can you go out for a run when your office
load stretches your workday from 8:00 A.M. to 8:00 P.M.? How
much time is left for running when the kids' activities turn you into
a chauffeur, or relationships tug at you after the workday?

The answer lies in finding a balance. It's not easy, I know. Just
when you think you've got the world in your grip, you realize it's
been the other way around all along. We all agree that the time
when we most need a workout is precisely the time it's toughest
to squeeze one in. But don't surrender to the pressure. You have
a responsibility to find a relaxing exercise time for yourself. I love
to play with my son, Christopher, and struggle to make time for
special activities with him. But I also know the requirements of my
own personal "bottom line": I need to run at least five times a

week for an hour or so. If I don't, I feel less of a person and I am sure I become less of a father. Few of us can take care of others unless we have also taken care of ourselves.

Running, therefore, must complement the rest of my life. Not the other way around. Running fits in. It enhances my days and weeks. It doesn't come first before everyone and everything else I care about. This is the balancing act, "the runner's triangle." It must be the cornerstone of any lifelong running program. Here are some ways you can make it work for you.

Family and Friends

When you start a running program or begin building up for a big race, you should try to make your family and friends a part of it. Share your interest in running with them; make them into allies, a support group. From the start, teach yourself and them to be flexible. Family and friends will no doubt be eager to support your running because they know why you got into it—to improve your health, to lose weight—and they recognize what it does for you.

All your family asks is that you be flexible—that's not an outrageous demand. They may find it more difficult to understand your interest in running if you start running right after work. That's also the time when they would like to have you around the house. Or at least not holding up dinner until 7:30 or later. You cannot expect their support if you use your running time as an excuse for shirking family responsibilities—from household cleaning to baby-sitting to weekend activities. Nor can you ask for support if you are using the running to get away from your family or friends, to put some distance between you and a relationship or a situation you want to avoid. You'd better turn around and face that one square on!

Are running and marriage compatible? An article in *Playboy Magazine*, of all places, states: "The more runners run, the more conflicts they experience with spouses or close relatives. A poll taken in the Boston area indicated that runners who averaged more than 70 miles a week were far more likely to have marital problems than occasional or moderate runners.

"Nearly half the full-time runners admitted that their partners felt neglected. In 40 percent of the cases, the friction from running was serious enough to lead to divorce."

Studies show that "running addiction" or overtraining starts during a period of increased emotional stress. Overexercisers frequently have family or personal problems they are trying to run from. They say to themselves: "I don't want to go home, so I'll go running instead." A study of compulsive runners, by V. A. Altshul, reported in *The Psychology of Running*, concluded that they start overexercising in response to a major emotional upheaval. That is, if "a lean, healthy man is consciously or unconsciously contemplating divorce, there is at least a 75% chance that he is or will be a compulsive runner," this study states. Running is seen as a pseudo-solution for avoiding problems or relationships in the runner's life. Compulsive runners overexercise because they are, literally, running from something: troubles at work or home, depression or anxiety.

Can you keep your significant other happy and also run? You are going to have to work just as hard at this as you do at running. Running can itself be an affair—a demanding lover that separates you from your friends, family, or loved ones. Psychologist Dr. Joyce Brothers received a letter from a thirty-five-year-old woman "married to an exercise machine that almost never is interested in making love to me." Instead, she competed constantly with her husband's love of running. "I never knew a man could fall in love with running. Can I sue his track shoes for alienation of affection?"

Dr. Brothers replied that such an addiction to running "is no laughing matter." These "exercise addicts" place their daily run above their job, family, friends. They continue even when advised by physicians or fitness experts that running will harm them. And what happens when they stop? They suffer from depression, anxiety, irritability, insomnia, fatigue—classic withdrawal symptoms.

Remember this if you have someone in your life who means a lot to you. Make a deal. Schedule time with that person the same way you schedule your running. Or, you could try forming a running partnership: both partners run together, which adds an activity and time to the relationship. Many romances begin when runners meet. The biggest problem, however, comes when runners try to outpace their mates, or when one partner runs and the other doesn't. A nonrunner who waits around for a running mate can become an unhappy person: He or she becomes a bored couch potato involved with a mate who has more self-confidence, independence, and running friends. He or she also looks terrific! One solution is to make your nonrunning mate into a cheerleader. He or she could have the bath ready when you get home, or supply you with replacement fluids at spots along the way in races. Never try to make your mate into a coach.

What about children and running? When baby Christopher arrived in my life in 1981, I suddenly found myself in many new roles: husband, father, breadwinner, coach, author, friend, and sometime runner. Today, both women and men try to balance marriage, career, and children; running is an added problem. Here again, shared responsibility and times might help. So face it, major adjustments will be needed. At least they are temporary: Kids do grow up.

Work

Your exercise program can allow you to be a more productive, cooperative employee. As I shall detail in Chapter 42, running may improve your creativity as well as your mood. The self-esteem that you gain with your running success will also result in more confidence in your career decisions. But it can work the other way, too. If you are late to work, leave early, or take too long a lunch break to get in your running fix, you may not be popular with your boss and fellow workers. If you are overtired from getting up early to run before work, or from your training—especially when building for a marathon—you may not be as sharp on the job.

One mistake many runners make at work is to talk too much about their running. Your boss and fellow workers may be impressed about your accomplishments—running your first mile, race, or marathon—and think more highly of you as a result, but if they think that the time and energy you spend running interferes with your dedication to the job, then they may think of your running, and you, in a negative way. In other words, even if you would rather be running than working (who wouldn't!), don't let on. Strive to give the impression at work that your running is in balance with your work and family life by being careful of your actions and statements. Your spouse is more likely to appreciate that you will be more energetic and less cranky if you run than your boss will. Then again, I've known runners who got so involved in their training and racing that they ticked off both their spouses and employers and ended up not only divorced and unemployed, but injured and unable to run.

One way to share your enthusiasm for running with fellow workers is to organize or participate on a company team in one of the many corporate running events that take place around the country. The Chase Bank Corporate Challenge, for example, in New York's Central Park attracts nearly 20,000 runners to each of a series of three races. After the race, the employees get together for company picnics in the park or go out to dinner together. These events provide a healthy way to balance running and work.

Most runners have their running schedules well integrated into other aspects of their lives and even making a positive contribution to their nonrunning side. But the line between positive and negative addiction is thin. Some runners lose perspective altogether. Running becomes an end, not a means. The final stage of this negative addiction occurs when running becomes your job, when friends and loved ones take second place in your life, or when you cannot stop running even when faced with serious injury. If you have reached any of these points, you need to reexamine why you run, and get your "runner's triangle" back into balance.

Part IX

Special Runners

TWENTY-EIGHT

Women on the Run

You may not believe this, but not long ago—at least as I now measure time—a woman out running in shorts was shocking, outrageous. Before the 1970s, when the running movement took off, a pregnant woman running in a city park was the focus of concern—or *laughter*. A woman running in the Boston Marathon and most other long-distance events was *illegal*.

Then the huge increase in running that started in 1978 along with the first edition of this book slowly welcomed women to join in. And join they did: first by the hundreds, then the thousands, and now millions. But the moment in history that finally assured women equality in the world of runners did not arrive until their acceptance into the marathon for the 1984 Olympics. Now, with this barrier fading into history, it is difficult to remember how extensive the restrictions on women runners were. But it is important to document the history, and to remember it.

In the early 1900s, women were allowed (by men) to whack a tennis ball in ladylike fashion, or even to swim—if properly covered. But British women who dared to run in any footraces were called "brazen doxies." Not until 1928 could women run in the Olympics, and when several untrained women collapsed at the finish of the 800-meter (approximately half a mile) race, the event was labeled—again, by men—as "frightful." Women were not allowed to compete at this long distance again until the 1960 Olympics; not until 1984 was the longest race for women extended beyond 1,500 meters—less than a mile. That year, women were allowed to compete in the Olympic 3,000-meter and marathon distances. In 1988, they could also run the 10,000-meter race.

The reawakening of the feminist movement in the 1960s—there have been such awakening feminist movements dating back to the 1820s—gave women the tools to fight for their athletic rights. One was the right to run as far and as fast as they could. One barrier women faced came from men, who thought long-distance running would make a woman's breasts sag and her muscles bulge. Chris McKenzie, a former world record holder in the 800-meter race, put that one to rest. She decided to convince American male race officials that women, not men, should control what happens to women's bodies. She arrived at their monthly meeting wearing only a bikini under her coat, and when the subject of sagging breasts and bulging muscles came up, Ms. McKenzie peeled off the coat and asked for opinions. She quickly gained official permission to run longer race distances.

Some men still didn't get it. In 1966, Roberta Gibb Bingay applied for the Boston Marathon and was denied entry. Race officials told her that women couldn't run that far because they would get hurt. So she hid in the bushes at the starting line, jumped in, and ran anyway. She finished the marathon in 3:21 and beat two-thirds of the male runners. Yet Boston officials still refused to recognize her accomplishment and claimed that she hadn't run *the* Boston Marathon; she had merely covered the same route as the official race while it was in progress!

The next year, in a particularly onerous and condemning episode that the Boston Marathon has still not lived down, Kathrine Switzer received an official entry number after she sent in her application as "K. Switzer." Race officials, thinking she was a he, let her run, or at least start. She was several miles into the marathon when Jock Semple, the fiery race director, discovered her noxious presence, caught up to her, and tried to rip off her number. Kathy's boyfriend deposited Jock on the curb, and because the action took place by the press bus the media couldn't miss the message. Kathy's plight and a particularly condemning photograph made newspapers throughout America.

Was Kathrine Switzer a new heroine? Don't bet your Boston Marathon T-shirt. A few days later she was thrown out of the AAU, the administrative body that governed long-distance running at the time. AAU officials gave four reasons: (1) she had fraudulently entered the Boston Marathon, (2) she had run longer than the allowable distance for women (1.5 miles), (3) she had run with men, and (4) she had run without a chaperone.

There's a nice irony here. Kathy Switzer finished the marathon in 4:20. In 1973, in her hometown of Syracuse, New York, she paced me to my first sub-3:30 marathon, which qualified me for —you guessed it!—the Boston Marathon. Actually, she and the legendary Syracuse Charger Arnie Briggs got me to the 20-mile mark when Kathy left us both in the dust. In 1975, after Boston finally opened to women, she was the first American woman across the finish line, running a 2:51:37.

Opening Boston wasn't easy, but in 1972 the race officials finally allowed women to run officially. The first woman winner of the Boston Marathon was my longtime good friend and heroine Nina Kuscsik of Huntington, Long Island, who completed the race in 3:10:21. The male-controlled AAU wasn't through playing games with women: Before the 1972 New York City Marathon, they suddenly decided that women would not be allowed to run with men. The women would run separately by starting their race 10 minutes ahead of the men. (Ladies first!) To get a complete idea of the pea-brained thinking here, realize how spread out the male and female runners would be anyway after 26 miles; women would be running with men regardless of when they both started!

Anyway, at the 1972 New York City Marathon, women were sent to the front of the race starting line. But when the gun fired, the women, led by Nina Kuscsik, sat down in protest and waited for the men's race to begin 10 minutes later. When the men started, off went the women—all of whom had voluntarily added 10 minutes to their official race times. (Nina was the leader of the women at the finish line, too, with time of 3:08:41.) This discrimination prompted a civil rights lawsuit against the AAU, which finally gave in and ruled that men and women could start "from a common line at a common gunshot"—but they would be scored separately and compete for separate prizes.

Until 1971, women were still trying to break the three-hour barrier for the marathon, which fell that year when Beth Bonner held off the challenge of Nina Kuscsik, 2:55:22 to 2:56:04, to win the

New York City Marathon in hilly Central Park. Some twenty-five years later, women are pushing hard against the 2:20:00 barrier. Historians of women and running should measure the accomplishments of Nina Kuscsik and Kathrine Switzer. Nina went on to complete more than eighty marathons and won many of them, including Boston and New York. She ran beyond that distance and set an American record for 50 miles. Perhaps more important, she continued to lobby governing bodies of the sport for equality in running for women and the inclusion of a women's marathon in the Olympics. At the same time, Kathrine Switzer was pushing back the barriers, too. She developed and directed the annual Avon International Marathon. The goal was to demonstrate that women everywhere could not only complete the marathon distance, but also run it fast.

The Avon International Marathons also played an important role in my coaching life. During these years I, too, made a commitment to women's running by forming the elite all-women's running team Atalanta, named for the Greek maiden who could outrun all men. From 1978 to 1983, Atalanta competed in all of the Avon International Marathons, from Waldniel, Germany, to San Francisco, from London to Atlanta to Ottawa, Canada. We placed second during our first year, and then reeled off five straight international titles.

By 1984, all these efforts by so many women—and men—paid off: Women were accepted into the Olympic Marathon. The first U.S. Olympic Marathon Trials were held in Olympia, Washington. To qualify, a woman had to run the 26.2-mile marathon distance in 2:51:16 or better, a cutoff time selected because it was the hundredth fastest by an American woman in 1983. (And almost exactly three minutes faster than Beth Bonner's record-setting New York City marathon time almost twelve years earlier!) A total of 267 American women, including six Atalantans, officially qualified. And there were some surprises. The youngest qualifier was Cathy Schiro, sixteen, who placed ninth at 2:34:09, a world record for junior runners. The oldest, and Schiro's roommate at the trials, was "the flying nun," Sister Marion Irvine, fifty-four, who ran an incredible 2:52:02.

I was at this exciting trials event (Atalanta placed second) and I still count it as *the* most emotional experience of my long career as a coach. It was an amazing weekend of celebration for women athletes. The climax of the trials came when Joan Benoit (now

Samuelson) crossed the finish line as the winner in 2:31:04 only a few weeks after undergoing arthroscopic surgery on her knee. She went on to win the first Olympic Marathon for women in Los Angeles in 2:24:52.

All of this history is surprising to recall. Today we see women running and competing everywhere. New studies and new information about women and running appear almost weekly. And we are finding that not only do women have a hard-earned "right" to exercise and run, but that it is important in terms of their health to do so. .

We discuss several aspects of women's running in separate chapters. For example, Chapter 24 describes important safety factors for women as they run; Chapter 18 details nutritional needs important to women, while Chapters 16 and 17 review shoe needs and clothing choices, respectively. These are things that men and women runners share. But there are some important differences, and these are detailed here.

The Woman Runner

Physical characteristics make men runners different from women runners. From this, one could conclude that having women run in separate competitions against themselves may indeed be fair. And there are some strong physiological reasons for this.

When comparing men and women of similar size, there are differences. Women have smaller hearts and lungs than men, but the structure and power of a woman's heart is essentially the same as a man's. Women also have smaller bones and less muscle than men, but nearly the same percentage of fast-twitch and slow-twitch muscle fibers. Approximately 45 percent of male body weight is muscle. In women, muscle amounts to only about 35 percent. They have more fat. This sex-specific fat cannot be eliminated by dieting or training. In fact, excessive attempts to lower weight and body fat percentage may lead to anorexia, weak bones, or other health problems.

Why are men faster runners? The male sex hormone, testosterone, increases the concentration of red blood cells and promotes the production of hemoglobin, an oxygen-carrying protein found inside red blood cells. Estrogen, the female sex hormone, has no similar effect. As a result, each liter of a man's blood contains 150–160 grams of hemoglobin—20 grams more hemoglobin and 11 percent more oxygen than the average for women. Men also tend to have a larger heart size and greater heart volume than women even if their body size is similar. Thus, men can more easily pump oxygen to the working muscles.

Body fat is another factor. The average body fat percentage for 30-year-old men is approximately 15–20 percent; for 30-year-old women it is approximately 23–26 percent. Elite male runners range from 4–8 percent body fat compared to 8–15 percent for women. Body fat acts as dead weight; it increases the energy cost of running. So the female runner has a distinct physiological disadvantage because of her smaller heart size and heart volume, and her higher percentage of body fat.

As a result, women also differ sharply from men in their maximal oxygen uptake (max VO_2)—that is, in their ability to consume, transport, and use oxygen. Extensive tests show that elite men and women runners differ by about 11 percent in oxygen uptake, in favor of the men—or about the same difference between men's and women's world records.

While men and women are physically different, they can train and run in similar ways. In this book, and in my classes and teams, I coach women the same way as men. Jack Daniels, an exercise physiologist and women's track coach at Cortland State in New York, agrees. "The basic physiological systems function in the same way in men and women," he says. "Likewise, training principles should be the same for both genders. Men and women can train and race at the same relative intensity." In fact, women recover faster. Research from Finland indicates that women recover about 92 percent of their muscle strength within an hour following a rigorous workout; men only recover about 79 percent.

Races over specific distances, however, reveal differences. I find that when we do short, fast workouts in my classes, most women cannot keep up with men who run similar 10K times. Men simply have more power for speed and can run away from most women. Still, women fare much better on the longer speed workouts and often beat the same men in the marathon.

For Women Only
Now that we've sorted out our differences and similarities, let's look at some of the issues particular to women runners.

Osteoporosis

More than 25 million Americans, 80 percent of them women, are affected by osteoporosis, a calcium loss that can cause bone structure to become fragile and increase the risk of fractures. Indeed, the disease leads to more than 1.5 million bone fractures each year—including my mother, who was seriously injured after falling on her brittle bones. The resulting complications often lead to significant alterations in lifestyle and loss of good health.

Women are more prone than men to this disease because the condition is influenced by the female hormone estrogen. Men also tend to have larger, stronger frames. The body continuously renews its skeleton by replacing old bone cells with new ones. But by age thirty-five or so, your bone mass reaches its peak and more bone is lost than replaced. The level of estrogen falls after menopause, resulting in even more acceleration of bone loss. Younger women who train heavily or who develop irregular or loss of menstruation are also prone to this disease.

Once bone loss has occurred it cannot be replaced. But the loss can be slowed. Rather than a natural consequence of aging, osteoporosis is a dangerous disease that can be prevented. It can be minimized by eating a diet rich in calcium, by estrogen replacement therapy after menopause, and by regular weight-bearing exercise. The disease can get an early start during childhood if your diet lacks sufficient calcium and vitamin D, which are required to build strong bones.

According to the U.S. Department of Health and Human Services, as many as three out of four American women fail to get enough calcium in their diets. While the recommended daily allowance is 800 milligrams for adults older than twenty-five, the National Institutes of Health have concluded from research that most adult American women need 1,000–1,500 milligrams daily. It is never too late to increase the calcium in your diet. To combat bone loss at menopause, doctors often recommend estrogen replacement therapy.

Weight-bearing exercise such as running increases bone density, which in turn helps prevent osteoporosis. It is also helpful in controlling the condition for those already afflicted. Running strengthens the bones in the legs but does little for the upper body. Weight training, therefore, may be effective to strengthen bones throughout your body. In sum, a diet rich in calcium combined with weight-bearing exercise, plus estrogen therapy for women after menopause, are all effective ways to minimize bone loss due to osteoporosis.

Heat

Most women will tolerate temperatures about one degree higher than men before they begin to sweat. Once women begin to sweat, their output of perspiration will be less and more efficient than that of men. Further, they have more blood flow to the skin surface, which also assists in cooling.

My observation as a coach is that women seem to tolerate heat better than men. This is supported by a study at Georgia Tech in Atlanta, which matched men and women by age, training, and aerobic capacity. These participants then ran more than 20 miles on a hot and humid day. They ran at the same speeds and drank the same amount of the same sports drink before and during the run. The result: The men and women had similar rates of sweating and lost about the same percentage of body weight during the run. But the women stayed cooler and had less blood plasma loss (and thus more blood circulating oxygen to working muscles) than the men. Conclusion: Women tolerate heat better than men.

Menstruation

Many women experience bothersome symptoms related to their menstrual cycles. These may include cramps, depression, irritability, backache, nausea, weakness, a feeling of "heavy legs" or of being bloated because of water retention. For some women, a heavy blood flow during the first two days of their menstrual period may make exercise impractical; severe cramping may make it uncomfortable.

Most doctors agree that exercise during menstruation is not only a good idea, but it may also be helpful in relieving these symptoms. Exercise that improves blood circulation and muscular strength and flexibility in the abdominal area is particularly beneficial. Ibuprofen or prescription drugs may help relieve some of these symptoms, but a conditioned body may simply be better prepared to handle the monthly stress of menstruation.

Most, but not all, women report that their menstrual periods do not affect their performance in races. One study of women Olympic athletes found that they won gold medals during all phases of their monthly cycle. Training may be more of a problem: The runner will overcome discomfort in the excitement of a race but not in the drudgery of practice. Some observers suggest that the most difficult time for women to run fast comes a week before menstruation begins since the female sex hormone progesterone is at high levels at this time, causing a faster rate of breathing while running. Most women runners find that running doesn't make menstrual cramps (dysmenorrhea) worse, but running may be slower during this time. They may suffer through sluggish runs or just wait until the symptoms ease before running. Other women find that cramping diminishes or disappears during their runs.

Between one-third and one-half of all American women between the ages of twenty and fifty suffer from varying degrees of premenstrual syndrome (PMS). PMS is usually experienced during the week or two before the onset of the menstrual period. Its signs include irritability, depression, change in sleep patterns, mood swings, breast tenderness, bloating, fatigue, and even hunger. According to Dr. Susan M. Lark, author of the *PMS Self-Help Book*, exercise relieves both the physiological and psychological symptoms of PMS. She writes: "Physiologically, premenstrual pain causes breathing to become rapid and shallow. Women also tend to contract their muscles involuntarily when they're in pain or anticipate pain. Both shallow breathing and tight muscles can decrease the amount of blood flow and oxygenation to the tissues, causing cramps and fatigue." Regular aerobic exercise can help with these symptoms by increasing blood flow and reducing water retention through sweating. A study at the Women's Exercise Research Center at George Washington University in Washington, D.C., showed that aerobic exercise for 45 minutes at least three times a week helped alleviate premenstrual depression and anxiety in the participating women.

Hunger also presents an unusual problem. Women may crave food because of hormone fluctuations and because their metabolic rate may increase premenstrually by 200–500 calories, the equivalent of an extra meal. Women athletes may suffer a double deprivation, states sports nutritionist Nancy Clark. They cut back on calories because they feel fat from premenstrual bloat and water retention precisely at the time when they need a higher caloric intake. The result is a strong craving for sweets. By adding more calories in the form of carbohydrates at breakfast and lunch, you can fight off the hunger.

Delay of menarche. Young women runners tend to experience their first menstrual period (menarche) at a later age than less active girls. Some do not begin until they are seventeen or eighteen years old. If a girl does not start menstruating by age sixteen, she should consult her physician.

Menstrual regularity. This condition bears careful watching. Some women runners report that running regulates their periods. Others experience the cessation of menstruation (amenorrhea). This occurs only in 2 to 3 percent of all women but in 25 percent or more of serious competitive women runners.

The cessation of menstruation is *generally* not considered harmful, and regular menstrual cycles reoccur when these women runners return to their original body fat levels or when they cut their mileage. The cause, however, is uncertain. Some studies indicate that amenorrhea is the result of high mileage and low body fat. Other studies show that it's the sudden increase in mileage, not the high mileage itself, that causes the problem. Still other studies don't point to mileage at all but to the intensity of training, of not eating enough calories and the right foods to support the level of exercise, and/or emotional stresses.

Still, there are some cautions. Doctors suggest that any woman who has vaginal bleeding more often than every twenty-three days or less often than every thirty-five days should be examined. Although some women welcome not having to deal with menstruation, if the condition continues for a long time it is potentially harmful. Amenorrheic women have a decrease in their bone mineral content, leaving them susceptible to stress fractures or the development of osteoporosis. In a study of college women athletes, 9 percent of those with regular periods experienced stress fractures; of the women with irregular periods, however, 24 percent had stress fractures.

The American College of Sports Medicine warns women who work out more than moderately of the dangers of "the female athlete triad": poor nutrition or an eating disorder, amenorrhea, and osteoporosis. The problem often starts with an unwise desire to lose weight. This may include eating too little and compulsive exercising. It may lead to amenorrhea, which in turn can result in osteoporosis. If you do train hard, stay alert to these dangers. Eat properly, exercise wisely.

There is another warning here: Pregnancy. Irregular menstrual periods do not mean you will not get pregnant. You can—as some women runners have discovered. Also, exercise has induced ovulation in previously sedentary women.

Menopause

This is the cessation of menstrual periods. It occurs when hormone levels change and signals the end of childbearing years. The whole process of menopause takes approximately five to ten years. During this time, a woman may suffer from hot flashes, depression, irritability, and a host of other side effects. Most women begin to show changes in their menstrual cycle between the ages of forty-five and fifty, though a few may begin as early as forty. Most women have passed menopause by age sixty.

Exercise may not help with hot flashes, but estrogen therapy is most effective. After menopause, women have lower estrogen levels, which accelerates loss of bone density (osteoporosis). With a diminished supply of estrogen, the hormone also believed to make arteries more supple, women become more susceptible to heart disease. Running can't reverse the loss of estrogen after menopause. Many women benefit from estrogen therapy combined with exercise, but for women who, because of potential health risks, do not choose to take estrogen, exercise is still beneficial. Check with your doctor for the best regimen for you.

Regular exercise will help with many of the side effects of menopause. But it also creates a challenge and provides a goal at a time when a woman may feel that her value and attractiveness are diminishing.

Christine Wells, Ph.D., and colleagues at Arizona State University in Tempe studied a group of masters-level women to look at the effect of menopause on fitness. They determined that although a woman's aerobic capacity declines with age (as does a man's), menopause had little or no influence on a woman's fitness. Menopause, like menstruation, may, however, affect fitness less directly. I've coached several middle-age women athletes who had to miss several days of training because of the side effects of menopause.

But this isn't the end of your life or your athletic career. And it certainly isn't the end of your fun. Take the case of Mary Ann Smith, a Key Biscayne, Florida, speech therapist, mother of two young women, and an enthusiastic rower and runner. Mary Ann took up rowing at age forty-five; by the time she reached menopause she was rowing in national meets from the Charles River in

Boston to the Columbia River in Portland, Oregon. And after rowing she loved to go out all night dancing! Running and weight training are important parts of Mary Ann's rowing training, and she rarely misses an exercise day—especially when she can go out and hammer her brother-in-law—the coauthor of a famous national best-selling running book—into the road. And Shepherd was certain menopause would slow Mary Ann down. Alas for him: Not a step.

Pregnancy

Should you continue running during pregnancy? Yes—if you have been running regularly for at least six months before becoming pregnant, *and* you are healthy, *and* you have no other medical or physical problems, *and* your doctor approves. Pregnancy is not the time to improve your cardiorespiratory fitness or to begin an exercise program. Maintaining your fitness should be the goal.

A study, at the University of Illinois, of women who had been running an average of three years before becoming pregnant showed that healthy women can safely exercise *throughout* their pregnancies. These women ran an average of 16.5 miles a week during their first trimester and then tapered off to 6 miles a week during their last trimester. Some even ran up to the day they delivered, without any problems. Studies at Penn State University College of Medicine compared exercising and nonexercising pregnant women and found that the exercising group didn't put on as much weight, but they did gain adequate amounts of body fat for a healthy baby. And the exercisers' babies weighed on the average only a half pound less, which wasn't any added risk and may have made delivery somewhat easier.

Dr. Gyula Erdelyi of Hungary studied 172 women athletes through their pregnancies and found that pregnant runners had fewer complications during pregnancy and 50 percent fewer cesarean deliveries. He also found that duration of delivery was shorter for the women runners. Other studies indicate that exercise during pregnancy brings more oxygen to the placenta, which in turn helps nourish the fetus. Exercise also maintains Mom's muscle tone and cardiorespiratory conditioning. It will give you increased strength and endurance during labor and delivery, and a more rapid recovery.

There may also be an additional psychological benefit. "Regular exercise during pregnancy allows women to have control over their

bodies at a time of profound bodily changes," states the Melpomene Institute (St. Paul, Minnesota), which researches women's
health issues. "It gives them a chance to relax and helps them maintain a positive self-image."

But before you run off, consult your obstetrician. Pregnancy
greatly alters your body, and you may have complications that
would make running inadvisable. Sadly, there are still physicians
out there who are antiexercise. If your physician tells you to stop
exercising because you're pregnant, ask for a reason. If the answer
is satisfying, respect the opinion. But if it isn't, seek another opinion from a sports-minded physician, one who will support your
desire to maintain a physically fit body.

How much should you run? In 1985, the American College of
Obstetricians and Gynecologists (ACOG) set conservative guidelines; vigorous exercise during pregnancy should last only 15
minutes and push the woman's heart rate no higher than 140 beats
per minute. Some experts called these "old lady limits." Many
women runners were annoyed when their physicians referred to
this guideline, and many physicians who understand the benefits
of exercise saw the guidelines as too narrow for a well-conditioned
woman to maintain her desired level of fitness throughout
pregnancy.

Ten years later, after reviewing new studies, ACOG issued a new
technical advisory: Women with uncomplicated pregnancies can let
their own stamina and abilities be their guide for exercising. In
such low-risk pregnancies, said the ACOG, "there currently are no
data to confirm that exercise during pregnancy has any deleterious
effects on the fetus."

The ACOG did caution women not to assume that they could
exercise at their prepregnancy levels. But in the absence of complications, determined by their physician, "Women who have
achieved cardiovascular fitness prior to pregnancy should be able
to safely maintain that level of fitness throughout pregnancy and
the postpartum period."

What level of fitness should you maintain? Dr. Shanegold recommends that you limit your workouts to 30 minutes or less at a
comfortable pace. Dr. Joan Ullyot notes in her book *Women's
Running* that "A general rule for any form of exercise during pregnancy is, 'Do what you're accustomed to, as long as it feels comfortable.' If you've been jogging five miles a day, keep it up. If you

find yourself getting tired more easily, cut down the mileage. . . . Using the 'talk test' while running, you will be assured that both you and the baby are getting plenty of oxygen."

But what about your training heart rate? Pregnant women will have a resting heart rate that is 10 to 15 beats above what is normal for them. Thus, their training heart rate will also be elevated somewhat. Further, studies show that heart rate doesn't match perceived exertion during pregnancy—that is, your heart rate may be higher than how you feel. Don't be too concerned if you are pregnant and you go slightly above your training heart rate range (detailed in Chapter 8) while running. Again, the recommendation is to run at a comfortable, conversational pace.

The ACOG admitted that there isn't scientific evidence showing a need for pregnant women to limit exercise intensity. However, Dr. Raul Artal, the lead author of these new guidelines, cautions, "In my opinion, there really is no point in exercising strenuously [above talk test range], since pregnant women can maintain cardiovascular fitness through mild to moderate exercise."

If you start to feel too uncomfortable at any point during your pregnancy, walk or swim instead. This creates less jostling. Most women runners instinctively cut back on their exercise by one-third to one-half during the last eight to twelve weeks of their pregnancy. Again, work closely with your sports-minded physician for a personal program that will keep you and baby fit.

Here are some additional tips:

▪ Don't forget to get hubby involved. When Pamela Mendelsohn Burgess became pregnant, she continued running with her husband, Peter. "We had always enjoyed running together," she wrote in *Jogger* magazine, "and I had wondered whether we would have to start going separately because of my slowness due to the added weight. Peter began carrying rocks of increasing size to slow him down. His last rock weighed in at twenty-eight pounds!"

▪ Don't get too hot. Body temperatures more than 101°F. may not be good for your baby. Check your temperature immediately at the end of your workouts. Do this once a week or so. If your body temperature exceeds 101°F., discuss this with your physician. Work out for a shorter time in warm weather, wear loose-fitting and reflective clothing, and be sure to drink plenty of fluids. Consider swimming or working out indoors in air-conditioning during very hot days.

■ Do not exercise if you have a fever.

■ Stretch carefully. During pregnancy, the body releases the hormone relaxin to loosen your joints and make room for the baby. At this time most pregnant women are more flexible than at any other time of their lives. But this may also increase the risk of an injury from overstretching if you try to make the same effort as before you became pregnant.

■ Run on a smooth track, paved road, or even trail. As your pregnancy advances, your center of gravity shifts. You are more likely to be unstable and to fall if you are running on uneven surfaces.

■ If you experience uterine cramping, pain, or bleeding while running, or if your water breaks, stop running and contact your physician immediately.

■ During pregnancy, fluid needs increase due to expanding blood volume. As you lose fluid in perspiration, blood volume is reduced, making it more difficult for the body to cool down. As a pregnant exerciser, you should drink at least twelve glasses of water a day.

■ Cool down properly after your run. This will help maintain adequate blood flow to your baby after you finish exercising.

■ You don't have to run every day to maintain fitness. Cutting back to three days a week or less, combined with walking or swimming, will help you keep fit.

■ Eat according to your appetite, your weight scale, and your physician's advice. Your total caloric needs will be greater, especially since you will be exercising and feeding yourself and your baby.

Most doctors recommend that you gain about 20 to 30 pounds during pregnancy. Pregnant women require more calories, protein, calcium, iron, and many vitamins. To ensure proper weight gain, you may need as much as a 20 percent increase in calories, compared to a sedentary woman, if you continue to exercise throughout your pregnancy.

Deborah De Witt began exercising regularly when she reached thirty. Her husband, a member of the New York Road Runners Club, convinced her that running was fun and healthy. Little did she know how healthy.

"I would typically run three times a week for a mile or a mile and a half," she says. "I am not a gung-ho runner by any stretch of the imagination, but I was getting to the point where I could run two miles with not much effort and some enjoyment. Then, we decided to have a baby. I consulted with my obstetrician, who assured me that I could continue running as long as 'everything was going well.' "

Everything went well and Deborah kept running. Six months came and went. She reported to her doctor monthly and told him she was still running. He encouraged her. "Since I felt good, I decided to continue. Of course, my pace was slowing because I was carrying a lot of extra weight, twenty pounds in all. And by the end, I was having swelling in my legs which frequently caused cramps during running, but I tried to get through. Since I was running three times a week regularly, I never had any sensation of a large belly swaying back and forth. But I was a sight at the YMCA track in my green man's extra-large T-shirt and my maternity shorts."

Deborah ran a 10-minute mile during her exercise class on a Monday, and on Wednesday began labor. She was in labor for eighteen hours with no medication. She gave birth to a 7-pound, 13-ounce boy. "If this sounds like a testimonial to running, it is. But it is a testimonial from an average, run-of-the-mill jogger, not a super athlete." Six weeks after her postpartum check-up, Deborah was out running again.

After the Baby Comes
Postpartum. Your physician may want you to wait two to six weeks or more after the baby's birth before you start running. Before then, you can do some stretching and other light exercises. "If you don't begin to use your muscles in the first week after birth," says Elizabeth Noble, director of the Maternal and Child Health Center in Cambridge, Massachusetts, "they won't recover

as quickly." You might try some special exercises to strengthen your abdominal muscles, which get stretched out of shape during pregnancy. Here are a few exercises you can start soon after delivery:

■ Pregnancy puts extra stress on the muscles supporting your pelvic organs. The pelvic tilt exercise is recommended the day following delivery. Lie on back with knees bent and feet flat on the floor. Press your lower back into the ground, contract your buttock muscles, hold for 3 to 5 seconds. Then release. Do five sets.

■ Another important exercise is the "Kegel." Often after childbirth, women experience "stress incontinence" or involuntary leakage of urine. The Kegel exercise is important because it will strengthen the perineal muscles, which control the flow of urine. It is a squeeze exercise. While urinating, stop the flow; do this repeatedly. Once you get the idea, you can repeat this contraction when not urinating, as an exercise. Do ten to twenty repetitions several times a day.

■ Walk before you run. Most women can start walking within a few days to two weeks following delivery. When you do start running, remember to alternate walking and running at first, just like a beginner runner. You probably won't have the energy you did, but you'll have something more: Baby can come along, too. See Chapter 31 for guidelines concerning baby carriage running.

Breast-feeding. Studies by Kathryn Dewey, Ph.D., and Cheryl Lovelady, R.D., M.S., at the University of California at Davis indicate that moderate exercise has little effect on the quality or quantity of milk in women who are breast-feeding. Nor does it affect infant weight gain. Moderate, sensible exercise that doesn't cause dramatic weight loss may actually enhance nursing, boost energy levels, and reduce the fatigue of nursing mothers. Nursing women may require about 500 calories more per day. Physically active women may have an increased appetite and thus consume enough calories to meet the demands of running and nursing. Women who are nursing should monitor their exercise and diets carefully. They do not have to wait a certain amount of time before or after feeding to run. A sports bra with wide, nonelastic straps is a must.

Dewey says that finding time to exercise is the greatest obstacle to new mothers. Exercise may not fit into their hectic schedules. "It is really important to realize that women who are breast-feeding babies," she says, "need a lot of support and help getting the time to exercise."

Postbaby running performance. In the early 1970s, Dr. Ernst van Aaken theorized that motherhood may help a woman's exercise performance. He studied more than fifteen champion German women athletes who bore children during their careers. He found that five gave up sports after childbirth, but that of the remaining ten, two were able to maintain their prepregnancy performance levels while eight improved measurably. All of the women runners agreed that after childbirth they were "tougher" and had more strength and endurance. A study of women athletes who partici-pated in the 1964 Olympics in Tokyo showed that half of those who continued athletic training after pregnancy improved their athletic performance within a year following delivery.

There is plenty of anecdotal evidence, too. Miki Gorman gave birth to a son when she was thirty-nine. Eight months later she finished second in the 1975 New York City Marathon. The fol-lowing year she ran her best-ever marathon in 2:39. Norway's In-grid Kristiansen won a marathon when she was five months pregnant. (She wasn't aware of it and said she wouldn't have run had she known.) Within a year after giving birth to a healthy child, she set a world record for the 5K and went on to set more post-pregnancy world records in the 10K and marathon.

Why is this happening? Dr. James Clapp III is an obstetrician in the reproductive biology department at Case Western Reserve Uni-versity in Cleveland, Ohio. He studied forty women runners who exercised six times a week for more than 30 minutes for two years; he tested them for aerobic capacity. Then, half of the women who planned on conceiving became pregnant. Fifteen months later, ba-bies carried and delivered, Dr. Clapp again tested the aerobic ca-pacity (max VO_2) of all forty women runners. He found that the max VO_2 of the women who had not become pregnant remained unchanged. But of the women who had babies, aerobic capacity had increased by 7 percent even though they had decreased their training by 40 to 75 percent.

How could pregnancy improve aerobic fitness? Dr. Clapp and his researchers theorized that pregnancy has a similar effect on the body as training. Both pregnancy and exercise, they suggested, increase blood volume, bone mass, and metabolic rate. Perhaps running and walking with added weight contributes to this, like exercising with a weighted vest. Other studies suggest that this added aerobic boost may continue for up to three years.

Psychologists also speculate that during pregnancy and labor women discover emotional and mental resources that carry over into their running. "No marathon has ever been as difficult as labor," says Joan Benoit Samuelson, the 1984 Women's Olympic Marathon winner. Mary Decker Slaney, the U.S. record holder for the mile, adds, "I've never experienced pain like I did during labor. Now I can push myself so much harder. I don't think women have pushed themselves as far as they can physically, which is why I believe women are going to run a sub-four-minute mile."

In sum, there is no reason for a mother (or father) not to run after baby arrives. Even lack of time can be overcome. All three can get their exercise. Tell Dad to watch the baby while Mom runs. But be prepared: Baby Christopher was so demanding that I lost sleep and this drained my energy for running. I adjusted by pushing him along in our Baby Jogger and by cutting back on my running until he would allow me to get adequate sleep. Now, of course, every runner who is a parent tells me their baby sleeps all night!

Resources for Women Who Exercise

For more information on women's health issues contact the following organizations:

Melpomene Institute
2125 East Hennepin
Minneapolis, MN 55413
(612) 378-0545
(The institute is named for the Greek woman who illegally entered the first Olympic marathon in 1896. It is a research and resource center for women.)

National Women's Health Network
1325 G Street, NW, Lower Level
Washington, DC 20005
(Provides referrals and educational materials.)

Women's Sports Foundation
342 Madison Avenue, Suite 728
New York, NY 10173
(800) 227-3988 or (212) 972-9170
(Brochures on health and sports topics for girls and women.)

TWENTY-NINE

Aging: The Masters Runner

If you remember the running boom of the late 1970s, you're getting old. That's when the first edition of this book hit the national best-seller lists. Now the runners of that era are over forty—in fact, most are over fifty! As this book goes to print, I'm running into my fifties and Shepherd is sprinting into his sixties. We've aged with the growth of running. Now we can report firsthand about the effects of exercise on aging and the benefits of exercise in slowing down the aging process. Keep in mind two important points: Exercise can help you live longer, but more important, exercise can help improve the quality of the years you have left.

Take the case of Noel Johnson of Pacific Beach, California. He ran his first marathon at age seventy-two—two years after he started running. He wrote a book about his experiences: *A Dud at 70; a Stud at 80*. On a typical training day he got up at 5:00 A.M., climbed onto the trampoline in his bedroom, and ran in place for an hour. "Up and down," Johnson said. "In the nude." Then he walked to his health club and ran on the treadmill and worked out with weights for an hour. At age eighty-four, Johnson completed his best marathon time: 5 hours, 42 minutes. When he turned ninety-two, he celebrated by running the New York City Marathon.

Unusual? Not any more. Ruth Rothfarb of Miami Beach, Florida, took up running at age seventy-two. "When I started running twenty years ago," she said at age ninety-two, "people said I was an old lady and that I'd drop dead doing it. But most of *them* dropped dead and I'm still running around." At ninety-two, Ruth was running and walking 10 to 15 miles a day. She worked out twice a day. And she was a party animal—she'd dance past midnight at the postmarathon parties! And she could really swing— as I can attest from dancing with her after a race she ran in her early eighties.

Older Americans are off and running—and America is getting older. The so-called baby boomers, born between 1946 and 1964, will all be at least forty by 2004. In that same year, half of the people in the United States will be more than fifty years old; 14 percent of us will be sixty-five years old or older. By the mid-1990s, the fastest-growing population group was Americans eighty-five years old and older.

Those Americans who exercise regularly are learning what Hippocrates knew more than 2,400 years ago: "Speaking generally," he wrote, "all parts of the body which have a function, if used in moderation and exercised in labours to which each is accustomed, become thereby healthy and well developed, and age slowly; but if unused and left idle, they become liable to disease, defective in growth, and age quickly."

In short, use it or lose it. Dr. Walter Bortz, author of *We Live Too Short and Die Too Young*, agrees. "Aging," he told *Runner's World*, "is a self-fulfilling prophecy. If we dread growing old, thinking it a time of forgetfulness and physical deterioration, then it is likely to be just that. On the other hand, if we expect to be full of energy and anticipate that our lives will be rich with new adventures and insights, then that is the likely reality. We prescribe who we are and what we are to become."

As we age, our perceptions of old age change rapidly. In fact, almost everything we have come to associate with growing old is wrong. "What we once considered to be marks of aging, we now know are the results of disease or disuse," Dr. Bortz says.

Disuse is the culprit. It accounts for about 50 percent of the decline in aerobic capacity that occurs between the ages of thirty and seventy according to a study of 1,500 NASA employees at the

Johnson Space Center in Houston, Texas. On the other hand, no matter when you start to exercise, improvements in functioning will occur. Dr. Roy J. Shephard, an expert on exercise and aging at the University of Toronto, explains, "You'd have to go a long way to find something as good as exercise as a fountain of youth. And you don't have to run marathons to reap the benefits. For the average older person who does little more than rapid walking for 30 minutes at a time three or four times a week, it can provide 10 years of rejuvenation."

Researchers at McMaster University in Hamilton, Ontario, matched by weight, height, physical activity, and occupation a group of previously sedentary men in their twenties with men in their sixties. They all exercised on stationary cycles for one hour, three days a week for twelve weeks. The result: "In older subjects, increases in aerobic power after endurance training are at least as large as in younger subjects."

Studies contradict the long-standing and widespread belief that the elderly cannot improve physiologically and at best may only slow the decline. These studies also show that remarkable athletic achievements by the elderly are not solely the result of "good genes" but also the result, says Dr. Herbert A. deVries, former director of the Andrus Gerontology Center at the University of Southern California, of "taking care of the genes they have through continued activity that promotes fitness."

Dr. Everett L. Smith, director of the Biogerontology Laboratory at the University of Wisconsin, adds, "Exercise is not an unending fountain of youth. Eventually, we all decline. But the quality of life is so much higher for the elderly who are physically active than for people who sit in a rocking chair waiting for the Grim Reaper."

Fortunately, instead of settling into their rocking chairs, aging Americans are exercising in record numbers. According to a report by the Fitness Products Council, the number of people aged 35 to 54 who exercise frequently (at least 100 times a year) increased 65 percent from 1987 to 1994; those over age 55 increased by 45 percent. Meanwhile their kids (see Chapter 31) exercised less frequently.

Adding Years to Your Life

In 1880, the average American life expectancy was forty-five years. Now it is more than seventy-five. Even better news: If you exercise, or start exercising now, you may extend your life. Take the famous

Paffenbarger study of 10,269 male graduates of Harvard University. Dr. Ralph Paffenbarger, a physician who directed the study, reports that those men who run 20 to 35 miles a week (or do other exercise totaling 2,000 or more calories per week) will increase their life span, on the average, by one to more than two years compared to sedentary males their age. Those men who exercise regularly beginning at age thirty-five enjoy a two-and-a-half-year gain in life expectancy. Those in the study who began exercising after age fifty lived one to two years longer. Since these are average figures, some of us may extend our lives even more as a result of exercising. And the good news goes on and on: If you also stop smoking and start exercising, for example, add an average of three years.

But if you're past the retirement age of sixty-five, should you retire from running? Is it too late to start exercising at this age if you've been inactive? According to Dr. James M. Rippe, associate professor at the Tufts University School of Medicine, "A person who reaches the age of 65 in our society has an 80 percent chance of reaching the age of 80. I think there's good data to support the idea that even in your 60s you can lower your risk of heart disease by becoming more physically active."

Research by Dr. Paul Williams of the Lawrence Berkeley Laboratory at the University of California at Berkeley found continued improvement in mortality rates in people studied as they ran more mileage up to 50 miles a week. He stated: "We estimate that, compared to men who run less than 10 miles per week, those who run 40 to 49 miles per week have a 30 percent lower risk of heart disease." He found similar results among women runners. Why did these men and women show such improvements in mortality rates? Both the men and women runners showed lower total cholesterol, higher levels of protective HDL cholesterol, lower body weights, and less high blood pressure.

But do you have to run 20 to 50 miles a week in order to live longer? In another research study, Steven Blair, P.E.D., and his colleagues at the Cooper Institute of Aerobics Research in Dallas concluded that even moderately intense activity such as walking and working around the house has mortality benefits. Participants in this study were assigned to groups based on their level of fitness. The lowest rate of death came in the group with the highest level of fitness. Conversely, the highest rate of death occurred in the group with the lowest level of fitness. Across all the groups, the rate of death gradually fell as the level of fitness rose. The largest drop in the death rate occurred between the least fit group and the next group. When men improved from being moderately fit to being highly fit, there was a 15 percent decline in mortality, but there was an even greater benefit—a 40 percent decline in deaths from all causes—among men who improved from being unfit to being moderately fit.

This suggests that even a small increase in fitness for the most unfit people brings a significant health benefit. The Blair study reports that simply by walking 2 miles in 30 to 40 minutes several days a week, you can create a fitness level that will significantly increase your life expectancy. The Centers for Disease Control and Prevention estimates that if every American who is inactive would walk or do other comparable moderately intensive exercise for 30 minutes a day, there would be an annual decline in deaths of about 250,000 a year.

As Dr. Paffenbarger, an accomplished ultra-marathoner, summed up, "A little exercise is better than none, but more is better than a little."

"Who Said Gettin' Old Was Fun?"

This old saw is now showing up on bumper stickers in trailer parks from California to Florida, and on T-shirts worn by masters runners. True, the aging process takes its toll. I can't run those fast 10Ks I once did. Shepherd finds his pace slowly increasing with time, but he keeps on jogging. The decline of old age can be dramatic and depressing. With each year after reaching maturity, your heart's ability to pump oxygen during exercise declines by about 1 percent. Now, that's a definition of slow death! By age sixty, blood flow from the arms to the legs is 30 to 60 percent slower than at age twenty-five. We lose our stride. Nancy Hamilton, Ph.D., of the Biomechanics Lab at the University of Northern Iowa videotaped sprinters aged thirty-five to ninety. She concluded that between those ages our range of motion in the knee declines by 33 percent; in the hip, 38 percent. The greatest changes in her test group occurred after age fifty in the knees and after age sixty in the hips.

We also wheeze more. The amount of air we can exhale after a deep breath lessens as the chest wall stiffens with age. This results in a decline in the amount of oxygen our body can use: 50 percent decline for men and 29 percent for women by age seventy-five. We lose strength. The number of muscle fibers decreases at the rate of 3 to 5 percent per decade after age thirty. This leads to a 10 percent loss of muscle power per decade after age fifty. The size of the muscle fibers also decreases with aging. The lost muscle is usually replaced by body fat and results by age seventy in a 10 percent lowering of the basal metabolic rate (your caloric need while at rest). The speed at which nerve messages travel drops 10 to 15 percent by age seventy. Flexibility declines 20 to 30 percent. Bone losses average 15 to 20 percent in men and 25 to 30 percent in women. And on and on. Dr. Roy Walford, author of *Maximum Life Span*, put it briefly and bluntly: "Your breasts will sag and your erections flag."

By now you're wondering, Why bother getting up in the morning? One good reason is that some of this can be slowed down and even, in some instances, reversed.

The Physical Benefits of Exercise

Exercising regularly will not only add years to your life, but it will also add quality to your years. It's up to you. You can control this. Inactivity, as research at Tufts University shows, definitely shortens your productive years—that is, stop exercising and you will be less able to do things and more prone to illnesses like heart disease, diabetes, and osteoporosis.

Drs. William Evans and Irwin Rosenberg at the U.S. Department of Agriculture Human Nutrition Research Center at Tufts University have identified what they call ten biomarkers of aging: physiological factors that are associated with aging but which regular exercise and a careful diet can help. Genetics plays a significant role in these biomarkers, but so does lifestyle. Controlling them, therefore, is largely up to you. The ten Evans and Rosenberg biomarkers are:

1. Muscle mass

2. Strength

3. Basal metabolic rate

4. Body fat percentage

5. Aerobic capacity

6. Blood sugar tolerance

7. Cholesterol/HDL ratio

8. Blood pressure

9. Bone density

10. Internal temperature regulation

A regular exercise program, say the researchers, will keep all the biomarkers in any body in the best shape possible.

Aerobic Fitness

The maximum level at which the body can utilize oxygen efficiently is called aerobic capacity (measured as maximum VO_2) This measure of aerobic fitness increases during children's growth years, peaks in the twenties or thirties, and then drops off as we age. Aerobic capacity generally decreases by about 10 percent per decade in relatively sedentary individuals. Active individuals have a rate of loss of about half that observed in sedentary individuals— even less for those athletes who train intensely.

In one of his early studies at the University of Southern California, Dr. Herbert deVries, an exercise physiologist now over seventy, put more than 200 men and women, ages fifty-six to eighty-seven, who lived at a California retirement community, through a fitness program of walking/running, calisthenics, and stretching three to five times a week. After just six weeks "dramatic changes" were seen: blood pressure among the men and women dropped, aerobic capacity increased, arm strength improved, and muscular signs of nervous tension diminished. "Men and women of 60 and 70 became as fit and energetic as those 20 to 30 years younger," deVries noted in his book *Fitness After 50*. He writes: "The ones who improved the most were the ones who had been least active and most out of shape."

Generally, an endurance exercise program such as running will result in a 20 percent increase in aerobic capacity. You can look at that as a twenty-year rejuvenation. That is, an inactive sixty-year-old who begins a vigorous aerobic exercise program can attain the same cardiorespiratory level he had two decades earlier—as an inactive forty-year-old. Are you interested in becoming twenty years younger aerobically?

Muscular Strength

As we age, two things drain us of physical strength. Our muscle strength declines an average of 30 to 40 percent over our life span, due in large part to a decline in the size and number of our muscle fibers. Most of this decline comes after age fifty. Second, our increasingly sedentary lifestyle as we age causes our muscles to atrophy even faster than if they were used regularly. The first to go are the fast-twitch muscle fibers (used for strength and speed), followed by slow-twitch fibers (used for endurance). "The fibers you lose are the ones you use the least," says David Costill, Ph.D., director of Ball State University's Human Performance Laboratory. "In normal daily activity, the fibers you use the most are slow twitch, so you retain those. The fibers you use the least are fast twitch. So to maintain muscle strength, it becomes a case of 'use it or lose it.' "

The cure is obvious. Weight training minimizes strength loss. And it is never too late to start. Studies at the U.S. Department of Agriculture's Human Nutrition Research Center at Tufts University found that frail men and women in their late eighties and early nineties can benefit from a limited program of mild weight lifting. In the study, 100 men and women who lived at the Hebrew Rehabilitation Center for the Aged in Boston were divided into two groups. One group did ordinary nursing home activities, while the other worked vigorously on exercise machines for 45 minutes three times a week to strengthen their legs. The exercising residents increased their walking speed by 12 percent and their ability to climb stairs by 28 percent. They were also less depressed and more likely to walk around on their own and take part in nursing home activities. "Our findings suggest that a portion of the muscle weakness attributable to aging may be modifiable through exercise," the researchers concluded.

Since running primarily exercises the lower body, runners lose muscle mass more quickly in their upper body. In addition, bone density decreases with aging but increases with exercise. But running only aids in lower body bone density. To improve upper body bone density you need to weight-train. I recommend that older runners include weight training as part of their exercise regime. (See Chapter 36 for guidelines.)

Flexibility

Along with increasing bone mass, maintaining flexibility is increasingly important as we age. Studies of exercise and flexibility also contain good news. Kathleen Munns, a researcher at the Biogerontology Laboratory at the University of Wisconsin, conducted a twelve-week study to test flexibility among the elderly. Her twenty participants, with an average age of seventy, participated in a stretching program. They were able to increase motion in their necks (by 26 percent), wrists (13 percent), shoulders (8 percent), hips and back (27 percent), knees (12 percent), and ankles (48 percent).

In a University of Michigan School of Public Health study, 100 men and women aged seventy-five to ninety-eight were given three months of low-intensity aerobics. These exercises emphasized flexibility and stretching twice a week for 40 minutes each time. The results were similar to the Wisconsin study: significant improvements in flexibility and better balance and ability to move steadily and quickly (which diminishes the risk of accidents). There were other benefits: All reported the exercises reduced arthritis pain. On average, the participants' blood pressure fell from 154/83 to 142/77. Equally important, they were in a more upbeat mood than evident in the preexercise psychological tests.

Immune System

The ability to ward off colds, infections, and serious illnesses—such as cancer—decreases with age as your immune system weakens. But if you exercise regularly you can dramatically slow that decline. Researcher David Nieman, Ph.D., compared the immune function of three groups of seventy-year-olds: highly trained women who had exercised vigorously for one and a half hours each day for the past eleven years, previously untrained women who walked for half an hour for twelve weeks, and sedentary women. In general, the immune systems of the highly active women was 55 percent higher than the two other groups. This suggests that a long-term commitment to a highly active, healthy lifestyle promotes superior immune functioning as we age.

Disability

An eight-year study comparing the health of 451 runners and 330 nonrunners, ages fifty to seventy-two, directed by Dr. James Fry at the Stanford University School of Medicine concluded: "Older persons who engage in vigorous running and other aerobic activities have lower mortality and slower development of disability than do members of the general population. This association is probably related to increased aerobic activity, strength, fitness and increased organic reserve." The nonrunners had three and a half times more disabilities as measured by such mobility tests as ease of walking, reaching and gripping objects, and ability to rise straight up from a chair. The runners, who averaged 26 miles per week during the study, had fewer disabilities than the nonrunners did eight years earlier, when the study began, and the gap between the groups widened throughout the study—refuting any claims that all that running will leave us crippled as we age.

Weight Management

Most Americans, including Shepherd and me, get heavier as they get older. So why the extra pounds? Two reasons: First, most people become less active as they get older, and thus burn fewer calories; and second, our metabolic rate (the rate at which the body uses calories) gradually slows with age. This rate tends to fall by 2 percent per decade after age twenty, which means that with each passing decade you need to consume 100 fewer calories per day. Even if you continue to exercise at the same level as you age, you'll still put on weight. If you exercise less, you'll gain even more. The only way to beat the system is to taper the caloric intake and stay active or increase your exercise as you age. I used to weigh 160 pounds no matter how much I ate, since I was always physically active. After I hit age forty, this was no longer true. I'll concede up to 5 pounds to aging, but no more. Like most of us, I, too, must now count my calories and keep on running.

Gastrointestinal Bleeding

A study at the National Institute on Aging shows that older exercisers are half as likely as nonexercisers to experience gastrointestinal (GI) bleeding—a common problem among older men and women. Study director and epidemiologist Jack Guralnik told *American Health* magazine: "Fit individuals deliver blood and oxygen to all their organs more efficiently, including the GI tract, and better blood flow equals healthier tissue. In times of physical stress, then, older people who are fit may have a greater margin of safety."

Cognitive Abilities

In a study of 300 men and women ages fifty-five to eighty-eight at Scripps College in Claremont, California, researchers Louise Clarkson-Smith and Alan Hartley found that exercise improves our cognitive abilities. Among the men and women in this study who exercised regularly, there was a measured improvement in their ability to remember, to reason, and to solve problems. As their level of activity increased, so did their level of cognitive function. As Hartley noted, "The practical application of this study is clear. If people want to maintain [their] mental abilities as they get older, they should exercise on a regular basis."

Osteoporosis Fighter

Perhaps no single event in aging—other than the specter of death itself—concerns the elderly more than falling and breaking a bone. This is often due to osteoporosis, a reduction of bone density and strength that often accompanies aging, particularly among women. A study by Gail Dalsky, Ph.D., at the Washington University School of Medicine in St. Louis, showed that exercise, including running, can increase bone mass and aid in the treatment of osteoporosis. This study measured the effects of weight-bearing exercise on lumbar (spinal) bone mass in thirty-five postmenopausal women ages fifty-five to seventy. After twenty-two months of exercise, the women had a 6.1 percent increase in bone mass. A nonexercising control group experienced a 1 percent decrease. To test their results, the researchers had the exercise group stop exercising for one year. When remeasured, their bone mass had reverted to preexercise levels. A program of running and weight training is recommended to keep bone density from deteriorating with age.

Age and Diet

One of the best weapons against aging is eating carefully. What we eat, and avoid, and how much and when we eat all have an impact on our longevity. Continuing research at the Human Nutrition Research Center on Aging at Tufts is finding that cutting back on our intake of fat and increasing other foods may help us live longer. As described in Chapter 18, changing your diet to include plenty of fruits and vegetables, avoiding alcohol and caffeine, and eating foods rich in calcium will help you to better handle the physical changes of aging.

Aging also affects diet and nutritional needs. More attention must be paid to the nutritional value of foods as we age. Older people need fewer calories to maintain normal body weight, yet the need for essential nutrients is as great as it is for younger adults. There is less room in an older person's diet for high-calorie, low-nutrient foods like sweets, alcohol, and fats.

A National Institute on Aging study indicates that 16 percent of Americans over age sixty-five who live alone eat nutritionally poor diets. Older men who have been widowed are the worst offenders, relying on package meals and takeout foods: 16 percent of men fifty-five to sixty-four and 25 percent of those over seventy-five who live alone have poor diets. The problem is not poverty, the study shows, but lack of motivation coupled with the process of aging itself: limited mobility, the decline of our taste buds and odor receptors, gum disease or the loss of teeth, various chronic ailments that necessitate bland or restricted diets, medications and diseases that decrease appetite or impair digestion, and so forth. Chronic depression also impedes good diet: 12 to 14 percent of America's elderly suffer persistent depression accompanied by progressive weight loss.

Here again, we can take control of our lives and live better. Combined with exercise, we can change our diets to include more beta-carotene, vitamins C and E, and selenium. All serve as anti-oxidants that neutralize free radicals. These are substances produced by our bodies in response to normal processes such as oxygen consumption, pollution, cigarette smoke, X-rays, and infection. Free radicals may damage the DNA and attack healthy cells, setting the stage for many age-related diseases. Vitamin D and calcium are also important in the prevention of osteoporosis.

Training and Aging

Okay, we've convinced you. Increase your exercise and change your diet. But there are several things you should do and be aware of after you return from the health-food store and before you run out the door. First, follow the basic training instructions in the first half of this book. Start slowly and step up your training gradually. "Easy" is a word that Shepherd and I have come to appreciate. Run easy. Take it easy.

According to Dr. George Sheehan, the famous doctor-runner-author, the principles for training are no different if you are a fifty-, sixty-, or seventy-year-old runner than they are for world-class runners in their twenties. Stress is applied, time is taken for the body to adapt, then a little more stress is applied. "What differs as we age," said Dr. Sheehan, "is the amount of stress the body can accept and the time your body requires to adapt. You have to listen to your body. You may not be able to do the same number of miles you did at age 50 when you are age 60. But you may be able to run for the same number of minutes."

Beginning

More and more men and women over the age of forty are exercising now than ever before. Yet too many Americans reach their fiftieth birthday and start shopping for rocking chairs. They should shop for running shoes instead. So what are you waiting for?

If you are more than forty years old—the age I start counting as middle-age—you can most likely follow the same guidelines for beginners that I set out in Chapter 10. By the time you reach age sixty, you may need to modify the program somewhat.

Here are some training guidelines:

- If you are over age forty and have been comparatively inactive, you should first get your doctor's approval before starting an exercise program. Don't just buy a pair of expensive running shoes and try to get your money's worth without medical approval.

- Start with low-intensity activity, such as an easy walking program. When you are able to walk for 30 or more minutes at a brisk pace, you will be physically fit. If you then wish to expand your fitness level and enjoy running, follow my beginner's running program.

- Be sure to stretch thoroughly and regularly. This is important for the older runner. You need to continue to improve your flexibility.

- Walk before running to warm up, and walk after running to cool down.

- Remember that older people take longer to recover from exercise, especially weight-bearing activity like running. Therefore, run only every other day when you are starting your exercise program. You may alternate running a few times a week with swimming or biking.

■ Be extra careful on hot and cold days. Older people are more vulnerable to heat-related illnesses and frostbite. As we age, we don't handle heat as well. For example, researchers at Penn State University compared the ability to handle heat in young women (ages twenty to thirty) and older women (fifty-two to sixty-two) exercisers. They found that the older runners sweated more in humid conditions, lost more water in their urine, experienced a greater drop in blood volume during exercise in heat, and had less thirst sensitivity. Older runners need to be aware of these conditions and be sure to drink more fluids before, during, and after running in the heat.

Recovery
Here are some tips to help you recover from your running exercise:

■ As we age, it takes longer to recover from hard days (long runs, fast workouts, races). The hard-easy system needs to be expanded to the hard-easy-easy, or hard-easy-easy-easy. More easy days will be needed following hard efforts.

■ Cross-training becomes more valuable as we get older and take more time to recover. On days when you are too sore or stiff to run, or to prevent soreness or stiffness, substitute a non-weight-bearing exercise such as swimming, biking, or the use of rowing or stair-climbing machines.

■ As we get older—and I can attest to this—it takes longer to recover from running on hard surfaces. Running on dirt, grass, synthetic tracks, or treadmills will help.

■ More downtime is needed. You may want to take up to two weeks or more, twice a year (or more), when you feel you can cut your running and racing way back to rejuvenate.

■ Pay more attention to stretching and flexibility training. This will help compensate for the natural loss of flexibility and stride as you age.

Masters Competition

Running is one of the few sports that rewards you for growing old. Most races compare times according to five- or ten-year "masters" age groups after age forty. I've coached a lot of runners who celebrated their fortieth, fiftieth, sixtieth, and even their seventieth birthdays with a big party because they crossed into a new masters level for racing and got to be the new "kid" in their age group.

Running has created a new pride in aging. We all get a new competitive life every five years. How many sports allow a sixty-year-old to compete against his or her peers for a trophy? I retired from serious competition in my early thirties when I was at my peak. Each time I move into a new age group I think I'm a "kid" again! I figure if I wait long enough some of those old rascals will die off.

One of masters runners heroes is Johnny Kelly. He practically owns the Boston Marathon. In 1991, at age eighty-three, he competed in this prestigious race for the sixtieth time! He's won the race twice; in 1945, he took it with his best time, 2:30:40. When he was in his eighties, Johnny Kelly ran the marathon in slightly more than five hours. As he pushed toward his nineties, Kelly was allowed to start his "marathon" at the 20-mile mark and finish from there. His starting line? A statue on the Boston Marathon course honoring him.

Toshi d'Elia is an inspiration. She started running in her late thirties because she was ashamed that she couldn't keep up with her mountain-climbing husband, Fred, then in his fifties. Toshi's first race was a 2-mile cross-country run that her twenty-year-old daughter Erica had pushed her into so that none of her friends would come in last. But Toshi finished third—only a few seconds behind the winner, Erica. She has been hooked on running ever since. At age forty-seven, Toshi came to me and asked if I would coach her. We're still together nearly twenty years later.

Toshi became the first woman in the world age fifty or older to break three hours for the marathon—running 2:57:21 at age fifty in the 1980 World Masters Championship in Glasgow, Scotland. Toshi still runs marathons, although in her sixties she completes them a half-hour or so slower than at her peak. "I can accept that I am slower," she says, "as long as I'm in good shape." And she is: Every five years Toshi d'Elia moves into a new age class and gets ranked near the top in the country. At age 65 she won the gold medal for the 65–69 age group in both the 5K and 10K in the World Veterans Track and Field Championships in Buffalo, New York. She has been nationally ranked for age groups 45–49, 50–54, 55–59, 60–64, and 65–69. And she's famous! Her auto-biography, *Running On*, became a hit in Japan, and a prime-time television movie was made of her life as an inspiration to Japanese women.

As Toshi d'Elia would admit, we peak as competitive runners between the age of twenty-five and thirty-five, and then go steadily downhill. But as her life also illustrates, we can hold our own. A long-term study at Washington University in St. Louis, Missouri, reports encouraging news: After testing competitive runners age fifty and older, researchers concluded that we don't slow down with age as fast as previously thought. The Washington research indicates only a 5 percent per decade decrease in performance after age thirty—if training is steady and vigorous. This compares to a 10 percent per decade decrease in people who are inactive.

Another study at the University of Wisconsin and, later, the University of Florida followed competitive runners ages fifty to eighty-two for ten years. This study also indicated that runners who continue to train at a high level of intensity showed no statistical loss of aerobic capacity despite aging ten years. Many of those athletes actually increased their training over the decade to com-pensate for some lost ability due to aging. Michael Pollack, an exercise physiologist who directed the study, suggests that to hold our performance longer we will need to maintain an intense train-ing level, not just run easy mileage.

Some of us will, like wine, actually improve with age. I've seen sixty-five-year-olds run faster times than they did when they were sixty. This is because they didn't have the training background and experience to run faster when they were younger. If you are new to competitive training and racing, you very well may defy age and continue to run faster times. But eventually we all slow down. When we do, we will have to adjust our exercise goals.

To stay motivated, try recording your personal records all over again with each five-year mark you pass. That will give you at-tainable goals and keep you motivated. Also, compare yourself to the times runners in your age group are doing, not to the faster times you ran when you were younger. This is the beauty of mas-ters running: You start over every five years. It even works for me—at age 49½, as I completed this chapter, I got fit again and started winning awards in my five-year age group. That motivates me to keep training. And I'm even looking forward to moving up to the age 50–54 race category.

Be proud that you look and feel good at your age. Join with other older runners to provide each other with support and motivation. Maybe you'd even like to join a club or form one of your own. Shelly formed a team of women runners over age fifty, called the Mercury masters. The spirit of the masters runners is very high. It is a great social scene. (One masters club that has a lot of fun and travels to events together has a great name: the Scarsdale Antiques.) You certainly won't be racing alone. In 1980, 28 percent of the runners in the New York City Marathon were over forty. By 1995, half of the 25,000 runners in that event were in the masters class.

Running may not add years to your life—although, as we've said here, evidence suggests the opposite—but it will add quality. That's a guarantee—from Shepherd and me. Think of the legendary Larry Lewis.

Larry was 106 years old when he died from cancer. Until his death, he ran 6.7 miles at 4:30 every morning around San Francisco's Golden Gate Park. He then reported to work as a full-time waiter at the St. Francis Hotel on Union Square. Sometimes he walked the 5 miles to work as well. He spoke for all of us in an interview for *Runner's World*, given shortly before his death:

"Never say a person is so many years OLD. Old means something dilapidated and something you eventually get rid of, like an old automobile or an old refrigerator. I'm not in that category. You may become mellow, but never old."

Running with Health Challenges

Many of us experience various health impairments or physical disabilities, which I lump together and refer to as "health challenges" in this book, that may affect our ability to exercise. But most chronic health conditions—asthma, cancer, diabetes, epilepsy, heart disease, hearing and vision loss, as well as orthopedic and neurological impairments—do not have to keep you from enjoying exercise or sports. We tend to protect and coddle adults and children afflicted with these conditions, yet most can enjoy physical activity. Generally, the benefits from exercise far outweigh the risks or disadvantages. Any limitations you have, I believe, should be seen as limits on your skill at a specific activity rather than on limits on your ability to participate in exercise.

My experience with men (myself included), women, and children with health challenges is that exercise programs specifically designed to fit their needs improves the quality of our lives. In fact, rigorous physical activity will increase physical fitness, enhance the ability to deal with medical conditions, and create a greater social and psychological independence in them.

I do admit to some limitations. Any exercise program should be based on what is medically acceptable to each person's particular condition. That condition and any limitations or medical guidelines should be clearly communicated to all coaches, teachers, and family members. This includes any risks to your self-image. If your physician is too quick to discourage exercise, perhaps a second opinion from a sports medicine specialist would be recommended. It's too easy for doctors, coaches, and family members to say "You can't." Positive support and reinforcement are very important to anyone trying to overcome a health obstacle. Many experts feel that the health challenged should be "mainstreamed" whenever possible into school physical education programs, sports teams, running clubs. You should try to achieve physical goals like everyone else.

The Achilles Track Club

When Dick Traum walked into my office in 1975, I was shocked. He was, at age thirty-four, typical of any other businessman: gaining weight and under increasing stress as his business grew. He wanted a fitness test so he could start my beginner's runner course. The problem? Dick had only one leg.

I tested Dick just like everyone else, with one exception. Instead of riding the stationary bike for the cardiorespiratory fitness test, I had him hop up and down on a bench. Dick scored about the same as other men his age: He was in fair to poor shape on every test. (In fact, he even scored better than Shepherd, who took the bike test the next day.)

Dick's biggest handicap wasn't the lack of one leg. He was 20 pounds overweight and lived a sedentary lifestyle.

"Can you run?" I asked him.

"Sure," he lied.

In fact, Dick Traum hadn't run a step since losing his leg in an automobile accident ten years earlier. But he was determined to start a fitness program, and he wasn't going to get turned down just because he was an above-the-knee amputee. That evening, he later told me, he practiced running and hopping with his prosthetic leg along the hallway of his apartment building. He waited until it was late so his neighbors wouldn't see him.

How could I help this man run? For one thing, Dick Traum was a determined man. He had decided to become a runner. He had come in to start a running program and he was willing to take some pain running with his prosthetic leg. In my class, Dick quickly progressed from beginner to advanced beginner to intermediate runner. I challenged him to start running outdoors and to enter a 5-mile race in New York's Central Park. He did—and finished last in 72 minutes. But when he crossed the finish line, the other runners loudly cheered him. He was hooked.

Dick trained for longer races, and got more cheers as he crossed more finish lines. One day he asked me if he could train for a marathon. I asked if he would settle for a half-marathon since he had only one leg. "Sure," he replied with a mischievous smile.

We ran the half-marathon together on a hot day and I poured plenty of water on him. Near the end, he said he felt okay but his leg was getting heavy. I assumed he meant his good leg. (Hey, both of mine were, too!) But at the finish line he pulled off his prosthesis and out poured at least a quart of water!

After that race, Dick got serious. He was determined to run the other half of the marathon. In 1976 he made marathon history by being the first amputee to finish the New York City Marathon. He started early and finished in 7 hours, 24 minutes. Newspapers across the United States featured a photograph of winner Bill Rodgers patting Dick Traum on the back as he passed him.

I wrote an article about Dick's experiences for the January 1977 issue of *Runner's World.* A twenty-two-year-old Canadian who was about to have his leg amputated above the knee in an effort to stop the spread of his cancer read the story just before his surgery. Encouraged, Terry Fox vowed to run across Canada to raise money to fight cancer. In 1980, he set out on his trans-Canada run and logged 3,339 miles in a personal "Marathon of Hope." In June 1981, however, two-thirds of the way to his goal, Terry Fox died from the disease. He had raised millions of dollars for cancer research, and the books and television movie about his life inspired many men, women, and children—able-bodied and disabled—to start a fitness program themselves.

After attending a Terry Fox benefit run in Canada in 1982, Dick Traum was back in my office. He had a radical idea, he told me. Dick wanted to start a fitness program for the physically disabled. "We just need to get the word out that through exercise many of the obstacles to leading a full life can be removed for the physically disabled," he said.

I selected the name for the program—Achilles Track Club—after the Greek mythical hero who had a powerful body but one weakness. This is the way I see health-challenged men, women, and children. Certain parts of their bodies may be impaired, but they can still exercise and benefit from it. And exercise can be used to help them build confidence in the other parts of their lives.

Dick got the New York Road Runners Club to sponsor the program. We were off and running. From two members in 1982 there are now more than 3,000 members in 105 chapters all over the world. The Achilles Track Club includes runners in China, Russia, Mongolia, South Africa, and Vietnam, to name a few. More than 200 members from around the world complete the New York City Marathon each year.

Achilles athletes can run, walk, or use wheelchairs. They represent a wide range of disabilities, from amputations, blindness, deafness, cerebral palsy, and paraplegia to epilepsy, diabetes, multiple sclerosis, cancer, traumatic brain injuries, heart disease, obesity, and arthritis. Dick's book *A Victory for Humanity* details the development of the Achilles Track Club and stirs all of us with success stories of health-challenged runners.

For more information on the Achilles Track Club and information on running for the health-challenged, contact:

Dick Traum
President, Achilles Track Club
One Times Square
New York, NY 10036
(212) 354-0300.

Fitness Guidelines

As I said, I treat everyone just about the same.

Rule one: You are either in shape or out of shape. Period. A health-challenged person may spend years being inactive, but so do other people. You may think you're out of shape because you cannot exercise. But you can!

Rule two: You should check with your doctor before exercising. He or she may set some guidelines for you. Find a doctor who believes in exercise, understands its value to you, and listens to you. Then you listen to his or her advice. You may have to adjust your training program by starting and progressing more slowly.

Here are some general guidelines about exercise for some specific disabilities and conditions. They are listed alphabetically for your convenience, but also check with organizations that specialize in your particular medical condition. They will have good additional information. Or call the nearest chapter of the Achilles Track Club.

Alcoholism

I know about a dozen dedicated runners who are recovering alcoholics and who participate in New York Road Runners Club events. Running, combined with Alcoholics Anonymous or other professional help groups, has put many men and women back on the road to healthy lives. A study reported in the *Journal of Studies on Alcohol* reported that almost 70 percent of those men and women who undertake a fitness program along with their alcohol rehabilitation remain abstinent. The researchers concluded that fitness training may make patients receptive to change, reorganize their leisure time, and help them deal with stress.

This was certainly true for one woman I know, who was hospitalized in an alcoholic rehabilitation center. Fired from her job and going through a divorce, she had been depressed and suicidal. After her release from the center, she started my beginner's running class. Gradually, she built herself to running 5 miles a day. Running gave her release from her stress and greatly improved her self-image—one day at a time, one step at a time.

Arthritis

What is arthritis and how can exercise help? Read on and discuss your desire to exercise with your doctor.

There are 109 kinds of arthritis affecting some 37 million Americans. Osteoarthritis, involving the degeneration of joints, is the most common form by far. While its specific cause is a mystery, it often accompanies aging and will affect almost all of us during our lifetimes—as I have recently discovered myself. Osteoarthritis involves the narrowing of the space between the bones of a joint as cartilage breaks down. This results in friction that causes irritation. Bone spurs often develop in response to inflammation and may further aggravate the condition. The inflammation may also involve ligaments and tendons and cause them to lose elasticity. The result is increasing pain and a gradual loss of movement in the joint. Most of these types of arthritics benefit from exercise, including running.

Rheumatoid arthritis is the second most common form of this disease and afflicts about 2 million Americans. It is a more widespread illness marked by general fatigue, muscle aches, loss of appetite and weight, fever, and swollen joints. Many forms of rheumatoid arthritis are inherited. Even this form of arthritis may be helped somewhat by nonimpact exercise, but running is generally not advised.

Running and other high-impact exercises were once thought to cause arthritis. Now we know that this is not only untrue, but that lack of physical exercise may also lead to arthritis. Steven Blair, director of epidemiology at the Institute of Aerobics Research in Dallas, sorted through data on nearly 5,000 exercisers and nonexercisers. He and fellow researcher Harold Kohl found no evidence of increased arthritis in knees or hips of recreational runners, even among those who competed at long distances.

The Journal of Rheumatology detailed a 1,400-person study by Marian Hannan, a researcher at the Boston University Arthritis Center. She found that there was no increase in the risk of knee osteoarthritis with increased physical activity in men and women. Studies by Dr. Nancy Lane at the University of California at San Francisco and by researchers at Stanford University Medical School reached the same conclusion. In fact, these studies go even further than proving that running doesn't cause arthritis. They compared runners and nonrunners aged fifty-five to seventy-seven who had arthritis. After five years there was no difference in the extent of the deterioration between the runners and the nonrunners. The conclusion: Running doesn't accelerate arthritis.

Lack of exercise, however, may actually contribute to the onset of osteoarthritis. Exercise lubricates the various joint components and allows the connective tissue to function at the highest level possible. Most parts of the body, including the heart and the joints, work better when they are used than when they are not used. Many experts now agree that weight loss and regular exercise are important to protecting against developing this degenerative disease. Dr. David Schurman, professor of orthopedic surgery at the Stanford University Medical Center, told *Runner's World* that "Lighter weight reduces wear and tear, while exercise, such as running, builds up muscles that help protect against the skeletal damage associated with common types of arthritis."

Exercise can help the arthritis sufferer retain maximum range of motion in the joints and allow the person to move less stiffly and with less pain. A study by Dr. Robert Ike and associates at the Michigan Medical Center on inactive arthritis patients confirmed this: After a program of biking, the patients reported that they were more fit and had decreased severity of arthritis. In fact, four out of five had reduced pain and swelling after exercise. Range of motion stretching exercises and strength training, combined with aerobic exercise, are recommended for most arthritics by the Arthritis Foundation. By improving the strength and flexibility of nearby muscles, you take some of the stress away from arthritic joints.

Runners with arthritis may have to take a few days off when it becomes bothersome; instead, substitute swimming or biking. When cold, damp weather causes my arthritis to flare up, I head for the hills on my mountain bike and return feeling much better. If arthritis exists in your joints, particularly the hip or knees, a weight-bearing exercise such as running may actually prove to be harmful. Dr. John Bland, professor emeritus of rheumatology at the University of Vermont's College of Medicine, warns that increased joint pain with running may be a sign that the exercise is doing more harm than good. A non-weight-bearing exercise such as swimming or biking may be less painful and help with the management of the arthritic condition.

There is another danger among arthritics: If you stop exercising after developing arthritis, then the whole body tends to deteriorate. Again the warning: Use it or lose it.

Asthma

As many as a quarter of all Americans are afflicted by this respiratory disease. The cause of asthma is unknown. Symptoms may appear at any age, but most often in childhood. They may also occur later in life, as in my case. Symptoms may appear suddenly or gradually, and they may disappear. Asthma strikes both the sedentary and the very fit: 67 of the 597 U.S. athletes competing in the 1984 Olympics had asthma. Of the 174 U.S. medals won at those games, 41 were awarded to asthmatics including 3 golds and a silver by swimmer Nancy Hogshead, author of *Asthma and Exercise*.

Asthma is a condition in which the airways are constricted and/ or obstructed as a result of sensitivity to irritants such as cigarette smoke, dusts, pollens, molds, cold and dry air, certain foods, fatigue, respiratory infections, emotional stress—even exercise. When an asthma attack occurs the bronchioles become narrowed resulting in symptoms that include coughing, wheezing, chest tightness, and rapid breathing. For years I suffered from a chronic cough, sore throats, and periodic flulike symptoms. Then, while running hard up a hill on a cold, dry day, I suddenly felt as if I were trying to breathe through a very narrow straw. After a series of tests, doctors concluded that I was suffering from a mild form of asthma made worse by allergies and cold weather. By running regularly, using my inhalant prior to running, and by wearing a face mask to warm the air I breathe when exercising on cold days, I am still able to run. In fact, running helps me cope with the asthma.

Asthma affects the exerciser in two ways. Those afflicted with the disease must learn to adjust their exercise program. For many, the illness is exercise-induced asthma (EIA). Not all asthmatics have EIA, but most do. I get both regular asthma attacks and the EIA variety. Approximately 10 percent of all people who exercise suffer from EIA.

Joseph Kolb, a sports medicine and rehabilitation therapy specialist, wrote in *Running Times*: "The exact causes of EIA are still unclear. The consensus is that it's caused by a cooling and drying of the respiratory tract from the increased air movement associated with exercise. This effect is heightened when the air is cool and dry, but EIA can also strike on warm, humid days when the atmosphere can be a storage tank for pollutants, pollen and mold. Whatever the weather, the ensuing inflammatory response results in a release of irritating chemicals, such as histamine, that cause bronchial spasms and fluid accumulation."

The result for runners and other exercisers is that they suffer from discomfort or fatigue 5 to 10 minutes into their exercise or after stopping the workout. The condition often discourages athletes from sticking to an exercise program, especially if they don't realize that the cause of their problem is EIA. It affects various people differently. Some may have asthma attacks only during certain workouts and not during others or they may face EIA every time they exercise.

Too many doctors still tell asthma sufferers to avoid exercise. This should not be the case. Alan R. Morton, Dr. Kenneth D. Fitch, and Allan G. Hahn wrote in *The Physician and Sportsmedicine* magazine: "Regular vigorous exercise increases fitness, enhances tolerance to attacks, and provides more social and psychological independence. . . . The development of protective medication has made such activity possible for many asthmatics."

Here are some tips for safety when combining asthma with exercise:

▪ Get fit. Studies indicate that people who are fit can tolerate higher workloads, thus offsetting the start-up of episodes. In addition, the higher your fitness level the less you will labor when breathing, thus decreasing irritation of the airways.

▪ If you are a beginner exerciser, start with exercise that is easier on the lungs—walking or swimming—before moving on to running.

▪ If you are fit but having a bad streak with asthma, back off the running and switch to swimming, which is considered the best exercise for asthmatics because of the warm, humid conditions of indoor pools. Using indoor exercise equipment is the second choice here.

▪ Eliminate triggers whenever you can. If you have allergies, check with an allergist for help. Stay indoors for your exercise if pollen counts are high or it's very cold. If you insist on running, wear a mask to help warm and moisten the air and screen pollen.

▪ Medications to help prevent EIA may be recommended by your doctor. Used properly, these medications will minimize symptoms in all but the rarest of cases. I use three types of inhalers. First, an inhaled steroid (such as Azmacort) to prevent inflammation. I use this medication only when faced with a persistent problem. It is usually reserved for more severe and chronic cases that are caused by more than exercise alone. I take cromolyn sodium medication (such as Intal) 20 minutes prior to exercising on cold days. It helps prevent drying of the airways and decreases the sensitivity of cell membranes that store histamine in the lungs, preventing its release. Finally, a beta-adrenergic inhaler (such as Brethaire) may be used to relax the muscles of the airways and open them up. I take this medication 10 to 20 minutes prior to exercise, after any hard workout, and at any time I'm experiencing symptoms. This type of bronchodilator should be carried with you to be used in case of a flare-up during or after your run. A few puffs may allow you to regain control of your breathing and complete your workout.

▪ EIA usually occurs after 5 to 15 minutes of strenuous exercise. Besides taking inhalants prior to exercise, you can minimize EIA by warming up properly. Warm up slowly with a brisk walk and slow jog before moving into your normal pace. If you still can't get by the 5-minute barrier without discomfort once you've started to run, just take walk breaks as needed. But by all means exercise.

▪ You might want to add a series of increasingly intense pickups (short, fast runs of 30 to 60 seconds) to prepare your lungs for any type of intense speed workout or race. By starting a warm-up 30 minutes before a competition or intense workout, you will get through the EIA attack that occurs 5 to 15 minutes after starting—if it does occur—and begin running your race with reduced risk. Typically, this warm-up would include a walking period followed by 10 to 20 minutes of slow running and then faster-paced running warm-ups 10 minutes prior to the start of the run or race. If this routine is properly followed, competitive athletes may take advantage of a "refractory period" of about 30 to 90 minutes during which you should be able to exercise without an asthma attack.

▪ Cool down gradually after your run to minimize EIA. A slow jog and then walk is recommended for 10 to 15 minutes. This will minimize sudden changes in the temperature of the air reaching your lungs, which could trigger an attack.

▪ Breathe properly. Avoid fast, shallow breaths and practice diaphragm breathing ("belly breathing"). As you inhale, your stomach should go out. During workouts and races, I often sigh or hum. I've had training partners ask if I play the trumpet since they hear me blowing out against pursed lips on cold weather runs. (Hey, it works for me!)

▪ Use a peak-flow meter. This device measures how fast and how hard one can exhale air from the lungs. It can be used to differentiate between symptoms of an attack and ordinary windedness. Peak flow rates will change from your normal rate if lung capacity is diminished. Try warming up gradually and using your inhaler. If that doesn't result in improvement, back off your exercise intensity and don't attempt to race.

▪ Use a heart rate monitor or manually check your pulse. By keeping your heart rate within your comfortable training range you will minimize triggering an attack.

▪ Drink plenty of fluids before and during the run, especially in dry conditions, to inhibit bronchial drying.

▪ Most of all, take consolation in the fact that you are not alone if you experience asthma. Remember those U.S. Olympic athletes and the sparkling three-gold-medal example of swimmer Nancy Hogshead.

Cancer

Cancer is a killer. Approximately one American dies every minute from this disease. Previously sedentary men and women who have developed cancer should consider starting an exercise program with the permission and cooperation of their doctors. The exercise gives them the strength and confidence they need in this big battle.

Some famous runners have struggled against cancer. This includes Fred Lebow and George Sheehan—two "founding fathers" of the running movement.

In February 1975, I arrived in New York City to start work as fitness director of the largest YMCA in the United States, the West Side Y. One of my first projects was to check out the running scene and some guy named Fred Lebow. Fred was promoting the sport through his organization, the New York Road Runners Club; it then had 200 members—it now numbers more than 32,000. Fred soon had me up to my running shorts in the NYRRC—and he took over the back of my Y office so he could move the NYRRC out of his apartment. Fred and I bounced ideas off one another—including his incredible move to shift the New York City Marathon out of Central Park in 1976 and run it through each of the city's five boroughs. That idea has shaped marathons across America and Europe—London, Berlin, Warsaw, and Paris, for example, now run through those cities' districts, admittedly direct copies of Fred Lebow's idea.

In February 1990—almost fifteen years to the day after we first met—I visited Fred under far different circumstances. He had just been taken to the hospital after feeling ill—memory loss and numbness in the right side of his body. I arrived just as he staggered into his hospital room and visited him regularly after he learned that he had inoperable brain cancer. At one point he was even told that he had three to six months to live.

But Fred kept telling me, and everyone else within earshot, that he was going to beat cancer and that running was going to help. We talked running as I sometimes walked with him on his one-mile course—eleven loops around the hospital hallways—three times a day. (Fred pointed out that the indoor track at Madison Square Garden also had eleven laps to the mile.) Next he started sneaking up to the roof of the hospital to run. Then came chemotherapy and radiation. "No matter how bad I felt," he said, "I walked and then ran. I believe it has helped my cancer."

During the treatment he threw up often and couldn't eat much. "Running was kind of a way out. I didn't throw up or get hungry while I ran. It was an oasis from the discomfort. I always felt better when I ran." After his treatment stopped, Fred began to eat more and started to increase his running. Then cancer struck again: His thyroid was removed. He started walking and then built up to running once again.

By the summer of 1991, Fred's cancer was officially diagnosed as in remission. The 1991 New York City Marathon was dedicated to him—with the theme "Fred, this run's for you!"—and more than one million dollars was raised for cancer research. In 1992, to celebrate his sixtieth birthday, Fred ran the New York City Marathon and finished in 5 hours, 32 minutes. He also wrote his book, *The New York Road Runners Club Complete Book of Running*, in which he said: "Pills, operations, doctors' guidance, and the love of family and friends all aid recovery. But there is something more, something crucial to overcoming the failure of the body, and that is physical fitness."

But within two years the cancer returned and despite his heroic struggle and persistent optimism, Fred Lebow died on October 9, 1994. His running had helped him cheat cancer for four years and had allowed him to live those years with enhanced quality. This book is dedicated to Fred for his friendship and his many contributions to our running world. One of his last contributions was the founding, with Jeff Berman, of the Cancer Support Group for Athletes. The group meets twice a month at the New York Road Runners Club to run, talk, and share information and feelings about cancer. "I'd never gone to a support group before," Fred said. "People need this. Has it helped me? Yes, definitely. It helps just to share experiences and hopes and fears."

Dr. George Sheehan also knew the struggle of cancer. The world-famous cardiologist-runner-philosopher battled cancer of the prostate for more than seven years before dying in November 1993. He, too, didn't give up running when he knew he had cancer. In fact, he competed for six years despite going through treatment for the disease. Shortly before his death, Dr. Sheehan was asked by Amby Burfoot, editor of *Runner's World*, how he was able to continue running and racing so long after his cancer had been diagnosed. "I did that because I was addicted to racing. I can't believe how many races I've run in my life. Even with the cancer, I kept going as long as I could. At one point, I even quit the cancer treatments because I thought my racing was getting too slow. I had lost a minute a mile, so I stopped taking my medication. I wanted to be able to run faster." And he did; in 1989 George Sheehan finished seventh in the World Masters Championships in the 800 meters (slightly less than a half mile) for the 70–74 age group with the amazing time of 2:48:23.

Priscella Welch, the woman's winner of the 1987 New York City Marathon at age forty-three and a dominant force in masters (over age forty) running, had a cancerous breast removed in 1993. Since then, she has participated in several "Race for the Cure" women's 5K events to raise money for breast cancer research. After her surgery, she told *USA Today*: "I want to race and have a blast. I don't want it known that she left the sport because she had cancer. I want it known that she had cancer, overcame it, developed her fitness and was in racing mode when she was finished."

As these cases attest, having cancer does not mean stopping running. In fact, exercise may help cancer patients feel and look better. It may also give them the strength and optimism to battle their disease. Moreover, if you are a regular exerciser who then discovers that you have cancer, you will bring a healthy body and spirit to the crisis.

But can you run away from cancer? A growing body of evidence suggests that physical activity reduces the risk of cancer, particularly colon and breast cancer. A study of 17,148 Harvard University alumni showed that regular physical activity cut the risk of colon cancer by half. A study of 1,090 Los Angeles County women ages forty and younger—half with newly diagnosed breast cancer and half without—linked exercise with the prevention of breast cancer. The study, at the University of Southern California School of Medicine, directed by Leslie Bernstein, a professor of preventive medicine, showed that "Even one to three hours of physical exercise per week reduces a woman's risk of breast cancer by about 30 percent." Better yet: Women who exercise an average of four hours a week over the course of their childbearing years run almost a 60 percent lower risk of breast cancer. The researchers summarized their findings: "Our results strongly support the need for educational policies that require participation in physical education classes and that encourage lifelong participation in exercise programs." Yet other studies indicate that only 20 percent of teenage girls exercise three or more times a week.

Most men and women who exercise regularly also do not smoke. They watch their diets and eat fewer fatty foods and meat. These factors help reduce risk of developing cancer. Regular exercise may also lower body weight and improve the immune system. Running does increase the risk of skin cancer, however, by exposing large amounts of skin area to direct sunlight. This can best be avoided by using a sunscreen with a UVA rating above 15 and running early or late in the day.

"Being physically active is only part of the picture," said a report in the *Harvard Health Letter*. "A comprehensive plan for cancer prevention involves eating properly, not smoking, avoiding cancer-causing chemicals and radiation, obtaining appropriate medical screening tests and listening to your body for warning signs. After all, when it comes to cancer, you can run but you can't hide."

Diabetes

About 12 million Americans suffer from adult diabetes (Type II); another one million have juvenile (Type I) diabetes. Exercise cannot cure diabetes or make insulin injections unnecessary, but it may help lower blood sugar and decrease the amount of insulin needed. Further, doctors recommend exercise because it does reduce body fat and decreases the risk of heart disease. Complications from diabetes are best controlled by taking the right amount of insulin, eating the appropriate kinds and amounts of food, and exercising regularly. Eighty percent of diabetics are obese; thus, a gradual approach to exercise is important. The overweight should start with a walking program or nonimpact activity such as swimming or biking.

Diabetic exercisers should coordinate their diet, medicine, and exercise under careful medical supervision. The best time to run is in the morning, after eating a normal breakfast. Morning exercise helps stabilize glucose throughout the day. It is not high blood sugar that is the danger during distance running, but the opposite—low blood sugar (hypoglycemia). To prevent this, many experts advise beginner exercisers and distance runners to reduce insulin intake. Also, eat a complex carbohydrate snack 30 minutes prior to running, and every 30 minutes during exercise. And because the threat of hypoglycemia continues for a few hours after running, you should snack following your runs. For these reasons, also avoid running just before bedtime.

Diabetics who use insulin prior to exercise should not inject it into the limbs that will be exercised (such as the legs for runners). The increased circulation in the exercised extremities may cause the insulin to be absorbed too quickly. Exercising in hot weather may also speed up absorption; exercising in very cold weather may slow down insulin absorption. Due to high blood sugar levels, diabetics often have poor circulation and reduced sensation in the legs and feet. Thus any foot problems that result from exercise, such as blisters and calluses, should be treated promptly to avoid serious complications.

Not only can exercise help a diabetic manage the disease, it may very well prevent it. A study conducted by Dr. Ralph Paffenbarger, D.P.H., and others at Stanford University Medical School and the University of California at Berkeley, of 5,990 men ages thirty-nine to sixty-eight detailed the protective benefits of exercise to adult-onset diabetics. They found that every 500 calories burned in weekly exercise—the exercise equivalent of about 5 miles of running or walking at a brisk pace—lowers the risks of diabetes by 6 percent. Compared to sedentary men, those who burned about 2,000 calories each week (about 20 miles of running), decreased their risk by about 24 percent.

Why? The researchers believe that regular exercise not only reduces body fat but also improves the body's ability to metabolize glucose, or blood sugar. The researchers stress that the key is to exercise regularly or the body will revert to a less efficient glucose metabolism. They also indicated that these results should hold for women, too. And a study at Brigham and Women's Hospital in Boston corroborates that opinion. Dr. JoAnn Manson and colleagues studied 87,253 women over an eight-year period. Their conclusion: Women who participated in regular vigorous exercise —long enough to produce a sweat at least once per week—reduced the risk of developing adult-onset diabetes by 33 percent.

Epilepsy

I have coached several epileptic runners in my running classes. I think epileptics, like asthmatics, are unnecessarily sheltered and protected. If you are an epileptic, I encourage you to be active and to run. In fact, running may even help lessen the effects of this disease. Scandinavian studies have shown that people who are in good physical shape are less likely to have seizures than sedentary people. But be sure that your exercise and medication program are coordinated and medically supervised.

Epilepsy is characterized by recurrent convulsions that range from body-jerking seizures (grand mal) with loss of consciousness to milder transient spells (petit mal). Epileptics who have seizures that are not well controlled should exercise with a partner. If you have to run alone, do so in a well-populated area that is free from heavy traffic. You should also wear identification that will alert others to your condition and help them respond quickly and correctly if you have a seizure.

Hearing Impaired

People with hearing loss or impairment may also be in poor physical condition for two reasons, said Toshi d'Elia, a world-class masters runner and a teacher at the New York School for the Deaf in White Plains, New York. First, they often don't breathe well. This may be caused by the fact that many hearing impaired people have never learned to breathe and vocalize. Second, they may have been overprotected and held back from physical activity for most of their lives. A hearing-impaired person may also not have a good sense of balance. They lack confidence to run, or even to move quickly.

To restore their confidence, I suggest a walking program that gradually moves to fast walking and then running. Running on a track is generally safe. Roads are not. Hearing-impaired runners, therefore, should train with runners who have normal hearing when running near traffic.

Orthopedically and Neurologically Impaired

These are men and women with conditions of musculoskeletal impairment like spina bifida and muscular dystrophy, or neurological impairments like cerebral palsy, multiple sclerosis, or impairments associated with trauma, like amputations.

As I said, no one should be barred from fitness workouts because of any impairment. Check with your doctor to discuss any possible restrictions to your exercise program. Special programs for everyone with a disability are increasingly available and as much as possible everyone with an impairment should be in a regular fitness and sports program. The orthopedically impaired, for example, can use artificial legs, as Dick Traum did, or crutches or wheelchairs.

And Traum is not alone.

Senator Robert Kerry (D.-Neb.) is an amputee who enjoys keeping fit. So does Edward Kennedy, Jr., son of Senator Ted Kennedy (D.-Mass.), who is a fitness enthusiast despite having had a leg amputated because of bone cancer. Daniella Zahner was a world-class skier from Switzerland who severely injured her legs in a car accident. She set a world record by running the 1991 New York City Marathon in 4:13—on crutches!

Linda Down is one of the original members of the Achilles Track Club. She has cerebral palsy. She ran the 1982 New York City Marathon on crutches and finished well after dark in more than eleven hours. But she finished. Her effort was documented on nationwide television and earned her a trip to the White House, where she received special congratulations from President Ronald Reagan. "I discovered I can stress my worst aspects—my legs and my body—and still be successful," Linda said. "And if I can take care of my worst aspects and be a success, then imagine what I can do with my best aspects. The focus is on what I'm able to do rather than what I can't do."

At one time Darlene Wojiski, who has multiple sclerosis, a progressive disease of the central nervous system, was numb from her shoulders down. Her doctor told her that she would never be able to walk without a walker. So she took up running, building to 20 miles a week. "People say I'm crazy to run," she told *Runner's World*, where she's employed. "Maybe so, but I believe staying healthy and fit will help my chances of not having another bad attack. . . . Sometimes I feel so tired, I could just shut my eyes and fall asleep. But running gives me energy. If I don't run for a couple of weeks, I feel terrible." Dr. Randy Shapiro, director of the Fairview Multiple Sclerosis Center in Minneapolis, adds, "Running won't improve the MS. But it does improve health, and when you're healthy you feel better and you perform better overall." This lesson also holds true for many other physical disabilities.

Visually Impaired

Partially sighted people can participate, with some limitations, in many exercise programs. Those who are totally or nearly sightless can also walk or run while holding a rope attached to a sighted running partner. Or they may walk and run close enough to touch or be touched by a sighted runner.

Mort Schlein, one of my sightless running students, started exercising in the stairwell of his apartment building. Now he says, "Most people think it's incredible that a blind man can run. I don't know why. Blindness doesn't affect my feet, only my eyes. I move my feet like everyone else."

Cyril Charles injured his eyes playing cricket in Trinidad at the age of nine. An excellent athlete, he could only see shadows. Ten years later Cyril learned of a race for handicapped runners sponsored by the Trinidad & Tobago Road Runners Club. It offered first-place prize money equal to two weeks of his pay, so he entered. Despite no training, Cyril took off in a sprint and held on to win. A few months later, Cyril ran his first New York City Marathon and finished in 3:47 with an Achilles Track Club guide to keep him on course. He moved to Philadelphia and every Tuesday took the train to New York to work out with the Achilles club. But Dick Traum was soon on the phone to me. "Cyril is too fast for us," he exclaimed. "Will you take him?" So Cyril Charles started running with our New York Road Runners Club classes—and was too fast for most of them!

In 1989, with the assistance of the Achilles Track Club and the New York Eye and Ear Infirmary, Dr. Richard Koplin, director of the hospital's Eye Trauma Center, volunteered to try to restore Cyril's eyesight. Dr. Koplin did a cornea transplant and the next day Cyril Charles could see clearly for the first time in nineteen years.

One evening two years later I was running in Central Park. I spotted Cyril and as he approached I instinctively called out, "Cyril, good to see you." Recognizing my voice, he flashed a large smile and said, "Bob, glad to *see* you!" I suddenly realized that after all those grueling workouts I had put him through, Cyril had never seen my face. Inspired by his determination, I offered Cyril a job. First he worked with our youth program. Now he coaches our beginner's running classes, and each year he serves as a guide in the New York City Marathon for a blind runner.

Cyril's story is inspiring—in fact, it has been in *Reader's Digest* and a television movie on his life is under way. But he would be the first to admit that the person with a health challenge has to go out and make things happen. You can't sit back and feel sorry for yourself or let someone else take over your life.

Yes, You Can

If you are health challenged in any way, and you are still sitting there thinking you can't exercise, read these stories again. These are real people, just like you.

It's almost impossible to have a physical disability so severe that you cannot exercise. For example, Robert Wiegand "runs" marathons despite having no legs. He picks up his body with his arms and moves it forward. Although he may take days, Wiegand finishes every marathon he starts.

Dan Winchester, who has a Ph.D. in developmental psychology, suffers from cerebral palsy and has impaired speech and hearing as well as limited use of his arms and legs. Yet he sits in his wheelchair and kicks at the ground with his feet to propel himself backward to the finish line of marathons.

One of my all-time favorite stories is about Pat Griskus. He lost a leg in a motorcycle accident and spent several years putting on weight, drinking too much, and feeling sorry for himself. Then he started lifting weights, then swimming, and then running. Despite a below-the-knee artificial leg, Pat could outsprint almost all the runners in our advanced competitive running classes. He went on to run fast times from the mile to the marathon. Pat even raced 8 miles up the road to the top of Mount Washington, the highest peak in the eastern United States. Tragically, while training for the grueling Ironman Triathlon in Hawaii, Pat Griskus was hit by a truck and died. His life is still an inspiration of grit, determination, and sweat overcoming handicap.

Or take my old friend Sandy Davidson, a Scotsman who works at the United Nations. Sandy was partially paralyzed by a stroke and walked with the aid of a cane. He took up running with the Achilles Track Club and completed the 1983 New York City Marathon in 10 hours, 15 minutes—accompanied by his proud wife, Wilma. Sandy ran with his own style: a brisk run-walk using his cane for balance. He returned the next year and ran the marathon a hour faster—without the cane! His doctors are still trying to figure out how he did it.

I've saved Zoe Koplowitz for last, but only because she finishes last every year in the New York City Marathon. Despite that, Zoe is a winner. She has had multiple sclerosis for more than twenty years. But during the first fifteen years she was getting worse and worse. Fed up with feeling frail and helpless, Zoe decided in 1988 to fight back. She began to train for the marathon. By 1994, she had finished the New York City Marathon seven times and placed last each year. Her slowest time was in 1993, at age forty-five, when she crossed the finish line in 27 hours, 45 minutes. More than three dozen runners from all over the world celebrated her remarkable achievement. As she crossed the finish Zoe was greeted by a group of elite French runners singing "La Marseillaise." Some Mexican runners, who had seen her run by their hotel, cheered wildly and gave her roses and kissed her. Grete Waitz, the Norwegian who has been the top woman New York City Marathon winner nine times, was there. The New York City Marathon record holder for most wins presented the record holder for most last place finishes with her race medal. They hugged and cried. For days after her marathon, Zoe Koplowitz was telling anyone who would listen that disabled people have the same needs, wants, and feelings as everybody else. "They just move at a different pace, that's all," she said.

In her bedroom, Zoe hangs a poster over her bed: "The race is not to the swift, but to those who keep on running." Whether your disability is MS or your sedentary lifestyle, running can keep you on the road to happiness and better health.

THIRTY-ONE

Kids on the Run

I like to see children exposed to running at an early age, but not forced into it. Be sure that this experience is positive, successful, and *fun*. Running is a natural extension of play for children. We need to encourage kids to enjoy running as play at a young age and continue running throughout their lifetime—for fitness and fun.

I learned a lot from running with my son. Chris's first exposure to running was captured by television cameras! I still have a tape of it, which he likes to watch with me every year on Father's Day—our running anniversary. He was one month old at the time and I convinced the New York Road Runners Club to add a "pee wee" race before its regularly scheduled race on Father's Day, 1981. It was a big hit for the age six and under boys and girls, but perhaps even a bigger hit with the parents. My dad and I walked and jogged the quarter-mile pushing Chris in his baby carriage. One of the local TV stations interviewed us and Chris was so excited about his "run" that . . . well, he fell asleep during the interview. Nevertheless, he seemed to like the movement that came with the exercise, so I became one of the first runners to invest in a Baby Jogger.

Now, that was great fun! Not only did I solve the problem of how to get in my run when it was my turn to be in charge of the baby, but Chris seemed to really enjoy it. He got plenty of fresh air and best of all, he was with his dad. As he got older he would laugh and giggle while I talked to him on the run. He would take in the sights and then doze off for his nap. Soon he began to take charge. He began to toss toys out as we ran along to see if I would stop running. Perhaps the funniest moments came when he began mimicking Dad, the coach. He would shout out at runners who passed us in the park, "Faster! Faster!" I'll never forget those precious times together, on the run. Eventually, not too long after his first birthday, he began to demand to get out of the Baby Jogger so he could play. Enough of this spectator sport stuff. So I began to take fitness breaks during my runs. We'd stop at grassy fields so he could get out and run around and explore the terrain his way.

I'm convinced that this initial, positive exposure through baby stroller running was good for him. At least it was fun for me. After all, I got to do my two favorite things at the same time: run and show off my son.

The next phase of his running was racing Dad. We played this game often. He loved to run to an object and back at full speed, always beating me. It was loads of fun! I would always play it up. Sometimes I would take the lead near the end and express shock that he outkicked me. Other times I would proclaim "Watch out, here I come," and sprint after him only to be nosed out at the finish line.

We moved on to "Tom Sawyer adventure walks." By then he was four years old. Like most kids, Chris loved to explore. Ask a kid "Who wants to go out and exercise?" and you won't get your desired response. Try saying "Who wants to go exploring?" instead and watch how your child's enthusiasm increases. Off we would go to Central Park, me (Huckleberry Finn) and my son (Tom Sawyer). Sometimes we'd bring along some of his friends and give them names, too. You need quite an imagination for this special type of "fartlek." We climbed up and down "mountains" looking for the treasure hidden by the pirates. Whenever we saw signs of pirates —such as discarded bottles of beer or whiskey and cigarettes (pirates enjoy things that are bad for you)—we would take off running. The game would go on and on as we explored the backwoods and trails of the park for distances ranging from 1 to 6 miles. We would return home with wild stories to tell our friends and a continuation plot to look forward to on the next adventure.

Next, the big deal was tag games. I'd round up a bunch of kids and off we'd go to a playground or park. The more obstacles—hills, slides, ladders, tunnels—the better. They would make up the rules (I never understood them) and I'd just cheer them on as they ran and ran, having fun.

Chris didn't run in a structured way until the first grade. His physical education teacher trained the kids by running a half-mile and then a mile in preparation for the school's annual 1.5-mile fun run around the reservoir in Central Park. This running was fun for Chris because he did it with his friends.

Let the child decide—like mine did, and still does—when and how often he or she wants to run. Don't push them. We cannot and must not force our kids to run with us. But we should encourage them to run. It's important that they enjoy running. Otherwise, they will quit this form of exercise. To keep them motivated, parents and teachers need to think like children. That may be my greatest advantage when working with kids. I'm always being told that I act like a six-year-old—well, okay, a two-year-old! I try to break the boredom of running for kids with their limited attention spans with walking, skipping, hopping, and other fun movement breaks. For very young preschoolers, brisk walks and a few dashes let their enthusiasm erupt.

The trick for any age—adults and kids—is to keep running fun. This may mean running with one's peers or as a family group. If you run with the kids, follow their lead, and when they want, chase them through fields, pick flowers, and play games along the way. Young kids don't think like adults. They could care less about the cardiorespiratory benefits of aerobic exercise or the value of 20 minutes of continuous running. They just want to explore, have fun with their friends and their parents, in bits and pieces, at their own pace, at their will—not yours.

Older children, like adults, enjoy talking during the run (or walk or bike ride) to pass the time. A good 30-minute conversation on the run is a great way to find out what your child is doing and thinking, and both of you will be surprised at how fast the time will fly. Running removes much of the stress and communication barriers that stand between parent and child, enabling both to open up and express their feelings in a more relaxed way.

Most kids will develop a positive attitude toward exercise if they're allowed to develop at their own pace. Don't push them. Make the early experience positive, successful, and fun. They might want to run for a few days and then move on to something else, returning on and off to running. As long as they are exercising and happy, you should be satisfied. Don't lose sight of the ultimate goal—that your child should run to meet his or her physical and emotional needs, not yours.

Here's a few tips for running with kids at various ages.

Baby Stroller Running

Back in the early 1980s, people would take our picture while I was pushing Chris down the road and exclaim, "Look at that family running together!" We were a novelty back then; now I see baby stroller runners every day in the park. I even organized a Baby Stroller Running Clinic and Fun Run for the New York Road Runners Club. We wanted to encourage families with babies to run together. We had a diaper drawing: The parents tossed a diaper with their babies' name on it into a baby carriage and the winner received a pair of Nike baby running shoes. It was a lot of fun. Best of all, between the clinics and my own experience pushing my son through miles of running, I learned a lot. Here are some of my tips for safety and training.

- If you have a baby, don't give up running. It might even be a good time to start. Put the little nipper in a baby stroller, and push him or her around your favorite running route. Baby stroller running is a great way for mothers who may have stopped running while pregnant to get back into the activity. Start with brisk walking while pushing the stroller. The resistance of the stroller will push up your heart rate. Then, alternate slow jogging with walking until you can run pushing the stroller for 20 minutes without stopping. You won't be able to run as easily since you can't use your arms to propel you along. Run at about the heart rate level you would run at without the stroller. This may mean slowing your pace by a minute per mile or more. Run at an easy pace so as not to overexert yourself. Once you are fit and ready for more of a challenge, push the baby and stroller up hills. You'll find that the increased weight will make you work a lot harder.

▪ Think first of the safety of your child, not your workout. Running at high speeds lessens your ability to control the stroller. Walk down steep hills rather than risk losing control. Walk or stop if any sign of danger appears, such as bikers coming toward you at full speed. Your best bet is to run in parks at times when they are not congested. Do not run on roads with car traffic.

▪ *Do not* run in races pushing your child in a stroller. Show him or her off before or after your race. Consider the following guideline:

> The Road Runners Club of America strongly recommends against the participation of baby strollers/joggers in road races and against race organizers creating baby stroller divisions.
>
> The reason for this recommendation is that the inclusion of strollers in races increases the potential for injury to race participants and the children.
>
> The RRCA has no objection to and does not discourage the safe and prudent use of strollers or baby joggers in training situations.

▪ Use only a well-made stroller with good shock absorption. Do not use lightweight, collapsible strollers with small front wheels that pivot. They are made for walking the streets, not running. The front wheels may catch in a crack and catapult both baby and running parent. Standard, sturdy baby carriages may be used but are heavy and awkward for running. Specially designed strollers are available for runners that are comfortable for both baby and parent. Among the companies offering these products: Racing Stroller (the pioneer in the field with the Baby Jogger), TRI Industries, Huffy, Weebok, and Run About.

▪ Dress your child more warmly than yourself. Your body temperature will rise as you run, but the child is sitting still. Further, the wind resistance will cause the baby to be cooler as well. Be sure to bring extra clothing with you to keep you both comfortable. Don't forget the diapers! Be especially careful in cold weather to protect the baby's skin from frostbite and in sunny weather to protect against the sun. Use hats and blankets as a shield and don't forget sunscreen. Accessories available include sun and rain shields, and extra carrying baskets.

- Bring along some toys to keep the baby occupied. You may want to tie them to the stroller. (Why didn't I think of that before?)

- The baby should be strapped in very securely. A full harness is best.

- Choose a stroller with a hand brake. It is a big help when you're trying to get your baby in and out, and it can help slow you down when you need to stop. A wrist tether is also recommended so that you and baby stay together.

- Most running strollers come with protective devices to keep little fingers away from moving spokes.

- Look for a stroller with easily adjustable handles to fit the height of both Mom and Dad. This is important to your running comfort.

- A key feature is how easy the stroller can be folded up for storage and transportation. You'll want to be able to stick it in the car for a drive to the park for a run.

- Pick a stroller that is easy to run with in terms of speed, maneuverability, and ruggedness. It should be lightweight but sturdy and able to roll smoothly over roads as well as easily make it over curbs and rough terrain. With practice you will master the steering. There are two methods of turning: stop and turn after popping a wheelie, or turn in a wide, gentle arc (the safest and the best choice).

- When in doubt, get the highest-quality stroller. It isn't hard to find someone who wants a used one.

- Increase the baby's comfort by shifting the child to different positions during the run. Be prepared to take breaks and let the kid out for his or her exercise.

- You'll find that the motion soothes the baby and often will put him or her to sleep. So if the kid is getting on your nerves, a run will do you both good. When the little one is getting cranky and is overdue for a nap, head out the door.

■ Talk to your child throughout the run, pointing out things of interest along the way. Build your parental bond by making baby, no matter what age, part of the run.

Preschool Runners

The best way for parents to introduce young children to running is to make it a natural part of their play. Encourage them to run with you and after you while playing baseball or soccer. Let them chase you up and down hills while playing hide-and-seek in the park. When the family walks to the playground or home from school, break into a jog occasionally for a change of pace. Don't force young children to run for long, as very few of them will enjoy nonstop running over any substantial distance. Instead, use your imagination to integrate running into all aspects of your child's play.

Most preschool kids think of running as nothing more than a playtime activity, and that's exactly the way it should be. Even at this age parents can get too involved and push their kids to compete against their peers. Let the kids exercise for themselves, not you.

I've had several experiences that illustrate the lack of competitive instinct in preschoolers. In 1973, I directed a youth track program in Rome, New York. One evening, we attracted hundreds of kids and adult spectators to a big meet. I had decided to add a new event—"the Pee Wee 440"—and anxiously awaited the results. This was my first experience with four- and five-year-old runners. About twenty kids fidgeted around the starting line of the one-lap race around the school track. They didn't understand the commotion, but they liked the excitement.

When the race started, many parents ran along cheering madly for their little ones. Less than 100 yards into the race, however, the lead runners caught sight of the long-jump pit beside the track. Naturally, they assumed it was a sandbox, and that pretty much ended the race. The kids veered off into the "sandbox" because it looked like more fun than continuing to run around the track.

Chris's first race as a runner was a pee wee event. He was five years old and I had been organizing pee wee runs for the New York Road Runners Club since he was two years old. He could have participated at that age but he didn't want to, and I didn't force him. Instead, he would go to the races and simply watch. He enjoyed that and I never suggested that he enter. Rather, because of my background and notoriety as a running coach and author, I played down running as an exercise option for him.

One day, Chris finally asked if he could enter a race to win a finisher's ribbon. He did and he loved it. I later gave him one of my old trophies with a new inscription: "Chrissy's First Race." It still occupies a cherished spot in his room.

He enjoyed his experience so much that he invited a few friends to our next pee wee run. At the start, Chris bolted off the line and soon was in second place. I was standing nearby, biting my tongue so I wouldn't start yelling for him, when he suddenly stopped and looked back.

Chris stood there, searching behind him, while more than half the field ran past. Finally, I saw him waving to someone, and I realized that his friend David Pena was jogging toward him. David was running his first race, and Chris was obviously concerned about him. The two of them held hands and ran together all the way to the finish. Later, I asked Chris why he had stopped. "I was worried that David would get lost," he told me, "and anyway it was more fun running with my friend." I was prouder of him at that moment than if he had "won" the race. Fellowship and fun takes priority over winning for youngsters, as it should.

If the kids want to run, encourage preschoolers to sprint short distances—maybe a few yards on the track to a sandbox. They may wish to build up to once around the local track or even around the block. Praise them for trying, no matter how fast or slow they run, how many times they stop. Run against them, letting them beat you to boost their self-esteem.

Our pee wee program with the New York Road Runners Club is designed to develop an awareness and joy of running for kids ages two to six. The program has attracted as many as 500 kids to the half-dozen events the NYRRC hosts each year, held prior to adult races. The pee wees are divided into groups by age: The two- to four-year-olds run between one and three blocks. Five- and six-year-olds run a quarter-mile—five city blocks. The kids all get cheered on by their parents and the adults waiting for their race. Thus, they develop a feeling that running is fun and something that adults encourage. At the finish line everyone is a winner; each kid gets a brightly colored participation ribbon!

Elementary School Runners

Kids pick up most of their attitudes about fitness and exercise during these years. This is the time to emphasize running for fun. The fact is, real fitness results can't be achieved by preschoolers. By adolescence, it is very difficult to change one's lifestyle, so good fitness habits should be established early on.

If your child volunteers to run with you, do so at his or her pace for as long as they remain interested. This could be once around the block or a few miles. If you run with your kids, here's a tip to keep them going: talk, talk, talk. This will keep their minds off the actual running. Discuss their favorite toys and movies, bring up the family's vacation plans, and, of course, make use of the time to catch up on your child's school and social activities. You'll have to jog and walk slowly to allow for all this chatter, but there's nothing wrong with that.

You can also encourage your child to participate in activities in which they do a lot of running without realizing it, such as soccer and tennis. Biking, skating, dancing, jumping rope, and swimming are other fun aerobic activities. Many kids enjoy riding their bikes or skating to accompany parents on the run. This can be a great way to get in your run while chatting with your kid. Establish a good motivation base for a lifelong interest in aerobic exercise, not just running.

As the pee wees in our New York Road Runners Club program, including Chris and his buddies, outgrew our age-six-and-under program, I organized a series of youth fitness runs that take place right after the little ones finish. The kids run out a quarter-mile and then turn around and head back to the start. One loop is a half-mile and two loops is a mile. Kids are allowed to stop at the halfway mark and get a finishers ribbon, but most are motivated to continue on to complete the mile. This is a fun run, not a race. If they choose to do so, the kids can look up at the finish line clock to see their time and compare it to the health-fitness standards for their age (see Figure 31.1).

Teenage Runners

You can't tell a teenager to do anything, let alone run 30 minutes, three times a week to prevent a heart attack in middle age. A better bet might be to tell them not to run. Then, they might take off running!

Encourage your teenager to do anything physical—swimming,

tennis, hiking. Encourage, make things available, but don't push. Fortunately, mountain biking and in-line skating are cool and acceptable to teens as this book goes to press. Chris enjoys those activities, but seldom runs. He will, however, bike along with me on some of my runs. At least he had a good experience as a preschooler and grade schooler and may even get back to it some time in the future.

Most teens exercise far less than younger kids. First, their interest in sports diminishes as school teams get more and more selective and competitive. Second, they feel self-conscious about being seen doing anything that doesn't conform. If you're lucky, your teen will join the school soccer, tennis, swimming, or track team and get plenty of exercise while having fun being with friends. The best sport in my opinion to build a love of running for teens is cross-country. Most cross-country teams welcome kids of all abilities. Unlike football, basketball, or baseball, cuts aren't necessary and everyone can participate. Encourage your teen to give the school team a try. On second thought, show very little interest in it but make sure they know about the option. After they join up and enjoy it, then you can safely jump in and show your support, as long as you don't try to tell them what to do. Don't be surprised if your teen is embarrassed to be seen running with Dad or Mom. Be patient (they tell me), it's just part of the growing up process.

Training

"Children are not miniature adults," says Greg Payne, P.E.D., professor of human performance at San Jose State University in California. "Physiologically and psychologically, the two differ dramatically." Kids won't keep running if it isn't fun. They don't care about the health benefits.

Various studies show conflicting results about the trainability of prepubescent children. A position statement by the American Academy of Pediatrics (AAP) states that kids can improve their aerobic fitness by running; however, improvement is likely to be half to two-thirds that of an adult. It's hard to compare exactly because, according to the AAP, the aerobic capacity of a child's body changes as he or she grows. Who cares! This is the position of Professor Payne. He stated, "From a practical viewpoint, we shouldn't care what our children's max VO_2 values are, only that they are healthy and physically active. I suggest parents downplay intense training for their children and focus instead on correct technique and fun. Kids will still improve this way, only less stressfully."

Indeed, I've found that kids could greatly improve their times for the one-mile run by only running once or twice a week for distances as short as a half-mile. But then these kids were active doing other sports and activities as well.

It would be ideal for kids to run or do other aerobic activity at least three times a week. Here's the general training program I recommend for various ages:

Grades K–3: Build gradually to 1 mile or 10 minutes of running.

Grades 4–6: Build gradually to 2 miles or 20 minutes of running.

Grades 7–12: Build gradually to 3 miles or 30 minutes of running.

There are many recommended training programs for elementary school kids and teens. Some work for some kids, but not for others. Parents and teachers should pick the system that best fits the kids you are working with. If it doesn't work, try it a different way. This isn't science. Remember, the goal is to establish a baseline of fun-filled fitness for a lifetime. Here are some methods that might work for your child:

Run for time. The adult beginner runner's programs detailed in Chapter 10 may work for many kids, especially teens. The goal is to alternate running and walking for a certain time period until your child can run the full time nonstop while smiling and talking. You might want to adapt the program to a 5- or 10-minute routine for younger kids, instead of my 20- or 30-minute program.

Run for distance. Many kids prefer a tangible goal. After all, you can't see 10 minutes but you can see what four laps of a track looks like. Pick distance goals to run, starting with a half-mile. The kids, for example, can run half a lap on a track (220 yards), and then walk the remainder of the lap. Then repeat it to complete a half-mile. When they feel ready, have them run a full lap followed by a half-mile walk, and then another full lap of running. Later, they will be ready to run a half-mile without any walk breaks. After two weeks, have them move up to running three-quarters of a mile (again, taking walk breaks as needed). A week or two after that, have them try a full mile. Following this system, your child may move up to 2 or 3 miles of running. But even running a half-mile or a mile a few times a week will help get your kid fit and prepare him or her for a lifetime of fun running.

Run intervals. Many kids are bored running slow and easy in a continuous workout. Add fast-paced intervals spaced by rest breaks and they'll have more fun and get in just as good—if not better—shape. The kids can run a certain time period (such as 1 or 2 minutes) at a fast pace followed by equal time as a recovery walk, or they can run a certain distance (such as half a lap or a full lap) followed by an equal distance recovery walk. Of course, you can mix up the distances and time periods run to add variety. You can also keep things interesting by interjecting skipping, hopping, running backwards, racewalking, and imaginative exercises such as "run like a monkey." If you have a group of kids, relay races can keep things moving and fun.

Play games. Who says running has to be structured. Remember the fartlek runs described in Chapter 15? Well, kids enjoy "speed-play," too. But you need to do it with the imagination of a child. The Tom Sawyer adventure hike described earlier is one example of a running game. Shelly-lynn has a favorite theme game she plays with grades K–2 students in our sports club programs. She calls it "Road Runner" after the TV cartoon bird that likes to run to escape the coyote. The kids follow her across a field in a slow trot pretending to run like the Road Runner as they chirp "beep, beep." Then she announces, "Here comes the coyote," and the kids sprint to the nearest tree for safety. The run goes on and on until they have completed at least a half-mile or more. Most of the kids couldn't have run that distance in a slow, steady run; they would have gotten bored and quit. Keep things fun and the kids will keep on running.

The One-Mile Health-Fitness Standards

The American Alliance for Health, Physical Education, Recreation, and Dance developed noncompetitive goal-times (Figure 31.1) for the one-mile walk-run for kids ages five to eighteen. Encourage your child to achieve these goal times, which represent "the fitness level required to allow children to move into adulthood full of

FIGURE 31.1: YOUTH FITNESS GOALS
One-mile walk/run: minutes

	FITNESS GOALS	
AGE	GIRLS	BOYS
5	14:00	13:00
6	13:00	12:00
7	12:00	11:00
8	11:30	10:00
9	11:00	10:00
10	11:00	9:30
11	11:00	9:00
12	11:00	9:00
13	10:30	8:00
14	10:30	7:45
15	10:30	7:30
16	10:30	7:30
17	10:30	7:30
18	10:30	7:30

energy and free of degenerative diseases associated with low levels of fitness."

You might try an incentive system. For example, promise a fancy new pair of running shoes, a mountain bike, or pair of in-line skates (choose fitness gifts) once they achieve these one-mile time goals. If they are way behind the standards at first, give them intermediate goals to gain some success.

Competition

The American Academy of Pediatrics (AAP) recommends that pre-adolescent children not run long-distance races held primarily for adults. I strongly agree. Let the kids run against each other, not adults. Kids may benefit from running along with adults if the event is basically a fun run, or if the parent and child run together in a race and treat it as a fun run.

How far should they run? My guideline is that it may be okay for kids aged six to nine to run in adult-oriented low-key races up to 5K (3.1 miles) in distance; up to 10K (6.2 miles) for kids ages ten to thirteen. But the kids should be properly trained, well supervised by an adult who is running with them, and they shouldn't try to race competitively. In addition, the adult running with the child should be there to provide support, not attempt to push the child to run faster. Run at the pace that the child chooses—and take as many walk breaks and water stops as the child wishes to make. One additional rule: Participation in the event should be the kid's idea of fun, not just the parent's.

I prefer that kids aged thirteen and under run youth-only races of a quarter-mile to 1.5 miles—typical distances for competition on the track and for cross-country for kids this age. A few running clubs exist for kids this age. Some are good, some are bad. Don't allow your child to join one unless he or she really loves to run and wants to learn how to compete. Make sure the competition doesn't get out of hand and that the coaches emphasize sportsmanship and self-improvement, not just winning.

You can be successful without being too serious. I enjoyed coaching a team for Chris and his friends at school. They ran with me once a week and with the school gym class twice a week. Twice as grade-schoolers—competing against teams that held regular, serious practices—they won the National Age Group Cross-Country Championship over the rugged 1.5-mile course in Van Cortlandt Park in the Bronx.

What about teens? They may choose to run distances from a quarter-mile to 5K on their junior high or high school cross-country or track teams and should be encouraged to do so. Others will choose to enjoy a few local road races rather than compete on a team. Older teens have increased stamina over long distances and may compete, in my opinion, on a low-key basis in road races up to 10K in distance. A select few may train wisely enough and be able to pace themselves appropriately in order to run half-marathons. I do not recommend marathon training and racing until the late teenage years or older, when young men and women are better able to handle the training and the race distance physically and mentally. This is why the New York City Marathon and many other marathons have a minimum age requirement of eighteen. The "Students Run L.A." program described below, however, demonstrates that some high school students can benefit from marathoning if properly motivated and supervised.

Cautions for Kids on the Run

▪ The AAP recommends that children, as well as their parents, should be screened by a physician before starting a running program.

■ According to Dr. Lyle Micheli, director of Sports Medicine at the Children's Hospital in Boston, "Children are especially susceptible to overuse injury because of the specialized growth cartilage in their extremities and spine. During growth, this cartilage is weaker than the rest of the long bones and is more easily injured than mature adult cartilage."

■ The AAP warns that a child's body is not as efficient as an adult's in controlling its temperature. They don't generate as much heat in the winter, and so are at special risk for hypothermia. In hot weather, kids don't sweat as easily, and so heatstroke risk is increased. Make sure your child learns the value of drinking plenty of fluids. On hot, muggy days play it safe. Go swimming with your child, not running.

■ Just like for adults, it is important to wear well-cushioned shoes and to warm up, stretch, and cool down properly to minimize injury. Also, gradually build up the training. Too much too soon can be just as damaging to a young body as an old one.

■ The longest-lasting injury to kids is psychological. A California study by Dr. Harmon Brown found that after two years, half the children who started a running program had quit. After three years, 75 percent had stopped, and after four years, 85 percent weren't running at all. Why? Most of them had taken up long-distance running because of their parents. The impetus, of course, must come from the child, and support and direction from the parent. Never force kids to run or race. *Never.*

The biggest danger to running kids according to the AAP? Pushy parents! Let the kids run for fun, for themselves, and they'll be more likely to be lifetime runners.

The Unfitness Revolution
It used to be the kids who ran around the neighborhood while the parents sat inside. Now, in many families—perhaps even yours—the reverse is true. The parents go outside to run around and the kids are left inside.

"We are under the impression that youth are the most vigorous segment of the population," wrote Dr. Robert Gold, project director of the National Children and Youth Fitness Study (NCYFS).

"However, young and middle-aged adults are probably as fit or more fit than what appears to be the case among schoolchildren."

According to figures from the President's Council on Physical Fitness and Sports, at least half of all U.S. school-age children do not participate in enough vigorous exercise. That is, most of our kids don't work up an aerobic sweat for at least 20 minutes, three times a week—the minimum recommended for their parents to maintain an effectively functioning cardiorespiratory system. Thirty percent of boys ages six to twelve and 50 percent of girls ages six to seventeen can't run a mile in less than 10 minutes—a feat accomplished by most middle-aged joggers, and many senior citizens. Not only are most of our kids below standard for aerobic fitness, they also score poorly in muscular fitness. Of kids ages six to twelve, 40 percent of boys and 70 percent of girls can muster enough strength to complete only a single push-up.

Kids don't follow good wellness practices either. Studies from the University of Michigan indicate that 50 percent of all children in kindergarten through grade twelve have at least one risk factor for heart disease. A study from the University of California's Center for Adolescent Obesity reported that nearly one-third, or about 20 million, school-age children are overweight.

Causes of Unfitness
What is causing this unfitness epidemic? There are four major areas of concern:

- Lifestyle

- School programs

- Community programs

- Parental role models

Lifestyle
The decline in youth fitness among American children today is directly related to the way we live. Technology and cultural changes have turned our children into watchers instead of doers, undermined their nutrition, and created a stressful, hectic lifestyle. We are paying a price for the conveniences our ancestors didn't have—and the price is the health of our children.

Our kids sit almost all day. They ride everywhere. As a kid I walked to and from school, but now kids in my neighborhood take the bus. I used to ride my bike to get around town, but today kids are driven everywhere by their parents for safety reasons. We have more highways and cars and this limits where our kids can run, bike, and walk on their own. The old ritual of rushing home from school so we could play outdoors has almost disappeared. In most cases, parents can't allow their children to play outside unattended by an adult for safety reasons. After school, too often children come home to a parentless house. They may be "latchkey" kids, who open the door to an empty home, or are looked after by a baby-sitter. Exercise is not high on anyone's list at that time of day; quiet inactivity is. Fewer parents are home, and fewer kids are allowed or urged outside to play. The (in)activity of choice is watching television or the VCR, or playing video and computer games.

Passive forms of entertainment compete with vigorous activity for our children's time, and take the place of exercising. Television is the most serious culprit, accounting for twenty-five inactive hours a week for the average kid. "Children are living vicariously," says Dr. Joseph Zanga of the American Academy of Pediatrics. "Instead of playing sports, they watch sports. Instead of dancing, they watch rock videos."

School Programs

Many parents assume that the schools and community programs take care of our kids' exercise needs. But according to the NCYFS study, only 36 percent of students in grades five through twelve, the years when kids are growing most rapidly, take physical education daily. Many kids have only one or two physical education classes per week. Some, incredibly, have none. When my son entered a public school in New York City in the sixth grade, I was shocked to find that they had no physical education program. The kids had no physical outlet for their stresses, no opportunity to have fun exercising and playing sports. So I volunteered to start a program. For a full year I went to his school and had fun working out with Chris and his classmates twice a week. In the meantime, I lobbied with the state government to force the school to meet the minimum requirements by law for physical education. The following year the kids were very pleased to have regularly scheduled physical education classes with a trained instructor. By the end of the year, due to budget cuts, the program was dropped.

Clearly, parents need to lobby to improve physical education courses in their schools and to get the programs to stress more lifetime fitness classes, such as running for fun and fitness, rather than primarily the traditional regime of competitive sports. The emphasis on competition, especially in high schools, means that the active few entertain the passive many.

"We have to conclude that not enough time is spent in school or outside school on activities that would maintain a high level of cardio-respiratory fitness, such as running, swimming, bicycling or walking," wrote Dr. Gold of the NCYFS study. "The majority of activities are team and competitive sports and informal games, which don't promote fitness and are not the kinds of activities that will be pursued throughout life."

The American Alliance for Health, Physical Education, Recreation and Dance (AAHPERD) recommends elementary school children receive 30 minutes of quality physical education and secondary school children receive 45 to 55 minutes every day. By quality physical education, AAHPERD meant vigorous activity directed by a qualified instructor.

As I've said, most of our kids don't get enough exercise at school. But this doesn't have to be the case. Despite the fact that budget cuts have affected the quality and quantity of many public school physical education programs there are options. Parents, physical education teachers, classroom teachers, and school administrators can make fitness a priority at their school and their hard work and dedication can pay off. Many schools build a fitness program around running. Here's a few examples of the good work being done around the country:

- Public School No. 6 in New York City has a part-time physical education instructor whose salary is paid by donations from parents. My New York Road Runners Club running classes are headquartered at this elementary school, so we give an annual donation to fund a school track team that services over 100 kids. The boys and girls in the program learn to run for fitness and also compete in area races.

- Harvey Pachter is an example of where one teacher can make a difference. His 1.5-mile "Minithon" in the South Huntington,

New York, elementary schools is the culmination of a full-year physical education program with running as a centerpiece. He started the annual program in 1978 because he wanted to convey to youngsters the importance of physical fitness, of working toward a goal, and of developing self-discipline and determination. The Minithon is held each year during the first week of June and students train for the event starting in the fall. The training, which is integrated into the physical education curriculum, comprises the first 15 minutes of each 40-minute class. Students in all grades participate in running and fitness activities but the Minithon event is reserved for sixth graders.

Pachter gets a lot out of limited time—he also fits in motor-skill training and introduction to team sports for each class period. Each session of the twice-per-week program (he would prefer having the kids daily) includes 4 minutes of muscular fitness and flexibility training, 6 minutes of running (indoors or outdoors depending upon weather), and a 2-minute cool-down. This is followed by a 3-minute discussion about fitness, nutrition, weight management, stress control, and other important topics.

The program focuses on the excitement of the New York City Marathon. The students run laps that are translated into miles and each student charts his or her miles on a large map of the 26.2-mile New York City Marathon course. These kids see themselves, in their daily workouts, inching along the marathon route. They are ultimately classified in and receive certificates for one of five fitness levels, according to the level of fitness they have achieved during the course of the year.

Prior to the big event, there are many activities that help build excitement for the kids, and get the parents and community involved as well. At the schools, lectures and workshops are held on the do's and don'ts of running. Parents are sent reports on their children's progress for the year, and are invited to join them on group runs. Race numbers, water stops, and other special effects line the course to simulate the New York City Marathon experience. The event is played on local cable television, reported on in the local papers, and the town supervisor proclaims "Fitness Week" in honor of the graduating sixth-grade fitness enthusiasts. Afterward, the students return to their schools for an award ceremony and a "pasta party" organized by the P.T.A. All participants receive T-shirts and all finishers—all the kids—

get a certificate. This is a fitness run, not a race. The kids can walk as much as they want. The goal is simply to complete the 1.5-mile distance. Awards are given not to the fastest finishers, but to the kids who come closest to predicting their time.

▪ "Students Run L.A." had its beginnings as a challenge from teacher Harry Shabazian to seven of his students at Boyle Heights High School in East Los Angeles in 1987. Searching for a way to reach the troubled kids from a very rough neighborhood, he invited them to train with him for the Los Angeles Marathon. The challenge spread and by 1990 it was promoted by the Los Angeles Board of Education to include all high schools in the city. Students are overseen by teacher-leaders who train with them, compete with them in progressively longer weekend road races, and run the marathon with the kids. Many of Shabazian's students come from broken, dysfunctional families about which he says, "The only things they have been recognized for are failures."

The goal of training for the marathon gives them a purpose; finishing means success. The experience has a strong influence on their lives: The graduation rate from the tough Boyle Heights school is better than 75 percent for his runners, which is more than three times the school's average. Shabazian barks to his congregation on race morning: "When you go home today after this marathon, you're going to make your parents proud of you, you're going to make your friends envious, you're going to prove something to the people who didn't think you could do it. And all of them are going to respect you. You've come too far not to finish and bring home that finisher's medal." Some 1,500 students each year—all wearing bright yellow "Students Run L.A." caps—start and finish the race. As Shabazian summed up his program in a feature story in *Sports Illustrated*: "I like to think of us as the biggest gang in L.A. A good gang, as in, 'How's the gang?' All of us are having a gang experience we'll remember the rest of our lives."

▪ Junior Bloomsday is the largest kids race in the country, with over 10,000 participants. Kids ages four to twelve run distances ranging from one-half mile to 2 miles. The race is part of a broader program in the Spokane, Washington, area school system designed to show kids that exercise can be fun. "Fit for

Bloomsday" includes a ten-week running program in which kids can earn patches and certificates by accumulating and charting training mileage. Programs at some 100 area schools are led by physical education and classroom teachers. All program supplies are given to the schools by the Lilac Bloomsday Association and its sponsors. The organization also runs the Bloomsday 12K race, which attracts over 50,000 mostly adult runners. Held three weeks after Junior Bloomsday, the parent race draws thousands of Junior Bloomsday kids as well.

▪ The Long Beach (California) Mini-Marathon started as a small fun event for spectators to watch while waiting for finishers to come in for the Long Beach Marathon. With over 5,000 kids in the 2.62K event, the race is now bigger than the marathon itself. The "Mini" is the culmination of a semester-long running program involving 25,000 elementary school youth. Consisting of twenty-five class sessions, it's become an integral part of the Long Beach Unified School District's and area private schools' physical education curriculum. Students progress from walking to be able to complete the noncompetitive 2.62K fun run. Certificates are awarded for participation and for achieving mileage goals. An extensive training booklet sponsored by the Long Beach Marathon and a local hospital is made available to all participating schools.

Community Programs
Children have plenty of time for exercise after school, on weekends, and during summers. But communities offer too few programs to keep the kids active. Sports leagues keep many of them involved, but traditional youth sports programs such as Little League Baseball offer little exercise and no lifetime fitness benefits. Without health-related fitness activities—such as running, swimming, biking, tennis—community programs fall short of what is needed to help improve the fitness level of young Americans.

The Y's, Scouts, religious groups, town recreation programs, and other similar organizations should include more fitness activities along with their usual sports offerings. Communities need to do more than erect a few playgrounds and ball fields. It can be done! When I was fitness director for the Rome (New York) Family Y in the early 1970s, we had thousands of kids, from toddlers to teens, working up a sweat all over the Y. We emphasized activities that included plenty of fitness. Swimming and gymnastics clubs and teams were formed as were karate and dance classes. I started a youth track-and-field program highlighted by a meet under the lights on a Friday evening at the high school football stadium that attracted 500 kids and plenty of enthusiastic spectators.

Parents and community groups can make a difference. Take the case of New York City's Asphalt Green, which developed out of one of the most seemingly hopeless situations parents face: no play space combined with astronomically high real estate values. Several years ago, when an asphalt plant closed down, developers planned to use the block it had occupied for more high-rise luxury apartments. Just what the city needed! But then Dr. George Murphy and his Neighborhood Committee for the Asphalt Green sprang into action. "This really is an oasis, with all these high-rises around," said Dr. Murphy, "and they wanted to take away our last open space. What a vulgarity."

The committee gained control of the land and raised the funds to develop a recreation center and a large, bright-green artificial field for sports and recreation. Later, they added an Olympic-sized swimming pool. Thousands of kids each year benefit from the many fitness-related programs offered at Asphalt Green. Of course, I was quick to organize a kids running program on their big green field.

Cosponsored by the New York Road Runners Club, City-Sports-For-Kids is a track-and-field program for boys and girls ages five to fourteen. The program is based on three goals:

1. Promote physical fitness for youth

2. Develop self-esteem through success-oriented sports

3. Build bridges of understanding through play between boys and girls of various races and religions.

Each year 1,000 kids, including my son, Chris, enjoy this unique program, which consists of three eight-week sessions—track and field in the fall and spring; basketball and running in the winter. Kids start off each session with stretching exercises and then they are grouped by age and rotated each week during track season through eight different events: sprints, hurdles, distance run, high jump, long jump, shot put, relays, and tug-of-war. After two weeks of practicing the events, we have a competition each session in a different event. Although we award ribbons to the top finishers to acknowledge excellence, the emphasis is on fun and participation. All kids receive a colorful participation ribbon each week. The spring program is highlighted by enthusiastic competition on Mother's Day between the kids and the parents. The fall program climaxes in the Junior Marathon. The kids race a quarter-mile or half-mile into the actual finish line of the New York City Marathon exactly a week prior to the big marathon. Since the finish line area is already set up for the marathon, the kids get to soak in plenty of the premarathon excitement. All finishers receive a replica of the same medal New York City Marathon finishers earn.

Parents

We parents have a dual obligation to our kids' fitness. First, we should be good role models by exercising regularly ourselves. Second, we should take time to have fun working out with our kids. The NCYFS survey found that fewer than 30 percent of parents exercise at least three times a week, and about 60 percent of parents never work out with their kids in a typical week. By making fitness a part of your life, you teach your child to value it. *The Family Fitness Handbook* includes plenty of guidelines on how to have fun exercising with your kids.

The Challenge

The President's Council on Youth Fitness and Sports states that "Every youth serving agency, institution and organization at all levels, federal, state and regional, in both the private and public sector, should look critically at their responsibilities to improve youth fitness. Families can also provide encouragement and motivation towards good fitness habits. Youth must be self-motivated to develop physically and learn how to maintain at least a minimum of fitness throughout life."

But fitness is a learned lifestyle. Parents cannot assume that children will exercise on their own. Nor can parents simply rely on the schools and community—on others—to teach their children the fitness habit. They must supplement this educational process with family fitness activities themselves.

Children have four potential sources for exercise: free play; school physical education classes; community after-school, weekend, and summer programs; and family activity. To reverse the tide of the "unfitness revolution," we need to improve the opportunities for our children in each of these four exercise areas. As parents, you can immediately make a difference in two areas—family exercise and free play—and your efforts, and those of other parents, can change the other two.

While the statistics on the fitness of our kids is depressing, there's much we can do to turn them around, and a great place to begin is to get the kids, and yourself, up and running. To make changes will take commitment, time, and effort. But the result will be improvement in the health of our children. The habit of exercise begun in childhood is the gift of a lifetime.

Part X

Illness and Injury

THIRTY-TWO

Illness

How can you avoid the common cold and the flu? Can you run away from these and other illnesses by enhancing immunity with exercise? Should you keep running if you get sick? The following guidelines pertain to colds and flus but will also apply to other illnesses that may affect your running—and your health.

Ninety percent of us come down with acute respiratory conditions, primarily the common cold and flu, each year. The Centers for Disease Control (CDC) estimates that more than 425 million cases of colds and flus occur annually in the United States, resulting in $2.5 billion in lost workdays and medical costs. Despite millions of dollars spent in research, doctors have yet to discover a cure for the common cold and flu. Decongestants, cough suppressants, antihistamines, and other medicines only relieve some of the symptoms. Many runners have their own remedies that they swear by: chicken soup, peppermint and elder flower tea, wheat germ oil, high doses of vitamin C, Mexican food, bee pollen, even acupuncture. None of these will hurt you in moderation, and they may even make you feel a little better. Annual flu shots may minimize the effects of that disease and are recommended for those with existing health conditions, such as sensitive bronchials like myself.

No matter what your mom told you, going outside with wet hair, damp feet, exposure to drafts, running in the snow or rain, or working up a sweat and getting a chill won't cause a cold or flu. Only a virus can do that. There are two ways you can be exposed: by air or by touch. The virus can be passed on by people who sneeze or cough it into the air we breathe, or it can get into your body when you touch a virus-contaminated surface and then rub your nose, eyes, or mouth.

To elude these viruses requires a simple change of lifestyle— avoid all people! More likely, you can shun crowds and obviously sick people. You can also avoid sharing water bottles, towels, or food with others who might be carrying the virus. You should even wash your hands frequently when exposed, since the virus is carried from hand to face. But you can only do so much. Whatever precautions you take, the surest way to catch a cold or flu is to work with lots of kids. I work with more than 1,000 kids each year in my sports programs. I'm almost a sure bet to get sick at least once during the cold and flu season.

Exercising in cold weather can dry out the lining of the nasal passages, which makes it easier for bacteria and viruses to penetrate. Drink plenty of fluids to ensure that your nasal passages and mucous membranes stay well hydrated.

Your best defense is a strong immune system. Dr. David Nieman, an exercise physiologist at Appalachian State University in Boone, North Carolina, is acknowledged as a leading expert in this field. "If the viral war cannot be prevented," he says, "a strong defense system may win the day. As the viruses enter the body, they encounter a legion of nearly one trillion highly specialized cells that have the marvelous ability to identify and destroy foreign substances. Keeping this army vigilant and healthy is where you can get involved."

Lack of sleep, quick weight loss, and not eating a well-balanced diet have been linked to a weakened immune system. So have mental and emotional stress. A study by psychologist Sheldon Cohen and colleagues at Carnegie-Mellon University in Pittsburgh indicated that almost half of those subjects who were experiencing high stress came down with colds (after being exposed to the virus in the study) while only a quarter of those experiencing low stress got sick. That's double the risk!

But what about exercise? Many runners and other aerobic exercisers insist that their increased fitness encourages resistance to colds and flus. In a *Runner's World* survey of 700 runners, 60.7 percent reported that they had fewer colds since starting to run; only 4.9 percent claimed they had more. Okay, so runners think their running protects them from colds and flus. But what do the research scientists have to say about this?

Exercise and Immunity

A number of studies point to the fact that exercise, in moderation, may minimize illness, especially colds and flus. Research by Dr. Greg Heath at the CDC in Atlanta reports that runners have an average of 1.24 upper-respiratory tract infections per year compared to 2 to 5 per year for the general population.

The immunological benefits of moderate exercise were also reported by Dr. Nieman. In one study he placed a group of sedentary women on a fifteen-week walking program (coinciding with the autumn flu season) and compared their rates of illness with those of a similar group that did not exercise at all. He found that moderate exercise, up to about 45 minutes a day, appears to minimize illness. The exercise group averaged five sick days per person during the fifteen weeks; the nonexercisers averaged eleven days— more than twice as many!

Why do exercisers improve their immunity to some diseases? It may be because they increase the number of white blood cells and antibodies circulating through the bloodstream when they exercise. This increase in circulation caused by the exercise makes it easier for these virus-fighting cells to do their job.

What about serious exercisers? Dr. Nieman studied a group of serious runners who had averaged two marathons a year over the previous twelve years and compared them to a group of nonexercisers. He found that the serious runners had far greater natural killer cell activity (an average of 373 Lytic units versus 237 for the nonexercisers). According to Dr. Nieman, "The natural killer cells are the Marine Corps of the immune system. They're the up-front, highly active cells that launch the first attack on any infection."

It seems that if you adjust to a mileage level—whether it be ten miles per week or fifty—that your body can tolerate, then you may continue to improve immunity. But if you push the mileage and intensity up too much, particularly as you increase your training as a marathon approaches, then you may overwhelm your defenses to illness.

Dr. Nieman's research shows that intense training may weaken the immune system and make us vulnerable to infectious illness. Dr. Nieman, a marathoner, surveyed a group of 2,300 runners who trained for the Los Angeles Marathon. He found that more than 40 percent had at least one cold or flu episode when at increased mileage levels during the two months prior to the race.

The lowest odds of sickness were found in runners who trained at less than 20 miles a week—not enough mileage to be well trained for the marathon. Those who ran more than 60 miles a week averaged twice as many colds and flus than the lower-mileage runners.

But what about the affect of racing itself? Dr. Nieman's figures show that 12.9 percent of the high-mileage runners got colds during the week immediately following the marathon. By comparison, only 2.2 percent of the runners who trained for the race but didn't run it became ill during the same period. Dr. Nieman concluded that "The risk of upper respiratory tract infections may decrease below that of a sedentary individual when one engages in moderate exercise training, but this risk may rise above average during periods of excessive amounts of exercise."

Marathon runners in the Nieman study experienced a drop of 30 to 40 percent in the overall activity of their immune cells almost immediately after the race. Their immune systems remained suppressed for six to eight hours. A similar result takes place after shorter races or hard workouts, although it appears that the marathon itself is significantly more taxing on the immune system. Dr. Nieman argues that "exercise training sessions that are intense, long and exhausting can depress the ability of certain immune cells to function properly." This depression, however, is usually short-lived.

The 10- to 20-mile-per-week recreational runner tends to get sick less often than elite runners or sedentary people. But they, too, will see their immunity decrease following any strenuous run or race.

Research by J. Duncan MacDougall, Ph.D., and colleagues at McMaster University in Ontario, Canada, demonstrated that sudden increases in mileage and, particularly, training intensity suppress the immune system. The result is an increased susceptibility to infection, especially for the first couple of hours after an intense workout.

How do you know when your exercise level no longer protects you from illness, but rather may set you up for it? Dr. Nieman's answer: "If you've been working out consistently and are feeling good, you're probably found the right combination of rest and exercise to give your immune system the boost it needs. If you've been training hard and are feeling run down or ill, you may need to cut back on both the time and intensity of your workout. It may be that you're doing your immune system more harm than good. As with most things, everyone is different. Only you can determine what is the right amount of exercise for you."

You can enjoy competitive training and minimize your chance for illness by taking a few precautions. "For those athletes who must exercise intensely for competitive reasons," states Dr. Nieman, "several precautions can help decrease the risk of sickness. These include spacing vigorous workouts and race events as far apart as possible, eating a well-balanced diet, keeping other life stresses to a minimum, avoiding overtraining and chronic fatigue, and obtaining adequate sleep." You should also avoid people who have colds and/or flu symptoms and you might consider getting a flu shot if you plan to train and compete hard during the flu season.

Dr. Nieman's immunity research indicates that by keeping blood sugar up during and after long runs or races by ingesting a sports drink or other easily absorbed carbohydrates, you will enhance your immune system. He tested marathon runners on a treadmill and compared those who drank a sports drink before, during, and after a 2½-hour run with those who drank a noncarbohydrate placebo. The postexercise blood tests revealed that the sports drinkers had significantly lower levels of cortisol, a substance in the body that suppresses our immune response. Keeping blood sugar levels up kept the cortisol levels down, resulting in a stronger defense against illness.

Your attitude about your exercise program may also be a factor in keeping you healthy. Dr. Randy Eichner, professor of medicine at the University of Oklahoma, writes in *The Physician of Sportsmedicine*, "Whether exercise enhances immunity or impairs it may, in fact, depend on whether the exercise is a joy or a stress."

Should You Run When You're Sick?

I am asked this question every day. And I always give the same answer: "That depends on the severity of your illness."

Shelly-lynn answered the question this way in the newsletter of our New York Road Runners Club Running Class:

Got a sniffle in your snout? A tickle in your tummy? Should you run it out or stick it out in bed?

Mild exercise during sickness with the common cold does not appear to cause further problems. So, ok, when your nose runs —generally if that's all that's bugging you, you can run.

But what happens when the peak race is only a few weeks away and you have the flu—complete with fever? Should you gut it out "like a real runner"? You know, pack in the miles despite the pain?

Nope.

Symptoms of systemic involvement including fever, extreme tiredness, muscle aches, swollen glands, etc. are definite stop signs to training. Hard training during real illness may even spread the disease within your body, including your heart.

Respiratory infections including the common cold and flu symptoms are all potentially serious. Stressing the body with vigorous prolonged exercise during the height of a viral infection —or soon thereafter—can cause permanent damage to the heart. So when you've had the flu and are finally back on the road again, give yourself two weeks before any heavy duty training, like speed work and long runs.

So if it is the common cold, a sniffle in your snout so to speak, mild running is ok. But when there's lots more involved and your whole system is on end, cutting back your training may speed you down the road to recovery faster than pounding in the miles.

As always, when in doubt—see your doctor. Your body is your asset. Treat your training like an investment, protect it.

There is no medical evidence that mild exercise aggravates a cold. In fact, one study indicates that military recruits who were given bed rest at the first sign of illness did not recover faster than those who were kept in basic training exercises. Research by Thomas Weidner, Ph.D., and colleagues at Ball State University in Muncie, Indiana, suggest that exercising with a cold may have no impact on either the cold's severity or duration. Further, they found that there was no difference in exercise capacity with or without a cold.

Dr. Randy Eichner, chief of hematology at the University of Oklahoma, suggests using the neck test since the common cold is usually confined to the head. If your symptoms are located above your neck, such as a runny nose, sneezing, a slight headache, or scratchy throat, it is probably all right for you to run, but with caution. He suggests that you run at a reduced effort for a few minutes. If that clears your head and you feel peppy enough and not in pain, it should be all right for you to finish the run. "But if your head pounds with every step, go home and rest," he advises.

The flu, however, is more serious, as it affects the whole body. If you have symptoms below your neck, such as a fever, vomiting, diarrhea, severe fatigue, muscle ache, loss of appetite, or a hacking cough deep within your chest, Dr. Eichner advises you not to run. What's the gain? Exercising when you are this sick may prolong your illness. It might lead to more serious problems, even a life-threatening condition. Moreover, what's the fun? It is difficult and often unpleasant to work out when you're feeling lousy. Go to bed, drink plenty of fluids, and come back tomorrow or in a few days.

Dr. James Rippe, a cardiologist, warns: "Running with a high fever (above 101 degrees) isn't a good idea because for every degree that your temperature rises above normal, your cardiac output goes up 10 percent. So if you're exercising with a fever of 101.6 degrees [F.], you can easily push your body temperature to 103.6 degrees [F.], which puts a tremendous strain on the heart."

If your temperature is more than 100°F., wait until your fever breaks before resuming your running. The rule of thumb is to expect to feel terrible as long as your fever lasts, and then take twice that time to overcome the flu symptoms. Remember, if you have a cold or the flu, cut back on your mileage (or don't run at all), slow down your pace and run within the limitations of your energy.

Coming Back from Illness

Each type of illness requires a different treatment and different training method for recovery. A slight cold may be helped by short runs at a slow pace. A bad cold or flu demands complete rest. Never begin a program of recovery until your illness is on the mend. Your temperature and breathing should be normal and most of your aches and pains and other symptoms should be gone. Take your time getting out for a run. In fact, a walking program for a week or so might be wise until your strength returns. Then start your runs slowly and return gradually. Drink plenty of fluids and get lots of sleep to aid recovery.

You will be surprised how quickly you can lose your endurance. After a cold or the flu, your comeback may be even slower than following an injury. When you resume exercise, if you don't notice any daily improvement in your health and running, stop and rest some more. Do not train hard until you have completely recovered.

Relapses are common, so be careful. If you don't take time off and care for that illness, your layoff may be longer. Or you may injure yourself in other ways. Sometimes a cold or flu is actually a blessing: It may be a warning sign of overtraining and the layoff may actually prevent an injury.

Dr. George Sheehan advised testing yourself to see if you are ready to run yet: "Start your runs very slowly until you reach the point where you start to sweat. This usually takes about six minutes. At this point, you should feel like running no matter how you felt at the beginning. If you don't and five more minutes confirms it, pack it in."

I advise a runner who returns after illness to start first with 20 to 30 minutes of alternating running and walking. See how that goes for a few days. Only exercise every other day. Once you can run for 20 to 30 minutes comfortably, increase those runs gradually to the distance you normally run each day. But continue to run one day and rest the next. As you gain strength, ease back into the program you followed before your illness. Give yourself one or two days of building up for every day lost to illness. All of your runs should be done at a conversational pace and well within your training heart rate range. If you are a competitive runner, after training for at least one week at your normal training mileage, ease back into speed training by doing half of your normal workout at a reduced but brisk pace. If this goes well, you should be able to return to regular competitive training the following week. I wouldn't advise racing until you have been able to train without difficulty for at least two consecutive weeks.

The three Rs here are rest, relax, and recover.

THIRTY-THREE

Injury

There may be nothing worse than an injured runner! Fuss, fuss, fuss. Whine, whine, whine. Why? Why? Why?

Injury is part of an active life, but the risks can be minimized. It is safe to say at some point every runner will face an injury. Some runners always seem to be hurt while others claim they've never been injured (I don't believe them!). Most of us fall somewhere in between. The key is to recognize problems early and to promptly deal with both treating the injury and eliminating its cause.

The most vulnerable body parts are tissues and bones. Tissue includes muscles, tendons (fibers that connect muscles to bones), ligaments (fibers that join two bones), and cartilage (cushions between two bones). Most injuries are one of two types: acute or overuse. Acute injuries occur suddenly when stress is applied too abruptly for tissues not prepared to handle it. Examples include trauma, overstretching a cold muscle, and running fast without proper warm-up. Overuse injuries are caused when tissues are repeatedly stressed too much over a period of time. These injuries come on slowly and usually give warning signs.

Running injuries can be called "diseases of excellence." While striving to improve our fitness or racing times we are more prone to some injuries than those who don't exercise. Follow the training guidelines in this book to minimize that problem.

Once a runner adjusts to 20 to 30 minutes of running three to five times a week, he or she seldom gets injured. Indeed, studies show that very few people who run 6 to 9 miles or less a week need medical attention due to injury during a year's time. But when a runner increases mileage, adds speed training, and begins to race, the risk of injury increases. Don't untie your shoe laces yet: All sports include this danger. Accept the fact that it is a part of your sport, but learn how to prevent it. Don't give up in frustration if you develop a nagging injury. Learn how to manage it properly and how to adjust your running to keep in shape while recovering.

Fortunately, there are few permanent injuries caused by running. Long Beach, California, podiatrist Dr. John Pagliano and orthopedist Dr. Douglas Jackson studied 3,000 injured runners and reported to the American College of Sports Medicine (ACSM): "Distance running is associated with a low incidence of disabling injuries. Although running places a heavy load on the musculoskeletal system, particularly the back and lower extremities, very few of the injuries sustained will preclude the runner's return to his or her desired mileage and training program."

Most studies show that an elevation in the risk of injury is associated with miles run per week. According to podiatrist Dr. Murray Weisenfeld, author of *The Runner's Repair Manual,* most of the injuries he sees in his practice appear after mileage creeps past 30 or 40 miles a week, especially for those training for a marathon.

What gets injured most? Several studies report different findings but most agree that knee injuries lead the way followed closely by the feet. Others ranking high in approximate order of incidence: Achilles tendon/calf, hip/groin, ankle, shin splints, quadriceps, hamstrings, lower back.

Most running injuries have one or more of four types of causes: inherited physical weaknesses, improper health practices, environmental influences, and, perhaps the most frequent cause, training errors. Few overuse running injuries are caused by a single factor or event, such as one particular run or race. Underlying the occurrence of shin splints, for example, may be several contributing factors, such as poor running form, a biomechanically weak foot, tight calf muscles, and worn down running shoes. Most running injuries do not occur suddenly, although you might think so. They are caused by a gradual and often predictable overstressing of a susceptible part of the body. Your body will give off warning signals that injury is likely to occur and that an injury is in its first stages. Two ways to prevent injury are to identify and eliminate the causes, and listen to the warning signs.

An important part of running is learning to prevent injuries. Seldom do injuries occur as a result of accident; most often they seem to happen for no reason at all. But there *are* reasons. You just have to ask yourself some questions.

Questions to Ask When Injured

These are some of the questions I ask runners who become injured. The goal is to discover the reason or reasons you developed your problem. Often more than one factor is involved. The basic question is, What have you done differently in your running or your daily routine that may have caused the injury or illness? Use the following to help you determine the cause of your problem or, better yet, to help prevent a problem from occurring:

1. Are your feet or legs structurally weak? (Your doctor may have to answer this for you.)

2. Do you have good flexibility?

3. Do you warm up and cool down properly for all runs?

4. Do you stretch properly?

5. Are your opposing muscles weak? (Abdominals, quadriceps, etc.)

6. Do you have any previous injuries that might make you vulnerable?

7. Did you return from an injury too quickly?

8. Is your running form proper?

9. Have you made any changes in the quantity or quality of your runs: mileage, speed, hills, surface?

10. Has running on snow or ice changed your running pattern or form?

11. Are you undertrained for the races you are running?

12. Are you racing too frequently?

13. Are you taking time to recover from races and hard workouts?

14. Have you changed running shoes, or are they worn down, or have you started wearing racing shoes?

15. Has your weight changed? Are you overweight or underweight?

16. Is your diet adequate for your training level?

17. Are you taking proper care of your feet?

18. Have you changed any daily habits, such as driving or sitting more?

19. Are you under additional stress?

20. Are you getting enough sleep?

21. Have you been doing other sports that might affect your running?

22. Have you changed running surfaces, or are you running on uneven or slanted terrain?

Causes of Running Injuries

Here are some of the most common reasons runners become injured.

Biomechanical: Weak Feet and Unequal Leg Length

Many runners, like me, have biomechanically weak feet. This means that the foot has some basic flaw that, aggravated by running, leads to foot, leg, or knee injuries. A runner's foot strikes the ground over 1,000 times during every mile of a run. The force of impact on each foot is approximately three or four times the runner's weight. With weak feet, the force exerted up each footstrike causes an abnormal strain on the supporting tendons, muscles, and fasciae of the foot and leg. Among the types of foot weaknesses are the extremes of overpronation, oversupination, completely flat arches, and extremely high arches. Arch supports (orthotics), either commercially made or custom fitted by a podiatrist, may help runners with biomechanically weak feet. It works for me!

If your legs are of different lengths, you may experience pain in your back, knee, or hip. In many cases, a runner can have unequal legs without injury. Somehow your body naturally compensates. This is true for me. On the other hand, unequal legs are often a major factor in injury. When it is a cause, the injury will occur first on the longer leg. Structural shortages may occur anywhere in the leg: the upper leg, the lower leg, and below the ankle. Heel lifts or orthotics to balance leg length often help; placed inside the shoe, they should not exceed a quarter inch.

Sometimes, structural weaknesses cause problems for beginning runners. Others may not have difficulties until mileage creeps up to a point where their body begins to break down. If you experience injury, have a sports doctor check you out for biomechanically weak feet and leg-length discrepancy. This is one of the most neglected causes of running injuries and one of the easiest to repair.

Poor Flexibility and Overstretching

Most runners do not allow enough time for stretching. Ask any runner how much he or she stretches and the most common reply is, Not as much as I should. From laziness or lack of discipline, we set ourselves up for injuries resulting from lack of flexibility. Tight or shortened muscles are more easily injured than flexible muscles. Concentrate particularly on improving flexibility in the lower back, calf and hamstring muscles, Achilles tendon, and the iliotibial band.

Overzealous or careless stretching can do more harm than good, and it has been blamed for many injuries. The fact is that stretching isn't to blame, but rather straining or improperly stretching. Don't stretch injured muscles. Often runners get injured and start pulling and tugging on the injured area in a frantic attempt to cure the problem. Instead, they may make it worse. Stretching an injured muscle may aggravate it and delay healing. Leave it alone until tenderness and swelling disappear, then work gradually to improve its flexibility. If you have a recurring problem such as back pain, don't do any exercise that aggravates it.

Chapter 37 details how to improve flexibility with safe stretching routines.

Incorrect Warm-Up and Cool-Down

Too many runners warm up and cool down improperly—if they do it at all. Overstretching or running too fast before muscles are warm sets you up for injury. So, too, does neglecting or rushing through the cool-down period. Chapter 7 discusses these important topics.

Muscle Imbalance

It is important that muscles be strong and have proper balance with opposing muscles. The prime contracting muscles (buttocks, hamstrings, and calf muscles) may become very strong and tight with running. Stretching exercises for these muscles combined with strengthening exercises for the opposing muscles are essential to restore muscle groups to proper balance. Otherwise, imbalances may lead to injury. Strengthen these opposing muscles: abdominals, shin area muscles, and quadriceps.

Old Injuries

Running may create a new problem from an old, forgotten injury. A person who suffered a severe ankle injury playing basketball a few years back, for example, may have latent weaknesses that may be aggravated by running. A previous running injury makes you vulnerable for future injury. In fact, studies show that half of all running injuries aren't new ones but rather recurrences of old problems.

Improper Injury Rehabilitation

Take your time! Allow an injury to heal before running hard or long again, and don't resume running too soon if you had to take time off. Guidelines for running with and coming back from injury are detailed later in this chapter.

Errors in Running Form

Technique is important for both fast running and healthy running. Among the form errors detailed in the following chapter that may contribute to injury: leaning too far forward or backward, running too high on the toes or hitting too hard on the heels, overstriding, swaying from side to side, and running too tense.

Overtraining—Too Much Mileage, Speed, or Hills

Any sudden changes in your running—increases in how far, how fast, how often you run or adding hills—may result in injury.

Even if you build up your mileage gradually, beyond a certain point you may be unable to handle more without injury. Increase mileage by no more than 10 percent from week to week and hold it at a level below that which causes problems until your body is ready to accept more training. Risks can be minimized by using common sense and moderation—in getting started, in increasing distances, and in judging how much running is enough for you.

Speed training helps you race faster. Unfortunately, it also increases your chance of injury. There is a very fine line between speed training that produces physiological benefits and that which causes injury. Ease into speed training. With experience, you will develop a feel for what is safe and still provides training benefits. Increasing the speed of your daily training runs may also result in injury. Be especially careful not to get pulled into too fast a pace when running with groups or other individuals. Run the pace that is best for you.

Beware of changes in the hilliness of your daily training runs. Be especially careful if you are a flatlander and suddenly find yourself in a hilly section of the world while traveling. Whether in training runs or speed workouts, let your body gradually adjust to the stress of running up hills. Running down hills places even more strain on the body. Avoid steep downhills in training—walk them if necessary. Practice good form when running downhill in training and races. The following chapter details good running form for going up and down hills.

Bad Weather

The main weather-related cause of injuries is poor footing during winter months. These often result from being tight when trying to guard against slipping. Tense muscles, whether consciously or unconsciously tightened, are more prone to strains and overuse injuries. Running in a few inches of snow forces you to work muscles normally not taxed. If your quadriceps become fatigued, knee injury could result. Beware of the obvious: If you slip and fall, try to land lightly and then immediately stop your run, get indoors to get warm and dry, and put ice on the injured area.

The most common winter running injuries are groin and hamstring pulls caused by slipping and sliding through snow and ice. You may also develop strains and pulls from slipping on rain-soaked surfaces—especially beware of wet leaves, which can be as slippery as ice. These nagging injuries require rest or they will stick around for a long time.

Running goes on, with or without dry surfaces. The best prevention is to make sure you warm up well, maintain good flexibility, and run relaxed, try not to tense out of fear of falling. When running on slippery surfaces, shorten your stride slightly and shuffle along, maintaining good balance. Walk if necessary rather than risk injury. Be especially careful on downhills and turns and when running in the dark, when you can't see where your feet are landing. Don't attempt fast running under slippery conditions—and this includes racing.

Chapters 21–23 detail other dangers of running in hot and cold weather and other difficult conditions.

Undertraining
You must have the mileage base and speed training to be prepared for races. If you put in only 20 miles a week and then run a marathon, you're asking for trouble. The same is true if you do all your running at 9-minute miles and then attempt to race at a much faster pace. Overtraining may cause you to break down before you reach the starting line. Undertraining may cause you to break down before you reach the finish line.

Overracing
You can stress yourself physically and mentally with too much racing. Select your races wisely, space them wisely, and allow yourself to recover before training hard or racing again. Don't race more than twice a month; seldom race two weeks in a row.

Inadequate Recovery
This is the principle of hard-easy training. Follow hard days—speed training and long runs—with at least one easy day or off day. You may need additional rest after very stressful runs. For beginners, a recovery day may be a day off following a day of easy running. Races require even more easy recovery time—two or three

days after a short race of 5K or less, up to two or three weeks after marathons. A good rule of thumb is to avoid hard running for one day for every mile raced.

Shoes

According to podiatrist Dr. Richard Schuster, running injuries vary year to year in response to the latest advances in running shoes. Changes in flexibility of the shoe and the rigidity of the heel counter, for example, may help some runners but cause problems for others. As shoes get lighter with the use of new materials, injuries may result from less support and cushioning. To minimize injury, shoes must offer flexibility, cushioning, support—and they must fit your feet. Monitor the wear of your shoes regularly. Uneven wear of the soles will cause injury, as this affects the angle of your footstrike. Also, check to see if the heel counter rolls inward as a result of pronation or outward as a result of supination. Midsoles wear out with use, leaving you with less cushioning. Replace shoes every 300 to 500 miles.

The type of shoe you purchase may be determined by the kind of injury you are susceptible to. For example, you may need a shoe that controls pronation or supination, one with a wider toe box or with more cushioning, or a shoe with increased flexibility. If you feel an injury coming on, suspect your shoes. Are they well worn? Have you recently switched to a different training shoe or to a racing shoe? Chapter 16 details what to look for in running shoes. Consult your running doctor and running shoe salesperson for assistance with your shoe-related injuries.

Body Weight

The more you weigh, the harder you pound the ground with each footstrike. A runner who is 30 pounds overweight slams the ground with 20 percent more force than when at a recommended weight. A heavier runner, whether overweight or just big boned, needs well-cushioned running shoes. Two recommendations: Lose weight to take some of the stress off your musculoskeletal system, and consult your running doctor and shoe salesperson for advice on shoes to minimize the pounding.

Inadequate Diet

Many running injuries are brought on by muscle fatigue in runs of one hour or more. A diet high in carbohydrates may help you avoid injuries, according to a study at Northern Illinois University. Adequate protein is also important since that is what builds and repairs muscles.

Improper Foot Care

Treat your feet like good friends. Prevent problems by following good foot care practices.

Athlete's foot is a fungus that occurs between the toes or on the sole of the foot. It can itch and burn and cause severe discomfort. Athlete's foot thrives in moist conditions—sweaty feet, socks, and shoes. To prevent it, wash your feet daily in warm water, dry them thoroughly, and sprinkle them with antifungus powder. Fungus also feeds on dead skin tissue, so clean your feet regularly with a nail brush, emery board, or pumice stone. It is also important to wear dry, clean socks every day, especially in summer. This means both your running footwear and your "civilian" socks. Take out your running shoe insoles after running and allow your shoes to dry. In hot weather, alternate running shoes to allow them to dry out more thoroughly. Wearing sandals in the summer to allow your feet to ventilate and keep dry is also a good idea. If you get athlete's foot, treat it immediately.

Blisters are perhaps the most common and least respected injury the runner faces. If not properly treated, they can cause just as much trouble as any damage to muscles or joints. They are caused by something rubbing—shoes that are too big or too small, abrasive or wet socks, faults in shoe or sock stitching, downhill running, etcetera. Beginner runners tend to get blisters because their feet are tender and need to be toughened gradually. You are more likely to blister in hot weather and in wet weather. Friction can be minimized by using petroleum jelly, talcum powder, or friction-reducing insoles and socks.

If a blister is small and not painful, leave it alone. If it is large and painful and interferes with your running, stop running until you no longer favor it. Favoring a blister has been known to cause knee and other injuries. If you develop a painful blister during a run, stop immediately and treat it or you may make it much worse. It may be better to take a few days off and give a blister time to heal properly.

Small blisters should not be punctured immediately. Keep the area clean and protected, and the skin may heal itself. If the blister gets bigger or is sore or painful, it must be opened to relieve the pressure. Use the following procedure:

1. Clean the area with a disinfectant such as alcohol or iodine.

2. Sterilize a needle or razor blade by heating it in a flame or boiling water.

3. Prick the blister in several spots with the needle or make a small slit with the razor blade. Make sure the holes and slits are large enough so the skin doesn't close over or the fluid will build up again. Do not remove loose skin—it is needed to protect the sensitive underlayer of skin.

4. Press lightly on the blister with sterile gauze to remove all excess fluid. Most of the pain will go away as soon as the fluid is released.

5. Clean the area with antiseptic. Gentian violet can be used to dry it. After it has dried, use an ointment to protect against infection.

6. Cover the blister. Use a square of gauze and tape it around the edges. Take it off at night or whenever you will be off your feet to let air at the injury.

7. You may cover blisters with a polyurethane film or hydrogel dressing (such as Spenco 2nd Skin) available at most running stores. They will protect the blister and may allow you to continue running.

8. If redness and pain are present and persist, you have a badly infected blister and should see a doctor immediately.

Calluses develop from the constant rubbing of the foot in the shoe and the pounding of the foot into the ground. They are usually found on the bottom and back of the heel, and under the ball of the foot. Calluses help protect the foot, but they can also cause painful problems if they thicken and increase pressure on underlying tissues and bone. Blisters can form deep under the callus, which can be very painful. Rub calluses regularly with a pumice stone or emory board to keep them from building up and getting crusty. Petroleum jelly or some other type of skin softener regularly applied keeps the skin moist and prevents buildup. Have a podiatrist remove thick calluses. Orthotics or metatarsal pads are sometimes required to eliminate the pressure on the foot that can cause persistent callus buildup.

Keep your toenails short; long nails can jam into the front of your shoes, causing black or ingrown toenails. Cut the nails straight across, not in a curve, to prevent ingrown toenail. Black toenail is caused by blistering under the nail. It is most often caused by nails that are long combined with shoes that are tight or slide too much because they're big. "Sanding" thickened nails with an emery board or pumice stone may help to prevent this condition. If your nails turn black but don't hurt, leave them alone. Eventually these blisters may go away on their own. But if they are painful, take action or you'll mess up your running form favoring this injury. Try cutting a slit in the shoe over the injured area to relieve the pressure. If the blister is out to the end of the toe, slit it with a sterile blade, soak, and use antiseptic. If that doesn't work, you may need to have a podiatrist drill a hole in the nail to relieve pressure and drain blood. I once put off treatment for a blister under my big toenail until it throbbed so much I had to go to the emergency room for treatment in the wee hours of the morning. Usually an injured toenail will grow back normally. Most runners experience black toenails. Consider it a badge of honor.

For basic foot care, apply moisturizing cream to your feet—especially the heels—in fall and winter to prevent drying and cracking, which can be quite painful. Also, corns, warts, slivers, ingrown toenails, and the like should be taken care of immediately by your podiatrist.

Poor Daily Habits

If you have pain, also look for nonrunning causes as a source of trouble. A sudden change in daily habits can cause the runner problems, especially back pain or sciatica. Be careful lifting and carrying heavy objects (including your kids); always use your powerful runner's legs to do the work and not your back. Sleeping on your back or stomach may also cause back problems. Comfort is the key to sleeping correctly, but the preferred position is on your side, knees flexed—the fetal position. The bed should be very firm.

Standing or sitting too much may cause problems made worse

with running. Many runners find that they have neck, shoulder, and back pain if they sit for long hours bent over—as in typing or writing. Make sure you have a good back support for your chair, elevate your feet so your knees are parallel to the floor or higher, and frequently change positions. Get up and move around and do some relaxation and stretching exercises often. While writing this book, I set a goal of getting up and moving around every 15 minutes. Every 2 hours I took a walk with the dog. Driving can also cause tightened muscles, strains in the back, and tension. Sitting combined with pushing the gas pedal or clutch for long periods can cause leg, knee, and back pain for many runners—especially me. You may want to put a small pillow behind the small of your back for support, and move the driver's seat forward or back to change your position. I never drive more than an hour or two without stopping to get out and walk and stretch. This minimizes injury.

Stress
Our emotions affect our muscles, and our muscles affect our emotions. Stress makes you more vulnerable to injury. During periods of unusual stress, cut back your running. But do some easy running for stress management.

Inadequate Sleep
Fatigue tends to accumulate quickly if you don't sleep enough, leaving you susceptible to injury. If you can't get enough sleep, back off your running.

Other Sports
Runners sometimes injure themselves playing other sports. Skiing, basketball, tennis, handball, soccer, in-line skating, and other activities, while fun, carry the risk of sprains and breaks that may take months to heal. Further, a minor injury that doesn't affect your sport may cause problems with the pounding of running.

Also, never do hard exercise in one sport, and then run hard that day or the next. Give your body time to recover. Don't play other sports in running shoes—they are not made for lateral movement, and you can easily turn your ankles and put strain on your knees.

Surfaces and Terrain

In your daily training, don't make sudden changes in the surface you run on, especially if switching from dirt or grass to hard pavement. Cement and concrete are harder than asphalt; you'll get less shock on the road than on the sidewalk. A medium-hard synthetic track, a dirt trail, or even level grass fields are the best training surfaces since they absorb more shock. If you must run on pavement—and most of us have little choice—be sure to wear well-cushioned shoes.

Most roads are banked or crowned for drainage. When you run on them, you are running along an incline; your upper foot is twisting inward with every step, and you're giving yourself a short leg. If possible, run in the middle of the road where it is more level, or cross the road every mile or so to change the slant. Of course, you also need to be aware of the danger of sharing your running path with cars, bikes, skaters, and fast-moving runners. Beach running also brings danger—the soft sand causes a pull on your Achilles tendon and the harder sand is slanted. Whatever the surface, be aware of obstacles—ruts, rocks, potholes, loose or uneven turf—that may cause injury.

Age

As we age, our bodies betray us. We recover more slowly from our runs, which leaves us more vulnerable to injury. Further, as we age, we become more brittle, more inflexible, and gradually lose muscle strength—thus, we are more injury prone.

Poor Advice

Everyone gives medical advice to runners. Your running friends, even your sedentary grandmother, will freely offer advice. Sports medicine "experts" pop up everywhere. Beware. There are no quick cures. Your best bet is to follow common sense and rest. If that doesn't work, go to a sports medicine specialist recommended by other runners.

Marathonitis

> **WARNING: THE SURGEON GENERAL HAS DETERMINED THAT MARATHON RUNNING IS DANGEROUS TO YOUR HEALTH!**

This statement, like those on cigarette packages, should be stamped across the toes of every running shoe. Too many people are training for and running in marathons before they are prepared. Ask any sports medicine doctor in a city with a big marathon—such as New York—and they will acknowledge the increase in patients for several weeks before and after a marathon. You can follow the training program in this book to minimize your chance of injury, but beware that injury risk does increase with marathon training.

Warning Signs for Injury

Many running-related injuries can be prevented either by minimizing the causes or adjusting to the warning signs our bodies send us. As Dr. George Sheehan warned us: "Listen to your body. It will tell you when you are doing too much." Here are some signals your body may give you:

1. Mild tenderness or stiffness that doesn't go away after a day of rest or after the first few minutes of your daily run. Be aware of any indications that your musculoskeletal system has been overtaxed.

2. A desire to quit or an unexplained poor performance in workouts or races. Also, an uncharacteristic lack of interest in running, or your life in general. This is what I call "the blahs."

3. A tired feeling after a full night of sleep. A sluggish feeling that lasts for several days. You may also have difficulty falling asleep, or may wake up often in the night and find it difficult to go back to sleep. An occasional poor night's sleep should not be a concern, but if it persists for two or three nights, take notice.

4. An increase in your morning resting heart rate of ten beats or more. Note any significant increases as a sign that you are not fully recovered from the previous day or days of stress— whether from running or from life.

5. Upset stomach, loss of appetite, constipation, or diarrhea. These are the most consistent warning signs of overtraining.

6. Increased irritability, feelings of tension, mild depression, apathy. I consider these sure signs of the overtraining syndrome.

Now that I have made you into a running hypochondriac, relax. Be sure to take these signs as nothing more or less than warnings. Most early warning signals will be mild. Don't panic, but also don't ignore them.

If the warning signs persist, respond by cutting back on the distance, frequency, and intensity of your runs. Also, get more sleep. Take a day or two off. Too many runners feel that cutting back, resting, or taking time off makes them seem weak. Or they worry that they will lose valuable training time.

The most obvious warning sign is *pain*. It is a sure signal that something's wrong. Pain should be heeded. Your body yells at you for a reason; if we didn't have the pain signals you would continue to run and more serious injury could result. Runners can push through discomfort; pain is different. Pain is a clear warning sign of injury and must not be ignored.

Don't stop running at every muscle twitch. Balance your observation. Act wisely. When in doubt, back off. Watch for what troubles you or gives you pain. If the symptoms persist, see your doctor as a precaution. Don't hesitate here. Seeking help early can prevent struggling with an injury or illness over a longer time.

A helpful aid in this is your training diary. It may reveal the cause of recurring injury or illness—and how you treated it in the past. Rereading your past experiences will help prevent future injury.

Keep in mind that moderation is the key to injury prevention. Run, rest, relax, recover.

Psychological Aspects of Injury

Most runners experience some psychological difficulty when they are injured and forced to stop running. They focus on their injury and become depressed from inactivity. Few injuries last forever, though, and a runner will recover more quickly if he or she backs off and doesn't "challenge" the injury. Taking time off from running will, over the long run of your athletic career, make no difference at all. In fact, it may make you physically and mentally tougher.

For many people, running has become an addiction, and when injured, they experience withdrawal symptoms: insomnia, irritability, depression, tension, constipation, headaches, or muscle twinges resulting from forced inactivity.

Stages of Adjustment for Injured Runners

Dr. Victor Altshul, who teaches psychiatry at the Yale University School of Medicine, wrote in *Running* magazine that those who must temporarily give up running because of an injury go through sequential emotional stages of loss similar to what one might experience with the death of a loved one. The five stages are:

Denial. Often runners will not accept their injuries and will continue to run in pain until it forces them to admit they should stop.

Rage. Runners know and acknowledge that they should stop running because of an injury, but they refuse and angrily subject their bodies to more abuse. Also, they take out their frustrations on others.

Depression. After the anger subsides, runners become depressed and experience feelings of helplessness.

Acceptance. Runners accept their injuries, and they contain training within their level of tolerance. They may choose to participate in an alternative aerobic exercise to ease their depression and helplessness. They develop an intelligent plan to return gradually to their preinjury fitness level.

Renewed neurotic disequilibrium. As runners begin to regain their fitness, they forget the cause of their injuries and neglect the warning signs of further injury. Too often they don't learn from their experience and once again attempt too much too soon or train for goals that are beyond their present physical and psychological capacity.

Psychological Guidelines for Dealing with Injury

All runners, whether strongly or marginally addicted to running, will experience withdrawal symptoms after one to three days without exercise. A Georgia State University study indicated that if habitual runners vary their schedules only slightly, negative effects result. The study revealed that when a habitual runner misses a day or two of running, he or she may feel guilty or tense.

Here are some guidelines to help you get over the blues associated with not being able to run:

Accept your injury. Analyze why it happened, and determine the causes. Treat the injury properly, seek medical attention if necessary, and develop a plan to ease back into shape.

Maintain your relationships. Don't reject your family, friends, or coworkers. Don't take out your frustrations on them or withdraw from them during your inactivity.

Think positively. Look at your injury as a scheduled rest period during your lifelong training program. Use this time to learn and enjoy alternative exercises. Many runners are pleasantly surprised to find after an injury that they have reached a higher level of fitness because they use the layoff time to develop upper-body strength or flexibility. They also learned to train sensibly to avoid injuries.

Take a break. Use the extra time to do things you couldn't do during your training. Take a trip with your family that isn't dependent on a big race, or go to a baseball game with your pre–running days friends.

Replace the habit, and keep active. Maintain an active life. Activity is a powerful antidepressant. The sooner you enter another aerobic activity, the easier it will be to defeat the depression of your enforced layoff and the better shape you will be in when you are ready to resume your normal running schedule.

Return to running with realistic expectations. Be patient and conservative. You won't get it all back right away.

Running Through an Injury

A runner cannot lay off every time he or she gets a minor blister, ache, pain, or sniffle. Yet by forcing yourself to continue at a high level of training, or any training at all, you may make things worse. Often a day or two off to allow a bad blister to heal, for example, will let you return sooner to quality training than if you had continued and aggravated the injury. However, total rest beyond a few days will not help many injuries. You may as well continue to run, but within certain limits. Gentle exercise will help you heal and will also help you maintain a base of fitness. The trick is to train enough to provide these benefits while allowing the injured area to rest by doing relatively less work that does not aggravate the injury. More serious injuries will require good judgment by you and your doctor about whether or not you should continue training or rest. Absolute rest from the stress of running for a few weeks (but not necessarily from other forms of exercise) may be required to allow some injuries to heal properly.

I use the following dozen rules to guide those who decide to run through their injuries:

1. Be aware of pain and other warning signals. Pain should protect you from overdoing.

2. Unless you can walk briskly with little or no pain for a mile, don't run.

3. Don't run if your pain makes you limp or otherwise alters your form. You may cause another injury, and it may be far worse than the one you already have. Bravely limping through a run is stupid!

4. You can run with discomfort, but not with pain. If the pain worsens as you run, stop. Beware! Your body produces its own painkilling drugs, which may allow you to run or race and forget your pain. But after the run, you will be in agony and may have further aggravated your injury. There is danger in pushing hard through workouts and races when you started in pain that disappeared after a few miles.

5. Never use painkilling drugs to allow you to run. You must feel the pain to adjust to it—either to continue or stop.

6. Avoid hills, speed work, races, long runs, and slanted or excessively soft surfaces that aggravate your injury and intensify your pain.

7. Analyze and treat the cause of your injury. Pain is a signal. If your pain lessens when you change shoes, for example, or

when you switch to the other side (and slope) of the road, you have learned its cause and can treat it.

8. After running, treat your injury by applying ice, and take aspirin or ibuprofen.

9. Warm up thoroughly and cool down thoroughly with each run.

10. Do specific exercises to strengthen or improve flexibility, if it helps heal your injury. Do not overstretch or stretch injured parts until they have recovered.

11. Adjust your training if need be. In more extreme cases, alternate days of running with days off, or alternate running with walking for each exercise session. You may find that you can't run more than a mile without having to stop. Try alternately running up to the edge of your capacity and then, before you feel pain, walking briskly. With this form of training you can exercise aerobically for 30 to 60 minutes, which is psychologically satisfying and can help maintain minimal fitness. These same rules can apply when coming back from a layoff resulting from injury.

12. Be patient, and persevere.

The key to running through your injury is to develop a feel for your limits. If during a training run you aggravate an injury or develop one that causes you to change your form and/or is painful, stop and take a cab home or call for a ride. Don't force yourself to get a few more miles in so you can keep on schedule. During a race or speed workout, if you feel an injury or tightness coming on, stop. Don't be foolish and feel you have to finish—you'll be a hero today and a painful fool tomorrow.

Distance runners sometimes develop high levels of tolerance for pain. All runners must develop a sense of their limits. This may mean, for example, running up to 2 miles before the knee acts up and later, as the knee strengthens, increasing to 3 miles. Since you are the one experiencing the pain, only you can determine how much training you can safely handle. You must balance the need to continue in order to build or maintain fitness with the need to prevent the destruction of your health—and thus your training. Better to play the limits wisely than to challenge those limits and risk long-term setback.

Detraining

According to David Costill, Ph.D., in his book *Inside Running*: "Unfortunately, the fitness gained from miles and miles of running is quickly lost when the runner stops all training." But how quickly? Costill answers: "In general, there is no loss for five to seven days. As a matter of fact, running performance may even be improved after two to five days of inactivity. Such rest periods allow the muscles and nervous system to recover and rebuild from the stress of training and provide the runner with improved energy reserves and tolerance of endurance exercise."

Thus it is okay to occasionally take up to a week off from exercise to allow an injury to heal or just take a break. But beyond that period we decondition quickly. Ed Coyle, Ph.D., studied detraining at the University of Texas at Austin. A group of highly conditioned runners and bicyclists were tested for fitness and then voluntarily quit training for three months (they must have gone crazy!). They were retested periodically. Two trends were observed: First, the more highly trained athletes lost the most fitness; and second, the greatest loss happened at first and then fitness lessened more slowly but steadily. Half of aerobic fitness was lost within twelve to twenty-one days, then half again in the next twelve- to twenty-one-day period. This pattern continued until all the athletes were completely detrained by three months.

So if you have to stop exercising beyond a week, beware. You could lose most or all of that hard-earned fitness rapidly. The sad truth is that you will lose fitness much faster than you gained it!

Detraining is greatly lessened if you are able to do at least a minimum amount of running. If you can't run, cross-training with aerobic alternatives such as swimming and biking will help you keep in shape. But these exercises do not use the leg muscles the same way running does; thus some loss of training will occur. Running in water is the best form of exercise to minimize detraining.

If you experience a long layoff from exercise and become detrained, take heart in the knowledge that most researchers believe that former runners can regain fitness faster than their sedentary friends can gain it. "The muscles may have some memory," says Costill, "or maybe we are smarter with our training the second time." However, Costill's studies show that even the most gifted runners are nearly indistinguishable from sedentary people after six to twelve months of inactivity.

Coming back from detraining does take patience, time, and common sense. Dr. Coyle estimates that two weeks of retraining is needed for every week lost. So if you do no exercise for a month, it may take approximately two months to regain your former fitness. You will shorten this time by maintaining some form of exercise—either a minimum amount of running or aerobic alternatives—while you have stopped or cut way back on your running whether due to choice, injury, or illness.

Coming Back

Coming back depends on how long you were off, what alternative workouts you have done, and what put you out in the first place. Each injury or illness has its own special road to recovery. When you are better, put together a recovery plan (see below), and start without any pain or changes in form. Losing a week or two may only require a week or two of gradually progressive training starting at one-half to one-third the preinjury distance. Longer layoffs for more serious injuries require a more conservative comeback. Return after long layoffs by following a program of alternating running and walking, just like a beginner's program except that you can progress more quickly since you can return in less time than you needed to build up the first time. Also take days off between running days. Start slowly: You'll feel side stitches, wobbly knees, muscle soreness, weakness. Beware: Veteran runners often find that their heart and lungs can return much faster than their musculoskeletal systems; you may be more vulnerable to muscle strain and injury than you realize.

After a long layoff, you might start with a 1- to 3-mile distance covered either with 3 minutes of walking, 3 minutes of normally paced running, or a half-mile of walking, and half-mile of running. Jogging very slowly may aggravate your injury or cause another. Thus, it may be better to run a fairly normal pace and take walk breaks to prevent continuous pounding. Slowly increase the running period and decrease the walking until you can run nonstop comfortably. Then slowly build back up to your normal training base. Don't attempt hills and speed work until you've run at least two weeks at your previous distance level.

Here are some further guidelines:

▪ Reach the base your body can tolerate, and stay there until you feel strong. That might be 10 or 20 miles a week instead of the 20 or 30 miles that caused the breakdown.

▪ If you lost a day or two to a minor injury, don't try to make them up. So what if you don't get in your 20-mile week? Proceed "at the rate of," and pick up where you can on your normal schedule as soon as it is safe. Making up may only set you back instead of getting you back on schedule.

▪ Since so many runners feel better going uphill, it can be part of rehabilitation. It is therapeutic because the body absorbs only about two-thirds the stress of running on the flat and only half the stress of downhill running. It is safer than doing speed work on a track and gives a similar training effect. But avoid hills if you suffer from lower-leg injury.

▪ You should also set goals well below your threshold of further injury. Avoid frustration. Give yourself the satisfaction of making slow and steady progress.

▪ Approach your racing goals differently. Run the first few races after your layoff only for "reexperience." Just get the feel again. Next, aim to approach your prelayoff times, and then match and exceed them. But don't be in a hurry.

▪ Reanalyze again and again the *cause* of your injury. The Chinese say: "Fool me once, shame on you; fool me twice, shame on me." Learn from your mistakes and don't repeat them.

Most runners stop running when they are injured, and those who don't often become ex-runners. When you can't run, you need an alternative way to stay fit. It is your choice how active you want to be. If you are patient and disciplined during your alternative training period, you will return to running with a toughened mental attitude about your ability to cope with training obstacles. See Chapter 35 for cross-training guidelines.

Injury, in fact, may be helpful. It can force you to back off and rest. It may also encourage you to condition neglected parts of your body, which in turn will help you to perform at a higher level later.

When to See a Doctor

According to Dr. Gabe Mirkin and Marshall Hoffman in *The Sportsmedicine Book*, you should consult a sports medicine specialist for:

"1. All traumatic joint injuries. All injuries to a joint and its ligaments should be examined by a sportsmedicine physician because these injuries have the potential of becoming permanent and debilitating if proper treatment is not administered.

2. Any injury accompanied by severe pain. Pain is nature's way of talking to you and when it speaks loudly, you had better listen.

3. Any pain in a joint or bone that persists for more than two weeks. These tissues are the ones in which the most serious injuries occur.

4. Any injury that doesn't heal in three weeks. All injuries that don't heal should be checked for a structural abnormality that may have caused them. Sometimes an injury may not heal because you won't rest it.

5. Any injury that you feel should be checked. If you are concerned about an injury, you should always ask for help.

6. Any infection in or under the skin manifested by pus, red streaks, swollen lymph nodes, or fever. Untreated infections may lead to serious complications, and since antibiotics generally bring relief quickly, it is foolish not to receive treatment."

Further guidelines:

▪ Dr. Weisenfeld's rule: If the pain is with you from the first step, the problem is usually not biomechanical. If it comes on into the run, after the run, or the next day, it's probably a biomechanical problem, and a sports medicine specialist should be consulted.

■ If pain doesn't diminish with a short (three- or four-day) layoff, or if it worsens during a layoff, see a doctor.

■ If an inflamed tendon (tendinitis) does not respond to rest or ice in ten days, see a doctor.

Choosing a Sports Medicine Specialist

Choosing the right specialist for your injury is often a problem. Whatever your injury, you are likely to get a different opinion from different specialists. A podiatrist is likely to say your hip hurts because of a problem in your foot structure, a chiropractor that you need your spine realigned, a physical therapist that you need special exercises to correct relative weaknesses, an orthopedist that you have a structural problem in the hip, a running shoe salesman that you need different running shoes, and so on. Your running friends may all recommend a different type of specialist. All of them may be right about your injury, or wrong. What should you do?

If you have an injury, you have two options in terms of medical treatment: Seek help from your family doctor or internist, or consult a "sports medicine specialist." Unfortunately, there is a problem with this term, and that is: Anyone, including some quacks, can claim to be one. Sports medicine is not a recognized specialty such as internal medicine or pediatrics. Until the fitness boom of the 1970s, few doctors exercised, and most of their patients were sedentary. The running revolution brought with it a demand for more than the traditional doctor's remedy: Take aspirin and stop running. Runners want to keep running and will seek specialists to help them cope with their injuries so they can.

Most individuals who become very good sports medicine specialists do so because of their special interest in sports, engagement in continuing education programs, and personal exercise experience. They keep up to date on the current state of knowledge in their specialty and its application to the athlete. Most important, they gain valuable knowledge with the experience of working with many runners over a period of years. They must know their treatment limitations and work with other specialists in an effort to provide the best possible service to the athlete. Runners may benefit from medical personnel from a wide range of specialties: The family practitioner, internist, orthopedist, neurosurgeon, podiatrist, acupuncturist, chiropractor, physiatrist, and osteopath are the most common. The practice of sports medicine is by no means limited to treatment by a doctor. Physical therapists, exercise physiologists, massage therapists, and others can work with your doctor to keep you running.

The following characteristics should be requirements for a sports medicine specialist for runners:

- He or she should be a runner, or at least a runner at heart.

- He or she should have experience treating many athletes, especially runners.

- He or she should have a good background—formal schooling and personal research—in general medicine and exercise. Although there is no separate field of sports medicine today, each medical specialty offers extensive courses on athletic injuries as related to it.

- He or she should be recommended by others: experienced runners, running organizations, your family doctor, and other respected sports medicine specialists.

Whoever you decide to use as your sports medicine specialist, give his or her treatment a chance. Few treatment choices result in immediate recovery. If orthotics are prescribed along with special exercises, for example, give them a good try. Many runners are impatient and don't follow a prescribed treatment properly; they then complain that it didn't work and search for another specialist. Remember, too, that every doctor can't cure every patient. Dr. Murray Weisenfeld states that he is happy if 80 percent of his patients are cured with his treatment. If a sports medicine specialist can't cure your ailment, he or she should refer you to another specialist who may be able to help you by looking at your problem from a different perspective.

Treatment
When injured, you can respond in one of four ways:

1. Ignore the injury and run through it, often making it worse.

2. Quit running and pray that it will go away.

3. Attempt self-treatment.

4. Seek medical help.

Most runners deal with an injury in that order: ignoring it, quitting for a few days, attempting self-treatment, and finally seeing a doctor.

Most running injuries respond well to RICE—rest, ice, compression, and elevation. Follow this procedure immediately after the injury occurs and continue for a few days. Rest is the easiest answer for most running injuries, but the hardest to accept by most runners. Cold treatment (cryotherapy) is the most common treatment for injured runners. It lessens pain, reduces inflammation, decreases blood flow, and brings down swelling and fluid buildup in the injured area. Cold treatment also may temporarily relieve muscle spasms because it numbs and calms the irritated nerve fibers around the affected muscles. It can be combined with compression and elevation for immediate treatment of many injuries, such as ankle sprain. Cold therapy is often used in combination with aspirin or ibuprofen, which also reduce pain and inflammation.

Ice is the most common form of cold treatment. Icing should begin immediately after an injury to minimize inflammation and frequently thereafter for at least twenty-four hours and throughout injury rehabilitation. I recommend always icing any injury that is bothering you immediately after your run. Do not ice for longer than 20 minutes at a time or you may cause increased circulation in the area rather than the desired decreased circulation.

There are several methods of applying cold:

Ice packs. Apply an ice pack for 15 to 20 minutes with compression and elevation. Then use for 15 to 20 minutes on and 15 to 20 minutes off for the first three or four hours after an injury. Later, apply the pack for 20 minutes, three times a day for up to a week. Continue to apply after running until there is no further pain or tenderness. Be prepared to reice if the injury starts to come back.

You can use various types of ice packs:

- Place crushed ice between two towels.

- Fill a plastic bag with ice and freeze it.

▪ Buy reusable commercial gel cold packs that are frozen in your freezer, or chemical bags that mix to produce cold.

▪ Freeze a wet terry-cloth hand towel, fold in a square, and wrap in plastic.

▪ My favorite: a bag of frozen peas—it molds to the body! This allows you to ice both sides of your shin, Achilles tendon, or your entire knee. Frozen peas don't melt like ice, and stay cold longer than frozen gels.

Ice towels. Soak a towel in ice water and place it on the injured area. As it warms up, resoak it. Continue that process for 15 to 20 minutes. An ice towel is good for large areas, such as the lower back and hamstrings.

Ice massages. The best method to apply cold to an injured area is ice massage. Physical therapist Ted Corbitt, a 1952 U.S. Olympic marathoner, recommends this technique: Freeze ice in a paper cup for easy application; using a rubber glove for comfort while applying, gently massage the area on and around the injury for 10 to 15 minutes. Be very careful not to allow the ice to touch bare skin for too long at one time. It is important to keep the ice moving to provide a massaging effect.

Specific Treatment

Following is a brief summary of the causes and treatment of the most common running injuries. Also included are recommended exercises to improve flexibility and strength that will help prevent the injury from happening again. Those exercises, as well as others that will help minimize injury, are detailed in Chapter 36 (Strengthening) and Chapter 37 (Stretching). For more detailed guidelines on treating injuries, consult Dr. Murray Weisenfeld's *The Runner's Repair Manual*. Remember: Extended treatment of all ailments, and early treatment of serious injury, should be administered by a medical doctor.

Achilles Tendinitis

Named for the mythical Greek warrior who was wounded at his only vulnerable spot, Achilles tendinitis, inflammation of the Achilles tendon, is one of the most common and difficult injuries to treat. This tendon connects the powerful lower leg muscles to the heel. If ignored in its initial inflammation stages, a tear or rupture may result. It often is stiff or painful when you get up in the morning and after sitting for long periods. You may also experience pain at the start of your run, but it eases up as you run.

Causes: Trauma, heel bone deformity, poor calf flexibility, overpronation or -supination, improper shoes or wear, constant rubbing of the back of the shoe against the tendon in poorly fitted shoes, running too high on toes or leaning too far forward, soft surfaces such as sand, high-heeled nonrunning shoes, overtraining—sudden changes in mileage, speed training and hills, overstretching.

Treatment: Correct causes above, completely rest or decrease mileage, avoid hills and speed until healed, anti-inflammatories, ice after each run, avoid stretching area until pain and swelling is gone, elevate heels in walking and running shoes with heel lifts, orthotics may be prescribed, surgery as a last resort.

Stretching exercises: Wall Lean, Kneeling Achilles Stretch.

Ankle Sprains

You are actually more prone to turning your ankle while playing other sports than running. In running, you are more likely to be alert about where you are placing your feet. Ankle sprains result in torn ligaments, broken blood vessels, and inflammation, accompanied by pain and swelling. If you twist your ankle during a run or race, don't keep going if it hurts. It is crucial to get off your feet immediately and treat the injury. If you keep running, it may get far worse. Recovery time can take from a few days to several weeks depending upon the severity of the injury and how quickly you treat it. Stay off the injured ankle until you can walk comfortably. Crutches may be needed during the first forty-eight hours to decrease weight bearing. Don't run until all pain and swelling have disappeared.

Causes: Trauma, running over uneven terrain, previous injury, inappropriate or worn shoes.

Treatment: RICE—rest, ice, compression, elevation; anti-inflammatories; taping the ankle or using ankle braces for support; use well-cushioned shoes in good condition; orthotics may be prescribed in some cases.

Strengthening exercises: Ankle Push, Towel Sweep, Ankle Band Exercises.

Stretching exercises: Ankle Roll, Standing Ankle Stretch.

Arch Pain (Plantar Fasciitis)
This is an inflammation of the fibrous tissue that runs from the heel to the heads of the metatarsal bones in the ball of the foot. It is caused by irritation of the fascia tissue and its separation from the heel bone. It is characterized by pain in the heel or arch when you get up in the morning and after sitting for long periods. You also experience pain at the start of your run, but it eases as you loosen up. It may lead to heel spurs.

Causes: Flat or high-arched or rigid feet, overpronating, poor flexibility in the hamstrings and calf muscles, soft surfaces, inadequate shoes, running too high on the toes, overtraining—too much mileage on hard pavement and sudden increases in speed training and hills.

Treatment: Correct the causes above, avoid hills and speed until healed, ice after running, anti-inflammatories, rest, friction massage, taping, heel lifts, orthotics, surgery as a last resort.

Strengthening exercises: Towel Exercise.

Stretching exercises: Plantar Fascia Stretch, Kneeling Arch Stretch.

Back Pain/Sciatica
This book was delayed for a year because I was disabled with this one. More than 80 percent of Americans are victims of back pain at some time in their lives. Lower-back problems are most frequent, but upper-back problems also trouble many runners. The sciatic nerve begins in the lower back and extends all the way down the leg to the ankle. It has been called "the longest river of pain in the body." Pain may occur in the back, hip, leg, or even the ankle and the two lesser toes. It may be a numbing sensation or a severe pain shooting from the back down the leg. Back pain and sciatica can

linger for months, or suddenly appear and disappear, only to reappear again.

Causes: Stress, inflexibility, muscle imbalances, leg-length discrepancy, overtraining, overstriding, slanted surfaces, misalignment of the spine, disk deterioration, biomechanically weak feet, overstretching, overweight, bad habits (lifting, sleeping, sitting, etc.).

Treatment: Treat causes above, relaxation exercises, massage, warm baths, anti-inflammatories, orthotics, surgery as a last resort.

Strengthening exercises: Crunches, Pelvic Tilt, Back Extensions, Alternate Extensions.

Stretching exercises: Knee to Chest, Cat Back, Fold-up Stretch, Seated Trunk Flexion, Modified Hurdler Stretch, Lying Hamstring Stretch, Towel Hamstring Stretch.

Pain in Ball of the Foot
Sesamoiditis, pain under the head of the first metatarsal (the big knobby bone behind the big toe), is usually caused by trauma. Pain under the second, third, and fourth metatarsal heads are called stone bruises, or just painful bruised bones. A burning, stabbing, or numbing sensation may also occur in the metatarsal area and extend into one or more toes. This is caused by the impingement of a thickened nerve sheath. Pain on the top of the forefoot over a specific area may be a sign of a stress fracture (although it may be caused by tying shoelaces too tight).

Causes: Overtraining, especially too much speed or hills; running too high on the toes and leaning forward; shoes too inflexible in ball of the foot or too tight in the forefoot; structural weaknesses in the feet; downhill running.

Treatment: Correct causes above, ice after running, anti-inflammatories, rest for a few days if running form is affected, pad around (not over) the bruise, no speed or hills until recovered.

Muscle Cramps
As Bryant Stamford, Ph.D., wrote in *The Physician and Sports Medicine,* "A cramp is a muscle contraction gone haywire, locking

the muscle into a painful and sustained spasm. You have no control over when a cramp strikes, and if you don't intervene, it will continue." Fortunately, this is a temporary condition rather than a long-term injury.

Muscle cramps are fairly common in beginner runners whose muscles are not used to exercising. But veteran runners are also vulnerable, especially when running hard races or workouts. Running farther or faster than you are accustomed, especially in hot weather, will make you prone to cramps. The calf muscles are the most frequent cramp location, but any muscle in the body may cramp. Some runners are more vulnerable than others. Recurrent cramps can be a symptom of more serious medical problems, thus a sports doctor should be consulted. No one knows for sure what causes cramps, but several factors are associated with them.

Causes: Overworked muscles for conditioning; slight muscle strain; dehydration; too little potassium, sodium, calcium, and magnesium in diet; exposure to extremes of temperature; inadequate warm-up; poor blood circulation; tight clothing; sudden change in shoes.

Treatment: Correct causes above, gently but firmly stretch the cramped muscle, massage it with your thumbs, ice.

Heel Bruises and Spurs

Heel bruises usually result from stepping on sharp objects, such as rocks, or hitting too hard and too far back on the heel while running. Heel spurs result from the plantar fascia pulling very hard at its attachment to the heel over a period of time. Many of the microscopic fibers of the fascia tear away and leave small droplets of blood, which eventually calcify. The spur then irritates the soft tissue and a "bursal sac" is formed. When this sac fills with fluid and you put pressure on it by standing or running, pain results. Heel spurs sometimes show up on X-rays.

Causes: Heel spurs have the same basic causes and symptoms as plantar fasciitis (see discussion earlier in this chapter).

Treatment: Same as for plantar fasciitis, also pad the bottom of the heel of both feet, cut a hole in the heel pad so the painful area will not be irritated, and have orthotics adjusted to take pressure off spurs.

Hip/Piriformis

A common injury for runners is "piriformis syndrome," in which the piriform muscle (which helps rotate your hips when you run) deep in the buttock is in spasm and pressures the sciatic nerve. The result may be pain not just in the hip, but also radiating up into the lower back and down into the hamstrings. You may also develop strains in other parts of the hip or possibly a stress fracture.

Causes: Prolonged sitting, sitting on your wallet, overtraining, leg-length differences, muscle imbalances, tight hip flexors, repeated rotations of the torso, tight low back.

Treatment: Correct causes above, ice, rest, anti-inflammatories.

Strengthening exercises: Side Leg Raises, Inside Leg Raises.

Stretching exercises: All Hip Stretches in Chapter 37.

Iliotibial Band Syndrome

The iliotibial band extends from the outside of the pelvis, over the hip and knee, and inserts just below the knee. It helps stabilize the knee during running. Pain occurs on the outside of the knee and up to the hip when the band is irritated.

Causes: Running on slanted surfaces or with broken-down shoes, overpronation, underpronation, inadequate warm-up or cool-down, too much too soon with mileage, a single excessive workout, bowlegs, excessive sitting, inflexibility, hills.

Treatment: Correct the causes above including stretching the iliotibial band, strengthening exercises for the structures that stabilize the hip, ice after running, anti-inflammatories, deep friction massage, decrease mileage, rest.

Strengthening exercises: Side Leg Raises.

Stretching exercises: Standing Iliotibial Stretch, Lateral Hip Stretch.

Runner's Knee

This is the number one most "popular" injury among runners. Runner's knee (chondromalacia patella) involves the softening of the protective cartilage under the kneecap caused by improper tracking: the kneecap is forced out of its normal "groove" and irritates the cartilage. Pain usually occurs beneath or on both sides of the kneecap.

Causes: Overpronation, weak quadriceps, inflexible hamstring and calf muscles, unequal leg length, knock knees, running on slanted surfaces, improper or worn shoes, overstriding, overtraining.

Treatment: Correct potential causes above, well-cushioned shoes, ice after running, rest, anti-inflammatories, knee brace, possibly commercial arch supports or prescribed orthotics, surgery as a last resort.

Strengthening exercises: Sitting Leg Extensions, Squats.

Stretching exercises: All Hamstring and Quadriceps Exercises Detailed in Chapter 37.

Runner's Nipple

This is one of those annoying problems that technically isn't an injury, but it is painful. Runners are usually more vulnerable in warm weather and when running for long distances. Chafing of the nipples results from constant friction between your skin and shirt. The result may be raw, painful, even bleeding nipples. To prevent this problem, choose loose, softer clothes. T-shirts or singlets with silk-screened designs across the chest can increase friction. Singlets with a soft-fabric panel across the chest will help minimize irritation. To prevent chafing, cover the nipples with petroleum jelly or a patch (Band-Aid, corn cushion, etc.).

Shin Splints

This injury is a painful swelling of damaged muscles and tendons along the front of the lower leg between the two bones, the fibula and tibia. The pain occurs noticeably during running. Shin splints may signal that a stress fracture is lurking so don't neglect this injury.

Causes: Tight calf and hamstring muscles; overpronation; muscle imbalance—weaknesses in the front of the leg compared to the backs of the legs; running too high on toes; overstriding; leaning forward while running; running shoes that are inflexible or have heels that are not thick enough; sudden change from soft to hard surfaces; slanted surfaces; sudden change in mileage; speed training or hill running.

Treatment: Correct causes above, well-cushioned shoes, anti-inflammatories, ice after runs, reduce mileage and pace or take off some time, avoid hills and hard running surfaces, elevate heels, taping, orthotics may be prescribed.

Strengthening exercises: Towel Sweep, Band Exercises, Foot Press, Toe Lift.

Stretching exercises: Wall Lean, Towel Calf Stretch.

Delayed Onset Muscle Soreness (DOMS)

Most runners develop muscle soreness at one time or another due to overuse. Sore quadriceps and hamstrings are especially common. Soreness doesn't necessarily mean you're injured, but it can make running uncomfortable, slow you down, and may increase the risk of injury. DOMS often makes walking down stairs or sitting very difficult. DOMS usually appears two to twenty-four hours after your exercise and may last from four to ten days. Peak soreness is usually twenty-four to seventy-two hours after exercise. DOMS is caused by microscopic damage to muscle fibers. Ease back or stop running while sore since damaged muscles need time to heal.

There are three types of exercise that cause DOMS:

1. Unaccustomed exercise. Beginner runners often develop this because their muscles are not used to the work. But any runner that runs significantly more or faster than normal is vulnerable.

2. Eccentric exercise. This involves contracting the muscle while it is being lengthened, producing muscle fiber damage. For example, your leg muscles are prone to this damage while running down hills. Beginners not used to running down hills are vulnerable as is any runner racing down hills. The Boston Mara-

thon, with its many downhill stretches, is well known for producing DOMS.

3. Long endurance exercise. You are especially prone to DOMS when doing long runs as you train for a marathon and after races of a half-marathon and longer. These runs cause damage to the muscle fibers that have been depleted of glycogen. If you want to see DOMS in action, go to any major marathon and watch the runners hobble around in the hours and days after the finish.

Other causes: improper warm up or cool down, inflexibility, improper recovery after hard runs, sudden increases in mileage or speed, hills, and shoes without adequate cushioning.

Treatment: Rest, or light exercise to pump blood to your muscles and help you recover (walking or non-weight-bearing activity such as swimming or biking)—but don't try to run if it's too painful and your form is altered; ice; anti-inflammatories, elevation, massage; run on soft surfaces; strengthen legs with weight training after soreness disappears.

Muscle Strains (Hamstring, Quadriceps, Calf, Groin)

These injuries are a result of an actual tearing within the muscle group and are most often accompanied by inflammation. A muscle that is suddenly jerked by a sharp action (slipping on ice, sudden bursts of speed, etc.) or hasn't been properly warmed up may pull at its tendon or connection with the bone.

Causes: Trauma, muscle imbalance, inflexibility, improper warm-up, leg-length discrepancy, shoes with uneven wear or that are inflexible, slanted surfaces, overstriding, running too high on the toes, overstretching, overtraining.

Treatment: Correct causes above, rest (don't run if you favor the injury), ice, anti-inflammatories, massage, orthotics may be needed; do not stretch injured areas until all pain has disappeared.

Exercises for groin

Strengthening: Side Leg Raises, Inside Leg Raises, Chair Press.
Stretching: All Groin Stretches detailed in Chapter 37.

Exercises for quadriceps

Strengthening: Sitting Leg Extension, Quarter Squats.
Stretching: Standing Quad Stretch, Lying Quad Stretch.

Exercises for hamstrings

Strengthening: Hamstring Curls.
Stretching: All Hamstring Stretches detailed in Chapter 37.

Exercises for calf muscles

Strengthening: Toe Raises.
Stretching: Wall Lean, Towel Calf Stretch.

The Stitch

This really isn't an injury, but there may be no pain that strikes a runner with the suddenness and devastation of the dreaded side stitch. This sometimes sharp pain is usually located in the upper abdomen or at the base of the ribs; almost always it occurs when you're running hard and ceases when you slow down or stop. It often strikes with no warning. The pain results from a spasm in the diaphragm—most often caused by faulty breathing, or sudden, hard running that jars and tugs on the ligaments that connect the gut to the diaphragm.

Causes: Faulty breathing (practice "belly breathing" as detailed in Chapter 34), stress, weak and tense abdominal muscles, running too soon after eating resulting in gas, intolerance to certain foods, running hard down hills, improper warm up, starting too fast, inadequate fitness for intensity of exercise.

Treatment: Correct above causes and try the following techniques to relieve the stitch:

- Decrease the pressure on the lungs and abdomen enough to let blood flow back to your diaphragm. To do this, stop running and empty your lungs by pursing your lips and blowing hard. This should release trapped air in your lungs. To relieve abdominal pressure, bend over and raise your knee on the stitch side while pressing your fingers deep into the painful area and tightening the abdominal muscles. The pain will usually disappear, and you can continue running. Or, just walk while belly breathing and the stitch will gradually subside.

If you don't want to stop when running or racing, try these:

- Slow the pace until the pain subsides, resume speed once you feel comfortable.

- Breathe out against a slight resistance—belly breathing—even if you groan a little or sound like you're playing the trumpet. Exhale deeply and noisily. Don't be shy. The clock is ticking at the finish line. Try Shelly's method: Breathe in like you are sucking air through a straw; noisily breathe out while pretending to blow up a balloon.

- As you run, bend over as much as you can and press the stitch with the fingers of your hand and tighten the abdominal muscles.

- A change in breathing pattern may help. Most runners breathe out as the same foot, usually the right, hits the ground. We usually breathe at the ratio of 4:1 or 2:1 footstrikes to breaths. Try breathing off the other foot to break the pattern. Some runners find that doubling their rate of breathing rids them of the dreaded stitch. Others raise their arms overhead, breathe deeply, expand their stomachs, and, as they lower their arms, exhale loudly and contract their stomachs. (This is not time to worry about appearances!)

- A few runners get away with not thinking about the pain, and continuing. Try thinking about something else or talking to another runner.

- You are always welcome to try my technique. When a stitch hits me in a race, I just pick up the pace and run harder and harder until the stitch goes away. It works for me—though everything else hurts! Then there is the technique developed by my former training partner Jim Ferris. His rather bizarre method was to do a quick somersault when bothered by a stitch during a race. It worked—and really "psyched out" the opposition.

Just remember that no one has ever died from a side stitch, although you may feel you are going to be the first. If you have tried all the treatments and eliminated all the causes and are still troubled by the stitch, check with a sports doctor. You may have internal problems that should be handled medically.

Stress Fractures

These are tiny, incomplete breaks or cracks in a normal bone caused by repeated trauma or pounding. It usually occurs in one of the metatarsals in the ball of the foot, or in one of the lower leg bones, but it may also occur in the upper leg, pelvis, and hip areas. Sometimes a runner can have stress fractures and not even be aware of it. Pain, if it exists, usually begins gradually and intensifies with running. If you can find a spot on the bone that hurts intensely when you press down on it, you may have a stress fracture and should consult a doctor. Stress fractures come on slowly. At first it may seem to be a bad case of tendinitis, but if pain persists X-rays should be taken. A stress fracture may not show up on X-rays for the first two weeks or so. A bone scan may be necessary to confirm a stress fracture.

Causes: Too much too soon—mileage, speed work, hills; switching to harder surfaces; too little recovery after hard runs; improper shoes for foot type; running too high on the toes; biomechanical weaknesses in feet.

Treatment: Rest—sorry, that's the only option. You must stay off a stress fracture and stop running for four to eight weeks, depending upon the location and severity of the injury. If you don't, more serious and permanent injury may result. Switch to nonimpact exercise while recovering—swimming, biking, and the like.

Part XI

Running Form and
Supplemental Training

THIRTY-FOUR

Running with Good Form

Running looks like the simplest, least technical of sports. Place one foot in front of the other and keep moving forward. What could possibly go wrong? Why should a beginner or intermediate runner be concerned with running form?

Every runner has his or her own form. I can spot a running friend at a distance. Some shuffle, some flow, some rock, and some roll. Runners have individual styles—their running "signatures." Many experts in the field say that little should be done to change the way you run. Others feel that improvements can and should be made, especially if you have obvious form faults.

Just observe runners going by in your local park for a few minutes. Some runners will have obvious faults in form, such as a pronounced forward or backward lean, high arm carry, bouncing motion, body sway, or flailing elbows. Others stand out because they prance up on their toes or grind away back on their heels. Still others run with quickly recognized quirks of habit such as a rolling head, or long-legged or short, choppy strides. A few of them just flow along like water in a fast-moving stream.

Running with good form is important for several reasons:

1. Sloppy running is less enjoyable than graceful running. Struggling against yourself isn't fun.

2. Poor running form wastes energy and detracts from performance. Whether you are trying to run your first nonstop mile, improve your 10K time, or finish your first marathon, you need to channel all your energy into efficient movement.

3. Injuries may be caused by poor form. For example, running high on the toes or leaning too far forward can contribute to shin splints or Achilles tendinitis. Leaning back too far or overstriding may contribute to back pain. Carrying the arms too high or swinging the elbows back too far can cause back and shoulder injuries. In fact, improved running form can help alleviate many injuries and prevent others.

4. If you learn good running form, you'll run more confidently. You might inch along with the speed of a turtle, but you'll feel better about your running if you look like a gazelle. Furthermore, once you learn to look like a gazelle, you'll be much more likely to run like one.

How can you improve running form? Use the following guidelines to check your running form and make a few adjustments, but don't worry about trying to run perfectly. Learn the basic principles of running form and concentrate on them off and on during your runs. These general principles apply to everyone, but no one form works for every runner. The main thing is to have the best biomechanical form and still run naturally with a relaxed, flowing, rhythmic style. Running, when done properly, should be a complete, flowing action that occurs unconsciously.

There are four basic parts to good running form:

- Footstrike

- Forward stride

- Body angle

- Arm action

Footstrike

As you move from walking to running, a few adjustments are needed in form. The difference between running and walking is that running involves a propulsive push and an airborne "float" before the next footstrike, whereas in walking one foot is always on the ground.

The suggested footstrike for the average runner is to land *gently* on the heel and then allow the forefoot to come down quietly as your body moves forward. The footplant ends as you push off the ball of your foot with a little spring. The toes should be pointing straight forward with your feet hitting the ground in a straight line as if running on a balance beam. You will notice that your foot first hits the ground slightly on the outside edge of the shoe and then rolls inward lightly to the ball of the foot with the knee slightly bent to absorb shock. The key is the impact. Allow the foot to caress the ground in a rocking motion, thus spreading out the shock over the whole foot. Since you hit the ground with the force of three times your body weight, it is essential that you learn to land gently.

Running shoes are thicker and more cushioned in the heel to accommodate this suggested footstrike. Many runners, observing that their shoes wear out first on the outside edge of the heel, incorrectly assume that they're doing something wrong. In fact, this is a normal wear pattern. If you roll inward too far, however, you may overpronate. Other runners supinate—their feet roll outward when they strike the ground. Both of these extremes of foot roll can cause injury. Chapter 16 details the importance of having a running shoe salesman check the wear pattern of your shoes. They can recommend shoes that will help minimize problems with your footstrike. A sports podiatrist may also analyze your shoe wear pattern and perhaps prescribe orthotics to help stabilize your footplant.

The recommended footstrike for beginner and intermediate runners is the heel-ball pattern. Some beginners run with a slow "flat-foot" technique. Their entire foot strikes the ground at one time, but as lightly as possible. The wide surface area cushions this footstrike, and it's also easy on the rest of the body. You cannot run very long or very fast using this style, however, and eventually you will shift to the heel-ball method.

Most of the fast runners up front in the races don't run heel-ball; instead, they run ball-heel. They land lightly on the back of the ball of the foot before touching down on the heel. They do this so swiftly and smoothly that it appears they are running on their toes. Running this way allows these runners to generate more speed. I run heel-ball in training and ease into ball-heel when racing short distances or doing fast speed sessions. I don't think you will benefit from the more advanced ball-heel footstrike until you can race at a 7-minute-per-mile or better pace. *The Competitive Runner's Handbook* describes how to make the transition to this form of fast running. For now, you can run more safely and still run fast enough using the heel-ball method.

The two most common errors in footstrike for beginner and intermediate runners involve using two types of footstrike to extreme:

Excessive toe strike. I call this runner "the bouncer." The runner lands high on his toes. This type of footstrike minimizes cushioning and increases the strain on the lower leg. You may quickly develop injuries to the shins, ankles, calf muscles, or forefoot. Running high on the toes results in too much bouncing as you run and, therefore, wasted energy. If you've played soccer or basketball you may have learned to run up on your toes to be prepared to change direction or jump quickly. If you were a sprinter you were taught to explode off the rear foot, the pushing foot, and land high on the ball of the reaching foot. When you run steadily for long periods of time this type of footstrike is neither safe and nor efficient.

Excessive heel strike. I call this runner "the grinder." Here, the runner hits the ground by jamming her heel into it and then slapping her forefoot down hard. This causes a shock to the body and may lead to injury. This type of runner is forced to run with a short, choppy stride. Again, energy is wasted.

Don't emulate "the bouncer" or "the grinder." Instead, touch down smoothly and gently and skim across the ground. Done properly, a slight rocking motion between heel contact and push-off ensures proper cushioning and strong forward propulsion. The result is a hitting and springing motion that is less jarring and increases acceleration. I call this runner "the glider."

Stride

As a beginner runner, you shouldn't worry about your stride. Just put one foot in front of the other and run. Once you're in better shape, you'll want to run a little faster and with more efficiency.

When you reach the intermediate level, proper stride form becomes more important. As you stride forward, the lead or reaching foot, after it has stretched forward and already started to swing back, should strike the ground more or less directly under your hips. If your foot hits the ground ahead of your center of gravity and before the knee begins flexing back, you're overstriding. That means you hit the ground with a straight leg, which transfers tremendous shock to the knees, hips, and back. A long, leaping stride is inefficient; you spend too much time in the air. Conversely, a short, choppy stride is wasteful; you spend too much energy to advance a short distance. This is understriding.

Runners with greatly pronounced or distorted knee lift or back kick are also wasting energy. A beginner will run with a low knee lift. Concentrate on lifting the knee just enough to allow your leg to swing forward naturally. Combined with a gentle heel landing, this will give you an economical yet productive stride. At first, the only time you need to focus on lifting your knees higher will be to help you run uphill.

As you grow more experienced, you can attempt to increase your stride length and stride frequency, the two ways of improving speed. Stride length is the distance you cover between each footstrike. Stride frequency is the total number of right- and left-foot ground contacts per minute. Running speed is the product of the length and frequency of stride. Therefore, there are only two ways to increase your speed:

Increase the length of your stride. You can improve stride length not by trying to stretch the lead leg out in front of the body but by increasing rear leg propulsion. You may need to lift your knees slightly higher and push off harder with your rear foot. Remember: Push with the rear foot, don't reach with the front one. Hill training, speed training, and weight training will improve leg drive. Increased flexibility will also help you lengthen your stride and improve running speed.

At any given pace, everyone has a stride length that is best for him or her; usually it is the most comfortable. Studies show that at least 20 percent of runners overstride. Stride length should not be copied from any other runner nor imposed by coaches. Arbitrarily adjusting your stride length would probably be counterproductive. There is no one optimal stride length for all runners. Be careful not to overstride. It is better to understrive than overstride.

Increase the frequency of your stride. Research shows that the stride frequency of elite runners is faster than the average runner: 90 to 95 strides per minute compared to just 80 to 85.

How do you know if your stride rate is quick and efficient? Peter Cavanaugh, Ph.D., director of Penn State University's Center for Locomotion Studies, suggests testing yourself while running at your regular training pace on a flat surface. Count the times one foot hits the ground per minute. If your strides per minute is less than ninety, you'll probably benefit from shortening your stride and increasing its frequency.

How can you improve stride frequency? There are several ways:

1. Weekly speed workouts, as detailed in Chapter 15, run at faster than race pace, will teach you to turn your legs over at a faster rate.

2. Run up and down a few flights of stairs to train yourself to take smaller, quicker steps. Do this once a week for a few weeks.

3. Exercise physiologist Owen Anderson, Ph.D., suggests practicing running at a steady pace at a faster stride frequency. First, count your current stride rate. Then, Anderson suggests running at a stride rate of ninety strides per minute or slightly faster. To do this in practice, he recommends running at that rate for 3 minutes while counting strides every 30 seconds. Adjust your stride rate—faster or slower—to keep on target. He recommends following this exercise until you have finished a total of four runs at your quicker pace. Between each timed 3-minute run, jog slowly for 3 minutes while not counting your strides.

Another of Dr. Anderson's tricks for increasing stride rate is to use a runner's watch that includes a pace beeper. It can be set to beep at a specific stride rate. Set it for your goal stride rate. Start your run at your normal tempo and then turn on the beeper. Keep pace with it for a few minutes at a time during your daily runs. Little by little, run at the quicker stride rate for more and more of your run. Eventually, you will be able to run your entire workout at a faster stride frequency without the assistance of the pacer.

The key to running faster then is to quicken powerful and controlled strides. Each runner usually finds a stride that naturally works best for him or her at a comfortable pace, and then "switches gears" to adjust power and speed for hills, speed training, and racing.

Body Angle

Too many runners worry about how they should hold their body as they run: erect, bent over, or whatever. The best advice is to relax. Allow your body to move as freely and with as little rigidity as possible.

Hold your head high, your eyes focused directly ahead, and keep your back as straight as comfortably possible. By "tucking in" your buttocks, you can run in an erect, comfortable position. An imaginary line drawn from the top of your head through your shoulders and hips should be perpendicular to the ground.

Leaning too far forward, one of the most common mistakes, places an extra burden on the leg muscles and can contribute to shin splints, Achilles tendinitis, back pain, and other injuries. If your upper torso leans too far forward, bending at the waist, you will force your hips too far back and drastically cut down on the length of your stride. More advanced runners use a slight forward lean to help them generate speed. But you aren't ready for that form yet. On the other extreme, leaning too far back has a braking effect, and it, too, places a severe burden on the legs and back.

I notice many beginner and intermediate runners chugging along with their head down, especially when tired. I also see runners of all levels in racing with heads down and feet churning. They think that by lowering their heads they can charge forward and gut out a faster time. Will it work? A study at Central Washington University in Ellensburg tested runner's oxygen uptake while running on a treadmill; they ran while looking at video displays of country road scenes placed straight ahead at eye level, and then while looking down at videos placed at ground level. The researchers determined that your running economy is more efficient by approximately 1 percent when you look straight ahead while running instead of looking down at your feet. What does this mean? The difference would amount to about 30 seconds in time during a 50 minute 10K run. Why? Your head will help keep you erect. If you look down as you run, you will start to lean forward which will ruin your efficient upright running style. This results in a loss of energy and a slower training or racing pace. Don't look at your feet; keep your eyes straight ahead.

Bring your head too far back, and you'll lean backward. Tilting your head to one side or the other will also throw off the efficiency of your movement. Your head weighs about 10 pounds (perhaps more for some of my thick-headed friends), so keep it centered on your shoulders in a natural, relaxed position. Envision that you are balancing this book on your head as you run.

Run relaxed. Your shoulders should hang loosely, parallel to the ground. Don't stick your chest forward or throw back your shoulders. Make sure you don't pinch your shoulder blades together. Tension collects first in the neck and shoulders. You can release any building tightness by occasionally letting your head roll from side to side, shrugging and lowering your shoulders, and dropping your arms loosely. By occasionally allowing your chin to lower and flap—as in talking—you can keep your jaw and neck muscles relaxed.

Maintaining good running posture is essential to good body mechanics. To maintain proper body angle while running for long periods of time requires strong postural muscles. Weight training to strengthen the upper torso and abdominal muscles is recommended. Otherwise your running posture will fall apart late in a run or race when you're tired.

Arm Action

In running, your arms are almost as important as your legs. They are not just along for the ride. If you use your arms properly, they will make your legs go faster by propelling your body forward. You will also maintain good balance and conserve energy.

The movement of your arms provides the rhythm that pulls you along. The faster your arm movement, the faster you will be able to move your legs and the easier it will be to make it up hills. "Pumping" the arms in powerful strokes is as important to the sprinter as a high knee lift. But the beginner and intermediate runner doesn't need to worry about vigorous arm pumping unless you are running up a hill, pushing yourself in speed workouts, or competing in a race. In everyday running you are interested in two important factors related to arm drive: body balancing and energy conservation.

Proper arm action is maintained by concentrating on the following:

Position
Your arms should hang loosely from the shoulders. If you carry them too high, the result will be a shortened stride, shoulder twisting, muscle fatigue, and tension in your shoulders and upper back. Arms carried too low contribute to forward lean or a side-to-side and bouncing motion. Too little forward or backward arm swing will result in a lack of proper forward drive, lift, and balance. Either flopping your arms or rigidly holding them in position contributes to inefficiency of motion.

Carry your arms between your waistline and chest. On the upswing, your hand should come close to your body at about your pectoral muscles. On the downswing, your hand should lightly graze the side seam of your running shorts. The arms naturally swing in front of your torso, but your hands should never cross the midline of your chest (such as the zipper line of your jacket). Arms moving across the body cause side-to-side motion and a shortened stride. Keeping your elbows unlocked and slightly away from your body will help maintain proper arm motion. Every runner will vary slightly in arm position. The main objective is to carry your arms in a relaxed and efficient manner.

Arm Drive
Arms balance the runner. Their motion helps propel you forward. Your arms should move in a vertical plane from front to rear, and should synchronize with the opposite leg. The arms act as a lever and balance for the leg drive and should move in the same plane as the leg. As the left leg pushes into the ground, your right arm is driven down at the same instant adding to the driving force. When the right leg drives into the ground, your left arm propels downward. The faster the beat the quicker the arms move.

You might want to practice arm and leg synchronization before a mirror, perhaps to the beat of music. First try your arm swing, and then synchronize it with an easy lifting of your legs, moving from heel to toe and back while standing in place. Get the feel of arms and legs in rhythm with each other.

For slower running, hold your arms in a comfortable, relaxed position and keep their action to a minimum. When you want to go faster, your arms should swing from the chest just past your hips. There should be a pulling action, as in swimming, or a snapping motion, as in snapping a whip, on the downward swing. Dr. Cavanagh's research indicates that proper arm motion "increases running speed by providing small amounts of 'lift' and 'drive.'" Arm action reduces the amount of force needed to lift the body from the ground, and also aids in propelling the body forward. Without using their arms at all, Dr. Cavanagh found, runners needed 4 percent more oxygen to run at the same speed than when using their arms. You can test the theory by running uphill first with your arms at your side, then using your arms properly.

Keep your arms and shoulders relaxed and strong. The success of your arm drive will be enhanced by improving your upper body strength. The use of weight training, and hand weights, will help.

Forearm and Elbow

When you swing your arms, concentrate on moving them from the elbow down, driving from the forearm. *This is the most important ingredient in proper arm drive.* Many runners swing from the shoulder, locking their arms at the elbow. This is a slow and inefficient method that requires a great deal of energy to move the large muscles of the shoulder and the length of the entire arm.

Imagine that you are cross-country skiing, and pushing yourself along the trail with your poles. The motion is very similar to running, and the movement is from the forearm down, which makes your elbow open and close with each swing. Do not lead with the elbow, but with the hands, wrists, and then forearms.

Don't lock your elbow; this common error makes the shoulders sway and dip and will not allow you to drive downward with the arm. The elbows should be "open" and should bend and straighten a little with each arm swing. They should neither point away from the body nor be tucked in close to it.

The Hands

Proper hand position is essential to correct arm drive. Percy Cerutty, the famous Australian coach, emphasized that "all natural running begins in the person's fingers and is transferred to the legs and feet." Your hands should be held loosely, so that your thumb and forefinger or middle finger just touch, "cupping." The thumbnail faces up. Fists clenched or fingers held stiffly create tension; hands hanging loosely cause the arms to flail. Both create an inefficient running motion.

The Wrist
The wrists should be relaxed and loose. At the top of the swing, cock your wrist slightly upward. At the bottom, flick your wrist as if lightly snapping a whip, turning your palm somewhat down and in. The snapping allows you to stay loose and rhythmic.

Putting It All Together
By driving the arms, maintaining proper body angle, and utilizing the proper footstrike and forward-stride techniques—all together—you will have arrived at near perfect form, for you. I encourage you to work at correcting the most common errors and strive to clean up bad habits. You can improve those areas that need work by concentrating on just one or two things at a time. Take a mental picture of the way you want to look when you run and gradually sculpt and model yourself until you approximate that image.

You may choose to have a coach analyze your form and offer suggestions for improvement. In my running classes I give our students an overview of good running form without telling them how to run every step. Then, I'll just allow them to start running naturally. I'll watch for obvious faults in their form and help them make corrections. But I don't overcoach. It's better that a runner feel comfortable than have perfect form. One of the best ways to know if you are running with good form is by watching yourself run. If you run on a treadmill in front of a mirror, you can check out how you look on the run. Or, have someone videotape you while running and review it. Film yourself from three directions—front, side, and rear. You may be surprised at the things you are obviously doing wrong.

Don't worry too much about having to remember all these points about running form. If you feel good when you run—relaxed and comfortable—you're no doubt doing far more things right than wrong. There's no need to become obsessed with attaining perfect form; nobody's got it, not even the world's best.

Changing Gears

Running at conversational pace involves one type of running form. If you choose to increase your pace in speed training or races, then you need to learn to "change gears." To go faster, remember the four "drives":

Drive off the back foot.

Drive up with the knee.

Drive forward with the hips.

Drive down with the arms.

As a result of emphasizing the four "drives," you will slightly increase your stride length (without overstriding) and increase your stride frequency. You will run faster. The best way to learn how to change gears in order to run faster is with speed training. These workouts will not only train you to run with better form when racing, but your form will also be enhanced for your daily training runs. By exaggerating your movements during speed training, it is easier to focus on them. By pumping your arms, lifting your knees, and driving off your back foot much harder in these workouts than you do in daily training or racing, it will be easier to maintain good form habits in all of your runs. Chapter 15 details speed training that will enhance running form. If you want more advanced guidelines on running and racing form beyond those included in this book, consult *The Competitive Runner's Handbook*.

Here's a "form drill" I recommend to help runners learn to run a little faster and to improve running form. Whether running for fitness or competition, this drill will benefit you by making you feel better about yourself. To enjoy it more, run with a few friends, and if possible, run on a quarter-mile track. If you can't find a track, look for a dirt trail or a smooth grassy field. Pick up the pace for a straightaway on the track—about 100 yards. Run briskly, not all out. Concentrate on the mechanics of "changing gears," not running hard. Then jog easily for the rest of the lap and pick it up again when you return to the starting point. Do four to six pickups total. Run this drill once a week.

In racing, you must concentrate on your form to maximize your potential. Efficient racing form will shave seconds, even minutes, off your time and give you an edge over your competitors who are not running relaxed and efficiently. Race technique involves the ability to maintain good form throughout an evenly paced race and to switch gears, making necessary alterations in form.

Uphill Form

Here's the moment all runners dread, whether a beginner or a veteran runner like myself. Hills. When you round the bend and see the Big Hill, don't wince. Prepare! Learn to shift gears—both mental and physical—and use proper technique to propel yourself up that hill. Attack the hill before it attacks you by changing your form; too many runners go uphill without using their arms and foot drive. Hill-running techniques can increase your comfort in getting up hills in training runs, and improve your racing time over hilly courses. Surprisingly, it is easier to run uphill quickly with good form than slowly in poor form.

For most hills, you should try to maintain, as nearly as possible, the rhythm and form you use on the flats. A few changes, however, are necessary to compensate for the incline and increased resistance.

- Keep a steady stride throughout the climb. First, increase your knee lift. If you don't, you won't be able to get your feet up and out in front of you. It's like climbing stairs: You want to pick up your feet more.

- Increase your stride rate slightly. Tighten your stride for economy. Shorten your stride length slightly to keep your center of gravity over or slightly in front of the drive leg. Consequently, your force is directed up and forward, which is the precise direction you want to go.

- Increase your arm swing slightly. By driving the arms a little bit more, you will overcome the pull of gravity. But don't exaggerate the arm drive. The faster the pace and steeper the hill, the harder you'll need to drive your arms.

▪ Push harder off the back foot. The faster you wish to run up the hill and the steeper the hill, the harder you push. Do not shuffle or bounce up the hill; drive up the hill. Try to look like an antelope gracefully gliding up the hill rather than an elephant awkwardly pounding up it.

▪ Lean into the hill slightly. This increased lean will help you keep your center of gravity forward; you lean forward slightly just to maintain an upright position relative to the pull of gravity. The steeper the hill, the greater your lean. Keep your hips slightly forward, chest forward, back straight, chin up, and eyes ahead. If you look down near your feet, you will bend forward at the waist, destroying your erect, efficient posture.

One other trick here: Focus your eyes on an object 10 to 15 yards ahead and watch it pass, then focus on another object. Psychologically, you can also pull yourself uphill with your eyes.

▪ Don't tense up. Don't bring up your arms to fight the hill, and don't tighten your neck, hands, forearms, or shoulders. This tension diverts energy from the real struggle of running uphill. Run relaxed.

Maintain an even, steady rhythm. The goal is to get up the hill with the minimum loss of energy. Attack the hills with finesse, not muscle, by steadily moving uphill with good form and reasonably controlled breathing. Practice switching gears when you approach hills during your daily training runs. Run the hills at a strong pace, but not all-out. Refer to the hill training workouts in Chapter 15 for guidelines on learning to run uphills at a faster pace.

Downhill Form

Downhill technique is ignored by most coaches—and most books. Uphill technique is more glamorous. But once you've passed 'em going up, don't let 'em pass you going down. Most runners think downhill running is easy: take off the brakes and roll. It is essential to let gravity do much of the work, but you must master the technique of letting yourself go while running in a controlled manner. This takes practice.

In an attempt to get down a hill as quickly as possible, some runners flail their arms and legs all over the place; they may get injured or lose their rhythm and speed. Others fight the downhill and lean back, shorten their stride, dig in their heels, and raise their arms to "brake" them.

You should develop a feel for downhill running. Some runners compare it to "throwing" themselves downhill; others feel like a mountain stream flowing smoothly with the hill. You can actually improve your race times more by perfecting your downhill technique than by perfecting your uphill technique. The speed with which you run downhill is regulated by the lean of your body and the length of your stride.

As you start downhill, try to keep your form as close as possible to that used on the flats. Allow gravity to do most of the work for you.

Forward lean. Keep your body perpendicular to the ground, back straight (don't bend at the waist), and your hips pushed forward over your lead leg. Your forward momentum will keep you from falling on your face. The angle of your lean helps determined how fast you go downhill. To maintain a steady pace, hold the angle of your body so that the center of gravity is over your lead leg. If you lean too far forward, you will pick up too much speed and be out of control; leaning back will cause you to slow.

Arm swing. Keep your arm swing under control. Unlike running uphill, downhill running uses the arms mostly to maintain balance and rhythm. There is no need to swing the arms hard; gravity is powering you downhill. Don't swing your arms wildly, windmilling all over the place as you go downhill; this causes you to lose balance and rhythm. Keep your elbows slightly away from the side of your body. Get your arms in rhythm with your legs.

Footstrike and stride. Use the same footstrike that you use on the flats. However, podiatrist Steve Subotnik suggests: "Concentrate on landing on the ball of the foot. If you're landing on your heels, you're overstriding. This is important because the foot and leg absorb shock much better when you land on the ball of the foot under a bent knee, than when you land on the heel in an almost straight-knee position." The ball-heel form absorbs shock and helps you hold forward motion as you run. But it may be uncomfortable. If you strike behind the ball of the foot, concentrate on lifting your feet quickly, hitting lightly, and pushing off against the slant of the running surface. If you are more comfortable running heel-ball, concentrate on hitting the heel very gently and quickly rolling your foot forward so you don't jam your heel into the ground. Most important, do not bounce on your toes or overstride by landing hard on your heels with locked knees.

Relax. Keep your arms, shoulders, neck, and chin relaxed. Practice will help alleviate tension. But as Dr. Subotnik warns: "I tell runners to master this downhill technique, then to avoid it whenever possible. That is, even if you are a great downhill runner, you should do as little of it as you can. No one can tolerate a lot of hard downhill running and no one should try."

Breathing

Many runners ask, "How should I breathe while running?" or "Should I breathe with my mouth open?" There is a theory that runners should breathe in through the nose and out through the mouth. This supposedly promotes relaxation and filters the air. But running calls for lots of air to satisfy the body's need for oxygen. You won't last long breathing in through the nose and out the mouth. Open up your mouth and suck in all the air you need.

Most runners breathe in time to their footstrike. They may inhale, for example, on every other left step, and exhale on every other right. Such breathing techniques may be relaxing during yoga exercises, but they would drive me nuts during a run, and I'm sure I'd get confused. If I had to blow my nose during the run, would it count as an exhale? What if I sneezed when I was due to inhale? Life is too short, and running too beautiful, to spoil it with rigid rules. My advice is to breathe when you feel like breathing. On the other hand, Shepherd, who will try anything once, has done special breathing exercises while running. He loves them. You decide what's best for you.

However, there are two basic rules. Breathing should be relaxed, and should follow "belly breathing" principles. Most of us breathe backwards. We tend to suck the stomach in, and breathe from the chest. With proper abdominal breathing, the belly expands as you inhale, and flattens as you exhale. The expansion of the abdomen indicates that the diaphragm is fully lowered, inflating the lungs to their fullest and allowing a more efficient intake of oxygen. Improper breathing can also cause the dreaded side stitch (see Chapter 33).

To understand how to belly breathe, lie on your back and place a book on your stomach. (Try this one.) Take a deep breath. If you are "belly breathing" properly, the book will rise as you inhale, and fall as you exhale.

Many runners hyperventilate, especially when running up hills or when excited during races. Instead of breathing in a slow, relaxed manner, they tense up and breathe in shallow, quick breaths. Keep your running form and your breathing under control.

THIRTY-FIVE

Cross-training

What is cross-training and why can you benefit from it? Cross-training is using one or more sports to train for another. It is a program that uses two or more types of exercises to promote total fitness—a combination of the three basic fitness components detailed in Chapter 2 (aerobic fitness, muscle fitness, and flexibility). Your fitness and running program can be enhanced by using other aerobic exercises.

Why Cross-train?

Running isn't the only way to promote fitness. In fact, it is just one of many options, although I rank it as one of the best. Whether you exercise for health and fitness, fun and fellowship, or competition, cross-training offers the following advantages for runners of all ability levels.

Total Fitness

Running is great for aerobic fitness and for fitness of certain leg muscles (hamstrings, calves). But it does little to improve the fitness of the muscles in the front of the legs, arms, shoulders, back, chest, or abdominals. Further, running does more to inhibit flexibility in the muscles and joints than it does to improve it. Runners can improve total fitness with a strength training program as detailed in the following chapter, but you can also work on your aerobic fitness while improving muscular fitness by cross-training. For example, following are key muscle areas developed with some cross-training activities:

Ankles	Swimming, deep-water running, snowshoe running
Shins	Biking (with toe clips)
Quadriceps	Biking, race walking, cross-country skiing, rowing, swimming, stair climbing, skating, deep-water running, snowshoe running
Upper body	Swimming, race walking, cross-country skiing, rowing, deep-water running
Low back	Swimming, rowing
Hip	Biking, race walking, cross-country skiing
Buttocks	Race walking, cross-country skiing, rowing, swimming
Abdominals	Race walking, cross-country skiing, rowing, swimming, deep-water running

No one activity can promote fitness in all areas of the body, including running. Swimming comes the closest to the perfect total fitness exercise; running would rank much farther down the list. Thus, the value of combining activities. The exercises that come the closest to mimicking running are deep-water running, cross-country skiing, and stair climbing.

Here's an example of how cross-training can bring total fitness. Running does a great job of strengthening the muscles in the back of the legs (hamstrings and calves), but does little for the muscles in the front of the legs (quadriceps and shins). Biking does the exact opposite. Combine the activities, and you get total fitness from the waist down. Add some upper-body weight training or an activity like swimming or rowing, and you've achieved a total fitness program! My advice for the ideal total fitness program would be the following:

1. Running three to five days a week for 30 minutes or longer.

2. Cross-training with another aerobic activity one or two days a week for 30 minutes or longer.

3. Weight training (see the following chapter) twice a week.

4. Stretching exercises daily for flexibility.

Increases Aerobic Fitness and Enhances Weight Control

If the goal is to improve endurance, then the runner most often keeps adding more and more mileage. When training for races, especially when marathon training, this buildup system is often used until race day or an injury occurs—quite often the latter. But since swimmers and bicyclists, for example, can train longer and harder due to the nonimpact nature of those sports, shouldn't runners adjust their training to take advantage of these and other cross-training sports?

Running ranks very high compared to other exercises for building aerobic fitness and burning calories. But you can only run so many miles in a week without risking injury. Cross-training can allow you to build your aerobic fitness even more and lose a few more pounds while you're at it.

Running Performance

Which cross-training activities are best for promoting racing performance? Exercise physiologist Owen Anderson, Ph.D., listed his top 10 in his newsletter *Running Research*:

1. Biking

2. Weight training/circuit training

3. Soccer

4. Deep-water running

5. Stair climbing

6. Cross-country skiing

7. Aerobic dance

8. Walking

9. Tennis, racquetball and squash

10. Swimming

Recovery on Easy Days

A great way to follow the recommended hard-easy approach to training is to follow hard running days (races, long runs, speed training) with a day of cross-training. Your tired legs will welcome the opportunity to exercise without being pounded, and the increased supply of blood will help flush out waste products and promote recovery. This is especially useful after a marathon. If you pound the ground on sensitive legs and blistered feet you're likely to cause injury. I advise runners to bike or swim for 30 to 45 minutes three straight days after a marathon before running a step. Beginner and intermediate fitness runners may benefit from alternating a day of running with a day of cross-training to maximize recovery from the running and minimize injury.

Injury Prevention

The spirit is willing but the flesh is weak. And for runners, the flesh always has the last word.

Specifically, it's the musculoskeletal system that betrays us. The heart and lungs—and the mind—have tremendous capacities for work. Swimmers and cyclists prove that by training hour after hour, day after day. But running, unlike those activities, is a weight-bearing sport, a stressful, pounding way to have a good time. The runner's training limit is reached sooner and enforced more strictly.

Cross-training decreases your risk of injury in two ways. First, muscle imbalance is a cause of injury and cross-training can strengthen key muscles not affected by running. Second, a non-weight-bearing activity such as swimming or biking can replace some of your running miles and thus eliminate some of the pounding that contributes to injury.

Recovery from Injury

Let's face the fact that every runner comes down with an injury at least once no matter how wisely he or she trains. When you can't run, or can only run on a limited basis, you most likely can still exercise aerobically. Chapter 33, "Injury," details how you can minimize fitness loss while injured by cross-training and how to use aerobic alternatives to come back from injury.

Obstacles: Travel, Safety, Bad Weather

For many reasons, you may not be able to get out the door for your run. When traveling, you may not have the time for a run or know where you can run safely, but you may be able to work out at your hotel's pool or exercise room. If you don't feel safe venturing out after dark alone, a good option is to work out at home or at your fitness club using exercise equipment. If the weather outside is horrendous—too wet, cold, or hot—you can still exercise inside. You also may need to escape to an air-conditioned exercise area if bothered by air pollutants and allergies. If snow and ice are the problem, you can turn that to your advantage by snowshoe running, cross-country skiing or skating. Too hot? Jump in the local pond, river, or outdoor pool for a good workout. Sometimes runners are forced to stay home and tend to a child or parent. No problem! This is another reason to put that exercise bike, stair climber, cross-country ski machine, or treadmill you have been wanting on your list for Santa.

No obstacle needs to stop a determined exerciser. Rumor has it that the great Czech Olympic champion Emil Zatopek stayed home with his very ill wife in the midst of training for some key races. He reportedly placed towels in his bathtub, filled the tub with water, and ran in place for hours at a time. (Wonder what he did with the rubber ducky?)

Competition

Some runners find that by experimenting with other sports they discover a talent for competition. You may decide to enter a few bike or swimming races, for example. Many runners take up crosstraining in order to compete in triathlons. These events usually consist of three consecutive races: swimming followed by biking, and then running. Many triathlons (and biathlons, which combine running and either biking or swimming) now attract hundreds of recreational athletes of all ages and abilities.

Change of Pace
Training for a big race, such as your first marathon, can become tiring. Give yourself some time off without guilt. Taking a day off, or even a week or two, for another aerobic exercise is an excellent idea. It will give you a chance to rebuild, regenerate.

It's Fun
Some runners never get tired of running. They won't even consider cross-training unless forced to by injury. I'll admit that even though I enjoy an occasional mountain bike ride or workout on a stair climber, I'm not much into cross-training. Just give me my running shoes and my trail through the woods and I'm happy.

Many exercisers get bored doing the same thing over and over, so the variety of cross-training can keep them motivated. Others feel that cross-training gives them a fresher approach to their running. It's also a good excuse to learn a new activity, such as in-line skating or mountain biking. And you can enjoy time exercising with nonrunning friends and family, as well as make new friends. You can schedule cross-training into your weekly schedule or just occasionally enjoy another sport. I do anxiously look forward to a good snowfall so I can head for my running trails on my cross-country skis or runner's snowshoes. And my son enjoys it when I go biking with him.

Properly used, cross-training will not take too much time and energy away from your running, but rather will increase your enjoyment of running and improve your performance. By varying exercises, your running muscles won't get strained and your enthusiasm for running won't get drained. It can combine the essential "three f's"—fellowship, fun, and fitness.

The Running Equivalent System
The only thing most runners respect is mileage—training mileage to record in log books, to count and discuss and overestimate. More mileage is the runner's solution to almost any problem, because miles are in the runner's language.

How, then, to speak that language and still stop runners from overtraining? Or to make injured runners appreciate the value of sensible alternatives to running? I developed a system that I call the "running equivalent" (RE), and detailed its value originally in a feature article in *Runner's World*. RE is not running, but it is expressed in miles and goes into the training diary. Runners are comfortable with it.

In the RE system, any high-quality aerobic activity can be expressed in terms of running miles. Simply replace running minute for minute with any vigorous aerobic alternative exercise. Approximate the distance you would have gone had you spent your exercise period running. If you normally run 3 miles in a half-hour, then 30 minutes of cross-training earns you 3 RE miles. Log them in your diary as such: "RE—3 miles." It works the same with speedwork: If injury, or just caution, keeps you from doing mile intervals, for example, swim or bike hard for as long as it would take you to run a good mile. Take the appropriate rest interval and go again. You may even choose to include a weekly RE speed workout when you are able to resume full training.

RE training works because the heart doesn't differentiate. The heart benefits almost equally from equal amounts of good aerobic activity, provided the heart rate is approximately the same. Aerobic endurance is improved when the heart rate stays in the training range (60 to 80 percent of estimated maximum heart rate) for an extended period of time. It doesn't matter what form of exercise gets it there. The goal in RE speedwork is to drive the heart rate up beyond the aerobic heart range. Again, if you work hard enough, it's all the same to the heart.

FORMULA FOR FIGURING OUT
RUNNING EQUIVALENT MILEAGE

1. Figure out your average training pace per mile of running (example: 10 minutes per mile).

2. Divide this figure into the number of minutes spent exercising with cross-training within your training heart rate range (example: 30 minutes on an indoor bike).

3. The result is your running equivalent mileage (example: 3 miles RE to record in your diary).

Guidelines for a Cross-Training Program

It's important to realize that you can simulate the aerobic value of running and even the anaerobic value of running fast, but no alternative activity uses the same specific muscle groups as running. You must still get out there and pack in the miles. Hour for hour, running is the best training for the runner. The ideal use of cross-training and RE mileage to prevent injury and enhance performance would be to limit it to 25 percent of your total aerobic mileage.

If you are coming back from an injury or trying to run through a nagging problem, simply lower your running mileage to a safe level and make up the difference with RE miles. Your goal should be to return gradually to running full time, but it's probably wise to reserve 10 to 25 percent of your aerobic training for RE miles in order to prevent further injuries.

If injury dictates that all your aerobic work be cross-training for a period, at least replace some of the running with cross-training to minimize detraining. You can maintain minimal fitness by cross-training three to five times a week for 30 minutes at a time. Ideally, try to replace running minute for minute with cross-training in order to maintain near normal fitness. Your RE mileage should be the same as or a little higher than your running mileage was. This allows you to replace the running habit psychologically, and although you'll lose some fitness, you'll be able to return to running in good shape.

Whatever your reasons for cross-training, don't just jump into it. You must plan your nonrunning exercise as carefully as you plan your program of running. Here are some guidelines for adding cross-training to your exercise schedule:

- Ease into the activity. Treat your new exercise just as you did running during your first few months: don't overdo it. Too much too soon will be worse than too little. If you have been running regularly, your cardiorespiratory system will be in great shape. You will think that you can do more than you should in your new activity. But you need to be conservative because different muscles will be used, or the same ones in different ways. Your muscles will be vulnerable to soreness and injury if you don't start your new activity gradually. You may feel fine while you are exercising, but the next day you are likely to be very sore and stiff if you overtax your muscles. Begin the new exercise slowly, and do it every other day, alternating with running if possible.

▪ Training principles that apply to running (see Chapter 6) also apply to cross-training, especially the principles of alternating hard and easy days and training without straining. Train with moderation: don't get carried away with the excitement of new activities and overstrain your body. A good warm-up and cool-down are also recommended. Don't neglect your stretching exercises.

▪ Perform your new exercise at a training heart rate, or perceived exertion, approximately equivalent to that of running. Take pains to keep the intensity level high enough to provide aerobic benefit. Don't coast, literally or figuratively. Don't cheat. Keep your heart rate in the training range.

▪ If your exercise is less demanding than running, do it longer. Examples may be walking or outdoor biking. An hour of outdoor biking (where you may coast down hills, etc.) may be equivalent to a half-hour of running.

▪ If you are using cross-training to supplement your running, establish your minimum weekly running mileage goal and build cross-training around it. For example, if you're training for a marathon and want to run 40 miles a week but feel that 30 is the safe limit for your body, schedule in your 30 miles and space 10 or more RE miles around it.

▪ If new techniques are required, take lessons (for example, in cross-country skiing). Learn the basics of your new activity from those who are familiar with it.

▪ Wear appropriate safety equipment (for example, helmets for biking and pads for in-line skating).

▪ Whatever you select as an alternative exercise for a change of pace, continue to run a few times each week to keep your "running legs." For example, if you go for a two-week biking trip, try to run a couple of times each week for at least 30 minutes.

This will ease the transition when you return to your running program.

- Choose activities that you enjoy. There are many to choose from, so there is no need to force yourself to do something you don't like.

Specific Aerobic Alternatives

Aerobic Dance

This is choreographed exercise to music. It might be an "aerobics class" at a fitness studio or a workout at home to a tape on your VCR. If you like to move to the beat of music, this may be your best bet for a fun cross-training exercise. Personally, I can't get my running legs into the rhythm! But aerobic dance does help develop balance, flexibility, and muscular fitness along with aerobic fitness. A good instructor will work your entire body. Be aware that aerobic dance that involves jumping, hopping, and bouncing is an impact activity, just like running. Be especially careful about the type of floor you are exercising on. You want one that has plenty of bounce. Instead of high-impact aerobics, I recommend low-impact aerobic routines that avoid the jumping around and instead emphasize upper-body movement to raise heart rates. Step aerobics is another popular option. It consists of movements to music in which you step on and off platforms. Basically this is a low-impact, vigorous exercise that is especially good for the quadriceps. Whatever program you use, be sure to wear shoes that are appropriate for the activity, not running shoes.

Biking

Running and biking complement each other since they strengthen opposing muscles in the legs—biking works the quadriceps and muscles in the shin area (if toe clips are used) that are neglected with running. It also helps increase flexibility in the hip and knee joints. Regular, intense biking workouts used as a supplement to running has been proven in several studies to boost running performance. Aerobic capacity may be improved by 15 percent, 5K race times by 3 percent, and 10K race times by 9 percent.

Biking outdoors offers fresh air and scenery, but you have the increased danger of accident. If you are injured falling off a bike you may still be able to bike, but the pounding of running may make the injury worse. Always bike defensively and wear a helmet and bright, reflective clothing. I'm strongly against biking anywhere near car traffic, but if you do, make sure you ride with traffic and obey all traffic laws. Outdoor biking requires you to really push the pace since it is easy to coast down hills. Uphill climbs will push your heart rate much higher than if you ran the hill. It isn't easy to find areas to bike where you can push the pace fast enough to get a good workout without the interruptions of slowing for turns, traffic lights, cars, pedestrians, and more. Although biking produces its own cooling breeze, you will still dehydrate, so bring along a water bottle. You will need to bike vigorously outdoors for 3 or 4 miles to equal a mile of running. As you become fit, you may enjoy participating in bike tours or even bike races.

Mountain biking has become increasingly more popular for a good reason: It's fun. You can explore trails and rugged terrain while working the whole body. All the pushing and pulling needed to control the bike strengthens the upper body as well as the lower body. I love zooming up and down steep hills on my bike, especially after dark with my floodlights. This was my preferred cross-training program when coming back from back injury. On tough trails, mountain biking is as challenging a workout as you can get.

Biking on an indoor exercise bike is safer and you can get a more consistent workout—just stay at a speed and resistance that puts you in your training range. You can easily monitor your heart rate. Indoor biking can be approximately equivalent to running minute for minute. But it can be boring. To make it more enjoyable, put your bike in front of the television as I do. I'll also spend the time reading or listening to music while sweating. If you have other people around or someone to talk to while pedaling, it helps a lot. That's why many people have more success biking at a fitness club. A good way to make your indoor biking less boring and more vigorous is to do intervals. Up the resistance and/or the pedaling rate for 1 to 3 minutes and then go easy for an equal time to recover. I enjoy the challenge of the computerized bikes that will automatically throw hills and speed changes at you. As you become more fit, you can move up to a more advanced program. Another challenging option are stationary bikes that include levers to pump with your arms while you are pedaling with your legs.

Biking simulates the leg motion of running. Pedaling a bike can be useful in helping you improve your leg speed and ability to run uphill. Try to bike at a pedal revolution per minute (rpm) similar to your running stride per minute, or to a faster rpm if you want to increase running leg speed. Switch to a lower gear or decrease resistance if necessary to keep this pace. Most competitive bikers pedal at a rate of 90 rpms, which is the recommended stride rate for competitive runners. A 90-rpm cadence may be too fast for most beginner runner-bikers, but at least strive for an 80-rpm pace. To keep this pace you may need to lower your gears or decrease the resistance on the bike. If you bike in too high a gear or with too much resistance, you will cause too much strain on your knees.

Make sure your seat height is appropriate to reduce strain on the knees. You should have just a slight bend in the knee at the bottom of your stroke. You will need to ease into biking to allow your shoulder and neck muscles, hands, and buttocks time to adjust to the work. Most runners find that their legs fatigue much sooner than they run out of breath when switching to biking. This is because the specific muscles needed for biking aren't trained as well as your running muscles.

Circuit Training

This total fitness workout involves rotating quickly through several strength training stations alternating with aerobic activities. Generally, a circuit uses approximately twelve to sixteen stations. It might be best to start with fewer stations and add more as you adjust to the workout. Also, start with one "lap" of the circuit and later build to three to five full circuits for a total workout lasting from 30 to 60 minutes.

Typically, at each strength training station you would use a weight machine, free weights, or do strength exercises such as crunches or push-ups. You would do about twelve repetitions of each and then move quickly to an aerobic station. Here you might run laps on a track, run in place, use aerobic fitness machines, or jump rope for 30 seconds to a minute. You can experiment and make up your own routine or consult with a fitness professional to design one for you. The goal here is aerobic and muscular endurance, not muscular strength. Thus, the key is the speed with which you move from exercise to exercise, not how much weight you lift. The faster you rotate stations and the more you keep your heart rate up into your training range, the better the results. But don't rush through the exercises, causing you to use improper form. For best results, alternate upper and lower body exercises, always spaced between aerobic stations. Be sure to warm up and cool down properly and ease into this workout.

An outdoor type of circuit training is called a par course. This is basically an obstacle course for adults. They are very popular in Europe and many U.S. communities have built them in their parks. The course is usually built along a running trail and consists of several stations set up over a loop of one-half to one mile in distance. Every 50 to 100 yards or so is an exercise station that consists of such activities as push-ups, sit-ups, chin-up bars, horizontal ladders for hand-over-hand crossing, and balance beams.

Circuit training and par courses can add some fun to your workouts, but be careful to ease into these rugged routines.

Cross-Country Skiing

Dr. Ken Cooper ranks cross-country skiing (also called Nordic skiing) as the number one aerobic activity because it involves all the upper- and lower-body muscles in vigorous activity. Elite cross-country skiers are considered by many to be the most fit of all athletes. The driving action of the legs strengthens those muscles, while the motion of using the ski poles to pull you forward uses your shoulders, arms, and abdominals. The gliding action stretches the muscles in your back and the backs of your legs. In one invigorating workout, you promote all the components of fitness: cardiorespiratory endurance, muscle fitness, flexibility, and body composition. Another big plus: You skim along rather than pound the ground, thus minimizing the risk of injury.

It's best to start with proper equipment and lessons. One problem: You need snow. I got all excited about this activity one winter and was just starting to get the hang of it when the snow melted. The next winter it only snowed once!

It will take you a few sessions to get used to it, but once you do you'll really get in a good workout. Besides skis and boots that fit properly, you will need poles that are the right height for you to allow proper arm drive. You can rent equipment to test the sport. If skiing outdoors, be careful not to overdress, since you will build up a sweat in a hurry. It is easy to get your heart rate up too high, so monitor it frequently. Do too much too soon of this exercise and I guarantee you'll be sore all over the next day. The easiest way to start is to go to a ski center that has prepared trails. Heading out in the snowfields to cut your own trail is a lot of fun but also a lot more work. You may also enjoy "citizen racing"—mass events that encourage participation as much as competition.

You can benefit from this total body workout all year by using a NordicTrack or other cross-country ski simulator at your home or gym. Again, get instructions on how to use the equipment and ease into it. It may take a while to get the hang of it, but once you do you'll get a great workout.

Racquet Sports

Tennis, handball, racquetball, and squash are excellent for developing muscle fitness and flexibility, but they depend upon a series of sprints and bursts of energy rather than continuous aerobic activity. You can increase your aerobic fitness benefits by playing singles rather than doubles. Play at as high a level of intensity as you can, with minimal resting between volleys. The better shape you are in, the longer and more intense the volleys. You can also wear down an opponent by being in better aerobic condition. Reserve doubles time for family fun. Don't play these sports to get in shape. Get in shape first, then play the sport as a fun option. Also, don't wear running shoes while playing these sports or you'll risk turning an ankle.

Rowing

This is Shepherd's favorite. He likes the machines with the funny computer games to keep you amused while sweating away. Whether you use an indoor machine or row on a lake or river, rowing is an excellent aerobic activity that places a minimum of strain on the bones and joints. It works the upper body as well as the lower body at the same time. It can be a very rugged workout. Competitive rowers have some of the highest aerobic capacity scores ever measured.

Rowing is a sport you have no choice but to ease into. A few minutes at first will exhaust you. Indoor rowing can get boring, so the use of intervals or computerized challenges make it more fun. Get tips for proper form to improve performance and minimize injury. Beginners are particularly prone to back injury if they use their back muscles too much at the start of the stroke and bring their knees up too much on the stroke recovery. Be sure to keep the back straight and avoid straining it by allowing your legs, arms, and shoulders to do the work. Canoeing and kayaking are two other similar and fun activities.

Skating

Dr. Cooper's research indicates that skating at a speed of 6 minutes per mile is the aerobic equivalent of running at a 12-minute-per-mile pace. In other words, you need to skate twice as fast as you run to benefit aerobically. Further, you need to keep skating nonstop with your arms and legs always in motion. If you coast along you'll lose fitness benefits. Skating strengthens muscles in the legs, ankles, buttocks, and, if you swing your arms vigorously, the arms and shoulders. Lessons and properly fitted skates are important.

There are many options for skating for fitness: old-fashioned roller skating, newfangled in-line skating, and ice skating. You can skate at roller- or ice-skating rinks or on in-line skating tracks. Many exercisers enjoy skating to music. If you choose to skate on the roads and sidewalks with runners, bikers, pedestrians, and cars—be careful! And *please*, don't weave in and out of traffic and buzz by us runners. It is wise to wear protective helmets and padding—knees, wrists, elbows. Skating is a nonimpact activity—until you crash and fall. Be careful, skating injuries and accidents are all too frequent and can be quite serious.

Snowshoe Running

I've tried all of the cross-training options in this chapter and enjoy most of them. But snowshoe running in my opinion is the best form of alternative training for runners. It is more specific than the other choices because it really is running—only more arduous and without much of the impact.

My favorite dirt trails through the woods were buried under one snowstorm after another during the winter as I was finishing this book. Unless I was willing to high step, slip, slide and risk injury, they weren't runnable for three months. The only options for running were pounding the cold, hard pavement while dodging cars on partially plowed roads, and getting nowhere fast running like a gerbil on the treadmill at my fitness club. But Santa Claus came to the rescue with a real neat toy: runner's snowshoes.

How can you run with those big, awkward things? It's easy. Even I can do it. (And I'll admit that I still can't get my cross-country skis to do what they are supposed to do.) The modern sport snowshoe is aluminum-framed, light and stable. Runner's snowshoes, such as those made by Atlas, Redfeather, and Tubbs, are less than two feet long and one foot wide, and weigh only about three pounds per pair. You just strap your running shoes into the snowshoe bindings and take off running. The rubber decking keeps your foot from sinking into the snow. Since your weight is distributed over a larger surface, you have more stability when running over uneven snow. You almost float over the surface with very little jarring. Steel cleats under the ball of the foot and heel provide excellent traction. No more slipping, sliding and falling on the run for me! I can even run hard on slippery downhills with my snowshoes.

Snowshoe running is a lot more efficient than running in snow and ice with running shoes. But it is also hard work! Your ankles and quadriceps will get extra work, which will make you that much stronger for running when the snow melts. You can also really push your heart rate up. I find that I can get a higher quality hard run at the upper limit of my training heart-rate range on my snowshoes than I could possibly manage in the winter with regular running. I can't push the pace on slippery roads enough in running shoes to get my heart rate up to where I can get it with snowshoe running. Further, I can train harder more often due to the lower impact. Most important, it is an exhilarating experience that provides a great change of pace in my training routine. Being able to run where few others are fit or brave enough to tread is rewarding. So, too, are the beautiful winter scenes that I am able to enjoy. I'm finding that all that snow is a blessing since I'm in better shape after several weeks of snowshoe running than I used to be trying to train with conventional running through the winter months. One other advantage: All the extra work keeps me warmer!

But be warned! Snowshoe running is tougher than regular running. Ease into it a few minutes at a time. If you normally run at a 10-minute per mile pace on bare roads, then you will probably run at about a 12-minute per mile pace on snowshoes over packed trails (much slower over deeper snow) for the same effort. If you really get fit and daring, you can enter snowshoe running races over packed courses. Tom Sobel of Leadsville, Colorado, holds the recognized world record as this book goes to press for the marathon with a time of 3:06:17.

You can also get in a great, fun workout hiking in snowshoes. You can go with the fancy, light ones over packed snow, or the larger, more traditional models for hiking over deep snow in backcountry.

Snow Shoveling

After spending several days this winter shoveling out after one snowstorm after another, I can tell you from experience that snow shoveling is a total fitness workout! Your upper body, abdomen, back, and legs will get plenty of muscular work whether you shovel or push along behind a small snow blower (which lessens the threat of back injury). Be sure to shovel with proper form and lift with those powerful runner's legs to minimize the strain on your back. Upper body work increases heart rate much faster than leg work. Researchers at William Beaumont Hospital in Royal Oak, Michigan, studied ten healthy sedentary men. After just two minutes of shoveling wet, heavy snow, their heart rates exceeded my recommended training heart-rate range limit of 80 percent of maximum heart rate. Notes Dr. Barry Franklin, director of cardiac rehabilitation at Beaumont, "On the basis of our study, we believe that men with a family or personal history of heart problems or who have one or more of the major risk factors for heart disease should think twice about shoveling snow."

If you aren't used to shoveling snow, work at a slower, steady pace so as not to strain your cardiorespiratory and musculoskeletal systems. Don't hold your breath as you lift. Instead follow the same guidelines as when lifting weights: exhale as you lift, inhale as you let go. If you have been sedentary or have any type of heart problem, look for a kid who wants to earn an extra buck and put him or her to work instead of risking your life. Far too many heart attacks are brought on by snow shoveling.

If you spend a steady half hour or more shoveling snow at a brisk pace, don't think you still need to go out and exercise that day. You certainly get as much aerobic and muscular exercise shoveling snow as with other cross-training activities. If I'm working hard in the snow for a long time period I just note it in my diary and take a running day off. Don't go out for a run when you are sore and tired from shoveling.

Soccer and Basketball

I've seen plenty of athletes with several years of background as soccer players develop into very good runners. Depending upon the length and intensity of play, a game of soccer may involve anywhere from two to six miles of stop and go running, including plenty of sprints. As a result it provides both a good aerobic and anaerobic workout. Shelly and I coach a unique baseball and soccer program for kindergarten through fourth-grade kids. Each session the young sports enthusiasts spend half their time playing baseball (which draws them to the program but provides no fitness benefit) and half playing soccer. They don't realize that we are luring them into a running and fitness program because they are too busy having fun with the game. Even adult beginner and intermediate runners can have some fun playing soccer while getting in a good fitness workout. But be careful not to overdo it. Another precaution: Wear shin guards or you may get accidentally kicked. That injury may keep you off the running trails as long as running-related shin splints.

Basketball is also a great conditioner that allows you to run around and have fun while not realizing that you are exercising. If you play full court basketball at a fairly intense level, you will get in plenty of aerobic work. You'll also get in some quality anaerobic work as you sprint up and down the court. I used to play basketball at a high level of play for one to three hours a day. That background enabled me to quickly ease into competitive racing.

Beware that activities such as basketball, soccer and racquet sports involve stop and go activities that may overstress your runner's legs and also increase the chance of ankle sprains. Further, running around playing sports is a weight-bearing activity that, combined with running for fitness or competition, could result in overuse injuries. Beginner runners should build up their aerobic fitness before attempting these vigorous sports.

Stair Climbing

Stair-climbing machines such as StairMaster have become increasingly popular, providing a similar aerobic benefit as running minute for minute but without the pounding that increases injury risk. It is a very similar action to running because you are lifting your center of gravity by using your leg muscles. Since you need to lift your knees high while exercising, stair climbing really strengthens the quadriceps, which don't get much work running on the flats. This improves your running stride length. Stride rate, however, isn't enhanced, since leg turnover is slower on a stair climber. On stair climbers you don't go airborne, so the weight load is shared by both feet. Also, the platforms "give" as you step on them to make this a nonimpact activity.

To get the most from your workout, pay attention to your posture. Don't lean forward or grip the rails. Pump your arms as you would if you were running to increase the work, but be prepared to grab the rails or slow the machine if you are having trouble keeping up with the pace. Stair climbers frequently overstrain their Achilles tendons. To minimize this, don't drive down on the ball of the foot as you would with running; instead, keep your feet flat on the step—envision yourself running flat-footed.

To increase your fitness challenge and decrease boredom you can follow computerized programs of interval work. At my fitness club I take on the challenge of "the Gauntlet" machine, which throws speed bursts and hills at me at paces equivalent to sub-6-minute running miles. When I'm done with this hard session I'm soaked with sweat but my muscles aren't beaten up like they would have been if I ran that fast on the roads or track. A challenging option is a hill-climbing simulator like Versa Climber, which adds levers that you pull down with your arms as you climb. You feel like a monkey climbing a tree, but it's a total fitness workout deluxe.

Swimming

This exercise may come as close as you can get to the perfect total body fitness exercise. It is especially valuable to runners because the upper body is the propelling mechanism. Therefore, swimming really strengthens the upper body, which is neglected with running, and stretches the hamstrings and hip flexor muscles, which are tightened with running. It also improves ankle flexibility. Further, the massaging action in the water helps tired muscles recover from the strain of exercise. Swimming is probably the least stressful cross-training choice, and therefore ideal after an injury. Water movement around the injured area has therapeutic benefits, and swimming seems to ensure more blood supply to injured areas and improve the possibility of quick recovery. When swimming, you must really concentrate on your breathing. The result is that you learn to inhale and exhale more completely and more rhythmically. This control of your breathing carries over into your running and helps you control the "panic breathing" that may occur in races.

Since your body is completely surrounded by water, which has a cooling effect, when swimming, you can exercise without fear of overheating—no matter how hot it is outdoors. Thus, this is a great option when running in heat and humidity is getting you down. Doctors recommend swimming, because of the humidity at indoor pools, as the best option for runners suffering from asthma.

There is little similarity between the action of swimming and that of running. Because of the cooling effect and pressure of the water, your heart will beat slower for the given effort by 10 or more beats per minute than with running. It's okay to let your heart rate fall off by that much, but not by much more. Keep your heart rate up by not gliding and by maintaining a steady kick. Just as in running, keep your arms and legs going. A good goal is to swim at a heart rate that is 60 percent of your maximum. Four or 5 miles of running is approximately equal to a mile of swimming.

Unskilled swimmers may find their heart rates rising quickly and it may be difficult for them to swim for long because of poor technique or unconditioned "swimming muscles." A few swimming lessons may be a good idea to help the novice swimmer get the most out of swimming for fitness.

Most runners are impatient people accustomed to running in interesting scenery and chatting with others on the run. You have to be patient and disciplined to train in the limited atmosphere of swimming. A 30-minute swim for a runner may seem to last twice as long as an hour's run. Personally, I hate swimming. For me it is *boring*. But many of my running friends love it. They like to get into a groove and just flow through the water. For variety and to work different muscles, vary your speed and use different strokes. It may help to break up the swim with different strokes per lap, or to alternate a hard swim lap with a brief rest interval rather than swimming one monotonous lap after another.

A word of caution: Always swim with a life guard on duty or at least swim with someone who is a good swimmer, especially when swimming in an ocean, lake, or river.

Treadmills

This really is not cross-training, but I get questions all the time about the value of treadmill running, so I'll include my answers here. First, running on a treadmill is of equal aerobic value to running outside as long as your heart rate is in its training range. On a treadmill you have the added advantage of being able to keep at an exact pace per mile or to add the resistance of hills at the touch of a button. Just as important, you can make the hills go away. Wouldn't that be nice when running a hilly race! If you run on a treadmill at your fitness club you don't have to worry about finding a training partner—you may be surrounded by a roomful of exercisers. You may even be able to converse with the person exercising on either side of you. However, treadmills are so popular that many clubs limit you to 20 minutes, so you may need to move on to another aerobic machine to complete your workout.

You don't have to deal with rain, snow, cold, or heat either. And you can keep fluids nearby for easy hydration. Also include a fan near the treadmill to keep you cool—you'll get warm in a hurry without a breeze. If the treadmill has good shock absorbing belts, it will minimize the pounding of your running. Also, treadmills eliminate the slants you encounter when you run on most paved surfaces. So this reduces injury risk.

Running on a treadmill is somewhat different from outdoor running. You do not experience air resistance as your body is not moving forward, nor do you encounter head winds. When your foot hits on the moving surface there is less braking action than when you hit on stationary surfaces. Thus, running on a treadmill requires less effort than running outside, so you may feel as if you are running much faster on the machine. If you want an equivalent effort in terms of pace, increase the incline approximately 1 percent. The pace per mile as indicated on computerized machines may be inaccurate. As long as you exercise within your training heart rate range, exact pace will not be important. Treadmill running may be an excellent way for beginners to get started running, since you don't have to deal with hot or cold weather and you can easily regulate pace and monitor your heart rate. Follow the same walk-run program as described in Chapter 10.

Many men and women prefer treadmill running, others find it too boring. Some runners think of treadmill running as going nowhere fast. To liven it up, listen to music, watch television, or keep varying the speed and elevation. Some choose to run on a home treadmill for convenience or safety reasons. I'll use a treadmill for a brisk speed workout when my track is covered with snow or it's too cold out to run hard. I also find that by running on a treadmill in front of a mirror I can work on improving my form.

To keep pace with the moving belt, runners tend to lean forward or run up too far on their toes. This combined with the slight pulling motion of the belts could cause lower leg and Achilles tendon problems. Concentrate on good form and be sure to warm up slowly before settling into your pace. The first few runs on a treadmill should be at a pace slower than what's normal for you to allow adjustment to the feel of the machine. You want to get used to the rhythm and gain confidence that you aren't going to fly off the back of the machine.

If you are a dedicated treadmill runner and intend to run some races on the roads, it would be a good idea to get used to this surface by running on it a few times a week. I actually get questions from runners who marathon-train on treadmills. I advise them to ease into long runs on the road to prepare them for the stress of the marathon, but to stay on the treadmill for most of their runs if that's what they enjoy.

Here's another treadmill option for marathoners to consider: Stu Mittleman, the world-class ultra-marathoner, overslept on the morning of a New York City Marathon and couldn't make it to the starting line in time. No problem, he hopped on his treadmill and started it up as he saw the race start on television. He ran the same pace for the same length of time he had planned to run and got to watch the race as well!

Walking
This is the most easily accessible exercise of all. You can walk almost anywhere, and at any age. My seventy-year-old father walks a very brisk hour each morning; his uncle Louie Snyder walked several miles at a fast clip every morning past his hundredth birthday. Hippocrates knew the value of walking 2,400 years ago when he said, "Walking is man's best medicine." Even walking at a moderate pace yields significant health benefits. It is a great way to slow down and see more, and it encourages curiosity about life going on around us. Oliver Wendell Holmes said, "In walking, the will and the muscles are so accustomed to work together and perform their task with so little expenditure of force, that the intellect is left comparatively free." Walking is also an excellent family activity since it requires no skill.

Walking is my recommended exercise to get in shape prior to starting a running program, and I promote walking breaks during runs for beginners. All runners would benefit from using walking as part of their cardiorespiratory warm-up and cool-down. The best shoes to use for walking according to most sports doctors are running shoes, not walking shoes, since they give the best support and cushioning.

The key to walking for fitness is to move along fast enough to produce a training effect. You may choose to measure your fitness with the walking test in Chapter 3. As you get more fit with running, the faster you will need to walk. This means really pumping the arms and striding along. To help keep the heart rate up to a recommended minimum of 60 percent of maximum, you can walk while using hand weights. By vigorously pumping weighted hands you will increase your heart rate quickly.

As you get in shape you may choose to try walking options for variety and challenge. Hiking may involve walking over rugged trails and up hills, even mountains. It is an activity that can be a lot of fun and provide fun for the whole family. You may enjoy participating in local "walkathons" for charity.

Racewalking is the most vigorous form of this type of exercise. This Olympic sport is a combination of running and walking without the pounding of running. You racewalk faster than you walk, but slower than you run. A top racewalker can walk sub-6-minute miles, but the average person will move along at paces ranging between 10 and 20 minutes per mile. Three miles of racewalking will be approximately equal to 4 miles of running.

Racewalking involves vigorously driving the hips and pumping the arms to propel the body forward, but a part of one foot is always on the ground. You don't have to race to enjoy racewalking, but you can compete if you choose. The New York Road Runners Club offers a racewalking class for injured runners and those looking for a change of pace. Racewalking strengthens areas not affected by running or regular fitness walking—muscles in the front of the legs, abdominals, buttocks, upper body, arms. Because racewalkers learn to drive their arms really powerfully, the runner who racewalks can also improve running form and gain an awareness of the value of arm action in increasing running speed. On the negative side is the fact that there are few racewalking coaches, and it is necessary to learn the proper form. In fact, racewalkers can be disqualified from races for errors in form. Racewalking form involves an exaggerated motion causing your fanny to wiggle as you walk down the street. If you can ignore the stares and comments from onlookers, racewalking is a great exercise.

Water Running

This activity mimics running better than any other exercise because you actually are running, but without the pounding. The New York Road Runners Club offers a deep-water running class that is popular with injured runners as well as those who wish to prevent injury while getting in a good alternative workout.

You run in deep water using a flotation device to keep you afloat. As you run, the resistance of the water makes your whole body work hard—even the upper body. This can be an especially tiring workout when you first try it, so start off conservatively. As with most exercise, it is a lot more fun when you water run with others—or at least with music.

If you don't have access to deep water or flotation devices, you can try shallow-water running. Just stand in water up to your waist and run widths of the shallow end of the pool (or parallel to shore) against the resistance of the water. Build gradually from a few minutes up to 30 minutes. You can also run in place in water up to your thighs, concentrating on raising the knees.

THIRTY-SIX

Strengthening

Whether your goal is total fitness or race performance, strengthening key muscle groups is important. Muscular fitness consists of muscular strength (how much weight you can lift or move) and muscular endurance (how many times you can lift or move a weight). Runners need a certain amount of muscular strength, but muscular endurance is more important. Throughout this chapter I refer to "strengthening" as exercises that improve both types of muscular fitness.

Runners can improve muscular fitness four ways:

1. Running itself strengthens many muscles, especially the calves, hamstrings, and buttocks. You can also strengthen your quadriceps by running hills on a regular basis. But for the most part, running does little for the opposing muscles—quadriceps, shin area, abdominals—resulting in muscle imbalances that can lead to injury. Further, running itself contributes little to upper-body muscular fitness. Thus, runners need to strengthen themselves with the exercises in this chapter.

2. A well-balanced cross-training program, as described in the previous chapter, can be used to promote total-body muscular fitness. For example, combine biking for the quadriceps and swimming for the upper body with your running program and most muscle groups will get plenty of exercise.

3. Strengthening exercises using your body weight for resistance (some call these calisthenics), such as push-ups and crunches, can be easily added to your prerunning or postrunning stretching routine.

4. Resistance training with free weights (barbells and dumbbells) and weight training machines (such as Nautilus) can be used two or three times a week to complement your running. This type of exercise is referred to as weight training.

Strengthening muscles in the upper body will improve your ability to run relaxed with efficient arm drive. Postural muscles in the abdomen, hips, and back need to be strong to hold you erect with good running posture throughout your runs. Specific strength exercises also will help you increase foot and leg drive. A well-balanced strength training program will allow you to improve your running form and efficiency. Thus, you will require less effort for running and, consequently, improve your speed.

Strengthening running-specific muscles is important to injury prevention. Podiatrist Dr. Joe Ellis, author of *Running Injury-Free*, wrote in *Runner's World*: "When a muscle becomes fatigued, it loses its ability to generate sufficient power for proper movement. Other, less-qualified muscles are recruited to 'substitute' for the fatigued muscles. This substitution phenomenon is the body's way of keeping you running. The substituting muscles have to do work they're not supposed to do and for which they are unsuited. The result is usually an overuse injury—usually to one of the substitute muscles."

Besides enhancing total fitness and athletic performance, and preventing injuries, muscular fitness is important to carrying out daily tasks. Loss of strength due to aging is slowed with a well-balanced strength training program. Weight training helps to maintain bone density and thus minimizes the development of osteoporosis and stress fractures. It also burns body fat. In a study at Penn State University, a group of college women from the tennis team weight-trained two to three times per week resulting in a loss of body fat from 23 percent to 18 percent.

Strengthening Exercises Using Body Weight

You can improve your muscle fitness without the use of weights with the exercises below. You may choose to use some of these key exercises on a daily basis along with your stretches. Or, you may set aside two or three days a week for 15 to 30 minutes to focus only on strengthening exercises. If you are vulnerable to certain injuries, be sure to include specific anti-injury exercises to help prevent problems. Don't try to do all of the exercises below. I've given you plenty to choose from for variety.

Guidelines

A few guidelines:

- Alternate muscle groups when doing these exercises.

- A set consists of a certain number of repeated exercises. You may do two or three sets of an exercise with a rest period in between. You may exercise another muscle group between sets. For example, I usually alternate sets of push-ups and crunches.

- Start with a few repetitions of an exercise at first and gradually increase the number you can do. If you adjust well to the exercise and wish to increase the workload you have two options: (1) do more repetitions or more sets of repetitions; or (2) increase the resistance, for example by gradually adding weights.

- The goal is to improve muscular endurance more than strength, so for most exercises you will do ten or more repetitions.

- Do the exercises with proper form and do them slowly and in a controlled manner. This way you'll work the proper muscles through a full range of motion. If you do the exercises too quickly, momentum will minimize the desired gains.

- Don't strength train muscles that are sore or injured. That invites further injury. Push through mild discomfort, not pain. If you are slightly sore, go easy.

Abdominals

These muscles are important to your posture—holding you erect while you run long distances. Weaknesses here combined with tight muscles in the hamstrings and lower back contributes to back problems.

Crunches (modified sit-ups): Lie on back with knees bent, feet flat on the floor, hands across chest, and elbows out straight. Do not anchor the feet or the hip flexor muscles will take work away from the abdominals. Slowly raise the shoulders and upper back about 6 inches off the floor. Hold for 2 seconds and then slowly lower to the starting position. Exhale as you sit up and inhale as you come down. Look at the ceiling as you sit up. Do two or three sets of 10 to 20 crunches as long as good form is maintained. Do not jerk the upper body or arch the back in an attempt to come up. Stay under control. To increase the work, place your hands on the sides of your head. To work the muscles on the side of the abdomen (the obliques), turn one shoulder toward the opposite knee as you sit up; then repeat on the other side.

Note that full sit-ups, in which you raise yourself all the way up to a sitting position, are no longer advised by fitness experts. They feel that this extra work does little to strengthen the abdominals and increases the chance of injury by stressing the disks in the lower back.

Reverse Sit-ups: Crunches work the upper abdominals (rectus abdominus), reverse sit-ups strengthen the lower abdominals (tranversus abdominis). Lie on your back with knees bent, feet flat on the floor, and arms at your side, palms down. Keeping the knees bent, bring your legs up until your knees are directly over your hips. This is the starting position for this exercise. Keeping your back pressed against the floor, tilt your pelvis up toward the chest in a small, controlled movement while exhaling. Don't raise your hips off the ground or rock the body. The range of movement is only about 6 inches; any more will strain the back. Release. Do two or three sets of 10.

Pelvic Tilt: Lie on your back with knees bent and feet flat on the floor. Tighten the butt muscles and abdominals at the same time while tilting the pelvis up and pressing the lower back into the floor. Concentrate on holding muscle contraction for 3 to 10 seconds while exhaling. Do this three to five times.

Ankles
Exercises to strengthen the ankles improve your foot drive and prevent ankle sprains.

Ankle Push: Provide resistance by pushing your hand (or use a bike inner tube or exercise band and pull) against the foot in four directions—inward, outward, downward, and upward—and holding each for 10 seconds. Do three to five times.

Towel Sweep: Sit in a chair and place one foot on a towel with the heel on the edge of it. Grip the towel with the toes and push the towel away from you to the inside in a sweeping motion while keeping the heel in contact with the ground. Do five times and then repeat while sweeping towel to the outside.

Ankle Band Exercises: Sit in a chair and tie a rubber exercise band or bicycle inner tube around your feet in front of the ankles (not too tight). While keeping your knees and ankles together, press outward with the front of the feet, and then relax. Do this ten times. Then, cross your ankles and tie the band around the feet. Push to the outside with one foot while keeping knees and ankles together. Relax and do opposite foot. Do ten times with each foot.

Arch
The following will help strengthen the muscles in the arch and prevent plantar fasciitis.

Towel Exercise: Sit or stand and place a towel under your foot. Curl your toes to pull the towel toward you (without moving your leg and keeping heel on the floor). Release it and pull again. Keep going until the whole towel has been pulled under you. Then reverse the exercise by pushing the towel away. Do this two or three times.

Back
Keeping upper- and lower-back muscles strong along with the abdominals improves posture and decreases propensity to back injury.

Back Extensions: Lie on the floor on your stomach with hands under shoulders in the push-up position. Slowly lift the chest off the ground by using the low back muscles while keeping hips on the ground. Assist only slightly with arms. Do not arch neck or overextend lower back. Exhale when coming up and pause briefly at top of exercise. Inhale while returning slowly to starting position. Do two or three sets of 10.

Alternate Extensions: Lie on stomach with arms extended in front of you, forehead resting on a rolled-up towel. At the same time, slowly lift one arm and the opposite leg. Hold for 3 seconds and then slowly lower to starting position. Repeat with opposite arm and leg. Do 10 of each.

Buttocks

You do more than sit on your butt. These muscles (gluteus maximus, minimus, and medius) stabilize the hip and help drive you forward.

Butt Raisers: Lie on your back with knees bent, and feet flat on the floor. With the heels supporting your weight, lift the pelvis an inch off the floor, keeping the abdominal muscles contracted. Hold for 10 seconds, release, and relax. Do 5 to 10 times.

Pelvic Tilt: Described under abdominals.

Squats: Described under quadriceps.

Calf Muscles

The powerful large calf muscles (gastrocnemius and soleus) attach to the knee and the Achilles tendon, which attaches to the heel. These muscles help power your runs. The following exercise helps minimize calf strains, Achilles tendinitis, and posterior shin splints (strains of the posterior tibialis muscles behind the shin bone that stabilize the ankle).

Toe Raises: Stand facing a wall or chair and place one hand against it for support. Slowly raise up on the toes and then slowly lower heels to the floor. Do two or three sets of 10 to 20 toe raises with a one-minute rest between sets. As you get stronger, gradually add weights that you can hold in your hands (or place barbell over shoulders behind the neck) to increase resistance.

Hamstrings

The "hammies" are behind the thigh and help to stabilize the hips and legs, extend the hip, and flex the knee. They provide much of the pushing action to help you run.

Hamstring Curls: Stand facing a table or other object that is thigh high so that you can put your hands on it for support. Bend one leg backward at the knee while keeping the thigh aligned with your upper body. Don't flex forward at the hip or bend backward. Slowly bring the foot up toward your buttock as far as you comfortably can and then slowly return to the starting position. Do two or three sets of 20 with each leg. Gradually add weight to the ankle to increase resistance.

Hips/Groin

These exercises strengthen the structures that stabilize the hip, thus improving the power of your push-off, range of motion, and preventing hip- and groin-related injuries including iliotibial band syndrome and piriformis syndrome. The abductor muscles on the outside of the upper thigh get more work with running than the adductors on the inside of the leg, resulting in a potential imbalance.

Side Leg Raises (for the abductors): Lie on your side. Align the upper leg with your body and bend the bottom leg. Lay your head on the outstretched bottom arm and bring the top hand across and place it palm down in front of your chest for support. Slowly lift the upper leg, leading with the heel, until you've reached as high as you can comfortably, then slowly lower it to the starting position. Don't allow your leg to move in front of your body, and keep your knee facing forward. Do two or three sets of 10 to 20 with each leg. You may choose to gradually add weight to your ankle to increase resistance.

Inside Leg Raises (for the adductors): Lie on your side with head resting on outstretched bottom arm and lower leg aligned with your body (don't flex your hip forward). Bend top leg and place foot on ground in front of lower leg. Slowly raise bottom leg, leading with the heel, as far as you can and then slowly lower it to the starting position. Do two or three sets of 10 with each leg. You may gradually add weight to the ankle to increase resistance.

Chair Press: Sit in a chair with knees spread apart and feet flat on floor shoulder width apart. Cross your arms and place right hand on the inside of the left knee and left hand on the inside of right knee. Slowly bring the knees together while resisting with the hands. Do 10 to 20 times.

Quadriceps

The "quads" are the large muscle groups in the front of the upper thigh. They stabilize the knee joint, extend the knee, and lift the leg upward as you run. These exercises prevent knee injury (by balancing strength with the hamstrings) and improve your ability to run faster and up hills.

Sitting Leg Extensions: Sit in a chair or on the edge of a table, straighten your leg, and tighten it, holding the kneecap parallel to the floor. Tighten the muscles and hold for 2 or 3 seconds in an isometric contraction. Do 10 to 20 times. Do the same with the other leg. As you get stronger, add a 2-pound ankle weight.

Squats: Slowly squat about one-fourth to one-third of the way down and hold for 2 or 3 seconds before slowly returning to the standing position. Do 10 to 20 times. Do not squat lower than halfway down (thighs parallel with floor). A good precaution is to do chair squats. Lower buttocks over chair.

Shins

The anterior tibialis muscle in the front of the shin helps control foot and leg action as you strike the ground. Weaknesses here relative to strong and inflexible calf muscles on the back of the lower leg contribute to shin splints. These exercises strengthen the muscles in the shin area, thus preventing shin splints and other injuries related to muscle imbalances with the calves.

Toe Lifts: Sit in a chair, extend your legs slightly with your heels resting on the ground about a foot beyond where they would be if they were directly below the knees. Then lower your toes until your feet are flat on the ground. Now, lift your toes slowly toward your knees while keeping the heels on the ground. When you feel the muscles in the front of the shins contract, hold that position for 3 to 10 seconds, then relax. Do 10 times.

Band Exercises and Towel Sweep: See ankle exercises.

Foot Press: While sitting, place one foot on top of the other. Pull up with the lower foot and resist with the upper foot. Hold for 10 seconds and switch feet. Do five sets.

Upper Body
Your arm drive is important to your running and you need upper-body muscle fitness to safely lift objects during daily tasks.

Push-ups (for the arms and chest): Follow form guidelines detailed in Chapter 3 for the one-minute push-up test. Do two or three sets of 5, taking breaks in between sets to do other exercises. Gradually increase to sets of 20 or so with good form. Set a goal to improve your score on the push-up test.

Reverse Push-ups (for the triceps at the back of the upper arm): Stand with your back to a well-anchored table or chair. Rest your hands on the table or chair and extend your legs out in front of you so that your weight is supported by your hands and your extended heels. Slowly lower your upper body toward the table, while keeping knees slightly flexed; return to starting position. Do 10 to 20 times. To make this more difficult, pick a lower object, such as a bench for your support.

The Car Push
If you want a real challenge of a strength exercise to work both the upper body and the legs, try the car push. Madina Biktagirova is a Russian Olympian who won the 1992 Los Angeles Marathon. Five times a week while training in Colorado, her coach would sit at the wheel of a 2,800-pound car and instruct her to push the car up a 600-yard hill. This was after running an hour and a half at high altitude. The pushy woman explains, "Pushing the car really helps me because I feel so strong, especially in my quadriceps."

Basic 8: Sample Strengthening Workout Using Body Weight

Here is an example of a strength training routine without the use of weights—using your body weight for resistance—that will help you prevent injury and improve performance. I've chosen eight exercises that work important muscle groups for runners. You may add or subtract from the exercises described in this chapter. Emphasize exercises that relate to specific injuries to which you may be vulnerable. You may choose to do all or some of these eight exercises before or after each run in addition to your stretching routine. I usually do two or three sets of crunches and push-ups alternating with stretching exercises most days of the week. You may choose to set aside two or three days a week separate from your runs to do your strengthening exercises. Your routine should start with large muscle groups first and then move on to smaller groups.

1. Squats (quadriceps, hamstrings, buttocks)

2. Push-ups (upper body)

3. Crunches (abdominals)

4. Sitting leg extensions (quadriceps)

5. Reverse sit-ups (lower abdominals)

6. Side leg raises (hip abductors)

7. Chair press (hip adductors)

8. Foot press (shins)

Weight Training

Whether you choose free weights (handheld dumbbells, or weight plates on barbells) or machines (Nautilus, Cybex, Universal, etc.) for your weight training, it is advisable to get qualified instruction on the proper and safe use of the equipment before starting. You will get more return for your effort if you take the time to learn how to do it right.

Which is best, free weights or machines? They are both beneficial and will offer more strength gains than exercises that use your own body weight. This is because they offer greater resistance.

Free weights offer an important advantage in that you can do most of these exercises at home with minimal equipment. To use weight machines, you would need to go to a gym or purchase a multistation machine for home. When I'm able to fit it in my schedule, I enjoy the atmosphere of weight training at a gym. For a minimal expense you can purchase sets of handheld dumbbells of varying weights that will allow you to do many of the key exercises without leaving home. I have a 15-minute routine of dumbbell exercises combined with body weight exercises that I use two or three times a week before I head out for my easy-day runs. If you have some extra space, you can also purchase a barbell, a set of weight plates, and a bench to expand your home exercise gym.

Many weight training experts favor free weights because, along with lifting and lowering these weights, you must also hold them in balance. This works the major muscles as well as their assisting muscles. But it's easier to hurt yourself using free weights, especially when using heavily weighted barbells. Free weights may be best if you know what you're doing and have a good training partner to help if you start to lose control of the weights.

On the other hand, machines offer an easier, safer exercise. You can move from exercise to exercise much easier in a room with machines (unless you have to wait in line to use them at a crowded club). They can better isolate the muscle groups you want to exercise without straining other muscles. Machines dictate the way your body can move, thus making it simpler and more efficient to do the exercises.

The bottom line: For all-around strength gains, use free weights; for safety, convenience, and time saving, use machines.

Guidelines for Weight Training
- Wear loose-fitting clothing and supportive shoes, such as your running shoes.

- Warm up properly before lifting. Walk briskly or bike, for example, for 5 to 10 minutes to get the muscles warmed up. Stretch thoroughly after completing the lifts.

- Alternate muscle groups as you lift so you don't overtax your muscles. Start your routine by exercising the larger muscle groups first (such as legs) and then the smaller ones. It is easier and less of a risk to work small muscle groups when fatigued near the end of a workout than big muscle groups.

■ Do eight to twelve repetitions of each exercise. This will take approximately 60 to 90 seconds of continuous muscle work per rep. Multiple repetitions with low weights builds muscular endurance without adding bulk. A set is a group of reps. Do at least one set, but not more than three, of each exercise. For novice weight trainers, the American College of Sports Medicine suggests "one set of 8 to 12 repetitions of 8 to 10 exercises that condition the major muscle groups at least two days per week is the recommended minimum." It may also be enough for all but the more serious weight trainers. Researchers at the University of Florida's Center for Exercise Sciences put a group of men and women (ages 20 to 49) through a 14-week strength training regimen in which they weight lifted two to three times per week. One group did three sets of 8 to 12 reps; another did only one set; and a control group didn't lift at all. The result: Both weight training groups recorded significantly higher strength levels than the control group, and the "one-set" lifters scored only three to four percent less than the "three-set" lifters. Noted Michael Pollack, Ph.D., the Center's director, "The message seems clear. Hammer yourself with the extra work [reps] only if those few little percentage points are important, or if you just want to burn up more calories. But if it's only a strong and toned body you're after, stick with single-set training, two or three times a week."

■ Although even doing three or four different exercises would be of help, you ideally should do more so that each major muscle group is included. As a runner you may choose more exercises that strengthen muscles neglected with running (such as the upper body and abdominals) and fewer exercises that work running muscles (such as the calf muscles and hamstrings).

■ Your entire weight training workout should take 20 to 40 minutes. That is enough to gain strength and improve fitness.

■ Rest for one minute between sets to recover. You may use this time to do stretching exercises or to do a set of another weight exercise using different muscles.

▪ Weight training is progressive, just like running. Start with low weights and gradually increase the weights as you become stronger. Increase weight by 2 to 10 pounds as you improve form and strength. After you can handle twelve reps of a weight, slightly increase it (about 5 percent) and restart with eight reps. You may cut back on the number of sets until you adjust. Pay attention to how you feel. You may need to decrease the weight some days if you are feeling tired or just "down." It is better to lower the weight than to decrease the number of reps you do.

▪ Lift at least two times a week but not more than three. Studies show that you will get almost as much improvement (70 to 80 percent) by doing weight training twice a week as you would by doing it three. Allow two or three days rest between each lifting session to allow your muscles to recover.

▪ Ideally, weight training workouts should be separate workouts from your runs. A good choice may be to run three to five days a week and lift on your nonrunning days. If you choose to run and lift on the same day, which should you do first? Experts offer conflicting advice. Running too long or hard prior to lifting will fatigue your muscles and thus your weight session won't be as effective. Running a few miles easy as a warm-up prior to lifting may work for you. If you run directly after lifting, go short and easy because your muscles will be fatigued. A more ideal combination would be to run in the morning and lift at least four hours later in the day—or vice versa.

▪ Always exhale as you lift the weight, inhale as you release the weight. Don't hold your breath. Besides making the lift harder, it will place a strain on the heart.

▪ Lift the weights with a slow, controlled motion. Then pause for 1 or 2 seconds at the peak of the lift, and slowly return to the starting position. If you work too fast you will build momentum, which will lessen the work of your muscles. The negative, or return, part of an exercise may actually be the most important part for developing strength. The lift should take approximately 2 seconds and the return approximately 4 seconds.

• The goal is to exercise the muscles through a full range of motion. This aids in increasing flexibility and permits muscles to be more fully exercised.

• Concentrate on proper form and posture. Especially be careful to provide support for the lower back. No jerking or bouncing! Cheating by using other muscles to help on a lift means that the muscles you are trying to strengthen will do less work. If you can't hold your form with each lift, you are lifting too much weight. Lifting for fitness should be fluid and graceful, not an awkward brute force heave.

• Use a spotter to assist you on difficult exercises when using free weights.

• Don't work muscles that are sore or injured. That invites further injury. Push through mild discomfort but not pain. If you are slightly sore, go easy.

The following exercises use free weights or machines to strengthen key muscle groups (Do one to three sets of 8 to 12 reps):

Abdominals
Abdominal Curl Machine: Sit erect on seat with ankles under or behind pads and upper chest against pads. Place hands behind back. Slowly bend forward pressing against upper-body pad until abdominals are fully contracted, pause, then slowly return to starting position. Keep head aligned with spine.

Weighted Crunches: This is the same as crunches but with a weight plate held across the chest. Lie on back with knees bent, feet flat on the ground. Slowly curl up until shoulders are 6 inches off the ground, slowly return to starting position. Keep lower back pushed against floor while sitting up.

Side Bends (obliques): Stand with a dumbbell in your right hand. Keep feet flat on ground, knees slightly bent, hips tucked. Slowly bend sideways to the left, pause, slowly return. After 8 to 12 reps, switch weight to the left and repeat exercise.

Back

Low-Back Machine: Sit in machine, hands crossed and relaxed on chest, knees flexed with feet on support to brace legs. Place upper back in contact with pad and slowly push backwards until legs are extended, pause, then slowly return to starting position. Keep head aligned with spine.

Back Extension Bench (low back): Place feet on the foot plate of a hyperextension bench and anchor the backs of the ankles under the bottom pads. Lean against the hip pad so that it is below the hip bones. Hips should be flexed so upper body hangs downward until approximately at a right angle to legs. Place hands across chest (behind head when stronger). Contract the muscles on both sides of the spine, then the buttocks, and slowly lift torso until it is just above a straight body line. To increase the work of the lower-back muscles, position yourself against the hip pad so that it is at waist level, above your hip bones. Instead of hanging the body with the torso down, start with the body in a straight line. Lift with just your lower back until you are just above parallel.

Pulldown Machine (upper back): See upper body.

Bent Over Row (upper back): Place right knee and right hand on bench for support. Place left foot on floor and grasp dumbbell in left hand with knuckles facing forward. Keep back parallel to the floor. Slowly pull dumbbell to chest while turning hand so palm faces inward, pause, then slowly lower to elbow-extended position (but not to floor until set is completed). Repeat to other side.

Buttocks:

Leg Press Machine: Sit or lay on machine with feet shoulder-width apart and flat against platform, knees bent at a 90° angle. Grasp handles for support. Slowly extend knees and hips until slightly before knees would lock in full extension. Slowly return to starting position without letting weights touch. Keep back flat against bench, do not arch.

Squats: See hamstrings.

Calf Muscles

Weighted Toe Raises: Use a spotter with this exercise. Stand with barbell resting on rear shoulders, gripping it with hands palms up. Feet and hands are about shoulder-width apart, eyes straight ahead. Slowly rise up on toes until calf muscles are fully contracted, pause, then slowly lower heels to the ground. This exercise may also be done on a machine.

Hamstrings

Leg Curl Machine: Lie or sit on machine and place ankles under pads. Push pelvis downward while gripping hand bars, and slowly lift pad until they hit your buttocks and hamstrings are fully contracted. Pause, then slowly lower to starting position. Do not let hips lift up more than a few inches.

Leg Press Machine: See buttocks.

Squats: Use a spotter with this exercise. Stand with barbell resting on shoulders using palm-up grip. Feet and hands should be shoulder-width apart, eyes straight ahead. Keeping your back straight, slowly squat until thighs are one-fourth to one-third of the way to the floor, then slowly stand back up. As you gain experience and strength you may squat halfway or until thighs are parallel to the floor. Don't go any further or you may strain your knees.

Lunges: Stand as in squats above with barbell resting on shoulder. Step forward with one foot (start with small steps and gradually lengthen with experience and strength). While inhaling, lower yourself until forward thigh is almost parallel to the floor and knee is directly over ankle. Keep your back straight and eyes looking ahead. Keep the bend of the rear leg to a minimum. Pause at peak of squat, exhale, and push off with front foot to return to starting position. Repeat with other leg.

Hips

Hip Abductor Machine: Sit in machine and place outside of knees and ankles against pads, hands on grips. Slowly push pads as far apart as possible, pause, then slowly return to starting position. Keep back supported by pushing into back pads.

Hip Adductor Machine: Follow same procedure as above except place inside of knees against pads and push them together.

Quadriceps
Leg Extension Machine: Sit with lower legs perpendicular to the floor and ankles under the pad. Place hands on grips. Slowly lift until legs are fully extended and shins are parallel to the floor. Pause, then slowly lower to starting position. Keep lower back supported at all times by pressing into back padding. If possible with machine, lift with one leg at a time and then repeat with the other leg.

Leg Press Machine: See buttocks.

Squats: See hamstrings.

Lunges: See hamstrings.

Upper Body (Arms, Chest, Shoulders)
Bench Press: Use a spotter with this exercise. Use barbells, dumbbells, or machine; strengthens chest, arms, and upper torso. Lie flat on your back on a bench, faceup, with feet flat on the floor (or bench). Place hands slightly more than shoulder-width apart on barbell and slowly lower it to chest. This is the starting position. Slowly press up until arms are fully extended, then slowly lower to starting position. Keep hips on bench and don't bounce bar off chest. Machines that use a sitting position are called a chest press.

Lateral Raises (for the shoulders): Stand or sit, feet shoulder-width apart, knees slightly bent, holding dumbbell in each hand, arms at sides, palms inward. Slowly raise arms straight out to the side from body to about shoulder height while rotating palms to the front and keeping elbows slightly bent. Pause, then slowly lower. This exercise may also be done on a lateral raise machine.

Shoulder Shrugs: Sit upright on a bench, but maintain a natural curve in your lower back. Keep chest lifted, shoulders down and relaxed. Hold a dumbbell in each hand, arms hanging down, palms in. Slowly pull shoulder blades up and together, keeping head up, eyes looking ahead. Then, slowly pull shoulder blades down and together, lifting chest slightly to help relax shoulders between repetitions. This completes one rep. Don't use too much weight; it's more important to have good form. To use a barbell, stand erect with palms inward and grasp barbell with hands about shoulder-width apart. Let arms hang down with barbell in front of thighs. Without bending elbows, shrug your shoulders to your ears. Pause, then slowly lower.

Biceps Curl Machine: Sit on machine with feet flat on the floor. Place upper arms on pads, palms up. Grip bars with both hands shoulder-width apart. Move the arms from an extended position to a flexed position, pause, then return to start. Begin with your arms almost straight and pause with hands almost touching shoulders.

Biceps Curls: Stand erect holding barbell using an underhanded grip with arms extended downward, barbell against thighs. Hands and feet should be shoulder-width apart. Eyes should be straight ahead. Slowly curl barbell to chin while keeping elbows at the side (do not lean back). Pause, then slowly lower to starting position.

As an alternate, use dumbbells from standing or sitting position. Curl up and lower with one arm, then the other to complete one repetition.

Triceps Machine: Sit on machine with feet flat on the floor. Slowly move arms from a flexed position to an extended position, pausing with arms straight, then return to start.

Triceps Extension: From either a sitting or standing position, hold a dumbbell with both hands behind the head. It should be vertical to the floor with palms against the top of the dumbbell head. Slowly raise overhead, elbows extended, then slowly lower behind the neck while keeping elbows pointed to the ceiling. Return slowly to starting position.

Pull-down Machine (chest, upper back, shoulders, arms): Sit with feet flat on the floor, knees anchored under support bars. Reach overhead and grasp bar with hands slightly farther than shoulder-width apart. Keep eyes straight ahead. Slowly pull down while leaning back slightly until bar is chest level, pause, then return to starting position.

Bent Over Row: See back exercises.

Basic 10: Sample Weight Training Workout

Here is an example of a strength training routine using weights for resistance. I've chosen eight exercises that work important muscle groups for runners. You may choose to add or subtract from the exercises described above, particularly emphasizing exercises that relate to specific injuries to which you may be vulnerable. I've chosen a mixture of free weight and machine exercises. You may choose to design a program using only one of each type. Start with exercises that use large muscle groups and then move to smaller muscle groups.

1. Squats (quadriceps, hamstrings, buttocks)

2. Back Extensions (lower back)

3. Abdominal Curl Machine

4. Pulldown Machine (chest, upper back, shoulders, arms)

5. Leg Extension Machine (quadriceps, hip flexors)

6. Bench Press (arms, chest, shoulders)

7. Hip Adductor Machine

8. Hip Abductor Machine

9. Triceps Extension

10. Biceps Curl

Summary of Strength Exercises

You may choose to do all of your strength training using your body weight, free weights, or machines for resistance, or you may choose a combination. Figure 36.1 summarizes some of the exercises that are available for you to choose from.

FIGURE 36.1

Muscle Group	Body Weight	Free Weight	Machine
Abdominals	Crunches Reverse Sit-ups Pelvic Tilt	Weighted Crunches Side Bends	Abdominal Curl
Ankles	Ankle Push Towel Sweep Band Exercise		
Arch	Towel Exercise		
Back	Back Extensions Alternate Extensions	Bent Over Row	Low Back Back Extension Bench Pull Down
Buttocks	Butt Raisers Pelvic Tilt Squats	Squats	Leg Press
Calf muscles	Toe Raises	Weighted Toe Raises	
Hamstrings	Hamstring Curls Squats	Squats Lunges	Leg Curl Leg Press
Hips/groin	Side Leg Raises Inside Leg Raises Chair Press		Abductor Adductor
Quadriceps	Sitting Leg Extensions Squats	Squats Lunges	Leg Extension Leg Press
Shins	Toe Lifts Band Exercise Towel Sweep Foot Press		
Upper body	Push-ups Reverse Push-ups	Bench Press Triceps Extension Biceps Curls Lateral Raises Bent Over Row Shoulder Shrugs	Bench Press Triceps Extension Biceps Curls Lateral Raise Pull Down

THIRTY-SEVEN

Stretching

Flexibility, the ability of the muscles to move a joint through its full range of motion, is an important component of total fitness. Flexible runners are able to run more efficiently with smoother form and may be less prone to injury. The key to improving flexibility, and maintaining it as you get older, is to stretch your muscles wisely and faithfully.

Some runners maintain they don't need to stretch. Indeed, I've known many elite runners who don't stretch at all. But these are mostly young, naturally gifted runners. As we accumulate mile after mile, year after year, and our young muscles age with time, most of us would benefit from flexibility training. Though no scientific study has validated the injury prevention value of stretching, it makes sense that flexible muscles are less likely to injure. Thus, most sports doctors encourage stretching for runners.

There are varying views as to when a runner should stretch. These include:

1. Stretch only after running. This is when the muscles are warm and very extensible, allowing for greater gains in flexibility and decreased risk of injury. With this system be sure to warm up with 10 minutes or more of walking before easing into running. Cool

down with a 10-minute walk after the run and then begin a thorough 10- to 20-minute stretching routine. This system is perhaps the safest and most convenient for most runners.

2. Stretch both before and after running. Warm the muscles with a few minutes of walking, biking, or jogging, then stretch. Then, walk or jog slowly again to warm up before running. This system may not be feasible or desirable for many runners. Others, myself included, feel tight for the first few miles of a run if we don't do *some* easy stretching prior to running. I usually walk the dogs at a brisk pace to warm up prior to my light prerun stretch; after stretching, I walk briskly again or jog slowly before getting into my steady running pace. I stretch more thoroughly after my runs. Since most of our students walk to class and thus are somewhat warmed up, we usually start with easy stretches before the workout and follow up with more stretching after running to help recover from the hard work. If you stretch prior to running without a good prestretch warm-up, concentrate on mild stretches and save more thorough stretches for after your run when muscles are warm.

Stretching Exercises

Guidelines for the warm-up and cool-down routines for runners are discussed in Chapter 7. Most runners stretch as part of these routines. But if your goal is to improve and maintain flexibility, stretching exercises can be done at any time as long as you first prepare the muscles with a good warm-up. Mild stretches can be done throughout the day to help keep you loose. I often do a few easy stretches at odd times: watching TV, talking on the phone, waiting for someone, taking breaks while writing books. Be careful not to overstretch in these cases since your muscles may not be warmed properly.

Stretching exercises that are properly executed will improve your flexibility, help you recover from workouts, and enhance your running. Improper stretching, however, may lead to injury rather than prevent it, and so is worse than no stretching at all. Most injuries related to stretching occur as a result of improper stretching procedures: inadequate warm-up prior to stretching, forcing stretches, poor form, performing high-risk exercises, and so on. If you strongly believe that you don't have the time to "waste" on stretching, or that stretching just isn't for you, then you probably are better off skipping it. If you don't value this type of exercise you are not likely to do it properly, and thus may do yourself more harm than good. For most runners, however, I highly recommend a regular stretching program to improve and maintain flexibility fitness. Remember that just like aerobic fitness, flexibility improvement is a gradual process. Frequency of stretching, not intensity, increases range of motion. Be patient, be consistent, and flexibility gains will result.

Stretching Guidelines:

▪ Easy does it. Do not force your stretching exercises. When a muscle is jerked into extension it tends to "fight back" and shorten. It may pull or even tear. When the muscle is slowly stretched and a comfortable position held, it relaxes and lengthens. Stretch easily to the point of mild sensation and hold the stretch for 10 to 30 seconds. This is called static stretching. Then relax for 5 to 10 seconds (or alternate with the other leg or another exercise) before repeating the stretch. Do each stretch two to five times.

▪ You should feel the stretching sensation in the belly of the muscle. Think about the muscles being stretched, focus on feeling the stretch. Properly done, stretching feels good.

▪ Concentrate on proper form and moving smoothly—both going into and coming out of each stretch.

▪ Do not bounce or swing your body against a fixed joint.

▪ Avoid the following common stretches, determined to be high-risk exercises by the American College of Sports Medicine and other experts: Straight-Legged Standing Toe Touch, Standing One Leg Up Hamstring Stretch (as in foot up on a bench), Hurdler Stretch, The Plow, Full Neck Circles, Cobra (back extension in prone position).

▪ Be especially careful about stretching in the early morning prior to running. Your muscles will be stiff and vulnerable to injury. It may be better to skip the stretching and instead walk briskly for 10 minutes prior to running and then concentrate on stretching after the run.

■ Breathe normally and in a relaxed manner. Do not hold your breath while stretching. Belly breathe while stretching just as you should when you run. Take an abdominal breath (stomach extends as you inhale) and let it out slowly. Emphasize the exhalation as you stretch.

■ You can injure yourself by overstretching. It is better to understretch than to overstretch. Always be at a point where you can stretch farther. Don't try to do more than your body is able to do.

■ Take your time. Do stretching step by step and thoroughly.

■ Many use the same basic routine every day so they feel comfortable with it; know it and stay with it. Others prefer variety. I'll give you a recommended daily routine as well as several options.

■ Introduce new stretches gradually. Ease into more advanced stretches.

■ Don't stretch injured or very sore muscles. This may aggravate them. Stick to easy limbering movements until the muscle is healed and ready to be stretched.

■ Don't overdo stretching after a hard workout or race when you may be especially tight.

■ Do not do stretches where your head is lower than your heart while your heart rate is still elevated from exercising briskly.

■ Be wary of overstretching before a race when you are nervous and may not be concentrating on proper stretching procedures. Look around you at races; most likely the majority of runners will be stretching impatiently and improperly.

■ Avoid exercises that aggravate pre-existing conditions, especially knee or back pain.

■ It is best to stretch on a firm but not too hard surface. If the surface is too hard, such as a bare floor or pavement, you won't be able to relax and stretch properly. If it is too soft, such as a very soft mattress, you won't get proper support and can strain muscles. I often stretch on my firm bed or the thick living room carpet, which are just right for comfort. You may choose to purchase an individual-sized exercise mat.

▪ Your environment for stretching is important. You can relax and thus stretch more thoroughly in a quiet, peaceful setting. Many find that stretching while listening to music is helpful. So is stretching while small kids and pesky dogs are napping! (Why do they think that while you are stretching is a good time to attack or play?)

▪ Wear loose-fitting, comfortable clothing to facilitate stretching.

▪ Stretch all major joint areas. Include areas most prone to running injuries: hamstrings, calves, Achilles tendons, and lower back. Be sure to include specific stretches that your doctor may have recommended to prevent recurring injuries.

▪ You may wish to add some strengthening exercises to your stretching routine before or after your run for a total fitness workout. You may include just one or two key exercises, such as push-ups and crunches, or a series of six to twelve strengthening exercises, such as those detailed in the previous chapter.

Following are more than fifty stretching exercises that will give you plenty of variety in your routine. If you are vulnerable to certain injuries, be sure to include specific anti-injury stretching exercises to help prevent problems. Follow the stretching guidelines detailed above. Remember to hold each stretch for 10 to 30 seconds, relax for at least 5 to 10 seconds before repeating, and do a total of two to five repetitions of each stretch.

Ankles
Ankle Roll: Sit cross-legged on the floor, or with right foot across your opposite knee if sitting in a chair. Grasp your right foot with both hands and rotate the ankle with slight resistance from your hands for 10 seconds, then reverse direction. Repeat with the other ankle. This is a good one to do while watching TV, as is the following exercise.

Standing Ankle Stretch: Stand with back flat against a wall with feet 1 to 2 feet away from it. Turn feet slightly inward and slowly lean forward while keeping knees straight.

Arches
Plantar Fascia Stretch: Sit on the floor with right knee bent. Flex the right ankle by pulling the toes toward the ankle with your hands. Keep the right heel on floor. This also stretches the Achilles tendon. Repeat with the left foot. You can also do this exercise while sitting in a chair: Cross your foot over the opposite knee and then pull on the toes.

Kneeling Arch Stretch: Assume a kneeling position. Kneel on hands and knees with toes curled under you. Slowly lower hips backward and downward until you feel a comfortable stretch in arches. Keep heels together.

Back
Knee to Chest: This is one the stretches I regularly do for my tight back. Lie on your back with knees flexed, feet flat on the floor. Slide left leg forward and slowly drop it to the floor. Raise right leg up toward your chest while keeping your knee flexed and your hands clasped behind the knee. Gently pull the leg toward your chest until you feel a mild stretch in your lower back, hips, and hamstrings. Keep head and lower back flat against the floor. Repeat with other leg. This stretches both lower back and hamstrings. To emphasize lower back, pull one knee up to the chest and then the other. Hug both knees, lifting feet off the floor but keeping lower back flat. Return feet to floor one at a time.

Cat Back: Assume a kneeling position, resting on your hands and knees. Arch your back like an angry cat, dropping your head at the same time. Then, slowly reverse the arch by bringing up your head and forming a U with your spine. (My dogs hate this one!)

Fold-up Stretch: In a kneeling position, lean forward and stretch hands forward, palms on floor. Reach forward while pressing chest into your thighs until you feel a comfortable stretch. Rest forehead on floor between arms while keeping buttocks on your heels.

Seated Trunk Flexion: Sit on a chair with your legs spread apart and arms crossed over chest. Tuck your chin and slowly curl your upper body downward. Relax and slowly return to starting position.

Trunk Twist: Sit on floor or chair with knees apart and flexed at 90 degrees. Clasp hands behind head and tuck chin to chest while tightening abdominals. Twist trunk to the right so left elbow is outside right leg (or dip shoulder between legs) until you feel a gentle stretch. Repeat on other side.

Full Body Stretch: This stretches the back as well as the total body. Lie on your back with hands stretched out overhead. Point your fingers toward one wall and point your toes toward the other. Elongate the whole body.

Upper Back Hang: Stand 3 feet from a supporting surface that is waist- to shoulder-high with feet together. Keep legs straight. Bend at waist while keeping back straight and grasp supporting structure. While keeping arms straight, position feet until you feel a gentle stretch in upper back.

Calf Muscles and Achilles Tendon
Wall Lean: I do this one every day in the shower with the water massage spraying my back. Stand 2 or 3 feet in front of a wall or tree with feet shoulder-width apart. Lean forward and place your palms chest high against the wall. Place one foot 6 to 12 inches behind the other while keeping your leg straight and toes straight ahead or turned slightly inward. Bend front knee and align over ankle. Lean hips forward while bending at the elbows. Keep both heels on floor and back straight until you feel a gentle stretch in the back of the rear leg. Repeat with other leg. You should feel this stretch in the upper calf. To reach the lower calf and Achilles tendon, assume the same position, but this time, when leaning into the wall, bend both knees slightly while keeping both heels on the floor.

Towel Calf Stretch: Sit with legs extended about a foot apart. Hold a towel or T-shirt at each end and loop it around the ball of one foot. Pull on the towel until you feel a gentle stretch in the calf muscles. Repeat with the other foot.

Kneeling Achilles Stretch: Kneel on left knee and place toes of right foot opposite left knee with heel flat on floor. Push forward with right shoulder until right heel raises slightly off the floor. Then try to gently push heel back to the floor as you lean shoulder against knee for resistance. Repeat on other side.

Groin (Adductors)

Sitting Groin Stretch: Sit with back straight (against a wall if possible for support), knees flexed and soles of feet together. Place your elbows on the inside of your thighs and grasp your ankles with your hands. Gently pull your feet toward your buttocks until you feel a gentle stretch in the groin.

Lying Groin Stretch: Lie on back with soles of feet together. Let knees fall apart and relax your hips while keeping lower back flat against the floor.

Inner Thigh Stretch: Stand with feet slightly wider than hip width. Point left foot forward and right foot toward the side. Place right hand on right thigh and left hand on left hip. While keeping left leg straight, bend right knee and put weight on right foot. Bend to the right until you feel a comfortable stretch in the groin. Repeat on other side.

Wide-V Stretch: Lie on the floor with your buttocks close to the wall if possible and your feet up along the wall. Let your legs slowly spread to form a "V." Spread until you feel a comfortable stretch and hold. You may wish to place towels under head and neck for comfort.

Hamstrings

Tight hamstrings relate to hamstring strains as well as knee, hip, and back pain.

Knee to Chest: See back exercises.

Sitting Toe Touch: Sit with legs extended and together. Slide fingertips of both hands forward on legs toward toes; keep knees slightly bent.

Modified Hurdler Stretch: Sit on the floor with both legs extended. Place left foot on inside of straight right leg at the knee (not with the left foot pointed away from the body as in traditional hurdler stretch) with toes of the right foot pointed toward the ceiling. With fingertips of both hands together, slide hands along leg toward toes on outstretched right leg. Lean forward from the hips with a flat back. Look straight ahead to a spot 8 to 10 feet in front. Repeat with other leg.

Lying Hamstring Stretch: Lie on your back with knees flexed and feet flat on the floor. Bring your right knee to your chest while you clasp your hands behind and below it. Slowly straighten this leg until knee is only slightly bent, then flex your ankle toward your knee. Repeat with the left leg.

Towel Hamstring Stretch: This is one of my most important daily exercises. But beware that the youngsters like to climb up your leg if they catch you doing it. Lie on your back with knees flexed and feet flat on the floor. Bring your right knee to your chest; grasp a towel, T-shirt, or rope at each end and place under the ball of right foot. Slowly raise and straighten the right leg while keeping your shoulders flat on the floor. Repeat with left leg.

One-legged Hamstring Stretch: Sit on the edge of a bed or bench with your right leg extended and parallel to the floor; your left foot should be flat on the floor. Keeping your back straight, bend forward from the hips and grasp your extended leg with your hands. Move your head toward your knee until you feel a gentle stretch. Repeat with other leg.

Table Hang: Stand facing a table with feet shoulder-width apart and one foot 3 feet behind the other. Bend forward at hips and place hands on table. Keep lower back and back leg straight. Keep front knee slightly bent. Position yourself until you feel a comfortable stretch on hamstrings and hold. Repeat on other side.

Wall Support Stretch: With feet toward a wall, lie on your back with your buttocks 12 inches from the wall, knees bent, and feet against the wall. Slowly slide your feet up the wall and straighten your legs. Move your buttocks farther away from the wall if you are unable to straighten your legs. You should feel a comfortable stretch in the back of the legs—do not force a stretch. Place a folded towel under your head and a rolled towel under neck for comfort. This is very relaxing. But beware, I've fallen asleep on this one and my legs went numb!

High Knee Stretch: Also stretches groin, front of hip and calf muscles. I do this several times a day while taking a break from the computer. Place ball of right foot on a raised surface such as a bench or table (knee- to hip-high). Keep hands on hips and left foot flat and pointed straight ahead. Bend right knee as you push hips forward. You should feel the stretch in the groin, hamstring, and front of hip. Repeat with other leg.

Hips

Standing Iliotibial Band Stretch: Stand with left side to a wall and support yourself against the wall with your left hand at shoulder height. Cross inside leg behind outside leg and place right hand on right hip. With most of your weight resting on the right leg and keeping the right knee bent slightly, lean your left hip toward the wall while keeping the left leg and left arm straight. You should feel the stretch along the outer thigh. Repeat with other leg.

Sitting Hip Abductor Stretch: A good exercise for piriformis syndrome, back, neck, and torso. Sit on the floor with right leg extended; cross your left leg over the right leg and place the left foot on the floor even with right knee. Place left hand behind body for support and extend right arm outside left knee. Use the right elbow to push your left knee to the right while twisting your body to the left and turning head to look over left shoulder. Slowly twist until you feel a gentle stretch on the outside of your left hip. Keep the hips in place. Repeat on other side.

Chiropractor Stretch: This is another of the exercises my doctor has me do two or three times a day to combat hip and back problems. Lie on your back with left leg extended and right knee flexed. Bring right knee toward your chest until at a 90° angle. Grasp it with left hand just above the knee and pull bent knee of right leg across the body and down toward the floor while keeping shoulders and back of head flat against floor. Gently push right knee across body until you feel a gentle stretch in the buttocks, lower back, and sides of the hip. Repeat to other side.

Hip Rotator Stretch: Also good for piriformis injury prevention. Lie on stomach with knees flexed at a 90° angle. Keeping knees together, spread your ankles apart until you feel a gentle stretch in the hips.

Lateral Hip Stretch: This is one of my daily stretches to fight off chronic hip pain. Lie on back with knees flexed. Cross left ankle to right knee, and grasp back of right leg with both hands interlocked. Gently pull both knees toward chest until you feel a comfortable stretch in outside of left hip. Repeat on other side.

Hip Cross: Lie on back with hands clasped behind head and knees flexed. Cross left leg over right leg and use upper leg to push lower leg toward the floor. Head, elbows, back, and shoulders should be flat on floor. Repeat to other side.

Hip Roll: Lie on your back with knees flexed and arms out to sides, palms down. With legs together, lower both legs to the right while keeping elbows, head, and shoulders flat on floor. Repeat on the left side.

Starter's Stretch: Assume beginning position for sprinter's start with both hands balanced on fingertips under the shoulders, front knee directly over the foot (keep front foot flat on floor), and ankle and back foot extended to the rear balancing on toe (or place back knee on a cushion). With weight supported by both hands, press hips forward until a gentle stretch is felt in hip flexors and groin. Keep back straight and hips forward. Repeat on other side.

Neck
Remember not to do full neck circles, which is considered a high-risk exercise.

Lateral Neck Stretch: While standing or sitting, place hands behind your back and grasp the right wrist with the left hand. Tilt head gently toward the left ear while gently pulling right arm to the left. Reverse hand positions and repeat stretch to other side.

Side to Side: While standing, sitting, or lying, slowly turn head to the right, center, and then left.

Ear to Shoulder: While standing or sitting, slowly lower head to right shoulder, return to center, lower to left shoulder. Keep shoulders relaxed. To increase stretch, provide gentle pull to side with hand outstretched over top of head.

Forward and Back: While standing or sitting, slowly move head forward, looking down. Don't put chin on chest. To increase stretch, clasp hands behind top of head and apply gentle pressure. Slowly return to start.

Quadriceps
Standing Quad Stretch: Stand on your left leg next to a chair, table, or wall and grasp or touch it with left hand for balance. Bend right knee and lift leg. Grasp right ankle with right hand and push back with thigh until knee points straight down to floor. Do not move the pelvis or the small of the back. You should feel the stretch in the front of the thigh. Repeat with the other leg.

Lying Quad Stretch: Lie on your stomach; bend right knee and grasp ankle with right hand (or grasp a towel wrapped around ankle). Keep body in a straight line and thighs together. Push hips into floor and squeeze buttocks as you slowly pull foot toward buttocks until you feel a gentle stretch in right quadricep muscle. Repeat to other side. If this position is too difficult, do it while lying on your side using the bottom arm for support and the top hand to pull the top leg back.

Upper Body: Chest, Upper Back, Shoulders
Stretch Tall: Stand and raise both arms over your head. Cross wrists and clasp hands together. Straighten arms and stretch upward while looking straight ahead and keeping feet flat on the floor. Stretch the whole body up to your wrists and palms.

Chest and Shoulder Stretch: Stand with the right side of the body next to a wall. Extend your right arm backward with elbow at a 90° angle, and place the palm of right hand against the wall at shoulder height. While keeping shoulder close to the wall, slowly turn your head over your left shoulder until you feel a gentle stretch in chest, shoulder and arms. Repeat on other side.

Side Reach: Stand with knees slightly bent. Place hands, palms inward, on outside of thighs. Reach straight up with left hand until arm is fully extended, palm facing away from body, and eyes looking up at outstretched hand. Lean to the right and brace body by pushing in with right hand against right thigh. Repeat on opposite side.

Shoulder Rolls: While standing or sitting, place hands on hips and slowly curl shoulders down and forward, then lift them up toward your ears. Then, stretch them downward and backward to return to starting position. This completes a full circle. Do for 10 seconds and then change direction.

Posterior Shoulder Stretch: While standing or sitting, place right hand over left shoulder and left hand on outside of right elbow. Keep right elbow up and parallel to the floor. Pull right elbow toward left shoulder with left hand. Repeat on other side.

Anterior Shoulder Stretch: Grasp hands behind back. With elbows slightly bent, push arms upward until you feel a comfortable stretch in the back of the shoulders and in the chest. This also stretches the biceps.

Backward Stretch: Stand facing away from a doorway or fence. Reach behind and place your hands at shoulder height on the sides of the doorway or grasp fence. Lean forward and let arms straighten as you feel the stretch in chest and shoulders. Keep chin up as you lean forward.

Triceps Pull: While standing or sitting, extend one arm straight up above your head. Then bend at the elbow and bring hand to rest behind the neck. With the opposite hand, gently pull the elbow backward. Repeat on other side.

Upper Back Towel Stretch: While standing or sitting, grasp towel in right hand and place behind your head. Place left hand behind back at waist level and grab bottom of towel. Gently pull. You may be able to do this stretch without a towel by grasping your hands behind your back. Reverse hands and repeat.

Pectoral Stretch: Resting on your hands and knees, slide both hands forward, bringing your elbows to the floor and then your arms. Keep your back and head straight, thighs perpendicular to the floor, hips up. Return to starting position.

Trunk Rotation: Stand with knees slightly bent and hands clasped behind neck. Slowly rotate upper body toward the right and hold at point of tightness. Repeat on other side.

Progressive Relaxation Exercises

Relaxation exercises are recommended by many fitness experts prior to prerun stretches to release tension from muscles and after postrun stretches to leave you feeling calm and energized. My mentor, Dr. Hans Kraus, is a leading proponent of the theory that muscles can't be properly stretched unless they are first relaxed. If you feel tense and tight, you should especially consider the relaxation exercises detailed below. Carrying tension with you on the run often results in a lousy workout and invites injury.

Sample Progressive Relaxation Routine. The purpose of this series of exercises is to tense each muscle group and then release tension throughout the body. "Feel" the tension escape as you let go on each exercise.

- Lie on your back, flex your knees into a bent position, feet flat on the floor, arms relaxed at your sides. Shut your eyes and take a deep breath in through the nose, letting your belly rise. Then, let go and breathe out through the mouth. Repeat two more times. Throughout the exercises below, continue to belly breathe; don't hold your breath while holding a position.

- Tighten the muscles of your face for a few seconds. Really make a contortion, and then let go.

- Hunch your shoulders up toward the ears and tighten muscles in neck and shoulders for a few seconds. Relax and let shoulders drop to original position.

- To loosen and stretch neck, slowly drop head to one side, return to center, drop to other side. Repeat.

- Push small of your back into the floor and tighten muscles in back and buttocks for a few seconds. Let go.

- Raise one arm a few inches off the floor, tighten fist and arm muscles, hold for a few seconds, and let go. Drop arm gently to the floor and repeat with other arm.

- Slide one heel along the floor and drop leg gently to the floor. Raise leg a few inches while keeping lower back flat on the floor. Crunch your toes under and tighten all the muscles in that leg, hold for a few seconds, and let go. Slowly return to starting position. Repeat with the opposite leg.

- As the final exercise when used as part of prerun stretch, do the Full Body Stretch as detailed under back exercises.

- As the final exercise at the completion of your postrun stretching routine, lie on back with eyes closed and take several deep breaths. Then, allow your body to go completely limp. Think of something very relaxing, like floating in warm water in the Bahamas. Rest, float for 30 seconds to one minute or more. You might even catch a short, refreshing nap like I often do with this routine. Slowly open your eyes and slowly get up, rising first to your hands, then knees, then one leg, then both legs but bent over, then slowly erect. You should feel very calm and refreshed.

Basic 12: Sample Stretching Routine

Here is an example of a stretching routine to use after you are well warmed up and/or after finishing your run. I've chosen a variety of exercises that improve flexibility in many of the key muscle groups that are important to runners. You may choose to add or subtract from the stretching exercises detailed in this chapter to add variety or to work on flexibility in an area where you may be vulnerable to injury. You may choose to follow the same routine each day for consistency. I've marked six of the exercises with an asterisk. At the least, do a basic series of these half-dozen stretching exercises daily if you feel you can't make time for more.

Do the routine in order from one to twelve prior to running; do in reverse order from twelve to one after running. This routine should take 10 to 20 minutes depending on how long you hold each stretch and how many repetitions you do of each stretch.

1. Progressive Relaxation Routine

2. Knee to Chest

3. *Chiropractor Stretch or Hip Roll

4. Lateral Hip Stretch

5. *Towel Hamstring Stretch or Lying Hamstring Stretch

6. Ankle Roll

7. Plantar Fascia Stretch

8. *Sitting Groin Stretch

Note: As an option, add alternate sets of Crunches, Push-ups, and/or Side Leg Raises (or other strengthening exercises) here, as detailed in Chapter 36. For example: one set of 10 Crunches, one set of 10 Side Leg Raises for each leg, one set of 10 Push-ups. Do two or three sets.

9. *High Knee Stretch or Modified Hurdler Stretch

10. *Standing Quad Stretch

11. *Wall Lean

12. Posterior Shoulder Stretch, Anterior Shoulder Stretch, or Triceps Pull

Part XII

Wellness

THIRTY-EIGHT

The Holistic Approach to Health and Fitness

You can be fit and not healthy. Despite following all the exercise guidelines in this book and passing all the fitness tests, you may still not be leading a healthful life.

"Fitness," said Dr. George Sheehan, "is only the ability to do physical work, like running or cycling. Health, on the other hand, is the prevention of unnecessary disease and premature death." Exercise makes us fit and improves our muscle function. Even someone who is sedentary may have excellent lungs and an adequate heart. Their body muscles, however, are weak. "Fitness makes our muscles more efficient," Dr. Sheehan stated, "but training alone will not make us healthy. The winner of this week's local road race may have a cholesterol level of 350 milligrams. A daily exerciser may still have high blood pressure or may even be overweight."

Exercise is essential to and part of good health, but it is only one facet of a wellness program. Dr. Kenneth Cooper, the aerobic expert, warns of the "myth of invulnerability"—the belief that the more we exercise, the healthier we become. We convince ourselves that we are impervious to coronary illness and other diseases that plague our stressful and sedentary society. But we need to combine fitness with good health practices.

We need a holistic approach to life to enjoy the benefits of fitness. A total wellness program is a marriage of fitness and good health practices. Wellness emphasizes the positive aspects of health and fitness, and it incorporates them into a lifestyle that contributes to an increased longevity and the improved quality of life. It helps to remove the risk factors of disease and prevent avoidable illnesses and premature death. Poor health practices and a lack of exercise result in the opposite of wellness: illness.

Dr. Lester Breslow, a professor emeritus at the School of Public Health of the University of California at Los Angeles, has conducted a long-term (since 1965) study of 7,000 Alameda County, California, men and women that has identified seven unwholesome health practices. According to the study, the more of these poor health practices people follow, the greater were their chances of dying within ten years. In combination, these poor health practices could double a person's chance of dying prematurely. On the other hand, those who followed the opposite of six or seven of these practices lived on the average eleven and a half years longer than those who did only three or less of them.

Further research in the 1990s by Dr. Breslow revealed that those whose lives were characterized by six or seven of these poor health practices were twice as likely to be disabled ten or more years later as were their neighbors with no more than two of these bad habits. Thus Breslow's "seven deadly sins" predict not only early death for many, but chronic and costly disabilities for those who survive.

The seven poor health habits:

1. Physical inactivity

2. Smoking

3. Drinking too much alcohol

4. Being overweight

5. Eating between meals

6. Skipping breakfast

7. Sleeping too little or too much

Why would numbers 5, 6, and 7 be associated with a risk for early death? According to Dr. Breslow, "I believe these poor health practices are indicative of a chaotic lifestyle and that people who follow them are likely to pay inadequate attention to their overall well-being." Sure enough, his data shows that snackers, breakfast skippers, and those who slept more or less than seven to eight hours a night were more likely to die prematurely or to suffer life-limiting disabilities.

I would thus recommend that you turn these "seven deadly sins" around into good health practices and I would add the following:

8. Take frequent time-outs from the stresses in your life.

9. Eat a low-fat diet.

10. Make relaxation (and fun) part of your daily routine. Have an optimistic attitude.

Another study, also from the University of California at Los Angeles, shows that Mormons have the lowest death rates from heart disease and cancer. Why? They never smoke. They avoid alcohol, caffeine, and drugs. They exercise regularly, and they have regular sleep habits. Moreover, they attend church weekly, with its good family and social support. As you will see in the next few chapters, several important studies now link lowered risk of heart attack, coronary artery disease, and cancer with, among other factors, support groups and relaxation or meditation. Worship and prayer are, of course, forms of meditation.

Unfortunately, few Americans are following recommended steps to wellness. This is proven by the lack of progress made in reaching the Healthy People 2000 goals established by the U.S. Surgeon General. The idea is to make significant progress in several key areas by the year 2000. This is how we measure up.

▪ The goal of cutting the percentage of smokers to 15 percent by 2000 does not seem achievable despite a significant drop to 29 percent by 1987 and a further drop to 25 percent in 1991. By comparison, more than 42 percent of Americans smoked in 1965!

▪ The goal for reduction of dietary fats was set at 30 percent of our diet by the year 2000. In 1980, that level was 36 percent; by 1991 it had only dropped to 34 percent.

▪ The goal of consuming only 10 percent of our calories as saturated fats does not look achievable by 2000. Between 1980 and 1991 the actual drop was only from 13 to 12 percent—a one percent decline in more than ten years!

Not only are these drops in consumption of health-damaging fats behind schedule, but there is also little reduction at all because Americans have increased their total caloric consumption.

▪ The goal of reducing the prevalence of inactivity to below 15 percent also seems doomed. The percentage of Americans who engage in regular light to moderate exercise increased only slightly, from 22 percent in 1985 to 24 percent in 1991. Those who exercise vigorously increased only from 16 to 17 percent. Meanwhile, those who are considered sedentary has remained at 24 percent since 1985. The result of increasing caloric consumption and not exercising enough? Simple: more overweight Americans. The number of Americans who are overweight (at least 20 percent above the weight that is desirable for optimal health) increased from 26 percent in 1980 to 34 percent a decade later. One out of every three Americans is now overweight!

A Wellness Program

This book so far has emphasized fitness and health-giving exercises that promote relaxation, improve flexibility, strengthen key muscle groups, and increase your cardiorespiratory endurance. Now we need to add wellness to that fitness component.

To do that, we must examine the health aspects of your life: stress management, nutrition, weight control, drug and alcohol consumption, smoking, sleeping habits, blood pressure, medical care, the concept of your self, and heredity. I consider you oriented toward wellness if you do most of the following:

▪ Meet the minimum fitness goals of this book—that is, exercise vigorously at least three times a week, with an emphasis on relaxation, flexibility, muscular strength and endurance, and aerobic conditioning.

▪ Work to balance the stresses and joys of work, exercise, friends, and family. Take minor upsets in stride. Seek support from friends or family, or professional help, to deal with more serious stress.

▪ Take frequent time outs—vacations, exercise breaks, regular family activities—to help overcome stress.

▪ Eat a balanced diet low in calories, fat, sugar, salt, and cholesterol but high in fiber and complex carbohydrates.

▪ Start each day with a healthy breakfast.

▪ Eat regular meals.

▪ Maintain a healthful weight.

▪ Do not abuse alcohol or drugs, and do not use tobacco in any form.

▪ Sleep seven to eight hours a night.

▪ Work to develop an optimistic attitude and a sense of humor.

▪ Have regular medical and dental exams.

Before starting a vigorous exercise program, have a thorough medical examination. You should know your medical history, especially any inherited heart risk factors. Your doctor should check for cholesterol and triglyceride levels, blood pressure, and body weight.

Some of the above are just good common sense. The point is that you should strive for a level of wellness where all of these points are commonplace to your life. You do them as part of daily living.

If you combine exercise with good lifestyle habits, you will take a major step toward total well-being, or wellness. This is not to say that you will live longer, although the studies cited in this book indicate that, statistically at least, you probably will. But the quality of the life you are given will increase.

Let's look at some specific guidelines. The following Wellness Quiz is published by the American Running & Fitness Association, a public service organization for which I serve on the board of advisers. The quiz is designed to help you evaluate the exercise and health practices in your life. You should take the quiz twice a year and use it to motivate yourself to lead a more wellness-oriented life.

Please understand that wellness, like fitness, does not happen overnight. You can reduce your health risks one factor at a time with gradual, partial changes. But do get started. You know the old saying: "A journey of a thousand miles starts with a single step."

Wellness Quiz*
Exercise:
1. How much time do you spend walking briskly, running, cycling, swimming, aerobic dancing, rowing, cross-country skiing, or doing other aerobic activities (nonstop, vigorous exercise) per week? To be considered, the activity must be done for a minimum of 20 minutes at a time, and must roughly double your resting heart rate (to around 120 beats or more per minute).
    (a) 150 minutes or more per week .... 18 points
    (b) 90 to 149 minutes per week .... 17 points
    (c) 60 to 89 minutes per week .... 16 points
    (d) 30 to 59 minutes per week .... 8 points
    (e) 15 to 29 minutes per week .... 4 points
    (f) 0 to 14 minutes per week .... 0 points

2. If you exercise regularly:
    (a) Do you stretch after you exercise?
        Always .... 2 points
        Sometimes .... 1 points
        Never .... 0 points
    (b) Do you exercise in spite of pain? .... −5 points
    (c) Do you alternate hard and easy (or rest) days?
        Always .... 2 points
        Sometimes .... 1 point
        Never .... 0 points

Nutrition, Diet:

3. Do you eat a wide variety of foods?
   (a) Every day ....   4 points
   (b) At least three times a week ....   2 points
   (c) Once a week....................................   0 points
   (d) Once in a while ....   −2 points

4. Do you limit the amount of animal fat (butter, fatty meats, fried foods) in your diet?
   (a) Avoid animal fat ....   2 points
   (b) Try to avoid, but occasionally have some .....   1 point
   (c) Never really pay much attention to this: don't try to avoid ....   0 points
   (c) Love fatty foods; eat frequently ....   −1 point

5. Do you limit the amount of refined sugar products in your diet?
   (a) Avoid refined sugar products ....   2 points
   (b) Try to avoid, but occasionally have some .....   1 point
   (c) Never really pay much attention to this; don't try to avoid ....   0 points
   (d) Love refined sugar products; eat frequently ...   −1 point

6. Do you limit the amount of salt or salty foods in your diet?
   (a) Avoid salt, or salty foods ....   2 points
   (b) Try to avoid, but occasionally have some .....   1 point
   (c) Never really pay much attention to this; don't try to avoid ....   0 points
   (d) Love salt or salty foods; eat frequently ....   −1 point

7. Do you eat a good breakfast (juice, cereal, and milk, for example)? Pick one that's closest to what you do.
   (a) Daily, with a light lunch and moderate dinner ....   2 points
   (b) Four days a week, with a light lunch and moderate dinner ....   1 point
   (c) Skip breakfast in favor of light lunch and heavy dinner ....   0 points
   (d) Eat snacks during the day and a heavy dinner ....   −1 point
   (e) Eat snacks plus heavy meals ....   −2 points

Weight:

8. Are you overweight? (To calculate your "ideal" weight: Men should take their height in inches, multiply it by 4, and subtract 128. Women should take their height in inches, multiply it by 3.5, and subtract 108.)
    (a) Under "ideal" weight by 11 or more
       pounds .... −3 points
    (b) Under "ideal" weight by 6 to 10 pounds ..... 0 points
    (c) Within "ideal" weight +5 to −5 pounds .... 8 points
    (d) 6 to 15 pounds overweight .... 0 points
    (e) 16 to 25 pounds overweight .... −1 point
    (f) 26 to 35 pounds overweight .... −2 points
    (g) 36 to 50 pounds overweight .... −3 points
    (h) 51 or more pounds overweight .... −6 points

Smoking:

9. Do you smoke?
    (a) Never .... 4 points
    (b) Quit two or more years ago .... 3 points
    (c) Quit within the last two years .... 2 points
    (d) 1 to 10 cigarettes or cigars per day, or pipe .. −1 point
    (e) 11 to 20 cigarettes per day .... −3 points
    (f) 21 to 40 cigarettes or cigars per day .... −6 points
    (g) More than 40 cigarettes or cigars per day .... −9 points

Alcohol:

10. Do you drink?
    (a) Never .... 0 points
    (b) Social drinker only .... 0 points
    (c) 1 to 2 drinks per day .... 1 point
    (d) 2 to 4 drinks per day .... −1 point
    (e) 5 to 6 drinks per day .... −3 points
    (f) 7 or more drinks per day .... −5 points

11. Do you get drunk?
    (a) Never .... 2 points
    (b) 1 to 3 times a year .... 0 points
    (c) 4 to 6 times a year .... −1 point
    (d) 7 to 12 times a year .... −3 points
    (e) More than 12 times a year .... −5 points

Drugs:

12. Do you use illicit drugs?
    (a) Never .... 2 points
    (b) Infrequently .... 0 points
    (c) Occasionally .... −1 point
    (d) Frequently .... −3 points
    (e) Regularly .... −5 points

13. Do you use prescription drugs?
    (a) Rarely needed .... 2 points
    (b) Used occasionally, as needed and prescribed by
        a physician .... 0 points
    (c) Don't follow prescribed dosage or schedule ... −1 point
    (d) Regularly use mood-altering drugs .... −3 points
    (e) Use mood-altering drugs combined with alco-
        hol or other drugs .... −5 points

Stress and Relaxation:

14. How much stress do you experience in your life?
    (a) Very little .... 2 points
    (b) Occasional mild tension .... 0 points
    (c) Frequent mild tension .... −1 point
    (d) Frequent moderate tension .... −2 points
    (e) Frequent high tension .... −3 points
    (f) Constant high tension .... −4 points

15. How secure and relaxed are you?
    (a) I'm always secure and relaxed .... 2 points
    (b) I'm usually secure and relaxed .... 0 points
    (c) I'm occasionally anxious or tense .... −1 point
    (d) I'm anxious or tense most of the time and have
        difficulty relaxing .... −1 point
    (e) I'm anxious, tense, and unable to relax most
        or all of the time .... −4 points

16. How much sleep do you get?
    (a) 7 to 8 hours a night .... 2 points
    (b) 8 to 9 hours a night .... 1 point
    (c) 6 to 7 hours a night .... 1 point
    (d) 9 hours or more a night .... −1 point
    (e) 6 hours or less a night .... −2 points

Self-Concept:

17. How do you feel about yourself?
- (a) I feel good about myself and generally am confident about my future and my abilities ... 2 points
- (b) I'm comfortable with myself and will probably do well in the future .... 1 point
- (c) I'm usually comfortable with myself, but have my ups and downs .... 0 points
- (d) I'm not too happy with myself and seem to make too many mistakes .... −2 points
- (e) I don't like myself and can't seem to do anything right .... −4 points

18. How do you feel about your job (housewives are professionals, too!)?
- (a) It's challenging and I enjoy it .... 2 points
- (b) It's sometimes challenging and I'm usually content with it .... 1 point
- (c) It's a living .... 0 points
- (d) I don't like my job .... −2 points
- (e) I hate my job .... −4 points

Medical Care:

19. How often do you visit a doctor for a checkup?
- (a) Once or twice a year .... 2 points
- (b) About once every four years or so .... −1 point
- (c) Rarely or never .... −4 points

20. Do you do breast self-exams/testicular self-exams?
- (a) Monthly .... 2 points
- (b) Occasionally .... 0 points
- (c) Never .... −2 points

To tabulate your wellness score, add or subtract the points to the right of each of your answers. If your total score is:

50 to 64	You take excellent care of yourself and are in excellent shape.
25 to 49	You take good care of yourself and are in good shape.

0 to 24   You take reasonable care of yourself and could be in better shape.

−31 to −1   You do not take good care of yourself and you are in risky shape.

−32 or less   Your lifestyle is hazardous to your health.

* Reprinted by permission of the American Running & Fitness Association.

Wellness and Health Care

Along with exercise, we need to pay attention to several other factors. Some of them—stress management, nutrition, weight management, bringing balance to your life (the runner's triangle)—are so important that we have devoted entire chapters to them. But there are other factors that are also important, that you can control yourself, and we discuss them here.

Smoking

Cigarette smoking kills. Shepherd and I can attest to this firsthand. As a young boy, I can remember my father lying on a couch in the living room struggling to talk to me after having surgery to remove a cancerous growth from his throat caused by years of cigarette smoking. I was scared. I was afraid he would die. His father had smoked so much that when he died from cancer his fingers and dentures were stained yellow. My father was luckier. His cancer has never returned. But his message was clear: He asked me never to smoke, and I never even tried.

Shepherd watched his sister, Sandra, die slowly from cancer. She had smoked two packs of cigarettes a day for about twenty years. She tried to stop but couldn't, and the cancer slowly consumed not only her lungs, but also her kidneys, heart, and finally, mercifully, her brain. Over the course of seventeen months she shriveled up from a stunningly beautiful woman to a skeleton sustained by medication and machines before dying in her sleep one morning.

We cite these family histories as warnings. You can tell us of people you know who have smoked for decades and are healthy as oxen. But, my friends, the odds are against you. All forms of tobacco—cigarettes, "smokeless" cigarettes, cigars, chewing tobacco—contain nicotine, tars, and carbon monoxide. They are killers.

In fact, cigarette smoking kills 1,000 Americans every day. That's one out of every six deaths daily. Cigarette smoking is one of the most significant predictors of coronary artery disease. If you smoke, your chances of dying from heart disease are *two to five* times that of nonsmokers, depending upon age. According to a study at the Imperial Cancer Research Fund in Oxford, England, it isn't just older folks that are killed by cigarettes. Smokers in their 30s and 40s are five times more likely to have a heart attack during those decades as nonsmokers their age. The researchers found that smoking causes four-fifths of heart attacks in smokers aged 30 to 49, two-thirds of attacks in smokers 50 to 59, and half of those among smokers aged 60 to 79. Cigarette smoking causes cancer of the lungs, mouth, esophagus, bladder, kidney, stomach, and pancreas. Moreover, if other risk factors are present—obesity, high blood pressure, and so on—then smoking increases the danger. Still, nearly one in four adults in this country smokes.

Passive smoking. This is the involuntary inhalation of tobacco smoke by someone other than the smoker. It is particularly dangerous to nonsmokers, whose lungs will absorb the smoke and its harmful ingredients faster than a smoker's already-damaged lungs, according to the medical journal *Lancet.* That's right, secondhand cigarette smoke harms people who don't smoke more than it does people who do!

Smoking kills nonsmokers. Researchers at the University of California at San Francisco and the American College of Cardiology have found that there is a 30 percent increase in the risk of death from heart attack among nonsmokers living with smokers. In 1990, passive tobacco smoke was declared a human carcinogen, a cancer-causing agent, by the Environmental Protection Agency. The EPA found that passive smoking causes 3,000 lung cancer deaths a year among nonsmokers and 1,500 lung cancer deaths a year among former smokers. A study by Dr. Stanton A. Glantz of the University of California at San Francisco estimated that 50,000 Americans die every year from diseases caused by passive smoking, two-thirds of them from heart disease. Passive smoking reduces the blood's ability to deliver oxygen to the heart.

Passive smoking ranks behind direct smoking and alcohol as the third leading preventable cause of death. Seventeen percent of all lung cancer cases occur among nonsmokers exposed to cigarette smoke at home, in the workplace, or in public.

Children in particular are victims of smoking. Like exercising nonsmokers, newborn infants have lungs that are particularly receptive to tobacco compounds and particles in the air. One smoking parent exposes his or her child to 60,000 hours of "passive smoking" by the child's twentieth birthday.

Studies show that infants in their first year who live in homes where parents smoke suffer twice as many respiratory illnesses as infants in nonsmokers' homes. The *American Journal of Epidemiology* reports that a person living with a smoker has a 1.6 times greater chance of getting cancer than a person who is not living with a smoker.

Studies also show that passive smoking decreases the ability of people to exercise. It increases the demands on the heart during exercise, and reduces the heart's ability to speed up during exercise. For people with heart disease, the decreased function may cause angina, or chest pains.

Addiction. Make no mistake: Tobacco is addictive. In fact, in 1988, Dr. C. Everett Koop, the surgeon general at the time, warned that nicotine is as addictive as heroin and cocaine. He stated that the use of tobacco in any form should be seen as a serious addiction rather than simply a dangerous habit. "Shouldn't we treat tobacco sales as seriously as the sale of alcoholic beverages, for which a specific license is required and revoked for repeated sales to minors?" he asked.

Stopping is difficult. "For many smokers," said Dr. Koop, "a genuine desire to quit and, if necessary, persistent and repeated attempts to quit may be all that is necessary. For others, self-help material, formal treatment programs, and nicotine replacement therapy may be needed and should be readily available." In a survey by the Centers for Disease Control and Prevention, 34 percent of the 46 million smokers in the United States try to quit each year. Just 8 percent succeed.

We nonsmokers can help by giving smokers who want to quit lots of love and support. That may mean a child's love and encouragement of his or her parent's efforts to quit smoking, or the love and support of spouses and good friends for one another. Sometimes, as Dr. Koop suggests, clinics are needed to help people stop smoking.

One of the best ways to stop smoking may be simply to change the way you live. Stop making cigarettes, cigars, or your pipe the focus of your daily life. Break the stimulus-response reaction—that is, eating and then smoking, reading and smoking, and so forth. My recommendation is to substitute exercise for smoking.

How? You could follow the fitness program detailed earlier in this book. As you slowly increase your fitness time or distance, you would correspondingly decrease your consumption of tobacco. Your health—wellness, if you will—increases as your unfitness (smoking) decreases.

Stopping reduces all the dangers of smoking and may return good health quickly. Cigarette smoking causes lower levels of high-density lipoproteins (HDL), the "good" guys, in your bloodstream. If smoking is stopped, however, the HDLs can return to normal levels. A study in the *New England Journal of Medicine* found that the death rate for older people who continue to smoke is 70 percent higher than that for people who quit smoking—that is, even older people with healthy hearts live longer if they stop smoking. "No matter how old you are, no matter how long you've smoked, there's a benefit to quitting," says Dr. John H. Holbrook of the University of Utah. "And as far as heart attack is concerned, the benefits begin to accrue within a few months."

Sleep

Almost half of all Americans are sleeping an hour to 90 minutes less each night than they should. By the end of the week they've missed the equivalent of a full night's sleep. At least 13 million of us sleep so badly that we cite it to investigators as a source of misery in our lives. "People cheat on their sleep, and they don't even realize they're doing it," said Dr. Howard P. Roffward, director of the Sleep Study Unit at the University of Texas Southwestern Medical School. "They think they're okay because they can get by on six and a half hours, when they really need seven and a half, eight or even more to feel ideally vigorous."

Without sleep, the body's homeostasis—its internal equilibrium—malfunctions. Lack of sleep interrupts the hormonal and metabolic processes that take place during the nocturnal hours. Sleep deprivation has both immediate and long-term effects. In the short term, performance suffers. We lose energy, have lapses of attention, cannot concentrate, and may suffer short-term memory loss. Sleepy subjects in research studies cannot distinguish between loud and soft tones, or see flashes of light on a board. In one study, college students deprived of 60 to 90 minutes of sleep every night performed poorly on psychological and cognitive tests. Sleep deprivation also decreases our ability to laugh at a joke or feel pleasure.

Over the longer term, our judgment may be impaired with a corresponding increase in automobile and industrial accidents. Sleepiness is second only to drunkenness as a cause of automobile accidents. The U.S. Department of Transportation states that at least 40,000 traffic accidents a year may be sleep related and that more than 20 percent of all drivers have fallen asleep at the wheel at least once. Further, sleep-deprived people are impaired by smaller amounts of alcohol than the rested, which also contributes to accidents. Finally, a public health survey in Alameda County, California, indicates that insufficient sleep simply diminishes our life span.

The sleep-deficit crisis probably began with the invention of the lightbulb in the late nineteenth century. Before then, the average person slept nine to ten hours a night; the best sleep habits were the result of having nothing to do in the evening, and going to bed shortly after it was dark.

By the mid-twentieth century, our sleep schedules had fallen to seven and a half to eight hours a night. Now pressures from work, family, friends, and exercise routines make sleep seem expendable. All-night television and sports entertainment, increased prevalence of shift work where men and women alternate between a day and night schedule, and the international workplace have also cut further into our sleep habits.

Even sleep disorders are becoming more prevalent and causing people to become wakeful. A National Heart, Lung and Blood Institute report estimates that 4 percent of Americans suffer from sleep apnea, a condition in which the sleeper frequently stops breathing for as long as 90 seconds or so during the night. This wakes the sleeper and creates a cycle of wakefulness, sleep, apnea, wakefulness.

Fortunately, there is a good way to improve the quality of your sleep: regular exercise. Scientists at Emory University and the Stanford Center for Research in Disease Prevention found that exercise improves sleep quality and shortens the time it takes to fall asleep. After a four-month exercise program, test subjects fell asleep faster than those in a control group (14.5 minutes compared to 24), slept almost an hour longer (6.8 hours compared to 5.9), and felt more rested in the morning.

The case for napping. Fortunately, the remedies for sleep deprivation are simple. Get more sleep. But when and how?

When our days are filled with stress that keeps our bodies and minds active, our nights must be filled with restful stress management. "Emerson," said Dr. George Sheehan, who was fond of quoting the essayist, "said we should put a solid wall of sleep between each day." Sufficient sleep, therefore, is a priority.

But what is sufficient? We should note that sleep researchers suggest that what is enough sleep in summer is not enough in winter: We need an hour more in the cold weather months, which may be our reaction to fewer hours of daylight. Also, studies show that when we have no access to sunlight or clocks, most of us sleep twice in a twenty-four-hour period, once for six to seven hours and again for one to two hours.

Ah-*ha!* Here is a case for The Nap. As early as 1975, scientists were proposing the radical notion that naps, preferably taken at midday, should be a natural part of the sleep cycle. I have suspected that highly successful men and women, especially those with impressive sofas in their offices, were sneaking extra winks right after lunch. Shepherd writes from early morning until noon, and he is certain that the most wonderful part of his day is a 30-minute blowout noontime snooze on the living room sofa in the sun with the cat curled on his chest.

Look around your office any afternoon and you'll see everyone trying to stay awake and work into the early evening. They forget the wisdom of Winston Churchill, well known for his naps, among other things, who said: "You must sleep some time between lunch and dinner. Don't think you will be doing less work because you sleep during the day. That's a foolish notion held by people who have no imagination. You will be able to accomplish more."

Naps are not only a good way to regain creativity and productivity at work, but it's also a good way to recover lost sleep on weekends. Instead of sleeping late, a better practice would be to get up at your usual time and then regain sleep with an afternoon nap. Guided by your own natural sleep rhythm, if you awaken around 6:00 A.M., you'll be ready for a nap around 2:00 P.M. The cat is optional.

How to sleep better. To determine how many hours of sleep you need, scientists suggest that you track your sleeping hours for a period from ten days to two weeks. Note whether you awaken feeling refreshed and able to be vigorous and concentrate throughout the day. If you feel good, you are getting enough sleep overall, and the average number of hours slept each night during the test period is probably close to what you need. If you need an alarm clock to get you up, or if you are sleepy doing sedentary work later in the day, like driving or sitting in a conference, try adding 30 to 90 minutes a night to your sleep time. Here are some other tips:

- To get enough sleep during the week, set a fixed bedtime and stick to it.

- Do not try to skate through days on too little sleep by using exercise or caffeine to overcome your sleepiness. This simply masks the problem.

- Exercise regularly, but do not do a hard workout within three or four hours of bedtime.

- Avoid sleeping pills. They are at best a temporary solution.

- Keep your bedroom at a comfortable temperature. Variations of hot and cold will interrupt your night's sleep.

- Reserve your bed for sleep and lovemaking, not for watching TV, talking on the phone, or eating.

- Eat dinner at the same time each night. If you snack before bedtime, keep it light. Your body will keep you awake while digesting a large meal.

- Go to bed only when you get sleepy. If you cannot sleep, get up and read or do something relaxing.

Follow these tips and easy steps. Remember, the road to wellness starts today. Begin with a regular exercise program and move on to a healthful lifestyle. You can move along that road at your own pace, and take control of your life.

THIRTY-NINE

The Heart-Lung Machine

Your heart and lungs work together to deliver oxygen and nutrients to your body and remove carbon dioxide and waste products from it. The cardiovascular system consists of your heart and its blood vessels, including arteries, arterioles, capillaries, veins, and venules. The respiratory system consists of two lungs—one on each side of the heart—and their bronchi, bronchioles, and alveoli.

A simplified way to look at these complex systems is to refer to them as "the heart-lung machine." The lungs provide the oxygen that drives the heart engine that drives the body. A strong heart-lung machine is essential to cardiorespiratory fitness, running performance, and good health.

As described earlier, cardiorespiratory (aerobic) fitness is the ability of the body to sustain exercise over extended periods of time. Aerobic exercises such as running promote the supply and use of oxygen and thus improve your cardiorespiratory endurance. Research shows that aerobic exercise strengthens this heart-lung machine and reduces the risk of heart disease.

How the Heart-Lung Machine Works

At the center of your chest—indeed, at the center of your life—is your heart. It is an extraordinary muscle about the size of your fist that weighs 8 to 10 ounces, beats an average of 70 to 80 times a minute while resting, or 4,200 to 4,800 times an hour, more than 100,000 times a day, more than 37 million times a year. Over the average life span of seventy-four years, your heart will beat approximately 3 billion times and pump about one million barrels of blood.

What about those who claim you only have so many heartbeats in a lifetime—and exercise uses them up? The opposite is true. Regular exercise lowers your resting heart rate so your heart has to work less all day long despite the increased heartbeats needed during exercise. A drop in resting heart rate from an average of 70 beats per minute to 60 beats per minute for a fitness runner—who exercises at a training heart rate range of 140 to 160 beats per minute for four 30-minute runs per week—would result in that runner saving over 6 million heartbeats over the course of a year. And this is despite needing an extra 600,000 or so extra beats to handle the added work of the exercise! If you want a stronger, more efficient heart-lung machine, exercise.

Your heart is composed of muscle tissue different from any other tissue in the body: Cardiac muscle has its own distinct appearance under the microscope. The heart is also one of the most adaptable muscular structures of our bodies, ready to improve its condition if we exercise it in a proper manner. This muscle pumps your body's entire blood supply (about 5 quarts) through your vascular system in less than a minute; during exercise, blood may travel through your arteries at speeds of 40 miles an hour!

The heart contains four chambers, two at the top (called atria) and two at the bottom (called ventricles). Each atrium is separated from the ventricle chamber below it by a valve. The right and left sides of the heart are separated by a wall of strong muscle. Each atrium is a holding chamber; each ventricle is a pump.

Here is how the heart works in conjunction with the lungs. We breathe in air through the mouth and nose. This air, carrying vital life-giving oxygen, enters the respiratory system through the bronchi, then through its smaller branches the bronchioles, and then finally it reaches the alveoli, the smallest respiratory units. The lungs contain millions of these tiny, balloonlike microscopic air sacs. Oxygen passes through thin membranes of the alveoli into the capillary beds of the lungs where the oxygen attaches to the hemoglobin of red blood cells.

This bright red oxygenated blood from the lungs next flows through the pulmonary veins and enters the left atrium of the heart. It is pushed through a valve into the left ventricle, where blood is pumped out of the heart into the aorta and into arteries that branch and divide and reach into all parts of the body. The arteries divide into arterioles, which in turn divide into the smallest units for carrying blood, called capillaries. At the capillary level, an exchange with the tissues takes place: Oxygen and nutrients are exchanged for waste products. The working muscles are nourished with oxygen.

After this exchange has taken place, blood from your muscles, low in oxygen and dark red in color, begins its return trip to the heart by capillaries to the larger venules to the larger veins. This blood, carrying waste products, flows through the veins until it enters the heart at the right atrium. It is pushed through a valve to the right ventricle, which pumps it back to the lungs via the pulmonary trunk. Exhale, and carbon dioxide is released. Inhale, and the cycle starts again.

Sounds complicated? Your heart-lung machine is an incredibly efficient system. To simplify how it works: inhale, and oxygenated blood goes from the lungs to the heart, which pumps it to the working muscles; waste products are then returned through the bloodstream to the heart, which pumps it to the lungs, where they are released as you exhale.

Like any machine, the heart-lung machine needs plenty of use to keep it running smoothly. Don't let it "rust" with a sedentary lifestyle. The stronger it becomes from exercise, the less it has to work to pump blood, breathe, and supply the body with oxygen. Exercise also makes the blood vessels more elastic (and less likely to clog) and uses more capillaries, thus making the heart-lung machine more efficient.

The Heart-Lung Machine During Exercise

At rest, the healthy heart and lungs maintain a steady rhythm. The average normal heart beats 70 to 80 beats a minute; a well-conditioned human heart beats fewer times. We inhale air through the nose or mouth into the lungs fifteen to eighteen times a minute. The lungs take in between 2 and 3.5 liters of air with each breath.

Start your warm-up. Your heart rate increases. Nerves that go directly to the heart and hormones in the blood speed up the heart in anticipation even before you exercise. As most aerobic exercise starts in healthy men and women, the heart rate rises steadily before leveling off within your training heart rate range.

As you finish your warm-ups, your heart is driving blood through your arteries to meet the new demands of your muscles for more oxygen. This is why warming up is important. It eases your heart into exercise.

During exercise, as much as 71 percent of the cardiac output is directed toward exercising muscles. Concurrently, other vessels that can temporarily compromise their blood supply constrict or "shut down." Blood flow to the stomach and intestines diminishes (one reason for not eating before exercising). Your kidneys, for example, take 20 percent of your cardiac output while you are at rest, but that drops to about 3.5 percent during the time you are exercising. Blood flow to your skin (to dissipate heat) and muscles (to supply energy) increases by almost four times. Your lungs and heart are being enriched and nourished.

As your exercise becomes more vigorous your body demands more oxygen; more blood must be pumped to the working muscles. The heart's output is determined by the rate of pumping (heartbeats or pulse) and by the quantity of blood ejected with each beat or stroke (stroke volume). Among the sedentary who attempt vigorous exercise, the heart beats more often and the stroke volume is less.

As a fit runner, your heart rate will accelerate at the beginning of your workouts much more slowly than untrained exercisers, and after about 5 minutes of vigorous steady-paced aerobic exercise your heart-rate plateaus, or stops accelerating. At this point you should be exercising at a steady state within your training heart rate range.

Now you are up and running. Your breathing has increased from eighteen to perhaps fifty breaths per minute. You are now breathing in greater amounts of air. In a single breath, the average trained runner can process a full liter of air more than the untrained person. The maximum breathing capacity per minute may reach 40 or 50 liters more than the untrained person. Your lungs have become stronger, better able to move air in and out at a faster rate. Your blood is carrying more oxygen.

Your exercise training has also increased your heart's efficiency. It grows stronger, and pumps more blood with each beat or stroke.

A conditioned person may have a resting heart rate 20 beats per minute slower than an unconditioned person. That means that you may be saving as many as 10,000 heartbeats during a single night's sleep. Even while running, your heart pumps blood and oxygen in a much more efficient manner than the unconditioned heart.

As your run ends, be sure to walk to cool down. The rate and depth of your breathing should return to normal, as do your heart rate and the stroke volume. An abrupt halting of all exercise after running can be dangerous because blood caught in your extremities (especially the legs) may "pool" there. The muscles need a cool-down period to return the circulatory system to normal.

Heart Disease and Exercise

How well you take care of your heart may affect how long you live. Consider these statistics from the American Heart Association (AHA):

- Every 34 seconds, a life is claimed by heart disease or stroke.

- Heart attacks are the single largest killers of Americans.

- About 1.5 million Americans have heart attacks every year and one-third of them are fatal.

- Over 56 million Americans (more than one in five) have some form of cardiovascular disease.

- More than two out of every five Americans die from cardiovascular disease.

Death rates from cardiovascular diseases have been declining since about 1970. According to the American Heart Association, deaths from heart attacks dropped by more than 29 percent between 1980 and 1990. Stroke deaths dropped 33 percent and deaths from high blood pressure fell 20 percent over the same decade.

Dr. William Castelli, director of the Framingham heart study, the nation's longest continuing study of heart disease, thinks the decrease in death rates from heart attacks and strokes may be due more to improved medical care and hospital efficiency than improved health. "We have to look at the whole picture, not just pat ourselves on the back because death rates have fallen. We have a long way to go in preventing these diseases." The Framingham study has followed 5,000 men and women since 1949, and their offspring since the early 1970s. The study of the offspring reveals that there is little or no improvement from one generation to the next in the important areas of high blood pressure, lack of exercise, diabetes, or obesity.

The AHA lists four primary factors that cause heart disease: smoking, high blood pressure, high cholesterol, and lack of exercise. The AHA didn't include lack of exercise as a primary factor until 1992; previously, lack of exercise was listed as only a contributing factor along with diabetes, stress, and obesity. They based this decision on the growing body of research that shows that exercise helps control cholesterol, obesity, diabetes, and high blood pressure—as well as being an important risk factor control itself. The AHA reports that coronary heart disease is 1.9 times more likely to develop in sedentary people than in active ones, independent of other risk factors. The Centers for Disease Control adds that "a sedentary lifestyle constitutes the greatest single risk to the collective hearts of America."

After reviewing twelve large clinical studies, researchers at Harvard University discovered that by changing the way you live, you can reduce your chances of heart attack. Their research is not surprising—much of it has been detailed elsewhere in this book. For example, by quitting smoking you may reduce your chances of a heart attack by up to 70 percent. Lowering your cholesterol may reduce those risks up to 60 percent; maintaining your proper body weight, up to 55 percent; treating high blood pressure with medication, up to 18 percent. And, as I've been preaching since 1978, regular aerobic exercise may reduce your risk of heart attack by up to 45 percent.

Women and Heart Disease

Since 1910, more American women have died from heart disease than from any other cause. Until recently, most physicians and researchers treated heart disease almost exclusively as a man's problem. As recently as 1964, for example, when the American Heart Association held its first public conference for women, it focused on how women could protect their husband's from heart disease.

Why the neglect? Previously, the focus was on premature heart attacks among males—those that strike the young or middle-aged rather than the elderly. But women tend to get heart disease ten to fifteen years later than men, after women pass menopause, which results in a drop in estrogen levels and the decrease of elasticity in their arteries. After they reach menopause, women have about the same average risk of heart attack as men. Women, however, have fatal heart attacks more often then men and die from a first attack more often.

Women can take at least two important steps to prevent heart disease. First, they can exercise regularly. According to a study of 2,802 women by Dr. Lars Ekelund of the University of North Carolina, women who do not exercise are three times more likely to die of a heart attack than those who do. Further, estrogen replacement therapy combined with exercise and a healthy diet are recommended for most women as preventative measures. The Harvard study indicates that women may reduce their risk for heart attack by up to 44 percent by using estrogen replacement therapy after menopause. Estrogen therapy, however, may involve health risks—consult your doctor.

Women of all ages are also facing far more stress in their daily lives. This is largely due to their increased roles in the workforce, especially at levels of high responsibility. Stress among all of us, men and women, is of course another important factor in causing heart disease.

Your Heart Disease Risk Factors

There are risk factors for coronary artery disease. Some, once you become aware of them, you can change, but others you have no control over. Here are some of the factors you *cannot* control:

- Age: The older we get, the greater our risk of heart disease and heart attack.

- Gender: Men are at a much higher risk than menstruating women, although this gap is narrowing. As discussed here, women increase their risk after menopause.

- Family history: Your risk is higher if you have a parent, sibling, or close relative who had heart disease. The risk is also increased if that relative developed the disease before age fifty.

Here are some of the risk factors you *can* control or alter:

- Blood pressure: High blood pressure is closely linked to heart disease and stroke. But blood pressure is also easily controlled by exercise, medications, or both.

- Cholesterol: The relationship between cholesterol in the blood and heart disease is strong. The type of cholesterol is important, as discussed in this chapter. Your cholesterol level can be controlled through diet and exercise.

- Diabetes: This disease and the development of coronary disease are strongly linked, especially when diabetes appears in middle age.

- Exercise: Regular aerobic exercise helps prevent heart disease and increases your chances of surviving a first heart attack.

- Smoking: Evidence linking tobacco consumption—smoking or chewing it—to heart disease continues to increase. If this addiction is broken, you can quickly reverse the negative effects of tobacco with diet and exercise.

- Stress: The role that stress plays in terms of heart disease remains unclear. But reducing stress is beneficial for a number of reasons—your mental comfort, for example, and blood pressure levels.

- Weight: Some experts believe there is little relationship between weight and heart disease, although most believe that obesity is a risk factor.

- Triglycerides: There is increasing evidence that this blood fat plays a significant role in heart disease. The relationship is still unclear, but here, too, you can control your diet and have an impact on the level of triglycerides in your system.

If you have several of the above risk factors, don't panic! Look at the risk factors you can control, and take charge of your life. You can start now to diet and exercise your way into a lower-risk category. You might also want to discuss these factors with your physician.

The primary risk factors are those that have been proven by significant amounts of scientific research to contribute to heart disease. They include high blood pressure, high blood lipid (cholesterol and triglycerides) levels, smoking and physical inactivity.

Hypertension or High Blood Pressure

Some 58 million Americans have hypertension, or high blood pressure, and 22 million take drugs to lower it. High blood pressure produces no symptoms in its early stage. It is a silent but known killer; it causes strokes and heart attacks.

Blood pressure is the force of blood pushing against the walls of your arteries. That force is caused by your heart pumping and resting. It is measured at the moment of the heart's contraction or pump (systolic pressure) and at the moment of relaxation (diastolic pressure). Systolic pressure gives an estimate of the heart's work and the accompanying strain on the arterial walls during contraction. Diastolic pressure provides an indication of the ease with which blood flows from the arterioles into the capillaries.

Using a cuff (a sphygmomanometer) around your upper arm, your physician can easily and quickly measure your blood pressure—which is read as millimeters of hemoglobin, or mmHg. A reading that is generally greater than 150 mmHg systolic and 90 mmHg diastolic is considered hypertension. Aggressive treatment with medication for patients with blood pressure readings above 150/90 has resulted in a decline of deaths from strokes of 54 percent since 1972. But side effects from the treatment—depression, sluggishness, impotence—are stimulating a lively debate over when treatment should start and what its effects on our lives might be. You should always check with your physican before starting an exercise program if you are on medication or have high blood pressure.

There is research evidence that endurance exercises like running actually lower blood pressure, especially in people with hypertension. A research team at the Columbia Medical Plan in Columbia, Maryland, and the Francis Scott Key Medical Center in Baltimore worked with a group of fifty-two sedentary men with moderate hypertension. They divided the group into three units, one given a placebo, one given beta-blocker medication, and the third given calcium blockers. All three groups followed a ten-week aerobic exercise and circuit weight training program. They also did aerobic exercise—walking, jogging, or cycling—for 45 minutes, three days a week.

The results? Blood pressure dropped on the average of 14 points per man in all three groups—even those given a placebo.

The American College of Sports Medicine did an extensive review of studies on exercise and high blood pressure. The result: They issued an official position statement supporting endurance exercise as an effective way to counter mild to moderate high blood pressure. The report pointed out that moderate to vigorous exercise for 20 to 60 minutes done three to five times a week can lower blood pressure by an average of 10 millimeters. They also pointed out that physically active people with high blood pressure have a lower death rate than sedentary people with the same condition.

Cholesterol and Heart Disease

More than half of all Americans have cholesterol levels that are too high. Knowing what cholesterol is, what raises your cholesterol level, and how to lower it can lead to a longer, healthier life.

Contrary to what many people believe, most of the cholesterol in your blood doesn't come from your diet but rather is manufactured by your liver. It is produced by the body because it helps to build membranes for new cells. It is also used in making bile, which aids digestion and assists in the manufacture of sex and adrenal hormones. Cholesterol is necessary for brain and nerve functioning and helps repair body tissues.

A certain amount of cholesterol is essential to life. The problem comes when the supply of cholesterol exceeds the demand for it. When there's too much lipid (fat including cholesterol and triglycerides) in the blood, a condition called hyperlipemia exists. Over many years, fat deposits may form in the inner walls of the arteries. This reduces their diameter and restricts blood flow. If the arteries to the heart muscle are blocked, a heart attack may result. If an artery to the brain is blocked, a stroke may result. High cholesterol may be the result of diets high in animal fats, particularly saturated fats found in red meat and high-fat dairy products. But high cholesterol may also be the result of heredity.

Numerous studies indicate that the higher your total cholesterol, the greater your chances of suffering from heart disease and/or stroke. The National Heart, Lung and Blood Institute recommends a total cholesterol count of under 200 milligrams per deciliter of blood. National health and nutrition surveys have revealed some good news: Average total cholesterol levels have fallen from 220 milligrams to 205 milligrams since 1960—a decline of about 7 percent—largely as the result of improved diet. Still, some 65 million Americans have cholesterol levels considered to be too high.

For years, health authorities concentrated on testing for total cholesterol as a key to predicting and thus preventing heart disease and stroke. Although these numbers are important, they don't tell the whole story. In fact, most heart attacks occur in men and women with only slightly elevated cholesterol levels. More recently, health authorities are beginning to agree that your total cholesterol reading is not the key. Rather, it is the ratio of so-called good and bad cholesterol that gives a more accurate prediction of heart disease and stroke.

Cholesterol circulates in the blood in combination with a protein coating. These are the lipoproteins that include high-density lipoproteins (HDLs), low-density lipoproteins (LDLs), and very low density lipoproteins (VLDLs).

LDL is the "bad" lipoprotein because it carries the most cholesterol, about 65 percent of the total, in the blood and is most likely to stick to the walls of your arteries. HDL, about 25 percent of the total, is the "good" cholesterol. It acts like a "scrubber" and fights artery disease by clearing away cholesterol from the artery walls. It returns cholesterol to the liver, where it is broken down and then excreted.

Numerous studies show a clear link between heart disease and elevated LDL levels in the blood. LDL readings below 130 milligrams are considered desirable, and LDL levels below 100 milligrams are probably ideal. The average American is between 150 and 160 milligrams.

Average HDL levels are 45 milligrams for men and 55 milligrams for women. Higher HDL levels for women may explain why they are less likely to get heart disease than men until after menopause, when their HDL levels start to drop off. HDL levels below 35 milligrams for both men and women are considered a risk factor; levels above 45 milligrams are desirable and above 60 milligrams ideal.

Your total cholesterol reading is in fact a composite of your HDLs, LDLs, and VLDLs. The average American male has a total cholesterol reading of about 215 milligrams—150–160 is LDL,

40–46 is HDLs, and 12–20 is VLDLs. Women have a similar total cholesterol number but their HDLs are about 10–15 milligrams higher.

What's in the numbers? We are now coming to understand that the *ratio* of the good guys to the bad guys is one indicator of possible heart disease. The National Institutes of Health reports that if your total cholesterol is high but your HDL levels are also high, you may be less at risk than someone with a lower total cholesterol level but also a lower HDL count. Dr. Castelli's work with the Framingham heart study shows that the ratio of HDL to LDL "is the single most effective predictor of heart attacks, and it's the number doctors should be checking." He notes that "in our study, there have been significant numbers of people with low total cholesterol readings who've had heart attacks anyway."

Dr. Castelli's data indicate that a person with a ratio of 4.5 or higher (for example, a total cholesterol of 225 divided by HDLs of 50) is twice as likely to have a heart attack, other factors being equal, as a person whose ratio is 3.5 or lower. A preferred range is 4.5 to 3.5; below 3.5 is ideal. According to the study, the risk of coronary artery disease decreases by 2 percent for every 1 percent increase in a person's HDLs.

The trick is to lower the bad stuff and raise the good. But how? To some extent your cholesterol levels—both HDL and LDL—are determined by genetics. But you can improve your numbers. One way to reduce LDL levels is to reduce fat in your diet to no more than 30 percent of your daily calories. (Diet and cholesterol are discussed further in Chapter 18.) Stopping smoking, keeping blood pressure low, and leading a less stressful life are all beneficial. Exercise also seems to lower the undesirable LDLs.

HDL levels are largely genetically determined, but you can raise them slightly through aerobic exercise, weight reduction, and not smoking. Once again, smoking is a significant factor: You may be able to increase your HDLs by 4 or 5 milligrams if you quit. Passive smokers suffer, too. Researchers at the Medical College of Virginia have found that kids whose parents smoke a pack of cigarettes a day have lower HDLs than children of nonsmokers. Postmenopausal women who take estrogen supplements may also increase their HDL levels.

A low-fat, high-carbohydrate diet can significantly lower your total cholesterol levels, but, unfortunately, it may also lower your

HDLs. That's why it is important to combine a low-fat diet with aerobic exercise. A vigorous exercise program may increase HDL levels by 10 to 20 percent.

As a last resort, drug treatment may be needed to lower your cholesterol to safe levels. Several of these new drugs can reduce LDLs by 25 percent or more while slightly raising HDL levels.

Still, the most important strategy in fighting cholesterol's role in heart disease and strokes is combining a low-fat diet with exercise. Dr. James Cleeman, coordinator of the National Cholesterol Education Program, points out that "three out of every four patients who need to modify their cholesterol levels can do it without drugs by changing their diets and starting an exercise regimen."

A study at Stanford University divided 300 moderately overweight men and women into three groups—low-fat diet, low-fat diet and exercise, and one with no diet change. The low-fat diet contained less than 30 percent fat and only 10 percent was saturated. Exercises began with aerobic movement and progressed to walking and running up to five times a week. After one year, the group that only dieted had greater benefits than the no-diet, no-exercise group. But those who dieted *and* exercised benefited the most: They lost more weight (men, 15 pounds; women, 12 pounds), decreased their LDLs, sharply increased their HDLs, and cut their overall heart risk (men by 34 percent; women by 23 percent). "Exercise seems to protect that HDL effect and, overall, it enhances the dieting benefits," said Dr. Peter Wood, director of the study. "You get more bang for your buck with exercise."

Several other studies indicate that you will benefit even from mild exercise. For example, people who walk at least two and a half to four hours a week have raised their HDL levels. What benefits come with running? Paul Williams, Ph.D., of the Lawrence Livermore Lab in Berkeley, California, studied 6,849 male runners with an average age of forty-five. His results, reported to the American Heart Association, show that increased vigorous exercise beyond the recommended minimum of 30 minutes or more four to six days a week results in additional gains in HDL levels. The researchers suggested that the first goal is to get sedentary people to do a minimum of exercise to raise HDL levels—30 minutes several times a week. Beyond that, running up to 50 miles a week offers increased benefits.

Even relaxing more may elevate HDLs. At Harvard Medical School, Dr. JoAnn Manson administered physiological and psychological tests to 349 heart attack survivors and an equal number of people who had no history of heart attacks. She found a strong link between low HDL levels and certain personality traits, such as a desire to get ahead and a preoccupation with time. Those Type A personality types had heart attack rates 50 percent greater than the others. The researchers theorized that uptight behavior increases the stress hormones such as adrenaline, which chemically lowers the ratio of HDL to LDL in the body. The recommendation: Increase exercise and stress management.

The National Cholesterol Education Program recommends that everyone should be tested for both cholesterol and HDLs starting at age twenty and then at least once every five years thereafter.

Exercise and the Heart

The lack of exercise is a leading modifiable risk associated with coronary disease or heart attack. Recent studies also show that sedentary people are twice as likely to die from heart attack as physically active people. The long history of research underscores the truth of this simple prescription: If you want to live longer, maintain a proper weight, stop smoking, and exercise aerobically three to five days a week for at least 30 minutes each day. Two separate and classic studies have concluded that men and women who exercise regularly are less likely to suffer from heart attacks.

The Morris Study

Some of the first studies were done in 1953, 1956, and 1967 by Dr. Jeremy N. Morris and associates of the Medical Research Council of London Hospital. Although somewhat flawed by modern research standards, the Morris studies set the foundation for further analysis of the relationship between activity, weight, smoking, cholesterol and heart attack and disease.

Dr. Morris reported that London Transport System bus drivers who sat all day had 1.5 times as much heart disease and twice the coronary death rate as the bus conductors, who climbed up and down the stairs of the double-decker buses collecting fares. A similar result was found among postal carriers compared to postal clerks, who did sedentary work.

Dr. Morris and his researchers in 1967 next studied 16,882 British civil servants, all of whom were sedentary at work and had similar coronary risk factors. They divided the group according to whether they exercised during their leisure time or not. Vigorous exercise included swimming, tennis, hill climbing, running, jogging, mountain walking, and fast cycling. By 1973, they had some interesting results: The vigorously active group had one-third the number of heart attacks as the less active group. By 1980, Morris and his group reported that, after thirteen years of study, the heart attack rate among the active civil servants was less than half that of their inactive coworkers. Most important, the heart attack rate among the active group remained the same even as they aged between forty and sixty years. But the rate in the inactive group more than doubled during those same years.

Morris and colleagues concluded that "vigorous exercise is a natural defense of the body, with a protective effect on the aging heart against ischemia and its consequences." (Ischemia is reduced blood flow generally caused by atherosclerosis or narrowing of the coronary arteries.)

The Paffenbarger Studies

Dr. Ralph Paffenbarger and colleagues have made major contributions to this field in their studies of two groups of men: those who were active in their work and those who were active in their leisure.

First, their long-term study of San Francisco longshoremen, published in March 1975, reached similar conclusions as the Morris research. Once again, vigorous exercise or activity was significant. Excellent medical data allowed the Paffenbarger team to study subjects whose medical histories covered up to forty years. Moreover, the San Francisco longshoremen could not select manual or sedentary work, because all of them had to perform manual labor at work for at least an initial five-year period. Most of them continued heavy manual labor for an average of thirteen years.

Among the 6,351 longshoremen studied over a twenty-two-year period, those who did the heaviest labor had the lowest incidence of heart disease. These men had only one-third the rate of sudden death from heart attack than men in less active jobs. The risk was reduced even in longshoremen who had other coronary risk factors. The researchers concluded that vigorous exercise was "a critical factor in cardiovascular well-being, especially as it would prevent sudden death from coronary heart disease." They reported similar findings in a follow-up study in March 1977.

A second long-term continuing study, first reported in November 1977, followed 16,936 Harvard University alumni. Dr. Paffenbarger was able to study subjects who had enrolled at Harvard as far back as 1916. This Paffenbarger study graded leisure-time activity according to stairs climbed, city blocks walked, participation in light sports or vigorous exercise. They found that each activity reduced the risk of a first heart attack: climbing fifty or more stairs each working day lowered risk by 20 percent; walking five or more city blocks lowered it by 21 percent; exercising vigorously dropped the risk by 27 percent. Dr. Paffenbarger reported that strenuous exercise, like running for at least 144 minutes a week, reduces the risk of first heart attack by 39 percent.

Furthermore, this research found that as men in the Harvard study exercised more, the risk of heart attack decreased—that is, men who expended fewer than 2,000 calories per week showed a 64 percent higher risk of heart attack than those who were more energetic. Those men who played "light" sports like golf, bowling, baseball, or recreational biking were no better off than those who were inactive. But men who walked regularly were better off than those who didn't, and men who exercised vigorously were better off than those who only walked.

Dr. Paffenbarger and his associates measured the incidents of heart attack versus energy expenditure in exercise. By doing so, they showed that about 3 or 4 miles of running per day three to five days a week was the minimum amount of exercise that will significantly reduce the risk of heart attack. Running 20 miles a week, or the exercise equivalent, makes you 64 percent less likely to have a heart attack than a sedentary person. Beyond 40 miles a week, you may have some small increments in additional protection. Periodic hard running also adds to your health benefits.

The Harvard study also holds out hope for men and women who start exercise programs long after they have left college (or college-age level). It determined that active college athletes who stop exercising after they graduate have no more protection than their sedentary peers. But men who, whether active during their college years or not, took up strenuous exercise later had a clearly reduced risk of heart attack.

Post–Heart Attack Exercise

Another area that supports studies linking vigorous exercise and lowered risk of heart attack concerns men and women who have already suffered from heart attacks. In the Harvard study, Dr. Paffenbarger found that those graduates who did have heart attacks but who were exercising vigorously had a 29 percent lower heart attack fatality rate than those who suffered heart attacks but did not exercise vigorously. Simply put, vigorous exercise lowered the chances of fatality from a heart attack.

Since 1967, Dr. Terrence Kavanaugh, medical director of the Toronto Cardiac Rehabilitation Center, has been encouraging his postcoronary patients to exercise. The program includes no smoking, special low-fat diets, and running. Some postcoronary patients build up to running marathons, but most of his patients run 3 miles or so a day. The results are impressive. "We have a 1.4-percent-per-annum mortality rate," Dr. Kavanaugh told the *New York Times*. "In groups that don't exercise, the comparable rate is 6 to 12 percent."

Exercise and Sudden Death

If exercise is so beneficial in preventing heart disease, why do athletes continue to die suddenly during their workouts, games, or races? This has created the paradox of vigorous exercise: While vigorous exercise like running lowers your risk of sudden death from heart attack compared to sedentary people, that risk increases dramatically *during* vigorous exercise.

This paradox has been questioned with increasing urgency and perplexity since 1909, when five prominent British physicians began inquiring about deaths during school and cross-country races of more than a mile for boys under the age of nineteen. The paradox arose again in the 1970s when the popularity of running as exercise and recreation boomed. The sudden death of Jim Fixx, author of a popular book on running, during his run in Vermont in 1983 refocused attention on sudden death among runners.

Is running the real culprit in these deaths? Some young athletes who die suddenly during exercise have genetically elevated blood cholesterol levels that may cause severe atherosclerosis. Others suffer from hypertropic cardiomyopathy, a thickening of the heart's walls. Still others smoke, use drugs, suffer from high blood pressure, or are physically inactive and have engaged in running or other vigorous exercise sporatically.

In the Jim Fixx case, he was at high risk because his father had died from a heart attack at a very young age (forty-three). Prior to starting a running program, Fixx had also been a smoker, overweight, and had high blood cholesterol. There is some evidence that he also had warning signs he ignored, such as tightness in his chest during exercise and shortness of breath.

Looked at another way, sudden deaths from heart attack during vigorous exercise may simply reflect deaths among those men who would have died anyway within days or weeks even had they avoided all forms of exercise, including walking. A large number of men and women die every day from heart attacks. Most of them were sedentary, smokers, with uncontrolled high blood pressure and elevated cholesterol levels.

Remember, too, that severe heart disease may be present even in persons who appear very fit. We know that while vigorous exercise seems to lower the risk of heart problems compared to sedentary folks, runners and other exercisers are not immune to diseases of the heart.

Further, research is indicating now that those who die suddenly during vigorous exercise almost always have experienced heart symptoms that they ignored, and preferred to keep exercising rather than seek medical advice. What are those signs? They include chest discomfort or squeezing, throat tightness, pain that radiates into the jaw or left arm. Heart disease can also cause abnormal heartbeats. Unusual fatigue is another signal that is often overlooked. If you find yourself feeling unusually tired after a workout, and are confident that it isn't related to another cause, such as overtraining or heat, mention it to your physician.

Some runners ignore these warning signals. Others actually increase their training after experiencing chest pain or shortness of breath in the belief that running will somehow save them. But it won't. One study of heart attacks and sudden deaths in marathons found that 81 percent of the runners who survived said they had had warning symptoms before the attack.

Thus we have the paradox of vigorous exercise. It has been well defined by a major study of sudden death among runners conducted by Dr. David Siskovick, a research cardiologist working at the University of North Carolina. During the 1980s, Dr. Siskovick and his research associates collected detailed information about all people who died suddenly from coronary heart disease during a one-year period in Seattle, Washington. Excluding those who had previous symptoms, Dr. Siskovick narrowed the group down to 145 people with no previous signs of disease who were healthy right up to the moment they suddenly died.

What this study concluded was that men and women who exercise vigorously on a regular basis have an overall risk of sudden death that is two-thirds lower than that of sedentary nonexercisers. But the risk of sudden death to those who exercised vigorously was also high, for the duration of their workout, above the risk of the nonexercisers. Thus, while all people who exercise vigorously reduce their risk of sudden death, a small group of exercisers with advanced heart disease who would ultimately die suddenly anyway are more likely to die during exercise than while at rest.

Prevention of Sudden Death

Is it possible to predict who might die suddenly during exercise? In addition to reporting to your physician the early signals of coronary problems stated above, you and your physician might want to discuss a series of possible tests. These begin with an electrocardiogram (ECG). This is usually given in your physician's office with you at rest.

If any abnormalities show up on that benign test, then you might want to discuss an exercise stress test (exercise electrocardiography). In this test, you have electrodes attached to your chest skin and you exercise on a treadmill while your heart's rate and performance are recorded. Sometimes abnormalities are picked up in this test, but there is a high rate of false positives—that is, an abnormality is shown where none exists. Runners have a high incidence of false positives on exercise electrocardiograms. Dr. Paul Thompson, a cardiologist at Brown University Medical School, who is a marathon runner himself, believes that a natural thickening of the heart walls occurs with endurance running. That means, if you are an endurance runner you are likely to have a false positive electrocardiogram.

Do you really need an exercise stress test? Should all runners with one of the risk factors of heart disease—family history, obesity, smoking, diabetes, high blood pressure, low HDL cholesterol—have such a test? Most physicians recommend a stress test to anyone over age forty-five who is starting an exercise program for the first time. Dr. Ken Cooper, head of the Aerobics Center in Dallas, also suggests that healthy men and women over forty have an exercise stress test once every three years. For exercisers with at least one of the above risk factors, Dr. Cooper recommends testing every two years.

FORTY

Stress Management

Stress is essential to life, but it's also a cause of death. It sweetens victory, and defines defeat. It relieves boredom and helps us maintain life, resist aggression, and adapt to changing external influences. It may be pleasant or unpleasant, damaging or helpful. Stress may result in either improved or decreased performance at work, school, or sports. Its effect, especially its negative impact on our bodies, may be long lasting, even occurring after the stressful event has passed.

Stress is everywhere in our lives. We may feel its characteristic signs immediately after someone's car nearly collides with our own, or before (and after) an important race, speech, appearance, event, or business meeting.

Stress, said Dr. Hans Selye, author of *Stress Without Distress*, "is essentially the wear and tear in the body caused by life at any one moment." It may come from work, school, family, play, or at home. There are various kinds of stress: emotional (caused by a family argument, the death of a loved one), environmental (caused by heat or cold), and physical (caused by physical activity or illness). There may also be perceived stress in our lives. How we see an event may make it more stressful than it inherently is.

Changes in our lives, whether good or bad, cause stress. Modern life gives us more change than ever before. And stress in response to change, whether good or bad, may impair the way we work, live, and feel.

What actually happens to us under stress? Imagine that you are facing a deadline. The boss or teacher tells you that what you've done so far is awful, third rate, and that you'd better get the job finished, in good shape and on time. Your body reacts to this stress and prepares for action. The stress excites your hypothalamus (a region of the brain near the base of your skull), which produces a substance that stimulates the pituitary gland to discharge the hormone ACTH (adrenocorticotropic hormone) into your blood. Signals begin rushing to all parts of your body, including the adrenal gland. Adrenaline pours into your bloodstream. The adrenaline increases your heart rate. Your heart demands more oxygen and there is an increase in your respiration. Now your heart is pounding, your muscles tense, your blood pressure is up, and your palms, armpits, or back may be sweating. You are ready to act.

Research in the early 1900s by Dr. Walter B. Cannon at the Harvard Medical School showed that animals used this physiological change to take action. When a wild animal fought or ran, it consumed this energy; later, when its muscles relaxed and its heartbeat and breathing slowed and returned to normal, its blood pressure dropped.

For us, however, the stresses of modern society aren't often short term and cannot be handled by fleeing or fighting. Yet our bodies still react to stress by preparing to run or fight. Instead of releasing the stress by enacting our inherent fight-or-flight response, we sit and fume—in traffic jams, in our offices, waiting in lines. As a result, our systems are flooded with hormones that respond to stress. The repeated suppression of this natural sequence of stresses strains our bodies and endangers our health. Illness often results.

"It's clear that our reactions to stress are no longer appropriate," Dr. Paul Rosch, president of the American Institute of Stress in Yonkers, New York, told *Running Times*. "But now something like running gives us a chance to mimic what the hormones released under stress are preparing us to do." We may not be able to run every time we are faced with stress, but we can go out for a brisk walk and later get out for a run. This will help. "The sooner you can take physical action when faced with stress," Dr. Rosch said, "the less the stress will negatively affect you."

Stress and Illness

And stress will affect you.

The impact of stress on us is significant and measurable. Stress changes us physically and can cause a variety of medical illnesses, some imagined and some very real, painful, even lethal. Studies show that 80 percent of all diseases are caused in part by chronic unrelieved stress. In fact, stress is thought to cost society $300 billion annually in health-related problems like absenteeism, lost productivity, and medical costs. Each period of stress, says Dr. Selye, especially from frustrating, unsuccessful struggles, leaves some irreversible chemical scars. When we become overburdened beyond our stress tolerance, we may become ill, develop emotional illnesses, or suffer physical breakdown. The list of diseases from negative stress is long and uncontested: high blood pressure, mental depression, anxiety, insomnia, sexual dysfunction, asthma attacks, ulcers, headaches, skin problems and rashes, overeating, various heart problems, and arrhythmias. "The relationship of stress and behavior to cardiovascular conditions is well documented," says Dr. David Jenkins, professor of preventative medicine and community health at the University of Texas in Galveston. "What is not widely known is that, through its ability to depress the body's immune system, stress probably also influences the development of cancer."

One of the earliest studies on the effects of stress was done by Lawrence E. Hinkle, a researcher in the 1950s, who determined that people do not become ill equally or randomly. His research of telephone company employees showed that 25 percent of them had half of all illnesses; another 25 percent had less than 10 percent of all illnesses. This was true regardless of how severe the illness. Hinkle also found that the illnesses occurred in "cluster years"— that is, one-third of the illnesses occurred in one-eighth of the time studied. The employees Hinkle studied became ill when they saw their life situations as negative, unsatisfying, threatening, overdemanding, or unchangeable. Hinkle concluded that the way we react to the events in our lives plays a significant role in at least a third of all our illnesses and their severity.

Our emotions affect our muscles; and our muscles reflect our emotional problems. Tense muscles restrict movement and are vulnerable to injury.

According to Dr. Hans Kraus, the internationally known back specialist, back pain occurs because we are underexercised and overtense. Our muscles, Dr. Kraus believes, are tensing for action but are not being used for anything all day long. Lower back muscles are prime targets of stress, as are less frequently the legs, thighs, and arms. Our underexercised and overirritated lives are especially bad for our children, who are even less active than their parents. They watch a lot of television, and as they sit before the screen they are both tense and motionless. Their predicament—tension and inaction—almost symbolizes our daily lives. Not surprising, Dr. Kraus has found that 60 percent of American children cannot perform the six basic Kraus-Weber tests that measure minimal physical fitness.

Stress can make our kids sick. Dr. Roger Meyer, a noted pediatrician, studied a group of healthy children and recorded the incidence of strep throat over several years. His throat cultures discovered that 30 percent of all the well children had streptococcus bacteria present in their throats at any one time, but showed no symptoms of the disease. Dr. Meyer concluded that "peaceful coexistence [between the child and the bacteria] is the rule, disease is the exception."

But what triggers the disease? Dr. Meyer discovered that 25 percent of the strep throat he and his researchers saw followed a family crisis. An ill child was four times as likely to have experienced a recent stressful episode as a healthy child. Stress, therefore, increased the probability of a child's getting a strep throat. Other studies have found that stress may be a significant underlying cause of *all* illnesses in children, and that stressful episodes, a family fight or school problems, double the possibility of illness in both mothers and children.

Stress also ages us. "We know stress has a powerful influence on aging," Joseph Brady of the Institute of Gerontology at the University of Denver told *Running Times*. "The hormones released by the brain during times of stress clearly speed the rate at which we age."

Stress and Behavior

Holmes/Rahe Social Readjustment Rating Scale
As we mentioned, life itself is stressful. Those stresses can also be measured, and if you know what is stressful in your life, you may be able to handle it better.

In what has become a classic study, Drs. Thomas H. Holmes

and Richard H. Rahe, psychiatrists at the University of Washington Medical School, ranked stressful events and their impacts on us. They interviewed 394 men and women and asked them to assign a relative number value—using marriage as the equivalent to fifty on their scale—to all kinds of life events. From this they devised a "social adjustment scale" of stressful events, which has proved to be a highly accurate tool in the statistical prediction of stress-related illness.

The Holmes/Rahe scale (see Figure 40.1) is helpful in measuring a stressful event and its *probable* impact on your life. An important part of stress-management is to realize that some life crises are predictable and even avoidable. It is important to keep in mind that life changes and crises, as reflected on the Holmes/Rahe scale, are for the most part normal in human development. The most stressful event we experience, according to the Holmes/Rahe scale, is the death of a spouse. Corroborating this, physicians have discovered that widows and widowers are ten times more likely to die within the first year after the death of their husbands or wives than all other people in their age group. The Holmes/Rahe scale lists divorce as the next most stressful event. Here, too, they found that divorced men and women, in the year following their divorce, had an illness rate twelve times higher than married people.

Type A and Type B Behavior
Stress works on our bodies in ways that we are only now coming to understand and measure. In a well-known study about heart disease and behavior patterns, conducted in the late 1960s and early 1970s, Drs. Meyer Friedman and Ray H. Rosenman of Mount Sinai Hospital in San Francisco examined about 3,500 men over a four-year span. Their landmark work created a phrase now in common usage, Type A behavior, and gave impetus to linking behavior and disease.

Drs. Friedman and Rosenman broadly divided the behavior patterns of their subjects into two categories: Type A and Type B. The Type A man was aggressive, ambitious, and success-oriented. He talked fast and was always on the run to meet deadlines; he competed against everyone and himself. Envy and hostility were characteristics of this person. The Type B man was calmer, working at his own pace, and under little self-imposed stress.

Not surprising, Drs. Friedman and Rosenman found that Type A men had 2.5 times more heart attacks than the Type B. They

FIGURE 40.1: THE HOLMES/RAHE SOCIAL READJUSTMENT
RATING SCALE

LIFE EVENT	MEAN VALUE
Death of spouse	100
Divorce	73
Marital separation	65
Jail term	63
Death of close family member	63
Personal injury or illness	53
Marriage	50
Fired at work	47
Marital reconciliation	45
Retirement	45
Change in health of family member	44
Pregnancy	40
Sex difficulties	39
Gain of new family member	39
Business readjustment	39
Change in financial state	38
Death of close friend	37
Change to different line of work	36
Change in number of arguments with spouse	35
Significant mortgage or loan	31
Foreclosure of mortgage or loan	30
Change in responsibilities at work	29
Son or daughter leaving home	29
Trouble with in-laws	29
Outstanding personal achievement	28
Spouse begins or stops work	26
Begin or end school	26
Change in living conditions	25
Revision of personal habits	24
Trouble with boss	23
Change in work hours or conditions	20
Change in residence	20
Change in schools	20
Change in recreation	19
Change in church activities	19
Change in social activities	18
Small mortgage or loan	17
Change in sleeping habits	16
Change in number of family get-togethers	15
Change in eating habits	15
Vacation	13
Christmas	12
Minor violations of the law	11

also discovered that, among other things, emotional stress and nervous tension play a relevant role in coronary heart disease. As John Hunter, who suffered from coronary disease, described it: "I am at the mercy of any fool who can aggravate me." The Type A man is also very good at aggravating others.

Some researchers have recently challenged whether or not Type A characteristics can actually lead to heart disease. But no one doubts that Type A behavior exists. The Type A person—and it can be male or female—gets angry driving behind a slow driver or standing in a bank line; he or she cannot stand being controlled by others or their environment. "A Type A person is someone who generally feels he has to do it all—and perfectly," Dr. Jerilyn Ross, a psychiatrist in Alexandria, Virginia, told *Runner's World*. "Type A's constantly push themselves. They always think more is better and they always want to be in charge. They always have the feeling that when they do something they could have done it better. Often, they reach a point where their system just says NO."

Dr. Thomas Tutko, Ph.D., professor of psychology at San Jose State University, believes there may be two Type A running personalities: a Type A–hostile, and a Type A–controlled. "The Type A–hostile," he told *Runner's World*, "has the pathological underpinning of compulsion and anger. He is the classic Type A guy. He has chronic anger, which he has been carrying for a long time."

Type A–controlled, however, is motivated by the excitement and reward of running. "He's like a kid in a candy store," says Dr. Tutko. "When he wants more, it's because he loves what he is doing." Both runners find that running reduces tension, but the Type A–controlled knows when to stop. He's happy with 5 or 10 miles. The Type A–hostile will run until he drops or gets hurt. "He cannot seem to put on controls," says Dr. Tutko. "Running will not help him; he gets too involved in it."

How can you tell if you are a Type A–hostile, Type A–controlled, or Type B? Dr. Tutko suggests that one way to tell the difference between his two Type A behaviors is to explore what emotions you have about running. "You are probably a healthy Type A if, as you are running along, you can enjoy the scenery. But if all you see is the strain, and if anger and frustration emerge, that's a pretty good clue that you are a Type A–hostile."

Will Running Relieve Stress?

Running is a form of relaxation for most of us, and gives us a way of leaving our stressful lives behind while we hit the road. We know that running releases endorphins and they have a calming effect; most runs are followed by a sense of peace. The social aspects of running also provide group support that may help combat stress. Finally, running makes us feel organized and in control of our lives, and helps build self-esteem—these are critical weapons against stress.

Dealing with Stress

How can you deal with the stress in your life? Here are three basic methods:

Control the way you live. To a large extent, you can control the pace of your life. There are several things you can do. First, eliminate the *minor* irritations in your life that cause chronic, negative stress. For example, if driving in rush-hour traffic makes you tense and angry, try riding public transportation or joining a car pool.

Second, evaluate the *major* stresses in your life. Look for ways to eliminate or minimize them. For example, it became stressful for me to live and work in New York City. The city was full of tension, noise, and obstacles. Even running in overcrowded Central Park became a stress. So I moved out of the city. I run with the deer and squirrels. I still commute into the city almost every day for various work projects, but when I'm finished with work I escape back into a less stressful environment.

Control your life. This sounds simplistic, but give it a try. What do I mean?

For one thing, you can get better control over your life with proper and careful planning. Don't crowd too much into your schedule (and remember to schedule time for your exercise). Plan time with friends and family. I find running friends particularly helpful—a chat on the run helps blow off stress.

Understand what makes you happy and gives you pleasure, and do these things. Build them into your daily life. Allow yourself time to "smell the flowers."

Take a break when you feel yourself getting stressed. Follow some of the exercises suggested in this chapter.

Distance yourself from your problems. Take them one step at a time. Shepherd runs an international program at the University of Cambridge in England. He has a staff of five and thirty-two Fellows scattered across two continents. He travels a lot and is under stress from his program, staff, Fellows, the university—and me, when he's slow in writing! He does two things: He writes all of his tasks and problems—the sources of his stress—on 3 × 5 index cards and tucks them into his shirt pocket. At the end of the day he goes through the cards scratching off tasks completed and ranking those to be done. If he can assign a task to someone else, he does so. Then he goes for a run.

When faced with stress, only you can decide how to react. You can get emotional, angry, upset, and let the health-destroying effects of negative stress build up. Or you can take a calmer approach.

Control your body. You know what I'm going to tell you: Eat properly, get adequate sleep, exercise daily. Physically fit people handle stress better than people who are not fit.

What is needed more than anything is balance. We need to control our stresses, even the stress from exercise, by doing several things. Hans Selye offers five important steps:

1. Identify the various stages of life, wonder about the type of person you are and the type of person you wish to be. Set realistic goals. Distinguish between healthy and unhealthy ambition, which is never satisfied.

2. Maintain a broad network of family and friends with whom you share interests, work, ambitions, and fun.

3. Engage in regular exercise in a gentle manner. This confers physical and psychological/emotional benefits on you, and provides diversity.

4. Vary your routines, create hobbies, take vacations to enjoy life, not to recover from it.

5. Continue your self-education and pursue further studies. Work to have compassion for others and for yourself. "The more we vary our actions," says Dr. Selye, "the less any part

suffers from attrition." The ultimate goal is to keep your muscles, organs, and brains healthy and active.

We cannot, and Dr. Selye and others argue that we should not, avoid stress. Stress is part of life, a natural by-product of the life well lived. What we must avoid is allowing stress to make us sick, weaken our resistance to disease, or kill us. We need to control the stresses we face. Here are some good methods to alleviate stress and to relax.

■ Modify your perceptions of stress. If an event is not stressful but you see it as stressful, try changing the way you look at that event, or at things in general. Is your glass half empty or half full?

■ Express your anger. But express it in an appropriate manner (not by striking someone). Verbalize your feelings.

■ Choose your fights. "Flee" by fantasizing, taking short walks, going away for the weekend. Talk to a friend. Give in once in a while instead of insisting that you are always right.

■ Plan a strategy to solve a dilemma.

■ Organize your time. Identify time wasters and try to eliminate or modify them. Pace yourself (here is a direct lesson from running). Stick to a plan.

■ Breathe slower. Dr. Jenny Steinmetz, a California psychologist who specializes in stress management, has her clients follow a relaxation technique that includes a 7-second inhale and an 8-second exhale. Do four of those in each minute, for 2 minutes. If you have trouble counting seconds, try Dr. Steinmetz's clever trick: Say a three-syllable word to equal one second. For example, one-el-e-phant, two-el-e-phant, and so forth.

Exercise and Stress
Research demonstrating the link between exercise and controlling stress is now flowing out of major universities in both the United States and Canada. At Concordia University in Montreal, Canada, for example, studies show that aerobic exercise shortens the time

it takes to recover from psychosocial stress and "promotes rapid recovery from an [upsetting] emotional experience." The same study found that aerobic conditioning of untrained subjects increased the speed of their recovery from stress.

A study at the University of Wisconsin demonstrates that aerobic exercise seems to lower your blood pressure and level of anxiety longer than simply resting. Another study from the University of Kansas discovered that aerobically fit men and women who experience a period of intense stress are less likely to get physically ill or depressed than unfit men and women under the same amount of stress.

Just the act of exercise itself may alleviate stress: It replaces the ambiguous psychosocial stress with a physical stress, it acts as a distraction, it channels anger and frustration into physical activity, and it drains off excess energy.

But running is not a panacea. Running itself can create two debilitating stresses: physical and mental. The physical stresses caused by running make our bodies create defenses against them. If the stress comes in small quantities and regularly, the body may adapt quite well. But if the physical stresses are too heavy and too repetitive, the body cannot cope, and exhaustion, sickness, or injuries may result.

Instead of relieving stress, for some men and women running adds to it. They make running obligatory, not optional and fun. While running may relieve stress, running may also manifest our stresses. The obligatory runner is no longer free not to run.

Relaxation Exercises

The ability to relax improves with practice. Medical studies at Harvard and other universities show that relaxation exercises can reduce tension and distress. They reduce high blood pressure and heart rates resulting from stress, as well as muscle tension. Relaxation exercises help "break" muscle tension that frequently causes injury. Moreover, a relaxed muscle stretches more easily. See Chapter 37 for a sample progressive relaxation exercise routine.

Two of the best forms of relaxation are meditation and yoga. These can be done regularly, and also before and after running. Experiments show that during meditation there is a marked decrease in the body's oxygen consumption, respiratory rate, and heart rate.

Meditation

A popular meditative technique, sometimes called "the relaxation response," employs the traditional four components of meditation coupled with some reassuring medical findings about reduced blood pressure. The following meditation was devised by Dr. Herbert Benson of the Harvard Medical School. It has four components:

1. Find a quiet environment, with no distractions, where you can concentrate.

2. Employ a mental device to shift your mind from the external, stress-filled world to your inner, peaceful world. Such a stimulus may be a sound, word, or phrase repeated silently or aloud; or an object.

3. Assume a passive attitude. This includes not worrying about your mind wandering, or about how well you are performing.

4. Be comfortable. Some people sit in the cross-legged "lotus" position. Shift around. Dr. Benson warns, however, that "if you are lying down, there is a tendency to fall asleep."

Relaxation is simply stillness, quiet, a word or sound repeated; you are awake and in control. You may be still, or on your run. You may want to link the two: Start with meditation, stretching, and then go on your run, repeating your sound or word through the entire process.

Runners at Harvard's Thorndike Medical Laboratory developed, with Dr. Benson, a variation on those four meditative components. Shepherd has tried them and thinks they're fantastic and beneficial. He sets aside 20 minutes every morning for a quiet meditative time, and tries to have 5 minutes of peaceful meditation before his runs to cleanse the tensions of the day. Here are some general guidelines:

▪ Find a quiet time and place and try to meditate six days a week for 20 minutes each day.

▪ Sit quietly in a comfortable position, close your eyes, and deeply relax all your muscles. One method Shepherd uses is the yoga massage: Begin by gently rubbing your head, and move slowly to every part of your body that you can reach, including your fingers and toes. Keep your muscles deeply relaxed.

- Close your eyes. Breathe through your nose. Pay attention to your breathing. Try some yogic breathing here: In one nostril and out, then in the same nostril but out the other (block the first with a finger), then in the second nostril but out the first. Continue for several minutes, alternating nostrils. Then, as you exhale, silently say the word "one." Continue for 15 to 20 minutes. You may open your eyes to check the time but don't use an alarm. When you finish, sit quietly for several minutes, first with your eyes closed, and then with your eyes open.

- Maintain a passive attitude. Permit relaxation to occur at its own pace. Ignore all distracting thoughts. Continue repeating the word "one" (or any other soothing word). Do not worry about whether or not you are achieving a deep level of relaxation.

- Your mind may wander. When it does, simply bring it back to your breathing. Try to focus on the complete breath: the full inhalation, the full exhalation, the pauses between.

- Don't expect to feel significantly different right away. The benefits come over several months and will be subtle.

There is some evidence for the ability of meditation to ease the symptoms of illness. In one study, the medical records of 2,000 people who said they meditated were compared with 600,000 non-meditators in the same medical insurance plan. David Orme-Johnson, Ph.D., a psychologist, found that over a five-year period meditators in their twenties and thirties went to physicians half as often as their nonmeditating peers. Meditators in their forties and older made one-third fewer visits.

Yoga

You may find that yoga appeals to you, and you may wish to incorporate some yoga exercises into your stretching routines. "The purpose," of yoga stretches, says Honoré Bonnet, French Olympic ski coach, "is to liberate the mind and relax the body." This is also why runners try yoga. The stretching should be gentle, smooth, nonpainful, and achieved over a period of time. It is also a good way to improve your flexibility.

One of the reasons we emphasize varying warm-up and cooldown exercises is that they are so important we don't want them to become boring or repetitious. Substituting yoga exercises is fun. Remember also to continue the deep breathing.

FORTY-ONE

Weight Management

As a nation, we are fat and getting fatter: A Harris Poll of Americans in 1984 showed that 56 percent of us age twenty-five or above were "over their recommended [weight] range" for their height, sex, and body frame. By the end of the 1980s that percentage had increased to more than 60 percent. By 1995, it had reached 71 percent.

All right, you say, so most of us weigh a few pounds too much. According to a National Center for Health Statistics survey, the average adult weighs nearly 10 pounds more than a decade earlier *at the same age:* An average forty-year-old man, for example, in 1995 weighs 10 more pounds than an average forty-year-old man did in 1985! The survey also found that one American out of every three—up from one in four in 1980—beyond the age of twenty is categorized as being overweight, a medical condition defined as at least 20 percent more than is desirable for optimal health. Overall, at least 60 million adult Americans are classified as overweight; more than 35 million of them need to lose 35 pounds or more. Many of them are considered obese, defined as being more than 25 percent body fat for men and over 35 percent for women. "Americans are the fattest people on earth," the survey concluded.

What's going on here? Despite reductions in cholesterol and fat in our diet, Americans are consuming more calories. We are also not exercising enough. Yet more than one American in every four says that he or she is on a diet. Clearly, the battle for maintaining a healthy weight is a significant challenge for many of us.

The next generation seems to be destined for fatness as well. A survey by the President's Council on Physical Fitness found that one American child in every three is overweight: That may be as many as 20 million kids! Obese children are three times more likely to grow up to be obese adults. The national problem of being overweight and obese really starts at home, with our kids.

Overweight and obesity are health hazards. They may lead to many illnesses, including heart disease, high blood pressure, breathing problems, arthritis, cancer, diabetes, orthopedic problems, and metabolic and digestive diseases. They also may lead to poor self-image and mental health problems. If all Americans weighed within 10 percent of their recommended healthy weight, our nation's skyrocketing health care costs would drop dramatically.

We would live longer, too. According to a Harvard University study of more than 19,000 alumni, those weighing the least had a lower mortality rate during their first three decades following graduation. According to Dr. I-Min Lee, an epidemiologist at the Harvard School of Public Health and the study's principal author, the most overweight Harvard men had a 67 percent greater risk of premature death than the thinnest. She found similar results for women. Dr. I-Min Lee's conclusion: Being as lean as possible, while keeping healthy, increases your defense against the major diseases.

Being overweight also affects your running. The overweight runner puts more stress on the cardiorespiratory and musculoskeletal systems. You cannot handle heat as well. You pound the ground with greater force, thus increasing the possibility of injury. And you cannot run as fast.

What can be done? First, let's agree on one thing: Diet and exercise go together. Many people who start running do so because they are overweight, or they want to hold their weight in check. Few can lose weight and hold that weight loss without exercise. And if you diet without exercising and manage to lose weight, the result may be a thin weak person in place of a fat weak person. Exercising improves muscle strength while reducing fat. Diets that do not combine physical exercise, says Dr. Peter Wood of the Center for Research in Disease Prevention at Stanford University, "are probably doomed to failure."

The Right Weight for You

Don't feel lonely if you weigh more than you did when you were more active. You've got lots of good company, including me. I always weighed in at 150–160 as a high school and college athlete. This weight continued through my twenties and into my thirties when I was a serious marathon runner. But then, as I marched toward the half-century mark, the scales somehow tipped 180! Of course, when I first noticed this I was visiting at home dining on Mom's good cooking. I told my parents that their scales were in error. Then I checked mine and they were off, too. I went out and replaced them and still no success: I couldn't lose weight by trading scales!

My running shorts and business suits didn't fit anymore unless I sucked it in and held my breath. Although I was far from being overweight, I didn't feel and look the way I wanted to, or should. Worse, when I ran, my legs and knees ached from the added weight and I was much slower. Despite appearing very fit to others, I felt more like an elephant on the run than an antelope. Then one day—this is a true story!—while running in Central Park, I was passed by an elderly lady wearing headphones and running while skipping rope. Then I knew it was time to take my own advice.

I hadn't really increased my food intake, but the stress of business combined with a continuing bout with asthma and a bad back reduced my exercise level dramatically. At the same time, I discovered that the research was true. You really do gain weight as you age because your metabolism slows down. As I was finishing this book I was committed to regaining my youthful weight and figure. I got back below 170 pounds and started racing well again. I could still lose more weight. So I invite you to lose a few pounds and run a few more miles along with me.

But what weight is desirable for optimal health? The problem here is that health experts have many theories and no one agrees on a single formula. Not only that, they keep changing their recommendations. Let's look at some of the tests designed to determine your ideal weight.

Your bone structure and metabolism largely control what is too much or too little weight for you. To determine your best weight, consider the following points. Use these guidelines to estimate the best weight for you. Confirm this with your physician. I'll start with the simplest tests.

■ *Want to take the nude jump test?*

I thought that would get your attention! Here is the moment of truth, your time in the ring with the great bull.

Stand nude in front of a full-length mirror. Don't cheat and suck in that big belly. Now . . . *jump!*

Holy Toledo! What was that? If your mirrors and furniture rattled and the room hit 7 on the Richter Scale when you landed, you've got a weight problem. Anything on you that shook (that shouldn't) is fat.

Still not convinced? Try running in place and look at the jiggles, especially your thighs and stomach. Go ahead and suck it in now. It's still gonna jump around. (How I did on this test is known only to my dogs, who thought I was trying to play with them!)

If you are like the majority of Americans, you will come away from this moment of truth with the conviction: I need to combine diet and exercise, just like ol' Bob Glover said. While you exercise, stay out of the ring with the bull in it for about six months. Then step back in front of the mirror and compare. You may be able to say "Olé!"

■ *How about the pinch test?*

Oooooh, this is gonna hurt—but not physically. Grasp the skin at the side of your waist (thought I was going to say the fanny didn't you?). Measure the fold. If it's more than an inch (no cheating!), it's time to lose weight. What you've got there, my friend, is a "tire"—and it's a spare. Trim it. (Whew, I passed that one—for now.)

■ *What did you weigh when you were young and tender?*

When we were eighteen to twenty-five, many of us were too active to get fat. Others, who were already fat at that age, will probably stay that way. Theoretically, we stop growing in our early twenties. No one should gain substantial weight as he or she ages. I will concede up to 5 pounds to decreased metabolism as we age, but no more.

Life insurance charts, which show that people weigh more as

they age, actually reflect what is happening, not what should happen. As mentioned, our metabolism slows as we age. To counteract this slowdown, there's a showdown: We should eat less and exercise more, thereby leveling off our weight rather than continuing to gain.

Estimating Ideal Body Weight

There are many ways to estimate your best weight. Let's see how I fit in at 6 feet 1 inch, 168 pounds. (Shepherd would have joined us, but he's been hanging out at the Red Bull pub in Cambridge, England, too much!)

One popular estimate, for example, is based on a mathematical formula. Men take their height in inches, multiply it by four, and subtract 128. That would put me at 164 pounds—I'll take it. Women compute their height in inches, multiply it by 3.5, and subtract 108. If you are large boned, you may add 10 percent. (To determine if you are large boned, try this simple test: Can you encircle your wrist with your thumb and middle finger? If you can, you are not large boned.)

Some of the most often used guidelines for determining your ideal weight follows.

Metropolitan Life Table. For many years, one of the most widely used guides for "ideal" weight was the Metropolitan Life Insurance Height and Weight Table. Indeed, the first two editions of this book used this table, with qualifiers. The table was revised in 1983 to show higher weights than the originals first used in 1959. For example, a 5-foot-10-inch male could weigh up to 172 pounds according to the 1959 table; this increased to 179 pounds in the 1983 table. These higher weights still fall below the average weights of the general population. What does this mean? The tables simply reflect the fact that Americans are growing heavier. Worse, they imply that it's okay!

Remember, too, that these height-weight mortality charts are based on what people who have the lowest mortality rates actually weigh, not what we should weigh to increase longevity. They do serve, however, as a general guide.

Once you have estimated whether you are small, medium, or large boned (see Figure 41.1), then simply find your height and ideal weight on the Metropolitan Life table (Figure 41.2, page 673). Okay, I'll take the medium frame, which means I can go up

FIGURE 41.1: HOW TO DETERMINE YOUR BODY FRAME BY ELBOW BREADTH

To make a simple approximation of your frame size:

Extend your arm and bend the forearm upwards at a 90° angle. Keep the fingers straight and turn the inside of your wrist away from the body. Place the thumb and index finger of your other hand on the two prominent bones on *either side* of your elbow. Measure the space between your fingers against a ruler or a tape measure.* Compare the measurements on the following tables.

These tables list the elbow measurements for medium-framed men and women of various heights. Measurements lower than those listed indicate you have a small frame and higher measurements indicate a large frame.

MEN

HEIGHT IN 1" HEELS	ELBOW BREADTH
5'2"–5'3"	2½"–2⅞"
5'4"–5'7"	2⅝"–2⅞"
5'8"–5'11"	2¾"–3"
6'0"–6'3"	2¾"–3⅛"
6'4"	2⅞"–3¼"

WOMEN

HEIGHT IN 1" HEELS	ELBOW BREADTH
4'10"–4'11"	2¼"–2½"
5'0"–5'3"	2¼"–2½"
5'4"–5'7"	2⅜"–2⅝"
5'8"–5'11"	2⅜"–2⅝"
6'0"	2½"–2¾"

* For the most accurate measurement, have your physician measure your elbow breadth with a caliper.

to 174 pounds. Many professional health organizations have refused to accept the heavier weights and so the 1959 table is still widely used.

Body Mass Index

The recommended guide for many health experts is the body mass index (BMI). This is a standard derived from height and weight measurements. Medical research shows that men and women do not differ significantly in terms of healthy weight-for-height ratios. Therefore, the BMI is an index of male and female weight in relation to height. It is determined by dividing your weight in kilograms by the square of your height in meters. You can use all sorts

FIGURE 41.2: 1983 METROPOLITAN HEIGHT AND WEIGHT TABLES

	MEN*					WOMEN†		
HEIGHT		SMALL	MEDIUM	LARGE	HEIGHT		SMALL	MEDIUM	LARGE
FEET	INCHES	FRAME	FRAME	FRAME	FEET	INCHES	FRAME	FRAME	FRAME
5	2	128–134	131–141	138–150	4	10	102–111	109–121	118–131
5	3	130–136	133–143	140–153	4	11	103–113	111–123	120–134
5	4	132–138	135–145	142–156	5	0	104–115	113–126	122–137
5	5	134–140	137–148	144–160	5	1	106–118	115–129	125–140
5	6	136–142	139–151	146–164	5	2	108–121	118–132	128–143
5	7	138–145	142–154	149–168	5	3	111–124	121–135	131–147
5	8	140–148	145–157	152–172	5	4	114–127	124–138	134–151
5	9	142–151	148–160	155–176	5	5	117–130	127–141	137–155
5	10	144–154	151–163	158–180	5	6	120–133	130–144	140–159
5	11	146–157	154–166	161–184	5	7	123–136	133–147	143–163
6	0	149–160	157–170	164–188	5	8	126–139	136–150	146–167
6	1	152–164	160–174	168–192	5	9	129–142	139–153	149–170
6	2	155–168	164–178	172–197	5	10	132–145	142–156	152–173
6	3	158–172	167–182	176–202	5	11	135–148	145–159	155–176
6	4	162–176	171–187	181–207	6	0	138–151	148–162	158–179

Weights at ages 25–59 based on lowest mortality. Weight in pounds according to frame (in indoor clothing weighing 5 lbs., shoes with 1" heels).

† Weights at ages 25–59 based on lower mortality. Weight in pounds according to frame (in indoor clothing weighing 3 lbs., shoes with 1" heels).

Source of basic data: 1979 Build Study, Society of Actuaries and Association of Life Insurance Medical Directors of America, 1980.

of formulas to calculate your BMI, but the formula below is probably the easiest method. Here's how to use it:

1. Weigh yourself without clothing and take your height.

2. To calculate your index, first divide your weight in pounds by your height in inches squared. Then multiply the result by the number 702.

Let's try this complicated formula on me. My height is 73 inches. To square that I multiply 73 × 73, which equals 5,329. My weight of 168 divided by 5,329 is .0315. I multiply .0315 times the number 702 and get my BMI of 22.13.

If you are male, your acceptable BMI weight category point on the BMI line should be approximately 22.7. (Hooray! I'm slightly under.) If you are female, your acceptable weight category should be approximately 22.4.

A good goal would be to score within 10 percent above or below these BMI target numbers. Studies have demonstrated that mortality increases significantly above a BMI of 25. According to the federal government's Dietary Guidelines for Americans, a BMI of 25 should be considered as the upper boundary of healthy weight. They suggest that a BMI of less than 19 may be unhealthy.

U.S. Government Guidelines

In 1990, the Department of Agriculture and the Department of Health and Human Services published a new weight table, based on the BMI. But they grouped men and women together and divided their table only by age: nineteen- to thirty-four-year-olds in one column; thirty-five years and older in the other. The government stated that their research indicated that individuals can be a little heavier as they age without increased risk to their health. This position met with mixed reactions: Those who were gaining weight as they aged (and were less active) were delighted; most nutrition and fitness experts criticized the guidelines for being too generous in the weight levels allowed.

Researchers took aim at the government position. Several studies refuted that position, including the one at Harvard University mentioned previously. This study revealed, for example, that women who gained as few as eleven pounds after age 18 had a 25 percent higher chance of developing heart disease than women who gained less as they grew older. As part of their Dietary Guidelines for Americans published in 1995, the government altered its position.

According to William Dietz, M.D., a member of the committee that formulated the guidelines, "There are now abundant data showing that no matter where you are in the life cycle, as weight goes up, so does the incidence of high blood pressure, diabetes, pulmonary problems, increased LDL cholesterol levels and decreased HDL cholesterol levels—all of which are associated with premature disability and death. The studies that confirm this finding are very large, often including thousands of people or more." The revised healthy weight chart eliminated the weight column for ages thirty-five and over and instead used the column that previously was for ages nineteen to thirty-four for all Americans of any age.

The healthy weight range chart (see Figure 41.3) is accompanied by the following statement:

"See where your weight falls on the chart for people for your height. The chart applies for men and women of all ages. The health risks due to excess weight appear to be the same for older adults as for younger adults. Weight ranges are given in the chart because people of the same height may have equal amounts of body fat but different amounts of muscle and bone. However, the ranges do not mean that it is healthy to gain weight, even within the same weight range. The higher weights in the healthiest weight range apply to people with more muscle and bone. Weights above this range are less healthy for most people. The further you are above the healthy weight range for your height, the higher your weight-related risk. Weights slightly below the range may be healthy for some people but are sometimes the result of health problems, especially when weight loss is unintentional."

So What Should You Weigh?

Confused? Amused? Frustrated? Let's sum up these tests and guidelines. I passed the nude jump test, and the pinch test. My weight at ages eighteen to twenty-five was around 160 pounds. The math formula put me at 164 pounds. According to the Met Life table my desirable weight range is 160 to 174 pounds. The government range is 144 to 189. As this book goes off to our friends at Penguin, I tip the scales at 168 pounds—down from 181 when I started it. So am I the right weight for me? What about you?

You can follow whatever guidelines you want. You know the truth about yourself if you are honest and face the facts. So pick your ideal weight. For me that is 165 pounds. I suggest that it is all right to go up to 10 percent above or below your target weight figure as long as you look and feel good and are in good health. This would give me a range from 149 pounds to 181. At the peak of my competitive marathon training I weighed 152 pounds. I was lean and mean, but also felt that any more weight loss would result in injury and illness. At the peak of my stressful out-of-shape and middle-aged life I weighed 181 pounds. I was starting to feel too heavy and not healthy. I was definitely getting too flabby (at least my wife told me so!).

Besides being concerned about being overweight, we also need to consider being overfat. A 6-foot-1-inch professional football player weighing 210 pounds would be overweight by any

FIGURE 41.3: HEALTHY WEIGHT RANGES FOR MEN AND WOMEN

HEIGHT*	WEIGHT (IN POUNDS)†
4'10"	91–119
4'11"	94–124
5'0"	97–128
5'1"	101–132
5'2"	104–137
5'3"	107–141
5'4"	111–146
5'5"	114–150
5'6"	118–155
5'7"	121–160
5'8"	125–164
5'9"	129–169
5'10"	132–174
5'11"	136–179
6'0"	140–184
6'1"	144–189
6'2"	148–195
6'3"	152–200
6'4"	156–205
6'5"	160–211
6'6"	164–216

* *Without shoes*   † *Without clothes*

Source: Derived from National Research Council, 1989, for adults.

of the measurements above. But his body fat percentage due to intense physical training could be lower than a skinny 168-pounder like me.

Body Composition: Fat vs. Muscle

One thing the charts and tables do not tell us is how much of our weight is in muscle or fat. Did you know that you can maintain or even gain weight and yet lose inches from your body? That's because muscle weighs more than fat but takes up less space. This is why some people trying to lose weight will see the inches decrease from, say, their waist before the scales show any weight loss. The objective of any weight-reduction program is to lose body fat while maintaining lean body mass (bone and muscle). Most research shows starvation and low-calorie diets result in large losses of water, electrolytes, and other components of lean body mass.

But there is minimal loss of fat. Without fat loss, weight loss is temporary and, as we will see, potentially dangerous.

Body composition refers to the percentage of body weight that is fat and is called your body fat percentage. It is determined by dividing your total body weight by the weight of your fat. Body composition can be measured in many ways. The most accurate assessment of body fat percentage is hydrostatic (underwater) weighing done by scientists in a laboratory. Skinfold tests measure fat under the skin using calipers; this may be almost as accurate as hydrostatic weighing. You can usually have one of these assessments done at your local fitness club or YMCA. High-tech fitness clubs may also offer computerized machines, sometimes called bioelectrical impedance, that send minute electrical currents through your body to determine your body fat percentage. Or, you can just save the money and do the nude jump test.

Why would we want to know about our body fat percentage? Body weight and body fat are closely linked. David Costill, Ph.D., director of the Human Performance Laboratory at Ball State University, has found that each pound of fat added or lost can result in an increase or decrease of body fat percentage by as much as half a percent. Some people may weigh within the standard ranges but have a high percentage of body fat. They are of standard weight but overfat. On the other side, some people, such as professional football players, weigh above the standard range for people their size, but because of their rigorous training program they have body fat percentages far below average. Their bulk is in muscle, not fat.

A person 5 feet 10 inches tall who weighs 150 pounds carries about 90 of those pounds as water and 30 as fat. The lean tissues (muscles, and with internal organs like the heart and liver, and the bones of the skeleton) comprise about 30 pounds. But this lean tissue and its water are vital to good health. To lose weight, you want to lose fat, not this critical lean tissue. To gain weight, you want to gain lean tissue and fat in proportion, not just fat. Normally, the ratio of weight gain or loss is approximately 75 percent fat and 25 percent lean tissue.

Average body fat is 15 to 20 percent for 30-year-old men and 23 to 26 percent for women. Elite distance runners will have a body fat percentage as low at 4 to 8 percent for men and 8 to 15 percent for women. Men with a body fat percent above 25 and women above 35 are generally considered overfat (obese). Women in general have more fat, and therefore a higher body fat percentage, than men. They store essential fat in their hips, thighs, and breasts, which is Mother Nature's way of providing a readily available source of nourishment for a fetus when a woman becomes pregnant. Fat isn't all bad. In fact, it performs a variety of important functions in the body and in the diet. Body fat supports and cushions vital body organs, is an essential structural component of cell walls and nerve fibers, helps make hormones and healthy skin, and insulates the body from the environment. Stored fats in the body are an important source of energy. As much as 70 percent of our energy at rest comes from fat, and during easy fitness running approximately half of our energy comes from fat. Most people think the less fat you have on your body and in your diet the better. This is only true to a point. All of us need a certain amount of fat for our bodies to function normally. For men, essential fat is 3 to 5 percent; for women, it's 11 to 13 percent.

Ideal Weight vs. Performance Weight

Ideal weight and the weight that is best for athletic performance may not always be the same. Competitive long-distance runners may be 10 to 20 percent below these recommended weight levels. They need a light chassis and a strong engine to run like the wind. If you move into competitive running, it may be fine to lower your weight somewhat to improve your performance. I once competed at below 160 pounds and was strong, healthy, and fast. As a masters competitor with less time to train, I need to stay below 170 pounds to be competitive.

In general, for every 1 percent reduction in total body weight, there is a 1 percent increase in running speed capacity. A 10-pound weight loss, for example, may result in an improvement of 2 or 3 minutes in your time for a 10K race, or approximately 30 seconds per mile in your comfortable training pace.

You still need proper nutrition and a certain amount of body fat in order to be healthy and to perform well. According to Dr. Edward Colt, an endocrinologist at New York City's St. Luke's Hospital, "The lighter you are, within certain limits, the less likely you are to become injured. The limits are set by your own constitution—each individual has an optimum weight below which he or she feels tired and becomes susceptible to infections." None of us should place too much value on thinness and loss of weight while sacrificing health and strength.

You Can Be Too Thin, Too

On any given day, about half of all American women and 25 percent of the men are on diets to lose weight. Most, but not all, of them need to diet. Many aspire to a weight and figure that is probably unrealistic for them. The pressure to be thin—to look good at all costs—is loose upon the land. In addition to the problems of being overweight, the drive to be thin also carries serious psychological and health costs. In a *Family Circle* magazine poll, 75 percent of the women said they diet to feel better about themselves. Almost nine out of ten American women who think they are overweight refuse to wear a bathing suit, half avoid pants and shorts, and 24 percent avoid sex. "The aesthetic ideal is unrealistically slim," says obesity researcher Kelly Brownell of the University of Pennsylvania. "People aspire to a body shape and size that is beyond where they need to be healthy."

One of the ways our obsession with being thin manifests itself is in eating disorders. Although many nonexercisers have eating disorders, athletes are at risk, too. Nancy Clark, the sports nutrition specialist, reports that one-third of women athletes in college have some sort of eating disorder, either anorexia (self-induced starvation) or bulimia (binge eating, followed by self-induced vomiting), laxative abuse, crash diets, or other unhealthy practices. The American College of Sports Medicine reports that as many as 62 percent of women competing in endurance sports suffer from some sort of eating disorder. Some men are similarly affected. Half of all dieters—and these are largely women—admit to having abnormal eating habits, being obsessed with food, or abusing food and exercise. Food for them is not fuel.

Gaining Weight

In some sports, such as hockey and football, a few extra pounds come in handy. Sometimes, runners and other exercisers get sick, or have surgery, or for other reasons lose weight and need to regain it. Athletes who are underweight may not have enough energy to work at their peak. Other athletes may have difficulty maintaining their weight. We've talked about taking it off. How about putting it on?

Piece of cake, you say. Sure. To gain weight, you have to eat more calories than your body burns. But gaining weight may not be easy; some athletes burn everything they eat, and more. To put it back, you simply have to add about 500 to 1,000 calories extra

every day. That should give you a weight gain of about 2 pounds
a week. How?

- Eat larger portions at every meal.

- Eat more often each day. Maybe increase the number of meals
from three to four.

- Snack between those meals, and before bed.

You should also increase the calories in the foods you eat. Be
sure to make those calories rich in nutrients, not the hollow calories found in junk foods and fatty foods.

To put on muscle, instead of fat, you still need to combine increased calories with exercise. Heavy muscular workouts, like
strength training, will stimulate muscle growth.

Calories, Exercise, and Weight Loss

That brings us to the terrible word no one who fails the nude
jumping test wants to hear: calories.

Our cells obtain and use nutrients through the body's three-step
process of digestion, absorption, and metabolism. Basically, the
foods we eat are broken down in the body to simpler forms, taken
through the intestinal walls and transported by the blood to the
cells. As mentioned earlier, our bodies require six nutrients: carbohydrates, fats, proteins, water, minerals, and vitamins. Carbohydrates, fats, and proteins are the three energy nutrients. All three
contain calories; water, minerals, and vitamins do not. Calories in
the form of fat build up easily. A gram of fat contains 9 calories,
whereas a gram of protein or carbohydrates contains 4 calories.
Thus, a diet that is high in carbohydrates and low in fat will be
less likely to contribute to excess weight. But even if you eat mostly
carbohydrates, too much food intake will still result in too many
calories and in excess pounds. Liz Applegate, Ph.D., wrote in her
Runner's World column,

Think of your body-fat level the same as you would your
checking account. Each time you eat (receive a paycheck), you
process food energy from protein, carbohydrate and fat. Then
you either burn it immediately as an energy source (spend the

paycheck) or store it for future use as body fat or glycogen (save the paycheck).

The catch is, not all fuel sources are burned or stored with the same efficiency.

Dietary protein mostly goes toward maintaining body protein in the muscles and elsewhere. The leftover gets burned for immediate energy with a tiny excess converted to fat and tucked away in fat cells.

Dietary carbohydrate gets used as an immediate energy source for the brain and muscles. That's because carbohydrate is such an efficient energy source. Most of the carbohydrate you don't immediately use goes toward replenishing spent glycogen stores in the liver and muscles. This leaves little carbohydrate to be converted to fat. And the conversion to fat is a relatively inefficient process.

When eaten, fat normally heads straight to fat cells for storage. And you guessed it, the conversion of dietary fat to body fat is extremely efficient—with hardly a calorie wasted. Returning to the bank-account analogy, it's as if a portion of your paycheck is earmarked for long-term savings before you have a chance to spend it.

Food intake is measured in kilocalories, more widely known simply as calories. A calorie is the amount of heat required to raise the temperature of one gram of water one degree centigrade. A pound of body fat stores about 3,500 calories. To lose that pound, you must take in 3,500 calories less than you use; to gain it, you must take in 3,500 calories more than you use. In general, a deficit or excess of 500 calories a day brings about a weight loss or gain, respectively, at the rate of one pound a week; a deficit or excess of 1,000 calories a day, 2 pounds a week.

The normal caloric intake is 18 calories per pound per day for men, and 16 for women. This differs from what your body needs, which is approximately 13 calories for each pound of body weight. This figure will vary according to your body composition, types of food you eat, and activity level. A recommended standard for calories required each day for a *moderately active* adult can be estimated by multiplying the adult's ideal body weight by 15. Most Americans consume far too many calories.

Three things contribute to burning off calories. First is your resting metabolic rate. Most of us burn off 60 to 75 percent of our total daily calories by breathing, thinking, maintaining body temperature, and pumping blood through our bodies. The speed of your metabolic rate depends on your body composition, and the more muscle you have the faster your metabolic rate. These rates drop as men and women age, partly due to loss of muscle mass. Women have less muscle than men of comparable size and activity level and thus have metabolic rates about 10 percent lower.

Second, calories are burned by physical activity that accounts for 15 to 35 percent of total calorie burning. This may be walking, running, working at your desk, mopping the floor, and such. Figure 41.4 shows the number of calories burned for 30 minutes of various daily activities and types of exercise. As you can see, watching TV doesn't burn off the calories you add if you eat while watching! Another warning: One high-fat dessert will eliminate the benefits of a 30-minute workout.

Running and other forms of vigorous physical activity not only boost calorie burning during exercise, but it also continues that calorie consumption afterward. Liz Applegate, the *Runner's World* columnist, says: "For up to 24 hours after a workout, your resting metabolic rate is faster than normal, burning anywhere from 50 to a few hundred more calories than usual. While this may not sound like much, it adds up. In the end, exercise afterburn could save you the equivalent of 2 to 5 pounds of fat over several months."

Third, and least significant, is the energy your body burns processing what you have eaten. This represents no more than 10 to 15 percent of total calories burned per day. But this thermic effect of food (TEF) can be significant over a period of time. A lower than normal TEF can contribute to weight gain.

Metabolism slows with aging. Thus, we need fewer calories as we grow older. A seventy-year-old generally needs 10 to 15 percent fewer calories than a twenty-year-old. Although regular exercise can boost the metabolic rate, most older Americans don't exercise enough. National Research Council data show that men and women over age fifty expend on the average 200 to 600 fewer calories per day than when they were younger. Most older Americans take in more calories as they age. For these reasons we need more, not less, exercise as we grow older.

Research by Dr. Ralph Nelson of the Mayo Clinic shows that a 154-pound man at age thirty who maintains a constant exercise level and eats the same amount will weigh more than 200 pounds by age sixty. To maintain that weight on the same amount of ex-

FIGURE 41.4: APPROXIMATE CALORIES BURNED FOR A 150-POUND PERSON PER 30 MINUTES

DAILY ACTIVITIES

Sleeping	35
Watching TV	35
Eating	50
Office work	90
Slow walking	100
Yardwork, housework	120

SPORTS AND RECREATION

Bowling	95
Softball	130
Calisthenics	150
Golf (walking)	170
Skating	175
Free weights	175
Brisk walking	200
Biking	200–300
Aerobic dance	210–270
Tennis (singles)	220–300
Lap swimming	220–300
Soccer	270
Basketball (brisk)	275–375
Slow running	325
Cross-country skiing	350–500
Brisk running	425

ercise, this man would have to reduce his caloric intake by 11 percent over the same period. Despite needing fewer calories as we age, your body still requires all the essential vitamins and minerals for good health. Those should not be cut back; they have no calories. As we age and face the calorie game, therefore, we have four choices:

1. Keep the exercise level constant and reduce caloric intake to maintain weight levels;

2. Keep the caloric intake constant and increase the number of calories burned with exercise to maintain a proper weight;

FIGURE 41.5: APPROXIMATE CALORIES EXPENDED PER 30-MINUTE RUN

WEIGHT (POUNDS)	PACE (MINUTE PER MILE)					
	11½	10	9	8	7	6
100	190	245	265	295	350	400
110	205	260	290	325	365	415
120	225	290	315	350	390	450
130	240	305	340	375	415	470
140	260	340	370	400	440	490
150	275	360	390	420	470	520
160	295	385	420	450	495	545
170	315	405	450	480	520	570
180	335	425	470	505	545	595
190	350	455	500	530	570	625
200	370	485	530	560	600	650

3. Combine the above (my recommended step) by cutting back somewhat on your caloric intake and increasing somewhat your exercise level to maintain a proper weight;

4. Keep your exercise level constant (or decrease it) and keep your caloric intake constant (or decrease it) and gain weight. This certainly is not my recommended step. I do not agree with all those charts that allow us to gain weight as we age. They are based on what average Americans do, not on what they should do.

Running and Calories

Running burns about 100 calories per mile depending on your weight and the intensity of your workout. At my weight of 168 pounds, I burn about 120 calories per mile at my brisk, but not too fast, training pace of about 7½ minutes per mile; I cover about 4 miles in 30 minutes. To lose one pound a week—a recommended goal—I would have to run about 30 miles per week while holding my caloric intake constant. The more you weigh and the faster you run, the more calories you will burn per minute. Figure 41.5 lists the number of calories you can burn by running at various paces for a 30-minute run. Remember to run at your "talk test" pace unless you are doing some speed training for racing.

What if I walk those 4 miles instead of run them? Running burns more calories than walking because the faster anyone covers a distance, the more calories are burned. I could burn more calories by running 4 miles at a 6-minute-per-mile pace than at 8 minutes per mile. Walking 15 minutes per mile would burn less. Not only that, running also creates more of an "afterburn." Studies at the School of Physical Education at the University of Victoria, British Columbia, for example, show that you continue to burn calories after stopping exercise and that the longer you exercise vigorously the longer your metabolism stays fast, burning those calories. Obviously, it is more valuable to exercise longer if your goal is to lose weight. Running 4 miles at a brisk pace will result in 20 to 25 percent more calories burned than walking, due to the combined effect of higher intensity and increased "afterburn."

But what about the "fat-burning zone" theory that has been promoted quite heavily? The idea is that slower-paced, lower-intensity exercise such as moderate-paced walking and very slow running is better for burning fat and losing weight than faster-paced, higher-intensity exercise. According to the theory, the fat-burning zone is between 50 and 60 percent of your maximum heart rate (MHR). Research at the University of Texas indeed found fat provides 90 percent of the calories burned when exercising at only 50 percent of your maximum heart rate. At 75 percent of your MHR only 60 percent of calories burned come from fat as your body switches to burning additional carbohydrates as you run faster.

Should you run slower in order to burn off more fat? According to the Texas study, running at the higher intensity, but still at a conversational pace, actually resulted in more fat calories burned. Why? The 50 percent intensity workout burned only 7 calories per minute while the 75 percent intensity workout burned twice that number. Further, researchers at Laval University in Quebec City, Canada, found that intense exercise resulted in a nine times greater loss of body fat, per calorie burned, than low-intensity exercise. Still, you will gain some valuable weight-loss benefits if you exercise at a slow to moderate pace rather than doing no exercise at all.

Some long-distance runners burn calories at the rate of 1,000 an hour, and they often eat more than their less active friends but weigh less. Dr. Peter Wood's study at Stanford Medical School indicates that people who run 6 or more miles every day eat about 600 calories more daily than nonexercising people. But they weigh

20 percent less! This holds true only for very active runners. You cannot jog around the block and then pig out on cake and ice cream. As all of us know, it is far easier to feed calories to the body than to burn them up. But it is important to emphasize that if you exercise you need a sufficient amount of calories in your diet to meet your energy needs. Those calories should come from a well-balanced diet high in carbohydrates and low in fat.

Dieting

Some 50 million Americans are dieting on any given day. Doctors believe that many of those dieters are not above a healthy weight and don't need to diet. Government studies show that only 25 to 30 percent of American women who are dieting are actually overweight. On the other hand, most of the men and women who do need to diet, don't. The National Center for Health Statistics studied America's fixation on dieting and concluded: "Weight reduction through caloric restricted dieting . . . which has associated expenditures estimated at $30 billion to $50 billion annually . . . ultimately is not very effective." Most diets fail. Why?

According to Dr. Kenneth Cooper, head of the Cooper Aerobics Institute for Aerobics Research in Dallas, "Any successful weight-loss program must include a whole lifestyle modification. If you don't have an exercise program, it won't be successful. It's estimated that 87 percent of people who lose weight with a fasting-type program will gain the weight back in two years. Low-calorie, quick-weight-loss programs do not work." It seems that most restrictive-calorie weight-loss programs are at best useless and at worst harmful.

Studies suggest, but others disagree, that losing weight on a low-calorie diet lowers the rate at which people burn calories, which makes regaining weight easy when they go off these diets, even if they don't overeat. Moreover, when people lose and regain weight, changes occur in the amount and distribution of their body fat. In the weight-loss phase of a low-calorie diet, a person loses both fat and lean muscle tissue. But when weight is regained, it is almost all fat. Worse, that fat tends to settle in the abdomen, a condition (as we have discussed) linked by medical studies to increased death rate as well as a raised risk of heart disease.

You should try to lose weight and hold that weight at the right level. You should not continue to lose weight until you are emaciated and in poor health. Nor should you lose weight, regain it, lose weight, and regain it—what some call "yo-yo dieting." Medical studies show that it may be equally harmful to lose the same 25 pounds over and over again as to lose 50 pounds and gain it back once.

"For the majority of individuals, diets clearly do not work," says John Foreyt, Ph.D., director of the Nutrition Research Clinic at the Baylor College of Medicine in Houston. "The goal, rather, is healthy eating and exercise." He suggests, and we agree, that most people will lose weight and keep it off if they exercise regularly and switch from their present diet to one patterned after the Food Guide Pyramid discussed in Chapter 18. Dr. Wayne Calloway, an endocrinologist and member of the Dietary Guidelines Advisory Committee of the USDA, agrees: "The emphasis should be on eating a healthful diet with an adequate amount of energy; then you plug in some type of exercise, whether it's building it into your daily activities or creating a formal exercise program."

A dramatic example of the wrong way and the right way to lose weight while dieting is contained in the story of one high-powered businesswoman. She made nationwide news by losing a large amount of weight following a low-calorie diet and then allowing the weight to creep back on until she peaked at 222 pounds. She was a yo-yo dieter and her efforts at controlling her weight failed. Worse, millions of television viewers had witnessed it.

She hired exercise physiologist Bob Greene to supervise a personal program. He started her off with healthy eating combined with running and weight training. Eight months later, she was under 150 pounds and training for her first marathon. She increased her running to 50 miles a week and completed the 1994 Marine Corps Marathon in Washington, D.C., without having to walk a step. Greene told *Runner's World*: "I like to think [that] her progress and her commitment will show millions of other people that they can improve their lives, too. Maybe they won't run a marathon. But they can run a 5K. Or they can lose the weight they've been wanting to get rid of. It's just so inspiring to watch someone transform herself, and that's what Oprah has done. She's a runner now for life."

If Oprah Winfrey can go from 222 pounds to the marathon finish line, why can't you?

Ten Tips for Healthful Weight Loss

Here are ten tips for a healthful weight loss:

1. Exercise. Three to six aerobic sessions per week consisting of at least 30 minutes of continuous, vigorous exercise within your training heart range will maximize weight loss. Running is a high-energy continuous burn-off. You burn approximately 100 calories per mile of running: 10 miles per week equals about 1,000 calories expended; 20 miles per week expends about 2,000 calories—a level associated with a much-reduced risk of heart disease.

If you are overweight, it may be wise to start with a walking program until some excess weight is lost.

Notice that Oprah combined her exercise program with weight training. Why? An effective weight-loss program should include two or three strength training sessions per week to increase muscle mass. Muscle is metabolically more active than fat: one pound of fat burns 2 calories a day to maintain itself while at rest; but one pound of lean body mass burns 30 to 50 calories a day. Weight training will help maintain muscle mass and help keep your weight under control. A recommended exercise program includes both aerobic exercise and strength training to reduce fat and increase muscle mass.

In contrast to widely held belief, exercise does not stimulate appetite. In fact, studies show that exercise will continue to suppress appetite long after you have stopped exercising.

2. Lose weight gradually. If you lose weight too rapidly it affects your body's metabolism. This may be a health risk and it may increase the likelihood that any weight lost will not only come back, but that you will also gain additional weight. A loss of no more than one-half to 2 pounds per week will help ensure that the loss is coming from body fat rather than lean muscle tissue.

3. Never consume too few calories. Men should eat at least 1,500 calories per day; women, 1,200. Below these levels, most dieters lose lean tissue and are hard-pressed to achieve adequate vitamin and mineral intake. Besides, if you get too hungry you'll be too tempted to give up. As I've said several times, restrictive calorie diets are dangerous and ineffective in the long run. You'll need more calories than these minimums if you exercise.

4. Control your negative caloric balance. The American College of Sports Medicine recommends a negative caloric balance of up to 500 to 1,000 calories a day—that is, to eat fewer calories than you burn by exercising. A suggested means of accomplishing this goal is to consume 250 to 500 calories less per day while burning off 250 to 500 calories more each day with exercise. A net loss of 500 calories per day over the course of one week is 3,500 calories, which equals one pound.

On the other hand, that formula can work the other way, too, which is how we gain weight. Err by a few calories each day on the wrong side of this balance and you will pay for it over time. For example, an excess of merely 30 calories a day will add up to 10 pounds of excess weight over three years or so. And this is exactly how many of us gradually but steadily become overweight. It creeps up on us.

5. Choose the right parents. Studies show that genetics may play a significant role in determining body weight. Take a look at the body types of your family members. Some of us are born to outweigh all those recommended ranges. This, however, is not an excuse to avoid losing weight or to not exercise. On the contrary, if you are among the "genetically challenged," get out there and exercise! You gonna let a little gene defeat you? But be realistic about your expectations if sleek bodies don't run in your family.

6. Consider professional help. Losing weight is difficult for most people. We do need to be more understanding of those who are overweight. The support of a trained professional can help you reach your goals safely. This may be a sports nutritionist, sports doctor, sports psychologist, fitness trainer, running coach, or a combination of experts.

7. Be consistent, patient, and disciplined. To succeed, you don't have to be perfect. You don't have to diet every day. Just try to be as consistent as possible by exercising and eating right. Set a reasonable goal, like 5 to 10 pounds off in two or three months. Remember, it took a long time to put it on; take your time in getting it off—but get it off!

8. Eat the right foods. Fats have more than twice as many calories per gram as carbohydrates and proteins. Switch to low-fat or nonfat dairy products, choose lean cuts of meat, skinless poultry, and lean fish. Fill up on vegetables and fresh fruits. Emphasize high-energy carbohydrates. Beware of snacks and desserts that are sold as low in fat; those fats are often replaced with sugar, which results in a low-fat but high-calorie cookie or snack. Switch to low-calorie items—water instead of soda, an apple or vegetable sticks (celery, carrots) instead of a candy bar. Cut out desserts and high-calorie, high-sodium snacks. Bavarian Chocolate Cake? *Out!* Chips? *Out!*

But do not reduce your fluid intake. No one loses weight permanently from sweating. You need to replace lost body fluids. But not with alcohol, which is high in calories.

9. Keep a nutrition log. Write down what you eat every day and analyze it to figure out your total fat, carbohydrate, protein, and calorie intake. To make it easier, try one of the nutrition software packages available for your computer. Periodically track your food intake for a few days. It may shock you. You may wish to have your diet analyzed by a sports nutritionist.

10. Change your eating habits. Learn to eat more slowly. Enjoy your meals and food. Try putting your fork down on the plate between bites. Eat until you feel comfortable, not until you are stuffed. Pass up those desserts. Do not do another activity while eating, such as reading or watching television. You will associate the two, and every time you read the paper or watch TV you will want to eat.

Keep those evening meals light, especially if you get home late from work or if you, like Shepherd, run late at night but before dinner. Nancy Clark, the dietician at Boston's Sports Medicine/ Brookline, warns: "Many runners diet at breakfast and lunch, drag themselves through a midday workout, are famished at dinner and eat everything in sight. They end up gaining weight."

Taking weight off should be done with a careful combination of dieting and exercise. Then, using the charts and suggestions in this chapter, maintain your best running weight with the combination of exercise and a healthy diet. You'll soon find that you've become a lean, mean running machine!

FORTY-TWO

Running Inside Your Head

"For every runner who tours the world running marathons," said Dr. George Sheehan, the late cardiologist, long-distance runner, and philosopher, "there are thousands who run to hear the leaves and listen to rain and look to the day when it all is suddenly as easy as a bird in flight. For them, sport is not a test but a therapy, not a trial but a reward, not a question but an answer."

John Donahue is over fifty years old, and works for a contractor in Rochester, New York. He runs 5 miles almost every day. Like a lot of other runners who have gotten into shape and run regularly, Donahue began running to lose weight. Now he continues because running gives him psychological benefits as well: "After about 35 or 40 minutes, it seems as if all sorts of tensions are relieved. It's almost like floating. . . . I am more mentally alert after I run. Things are more noticeable, clearer—imagine lots of cobwebs that you have just cleared away. Problems can be sorted out a lot easier."

Dick Traum is the New York businessman who runs using an artificial leg: "I really enjoy the opportunity to organize my thoughts away from business interruptions. Sometimes I just 'tune out' for hours and release tension. It takes about half an hour to completely unwind, at which time I feel very high, as if I were running without any effort whatsoever."

Mary Beth Byrne, a financial librarian in New York City, sorts through her attitudes toward her job on the run: "Running helped me find more satisfaction in my work. It gave me courage and strength to make several major decisions in my life.

"Running allows me to think of positive things, and to solve problems. I can think things through on the run and later I can make a better decision. Sometimes I just go blank. I get great freedom—sometimes just looking at the trees and scenery, and not thinking about anything at all. It has been a very personal thing for me, allowing me to be more optimistic. The act of running combines body and mind in a way that is very satisfying."

Dr. Sheehan spoke of a "third wind" and a "peak experience" when he was "completely at peace with things" while running. "At two minutes over my race pace," he wrote, "my body is virtuoso. It requires no guidance, no commands, no spur. It is on automatic pilot. My mind is free to dissociate, to wander on its own. On some days, this brings on another type of high—a creative one. My mind becomes a cascade of thoughts. The sights and sounds, the touches and tastes, the pains and pleasures of my entire life become available to me."

Runner's World's Joe Henderson calls the experience "meditation on the move." Others term it "attentiveness training," which keeps you focused on the present, just as meditation does. If you are running more than 5 miles a day, more than four days a week, you may have experienced it: the flow of movement, the second wind, the creativity, the euphoria, the "third wind," and even a meditative high. Dr. Sheehan called running at this level "the opening of the creative side of your brain." It doesn't always happen, but when it does, he said, "I seem to see the way things really are. I am in the Kingdom."

Scientists for decades observed that physically active men and women seemed less depressed and anxious than inactive people. Since the beginning of the current "running boom" in the mid-1970s, psychologists and medical researchers have corroborated what runners were saying all along: Exercise makes us feel good. More than 1,000 research studies have investigated whether exercise actually results in measurable improvements in depression, anxiety, intelligence, self-esteem, decision making, and other psychological issues. The answer is a strong "Yes!"—but no one knows exactly why.

"I would like to suggest," says William Morgan, Ph.D., past president of the American Psychological Association's Division of Exercise and Sport Psychology, "that running should be viewed as a wonder drug, analogous to penicillin, morphine and the tricyclics. It has a profound potential in preventing mental and physical disease and in rehabilitation after various diseases have occurred." Dr. Tom Stephens directed the evaluation of data from four national surveys of runners in Canada and the United States. "The inescapable conclusion," he told *Women's Sports & Fitness*, "is that physical activity is positively associated with good mental health, especially positive mood, general well-being, and less anxiety and depression."

Most runners agree with this conclusion. For example, a survey of 424 runners in Columbia, Missouri, by the University of Missouri's K. E. Callen and reported in the journal *Psychosomatics*, indicated that 86 percent of the runners believed that running relieved tension, 75 percent had a better self-image, 75 percent felt more relaxed, 66 percent were in a better mood as a result of running, and 64 percent were more confident. Anywhere from 53 to 58 percent also felt better, more alert, less depressed, more content, and could think more clearly.

The International Society of Sports Psychology (ISSP) reported in a position statement ("Physical Activity and Psychological Benefits"):

> Individual psychological benefits of physical activity include positive changes in self-perceptions and well-being, improvement in self-confidence and awareness, positive changes in mood, relief of tension, relief of feelings such as depression and anxiety, influence on premenstrual tension, increased mental well-being, increased alertness and clear thinking, increased enjoyment of exercise and social contacts, and development of positive coping strategies.

The ISSP paper recommends that "although 20 to 30 minutes of exercise may be sufficient for stress reduction, 60 minutes may result in even more psychological benefit."

Depression and Anxiety

As many as one out of four Americans suffer from mild to moderate depression, anxiety, and other emotional disorders. Many of them might benefit from vigorous exercise. *Runner's World* noted that "depression is the single most definitive personality factor that distinguishes physically active from sedentary middle-aged American men."

One of the first pilot studies comparing the effectiveness of exercise and psychotherapy was conducted by Dr. John Greist and his colleagues at the University of Wisconsin. Greist and company studied the effects of running on clinically depressed patients. During a ten-week program for eight patients, six found relief from depression by walking or running two to seven times a week, both alone and in groups. Most recovered from their depression, Dr. Greist reported, within three weeks of running, and maintained the recovery. After a year, "most patients who were treated with running have become regular runners and remain symptom-free," Dr. Greist noted. When he later expanded his research, the recovery rate for depressed patients who ran was 80 percent. In his analysis of the Greist studies, Keith W. Johnsgard, Ph.D., a psychotherapist and professor of psychology at San Jose State University in California, concluded: "Exercise therapy not only guarantees immediate postsession mood elevation, but, practiced regularly, also helps most clinically depressed individuals become symptom-free within three to five weeks. These are significant, indeed, nearly astounding, findings."

Today, scientific studies seem to tumble in from all corners of the continent:

- Duke University researchers found that adults who performed ten weeks of walking and running for 135 minutes a week had low levels of anxiety, depression, and fatigue and elevated vigor.

- Dr. George McGlynn of the University of San Francisco showed that exercising adults who ran for fourteen weeks at about 8 miles per week significantly decreased their levels of anxiety and depression compared to similar nonexercising adults.

- Dr. Herbert deVries, a physiologist in Los Angeles, tested patients suffering from severe anxiety and tension. One group was given tranquilizers. The others went on regular vigorous walks.

Dr. deVries found that those taking the 15-minute walks on a regular basis were calmer—that is, the exercise had a greater calming effect than the tranquilizers. In further studies, Dr. deVries reports that rhythmic exercises such as walking, running, cycling, and even bench stepping from 5 to 30 minutes will elicit a calming, tranquilizing effect.

Adults may benefit from exercise. But what about our children? The National Institute of Mental Health estimates that up to 1.5 million American kids suffer from depression. Here, too, the reports are good.

For example, Drs. James MacMahon and Ruth Gross investigated the effects of aerobic exercise on sixty-nine delinquent teenage males. For three months the young men either worked out in an aerobic program (running and basketball) or in a limited exercise program. The results: Tests showed that the aerobic group were happier, had greater improvement in self-esteem, and were less depressed. "We found that aerobic exercise may be more uplifting—physically and mentally—than previously thought," said Dr. MacMahon. "The average improvement was significant. By studying a group that was very prone to depression we were able to describe a phenomenon that is available to everyone, regardless of severity of depression."

Self-esteem

Clearly, running and other forms of vigorous exercise allow us to discover our bodies and our selves. Such exercise has an immediate and long-term effect on our self-esteem. According to research at the University of Rhode Island:

- Runners have developed a sense of success and mastery over a particular task and their environment. Establishing goals and then reaching them on a regular basis results in feeling of control over one's life—an important sense in a society that too often feels like it is controlling us.

- Runners find that they can change themselves for the better in terms of health, body image, self-confidence, and self-acceptance.

- A runner's sense of confidence flows into other areas where he or she also experiences success. I have known runners who after running their first nonstop mile or conquering the marathon have felt confident enough to take on significant business and personal challenges.

▪ Running is seen as a positive activity that replaces negative or neurotic behavior and habits.

Creative Thinking

A study at Baruch College in New York City substantiated what runners have known for decades: that along with the euphoria, runners may become more creative while running and are therefore better equipped to solve problems. "Running helps clear confusion," says Joan Gondola, Ph.D., the Baruch College researcher. "It can induce an alpha state, or a relaxed brain state. Your thoughts are thrown together randomly, and new ideas can emerge. You actually begin to process information differently, and it frees you up. By the time you finish your run, the answers seem to fall right into place." A study at the Sunflower Mental Health Center in Kansas found that 92 percent of all runners reported improved problem-solving abilities when running than when not running. A Purdue University study showed that improved decision-making skills in its subjects, who worked out for six months at a moderate pace, went up 70 percent.

Add memory enhancement to that list. A study directed by Kathleen Beckman Blomquist, Ph.D., at the University of Kentucky School of Nursing, placed middle-aged adults on an indoor bicycling program. Those who showed 15 percent or more improvement in their fitness levels also improved more on memory tests than a control group.

Another study, by Alan Hartley, Ph.D., at Scripps College in Claremont, California, reached similar results. The Scripps researchers followed 300 adults ages fifty-five to eighty-eight and found that those who exercised regularly had better memories than those who did not. The exercisers were also better able to reason and solve problems. Moreover, the higher the level of physical activity among those studied, the higher they ranked in cognitive ability.

The Runner's High

One group of runners and researchers thinks the whole concept of euphoria from running is nonsense. "There is no such thing as a runner's high," wrote Dr. David Levin, a marathoner and radiologist, in the *Journal of the American Medical Association*. "Anyone expecting a high or mystical experience during a run is headed for disappointment. I don't attain them, nor do the marathoners with whom I am acquainted." Is Dr. Levin just a spoilsport? He runs 60 miles a week, he claims, has completed at least seven marathons with a PR of 2:38.

Agreeing that not *all* runners experience euphoria, Dr. Sheehan offered an interesting explanation. "I suspect that dogged, determined, 60-mile-a-week marathoners are actually the last ones to ask about mystical experiences. For them, running is indeed tough, tedious, tiring, and often painful. But for those of us who do half that mileage, who train at two minutes over our race pace, who run to think, and reserve pain for the race—for us, the runner's high is an integral and essential part of our lives."

Indeed it may be. Callen's study noted that 69 percent of the 424 male and female runners surveyed experienced a "runner's high." This was described as a feeling of euphoria with a lifting of spirits, increased creativity and insight, and a sense of well-being. This feeling occurred more often in those who ran more than 20 miles a week and had been running for more than fifteen consecutive months. These feelings occurred about every other run on the average. Descriptions of an exercise high—other aerobic activity can promote this feeling and weight lifters have also described it—vary from person to person.

Some 56 percent of the surveyed runners experienced at times something more profound—a trance or altered state of consciousness during running. Long, slow aerobic running, writes Dr. Thaddeus Kostrubala, a San Diego psychiatrist, can "produce an altered state of consciousness. A non-ordinary avenue of perception does seem to open up." The experience is often dreamlike, but remembered by the runner and there to be considered, and sought again.

Dr. Kostrubala, author of *The Joy of Running*, is very clear about what he thinks we runners are experiencing. "The slow long-distance runner experiences a part of his unconscious." His or her running achieves

an altered state of consciousness that can be called a kind of Western meditation. . . . It's a distinct euphoria with feelings of excitement and enthusiasm. . . . I call the period of 40 to 60 minutes the "altered state of consciousness" that must be similar to the catalytic experience of drugs or religion that allows us to alter our lives from within. It's an opening to the unconscious. . . . The thought process is altered. Problems become irrelevant or annoying, and are let go. And, like some inner consultation, a random jumble of ideas flashes through the field of consciousness.

So it seems that there may be two basic types of feelings that come with running. One is the sense of feeling good that may occur during or after your run and is attainable on most runs by most conditioned people. But a more mystical experience may also occur.

Personally, I usually feel good about 2 miles into my run and I almost always feel a postworkout glow afterward. If I've ever had a "catalytic experience" or entered the Kingdom—someone forgot to tell me! (But you can bet Shepherd has done all that!)

Running inside your head usually involves distinctive stages. The first 20 or 30 minutes may cause you to ask: What am I doing here? You may feel sluggish and uncomfortable. Mild euphoria may start after 30 minutes or so. Tensions may drain away. You may be lulled by the rhythm of your steps or your breathing. New thoughts may enter your head. Ideas may flash in and out of your mind from the periphery of your consciousness. After an hour, a form of meditation may take effect, in which colors and thought patterns may be sharper and flow easily through your consciousness.

Why Does Exercise Make Us Feel Better?

Over the last two decades, scientists have discovered that the hypothalamus section of the brain produces a chemical that, when released into the bloodstream, acts like the drug morphine. The chemical was named endogenous (meaning naturally produced by the body) morphine. Scientists call them endorphins—from *endog*enous and m*orphin*e. The human brain is known to produce at least nine types of related endorphins.

"Endorphins have many effects," exercise physiologist Owen Anderson, Ph.D., wrote in *Runner's World*, "but their key role is to control pain and elevate mood. Stress—either emotional or physical—triggers their release."

Running, a physical stress, may release a flood of endorphins into your system. The endorphins then "hook" onto receptors of nerve cells and block the transmission of pain messages to your brain. The result: You feel no pain. On the contrary, you may feel comfortable and relaxed. Some say they feel as if they could run forever.

Research is telling us that more than two-thirds of all runners may achieve some sort of enhanced natural feeling during and after exercising at a vigorous pace for at least 30 minutes. Studies at the University of Richmond, in Virginia, showed a 112.5 percent increase in blood levels of endorphins in competitive runners tested on a treadmill. They found virtually the same increase for competitive bicyclists tested on a stationary bike. When the bikers were asked to run, however, the researchers then found only a 71 percent increase; when the runners were asked to bike, they found only a 47.5 percent increase. Their conclusion was that the body needs to be familiar with the activity to maximize the release of endorphins.

Some scientists are skeptical of the endorphin high. "The high many athletes describe," says Emory University neuropharmacologist Michael Owens, "may not be an opiate-induced euphoria, but rather a deep sense of relaxation and well-being."

How to Get a Runner's High?

We all know that simply trying and succeeding at something is good for your emotional health. Men and women who exercise regularly make plans and succeed at them: they run a set amount so many days every week; they plan and train for, and then enter, competitions. James Brown, Ph.D., author of *The Therapeutic Mile*, writes that during a run our bodies become more relaxed, our minds more focused. Running requires little concentration. Our minds can wander and fantasize—in fact, studies show that some runners fantasize routinely as they put in their long runs. During this heightened state of awareness, our minds cast off stress and become more receptive to ideas and thoughts. This state opens us up to being creative and to making plans and decisions.

Joe Henderson, author of *The Long-Run Solution* and other books, suggests five steps that are good general rules for vigorous exercise as well as reaching a meditative state during running. First, he says, start your run without an end in sight. It will take 20 to 30 minutes to pick up the flow, and by then you'll know how much you can do. Second, if the run goes badly, stop and try again tomorrow. Remember, any running is better than none at all. Third, let your pace find itself. You will usually run along the edge between comfort and discomfort. Fourth, run for yourself; don't look ahead or behind you thinking you might "reel in" that runner up there or be passed by someone you hear coming up. And fifth, run for today; don't compete with yesterday or tomorrow. Take pleasure in yourself and your own running, and accept being less than the best. Everybody is downhill from someone else.

There are several things that will inhibit or facilitate "penetration into one's inner world" while running. On the negative side:

- Competition, or the obsession with running miles.

- New surroundings that distract you. Some runners argue that new surroundings take your mind off your run during those first, often uncomfortable, 30 minutes.

- Other people and the noisy chatter of group runs; valuable for fun and sociability, group runs are out if you wish to reach a meditative state.

- Conversation, with someone else or with yourself, will misdirect your concentration; some runners like to talk to themselves to pass through stages of their runs. Don't talk, either to yourself or to others, if you are trying to reach a meditative stage.

By avoiding these four circumstances during a run, and by running at a steady, nontiring pace and letting your mind spin free, with ideas flowing through it like the water of a mountain stream, you can encourage the meditative stage.

Should you let your mind wander (dissociate), or should you key in (associate) on your running—your stride, footstrike, breathing, aches and pains? A study at the University of Alabama at Birmingham by psychologists Kathryn Goode, Ph.D., and David Roth, Ph.D., of 150 recreational runners confirmed what many of us find ourselves: It is better to think of other things besides running while on the run. (In a race, however, you'd better monitor your body, with occasional mental breaks.)

Goode told *Runner's World*: "We found that runners experienced more vigor if they focused their thoughts away from their bodies and more on daily concerns such as relationships with other people, the scenery round them, their jobs, even the hassles of daily life. Not only did these dissociative thoughts help runners feel more energetic as they ran, they helped them feel more invigorated after their runs as well."

Indeed, much of this book was written with energy gained on the run. I would brainstorm various concepts of the book while on the run and when I returned full of energy I'd head for the computer.

To get their minds focused, some runners sit and chant a mantra—a repeated word or sound—and then run. Others relax, begin running, and meditate on their steady breathing or the sound of their feet. Shepherd finds that humming a song is a wonderful way to get into a meditative state on the run. Chant a phrase or childhood prayer like "Matthew, Mark, Luke, and John, bless this bed I lie upon."

Bud Winter, a sports psychologist at San Jose State, suggests creating a state that is the opposite of tension. Keep unused muscles relaxed, and remember the chant of the long-distance runners: "Let the meat hang on the bones." Set your mind by making up a short phrase that expresses the attitude you want to carry as you run. Repeat the slogan or phrase over and over. Winter suggests "Calm," as in "caaaaaaallllllllmmmmmmmm."

The following are some methods you might want to try for reaching a mediative state on the run. Since I believe that running should be fun, I've included some wild ideas.

Visualization is a good method to reach a meditative state on the run. Sit quietly and alone near your running path. Close your eyes or focus them on the ground immediately before you. Concentrate on your breathing. Count your breaths. Count ten exhalations; start over and count ten more. Do this for about 15 minutes. As you feel yourself relax, start "imagery"—the technique for becoming proficient in any sport. Visualize yourself running well. Vividly picture yourself running the way you've always wanted to run: relaxed, smooth, powerful, easy. Create visual sensations of yourself. After visualization, rise slowly and start walking. Focus on your feet hitting the ground. Listen to your breathing. Focus on your body. Begin a slow shuffle, and then a slow run. Bring the meditative state into your running by counting breaths or steps, or by repeating prayers, a mantra, or numbers. After 30 minutes of running, let your mind wander free. Let ideas, fantasies, colors, smells flow through you. Be receptive, open to internal and external stimuli. And, as New York City psychiatrist Dr. Leonard Reich urges, "make your body rhythm so graceful that it enters the rhythm of the universe."

During the 1980s, Mike Spino of the Esalen Institute and James Hickman, a San Francisco research psychologist, devised several mental exercises. One of the most interesting is called a "witness meditation." First, you assume the standard Zen lotus sitting position, fingers curled, the left hand in your right palm, thumbs touching gently. Place your hands in your lap, and close your eyes. Breathe deeply into your abdomen. Proceed gently and slowly, and relax. Inhale deeply, filling the cavity, and as you exhale, release tension. After 2 minutes or so, switch and breathe deeply into the upper chest and lungs. Fill your upper chest. Exhale slowly and relax. Inhale and exhale in long draws, relaxed and rhythmical. After another 2 minutes or so, combine the two exercises: inhale, filling your abdomen first and then your chest. Exhale from the chest and then the abdomen. Inhale, filling the abdomen and then the chest; exhale from the chest and then the abdomen. Try it and you'll catch on. Spino and Hickman suggest that you next "visualize a light about the size of a halo directly over your head," then, while inhaling slowly, "draw light from this halo into the body." This "light" should relax and calm you. As the light fades from sight, you have "a personal energy source."

Okay, okay. Remember, these guys are Californians.

So, does a "runner's high" exist? I believe that a sense of euphoria comes with four types of runs, all of which are important:

1. The competition high of running fast at the edge of your physical limits

2. The social high of running with friends, of fellowship

3. The contemplative high that allows us to solve problems and to be creative (and write books)

4. The meditative high from running alone at a reflective pace which may, for some runners, become a mystical experience.

I don't get mystical highs from running, but I often feel a sense of euphoria during and after my runs. For Shepherd, the meditative techniques described here are appealing and fun; for him and for other runners, they are important and produce benefits.

To this list George Sheehan added the "contemplative high" of the philosopher. Dr. Sheehan was as delightfully looney as any runner. He ran around quoting Thomas Aquinas, Emerson, Thoreau, and even Marcus Aurelius Antoninus, who, the good doctor claimed, told us runners "it is in thy power whenever you shall choose to retire within thyself." That's what good meditative running is, retiring inside ourselves as we run. "Our destiny," wrote Thomas Aquinas, "is to run to the edge of the world and beyond, off into the darkness."

Appendix

RUNNER'S PACE CHART

(1–10 miles)

1-MILE	2-MILE	3-MILE	4-MILE	5-MILE	10-MILE
7:00	14:00	21:00	28:00	35:00	1:10:00
7:10	14.20	21.30	28.40	35:50	1:11:40
7:20	14:40	22:00	29:20	36:40	1:13:20
7:30	15:00	22.30	30:00	37:30	1:15:00
7:40	15:20	23:00	30:40	38:20	1:16:40
7:50	15:40	23:30	31:20	39:10	1:18:20
8:00	16:00	24:00	32:00	40:00	1:20:00
8:10	16:20	24:30	32:40	40:50	1:21:40
8:20	16:40	25:00	33:20	41:40	1:23:20
8:30	17:00	25:30	34:00	42:30	1:25:00
8:40	17:20	26:00	34:40	43:20	1:26:40
8:50	17:40	26:30	35:20	44:10	1:28:20
9:00	18:00	27:00	36:00	45:00	1:30:00
9:10	18:20	27:30	36:40	45:50	1:31:40
9:20	18:40	28:00	37:20	46:40	1:33:20
9:30	19:00	28:30	38:00	47:30	1:35:00
9:40	19:20	29:00	38:40	48:20	1:36:40
9:50	19:40	29:30	39:20	49:10	1:38:20
10:00	20:00	30:00	40:00	50:00	1:40:00
10:10	20:20	30:30	40:40	50:50	1:41:40
10:20	20:40	31:00	41:20	51:40	1:43:20
10:30	21:00	31:30	42:00	52:30	1:45:00
10:40	21:20	32:00	42:40	53:20	1:46:40
10:50	21:40	32:30	43:20	54:10	1:48:20
11:00	22:00	33:00	44:00	55:00	1:50:00
11:10	22:20	33:30	44:40	55:50	1:52:40
11:20	22:40	34:00	45:20	56:40	1:53:20
11:30	23:00	34:30	46:00	57:30	1:55:00
11:40	23:20	35:00	46:40	58:20	1:56:40
11:50	23:40	35:30	47:20	59:10	1:58:20
12:00	24:00	36:00	48:00	60:00	2:00:00

Note: Times are averaged and rounded off—they are not exact to the second

RUNNER'S PACE CHART

| | | (1 MILE–MARATHON) | | |
1-MILE	5K	10K	HALF-MARATHON	MARATHON
7:00	21:45	43:30	1:31:42	3:03:32
7:10	22:16	44:32	1:33:53	3:07:54
7:20	22:47	45:34	1:36:04	3:12:16
7:30	23:18	46:36	1:38:15	3:16:39
7:40	23:49	47:38	1:40:26	3:21:01
7:50	24:20	48:40	1:42:37	3:25:23
8:00	24:51	49:43	1:44:48	3:29:45
8:10	25:22	50:45	1:46:59	3:34:07
8:20	25:53	51:47	1:49:10	3:38:29
8:30	26:24	52:49	1:51:21	3:42:52
8:40	26:56	53:51	1:53:32	3:47:14
8:50	27:27	54:53	1:55:43	3:51:46
9:00	27:58	55:55	1:57:54	3:55:58
9:10	28:29	56:58	2:00:11	4:00:22
9:20	29:00	58:00	2:02:22	4:04:44
9:30	29:31	59:02	2:04:33	4:09:06
9:40	30:02	60:05	2:06:44	4:13:28
9:50	30:33	61:07	2:08:55	4:17:50
10:00	31:05	62:09	2:11:07	4:22:13
10:10	31:36	63:12	2:13:16	4:26:32
10:20	32:07	64:14	2:15:25	4:30:50
10:30	32:38	65:16	2:17:33	4:35:06
10:40	33:09	66:18	2:19:44	4:39:28
10:50	33:40	67:20	2:21:55	4:43:50
11:00	34:11	68:22	2:24:05	4:48:12
11:10	34:42	69:24	2:26:15	4:52:30
11:20	35:13	70:26	2:28:26	4:56:52
11:30	35:44	71:28	2:30:39	5:01:18
11:40	36:15	72:30	2:32:50	5:05:40
11:50	36:46	73:32	2:35:01	5:10:02
12:00	37:17	74:34	2:37:12	5:14:24

Note: Times are averaged and rounded off—they are not exact to the second

MILE-KILOMETER TIME COMPARISONS

Min/ Mile	Min/ Kilometer	Min/ Mile	Min/ Kilometer
6:00	3:43.74	8:10	5:04.53
6:10	3:49.95	8:20	5:10.75
6:20	3:56.17	8:30	5:16.96
6:30	4:02.38	8:40	5:23.18
6:40	4:08.60	8:50	5:29.39
6:50	4:14.81	9:00	5:35.61
7:00	4:21.03	9:10	5:41.82
7:00	4:27.24	9:20	5:48.04
7:20	4:33.46	9:30	5:54.25
7:30	4:39.67	9:40	6:00.47
7:40	4:45.89	9:50	6:06.68
7:50	4:52.10	10:00	6:12.90
8:00	4:58.32		

How to Use

It is easy to figure out what your pace per mile is for an odd running distance in miles, such as 7 miles. Just divide your time by your mileage—in this example, 7. But for odd running distances in kilometers, it isn't as easy. This chart shows you what a pace per mile is equivalent to per kilometer. If you race an 8-kilometer race, for example, in 48 minutes, divide this time by 8 to determine the pace per mile for 1 kilometer. Then look to the left-hand column to see what your pace per mile was for 8 kilometers. Forty-eight divided by 8 equals a pace of 6 minutes per kilometer, which is a pace of 9:40 per mile. You can also figure it the other way. If your goal is a 9:40-per-mile pace, you should hit each kilometer split in slightly over 6 minutes—for example, you would hit 2 kilometers in 12 minutes.

(Times on this chart are in minutes:seconds.tenths of seconds. Example: 2:47.80.)

RUNNING-DISTANCE CONVERSIONS

ENGLISH TO METRIC		METRIC TO ENGLISH	
ENGLISH	METRIC	METRIC	ENGLISH
220 yards	201.168	200	218y, 2'2" (0.124 mi)
440 yards	402.336	400	427y, 1'4" (0.249 mi)
880 yards	804.672	800	874y, 2'8" (0.497 mi)

RACE	CONVERSION	RACE	CONVERSION
1 mile	1,609 meters	1,500 meters	0.93 miles
2 miles	3,219 meters	3,000 meters	1.86 miles
3 miles	4,828 meters	5,000 meters	3.11 miles
5 miles	8,047 meters	8,000 meters	4.97 miles
6 miles	9,656 meters	10,000 meters	6.21 miles
10 miles	16,193 meters	15,000 meters	9.32 miles
Half marathon	21,098 meters	20,000 meters	12.43 miles
15 miles	24,140 meters	25,000 meters	15.53 miles
20 miles	32,187 meters	30,000 meters	18.64 miles
Marathon	42,195 meters	Marathon	26.22 miles
30 miles	48,280 meters	50,000 meters	31.07 miles
50 miles	80,467 meters	100,000 meters	62.14 miles

PACE CHART FOR TRACK RACES AND WORKOUTS

1 MILE	220 YDS (1/8)	440 YDS (1/4)	660 YDS (3/8)	880 YDS (1/2)
6:00	45.0	1:30.0	2:15.0	3:00
6:10	46.25	1:32.5	2:18.75	3:05
6:20	47.5	1:35.0	2:22.5	3:10
6:30	48.75	1:37.5	2:26.25	3:15
6:40	50.0	1:40.0	2:30.0	3:20
6:50	51.25	1:42.5	2:33.75	3:25
7:00	52.5	1:45.0	2:37.5	3:30
7:10	53.75	1:47.5	2:41.25	3:35
7:20	55.0	1:50.0	2:45.0	3:40
7:30	56.25	1:52.5	2:48.75	3:45
7:40	57.5	1:55.0	2:52.5	3:50
7:50	58.75	1:57.5	2:56.25	3:55
8:00	1:00.0	2:00.0	3:00.0	4:00
8:10	1:01.25	2:02.5	3:03.75	4:05
8:20	1:02.5	2:05.0	3:07.5	4:10
8:30	1:03.75	2:07.5	3:11.25	4:15
8:40	1:05.0	2:10.0	3:15.0	4:20
8:50	1:06.25	2:12.5	3:18.75	4:25
9:00	1:07.5	2:15.0	3:22.5	4:30
9:10	1:08.75	2:17.5	3:26.25	4:35
9:20	1:10.0	2:20.0	3:30.0	4:40
9:30	1:11.25	2:22.5	3:33.75	4:45
9:40	1:12.5	2:25.0	3:37.5	4:50
9:50	1:13.75	2:27.5	3:41.25	4:55
10:00	1:15.0	2:30.0	3:45.0	5:00

How to Use

This chart can be used to select even-paced splits for races or speed workouts on a quarter-mile (440-yard) track:

1. If you wish to run a 9-minute mile, for example, you can determine that your splits should be: 1:07.5 at 220 yards, 2:15 after one lap (440 yards or 1/4 mile), 3:22.5 at 660 yards, and 4:30 after two laps (880 yards or 1/2 mile). To find your splits at 220-yard or 440-yard intervals beyond 880 yards, add the time under those columns to the 880-yard time. Example: the split for 3/4 mile for a 9-minute mile is 6:45 (4:30 + 2:15).

2. If you did a speed workout on the track and wish to determine your pace-per-mile average, locate your average time for that distance and refer to the left-hand column for your average pace per mile. Example: 6 × 440 yards averaging 2:15 each is a pace of 9:00 per mile.

Note: Since 400 meters is very close to 440 yards, this chart can also be used for approximate pacing for 200 meters, 400 meters, 600 meters, 800 meters, and 1,600 meters.

(Times on this chart are in minutes:seconds.tenths of seconds. Example: 1:07.5.)

Index